T0146167

Providing for the Casualties of War

The American Experience Since World War II

Bernard Rostker

Prepared for the Office of the Secretary of Defense
Approved for public release; distribution unlimited

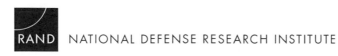

NATIONAL DEFENSE RESEARCH INSTITUTE

For more information on this publication, visit www.rand.org/t/RR2823

Library of Congress Cataloging-in-Publication Data is available for this publication.
ISBN: 978-1-9774-0470-1

Published by the RAND Corporation, Santa Monica, Calif.
© Copyright 2020 RAND Corporation
RAND® is a registered trademark.

Support RAND
Make a tax-deductible charitable contribution at
www.rand.org/giving/contribute

www.rand.org

Foreword

As a follow-up to *Providing for the Casualties of War: The American Experience Through World War II*, this volume continues the history of military medicine and how it has evolved during U.S. conflicts since World War II. As battlefield tactics and weaponry have changed, so has casualty care, from the battlefield to more definitive care to rehabilitation. The use of advanced technologies, such as hemostatic agents; new ways to use old procedures, such as tourniquets; and rapid evacuation have increased survival to unprecedented rates. However, as this book describes, there is a greater need not only for rehabilitation but for disability programs, so the interaction between the military medical services and the VA has taken on greater importance.

Some of the most significant consequences of recent conflicts, however, were unexpected and hold several lessons. Among them, the recognition of diseases caused by Agent Orange and Gulf War illness and the challenges of the military and VA disability systems are described in detail.

Dr. Rostker captures all of this beautifully, laying out the evolution of the VA's role and the military's reluctant dependence on it. He also puts in historic context how recognition of the invisible wounds of war—posttraumatic stress disorder and traumatic brain injury—came about and what is being done about them.

As Surgeon General and at Walter Reed Army Medical Center, I was involved in many of the changes described, especially Forward Surgical Teams, training in civilian trauma centers and the establishment of the Tactical Combat Casualty Care (TCCC) committee, which has allowed lessons learned from the battlefield to be assessed and doctrinal changes to be rapidly incorporated into casualty care. These and many other policy changes of significance are well covered, including new programs for families and caregivers.

This is a book for senior leaders in military medicine and the VA. Line commanders will find it of interest as well. For those who deal with casualties and the follow-on issues, it is a must read. For others, it is a terrific history, comprehensive, detailed, and fun to read!

LTG Dr. Ronald R. Blanck, U.S. Army (Ret.)
Former Surgeon General of the Army

Preface

The current and future care of the casualties of war—those who have been wounded or injured or who are mentally or physically ill as a result of combat—is a high priority for the military and civilian leadership of the Department of Defense and the Department of Veterans Affairs.[1] As highlighted in the 2010 *Quadrennial Defense Review Report*:

> Apart from working to prevail in ongoing conflicts, caring for our wounded warriors is our highest priority, and we will strive to provide them the top-quality physical and psychological care that befits their service and sacrifice. Providing world-class care and management, benefit delivery, and standardization of services among the Military Departments and federal agencies continues to be the focus of the Department's most senior leadership. Our wounded, ill, or injured service members deserve every opportunity to return to active duty following their recovery, or to make a seamless transition to veteran status if they cannot be returned to active duty. (Gates, 2010, p. 49)

As with every other aspect of the military, the relevant policies have evolved over time, and having a basic grasp of their roots and evolution should improve understanding of today's policies. This volume is the second of a two-part historical account that began with the ancient and European roots of care for fallen soldiers and continued through America's own wars, describing how the U.S. government arrived at its current set of policies for caring for its injured and ill soldiers and veterans. This volume covers the Korean War period, which started on June 25, 1950, through the present conflicts in Iraq and Afghanistan. The first volume, *Providing for the Casualties of War: The American Experience Through World War II* (Rostker, 2013), covered the historical antecedents of American policy and how that policy evolved through World War II and just after, before the beginning of the Korean War.

As with the first volume, the focus is on the medical care that combat casualties of the U.S. Army receive. While all the military services share some common history, they are distinct organizations with their own stories to tell. Sorting out the areas of

---

[1] As used here, the term *care* is limited to medical assistance rendered on the battlefield, in military hospitals before separation from the military, and health services provided or paid for by the Department of Veterans Affairs after separation from the military.

overlap and paying each service the same degree of attention as the Army receives here was beyond the scope of this effort.

This research was sponsored by the Office of the Under Secretary of Defense for Personnel and Readiness and conducted within the Forces and Resources Policy Center of the RAND National Security Research Division (NSRD), which operates the National Defense Research Institute (NDRI), a federally funded research and development center sponsored by the Office of the Secretary of Defense, the Joint Staff, the Unified Combatant Commands, the Navy, the Marine Corps, the defense agencies, and the defense intelligence enterprise.

For more information on the RAND Forces and Resources Policy Center, see www.rand.org/nsrd/frp or contact the director (contact information is provided on the webpage).

Contents

Figures

Tables

Boxes

Acknowledgments

Originally, the study from which this book emerged was one of four tasks in a project called *Implications of a Paradigm Shift: The Management of War Wounded Under the All-Volunteer Force*. The purpose of the original project was to examine the implications of what the research team believed to be an ongoing paradigm shift in the management of war wounded under the all-volunteer force. Each of the four tasks was to assess the paradigm shift in one specific area: changes in policy; medical treatment; support for the wounded and their families; and the organizational and institutional implications of reintegration of severely wounded soldiers, primarily amputees, back into the Army. I was responsible for the first task, with Terri Tanielian, Laura Miller, and Ralph Masi each being responsible for one of the other tasks.

An initial review by Donald Temple soon made it clear that, while care for the wounded was very important, the premise of the study—that there was a paradigm shift uniquely associated with the all-volunteer force—was too simplistic. A further review of the literature, by Melanie Sisson, showed that much of what appears new and innovative was actually rediscovery of what had gone before and that care for today's casualties was more of an evolution than a revolution. As a result, with encouragement and support of Jeanne Fites, the former Deputy Under Secretary of Defense for Program Integration, and Norma St. Claire, the Director of Information Management, this task was expanded into a separate project to provide a more-detailed look at how care had evolved overtime. Mrs. St. Claire was particularly concerned that decisions were being made with little knowledge of what had gone before and that a fuller account of history would provide information that would lead to "better" decisions by building on the successes and failures of the past. Their support was instrumental in the publishing the first volume, *Providing for the Casualties of War: The American Experience Through World War II*.

In preparing this second volume, which focuses on events after World War II, I am indebted to former Acting Under Secretary of Defense Brad Carson for providing financial support; Charles Scoville, Program Manager, U.S. Army Amputee Patient Care Program, Department of Orthopedics and Rehabilitation, Walter Reed Army Medical Center, for making available a variety of documentation on the evolution of the Army's amputation rehabilitation program since 9/11; Sandra Meagher for materials from the Department of Defense archives and Mrs. St. Claire for the backup books from the Office of the Under Secretary of Defense for Personnel and Readiness; Michael J. Carino of the Office of the Surgeon General of the Army for contemporary data on recent medical operations; and Sanders Marble, Senior Historian, Office of Medical History, Office of the Chief of Staff, U.S. Army Medical Command for his many suggestions and encouragement during the research of both volumes. The support I got from the RAND library team was outstanding, as usual. I was particularly fortunate to have the assistance of Kayla Williams in distilling the materials from the Amputee Patient Care Program and of Gail McGinn for making sense of the various efforts at the Department of Defense that developed after the terror attacks of September 11, 2001.

Susan Hosek, Kristie Gore, and Robert Goldich carefully reviewed the manuscript and provided valuable suggestions concerning the myriad of topics covered. Phyllis Gilmore edited both volumes, completing the herculean task of making them more readable while allowing my voice to come through.

Abbreviations

AC	active component
AE	aeromedical evacuation
AFB	Air Force base
AFQT	Armed Forces Qualification Test
ALS	amyotrophic lateral sclerosis
ARCENT	U.S. Army Central Command
ASTP	Army Specialist Training Program
ATTC	U.S. Army Trauma Training Center
ATLS	Advanced Trauma Life Support
AWOL	absent without leave
BCT	brigade combat team
BHO	behavioral health officer
CAT	combat application tourniquet
CBPSS	Chemical Biological Protective Shelter System
CCATT	Critical Care Air Transport Team
CCF	Chinese Communist Forces
CHAMPVA	Civilian Health and Medical Program of the Department of Veterans Affairs
CIA	Central Intelligence Agency
CNA	Center for Naval Analyses
COIN	counterinsurgency
CONUS	continental United States

CSC	combat stress control
CSH	combat support hospital
CSR	combat stress reaction
CY	calendar year
DARPA	Defense Advanced Research Projects Agency
DES	disability evaluation system
DHHS	Department of Health and Human Services
DMDC	Defense Manpower Data Center
DoD	U.S. Department of Defense
DoDTR	DoD Trauma Registry
DOW	died of wounds
DSM	*Diagnostic and Statistical Manual of Mental Disorders*
DVA	U.S. Department of Veterans Affairs
DVBIC	Defense and Veterans Brain Injury Center
EMT	emergency medical technician
EO	executive order
FM	field manual
FRC	federal recovery coordinator
FRCP	Federal Recovery Coordination Program
FST	forward surgical team
FY	fiscal year
GAO	U.S. General Accounting Office until July 2004, then U.S. Government Accountability Office
ICU	intensive care unit
IDES	Integrated Disability Evaluation System
IED	improvised explosive device
IG	inspector general
IOM	Institute of Medicine (now known as the National Academy of Medicine)

JP	Joint Publication
JTS	Joint Trauma System
JTTR	Joint Theater Trauma Registry
JTTS	Joint Theater Trauma System
KIA	killed-in-action
KTO	Kuwait theater of operations
MAMC	Madigan Army Medical Center
MASH	mobile army surgical hospital
M*A*S*H	The television show
MEB	medical evaluation board
MEDCAP	Medical Civic Action Program
medevac	medical evacuation
MHAT	Mental Health Advisory Team
MRAP	Mine-Resistant, Ambush-Protected
MSIC	Military Severely Injured Center
mTBI	mild traumatic brain injury
MTF	military treatment facility
MUST	Medical Unit, Self-Contained, Transportable
N/A	not applicable
NAS	National Academy of Sciences
NATO	North Atlantic Treaty Organization
NC	not comparable
NCO	noncommissioned officer
NDAA	National Defense Authorization Act
NPR	National Public Radio
NVVRS	National Vietnam Veterans Readjustment Study
OASI	Old-Age and Survivors Insurance (also known as Social Security)
OEF	Operation Enduring Freedom

OIF	Operation Iraqi Freedom
OIR	Operation Inherent Resolve
OND	Operation New Dawn
OSAGWI	Office of the Special Assistant for Gulf War Illnesses
OSD	Office of the Secretary of Defense
PAC	Presidential Advisory Committee
PDHA	Post-Deployment Health Assessment
PDHRA	Post-Deployment Health Reassessment
PEB	physical evaluation board
PIES	proximity, immediacy, expectancy, and simplicity
POW	prisoner of war
PTSD	posttraumatic stress disorder
Pub. L.	Public Law
QDR	Quadrennial Defense Review
RC	reserve component
RCP	Recovery Coordination Program
ROTC	Reserve Officer Training Corps
RTI	Research Triangle Institute
SABO	Seeb Air Base Oman
SEAL	Sea-Air-Land (Navy SOF)
SF	Special Forces (Army SOF)
SIPP	specialized intensive PTSD program
SOC	senior oversight committee
SOF	special operations forces
SSRI	selective serotonin reuptake inhibitor
TBI	traumatic brain injury
TCCC	tactical combat casualty care
TCDD	2,3,7,8-Tetrachlorodibenzodioxin, commonly known as dioxin

TDY	temporary duty
TDRL	Temporary Disability Retired List
TO&E	table of organization and equipment
TRICARE	a health care program of the United States Department of Defense Military Health System
UN	United Nations
USARV	U.S. Army, Vietnam
USASCV	U.S. Army Support Command, Vietnam
U.S.C.	U.S. Code
USCENTCOM	U.S. Central Command
USSOCOM	U.S. Special Operations Command
USUHS	Uniformed Services University of the Health Sciences
V-E Day	formal surrender of Germany in World War II (May 8, 1945)
V-J Day	formal surrender of Japan at the end of World War II (September 2, 1945)
VA	Veterans Administration (Department of Veterans Affairs)
VBA	Veterans Benefits Administration
VCP	Veterans Choice Program
VHA	Veterans Health Administration
VVWG	Vietnam Veterans Working Group
WIA	wounded-in-action
WRAMC	Walter Reed Army Medical Center
WTB	Warrior Transition Battalion
WTU	Warrior Transition Unit

CHAPTER ONE

Introduction: Looking to the Past for Lessons to Apply in the Future

War has been part of the human experience since before recorded history (see Keeley, 1996). Sigmund Freud suggested that this may be an inherent trait, that "conflicts of interest between man and man are resolved, in principle, by the recourse to violence" (Einstein and Freud, 1931–1932). Although people have not been able to overcome their essential proclivity to make war on one another over the millennia, there has been some progress in how the casualties of war are treated. Early efforts to care for those maimed in combat were established for four reasons. First, the wounded represented a valuable asset that, with proper care, could be returned to duty and could continue to serve. Second, without proper care of the wounded, the morale of the troops would suffer. Third, for those unable to return to duty, this was a way to deal with the potential problem of disabled veterans who were unable to work resorting to theft and other unruly behavior. Fourth, without guaranteeing some degree of care for the injured, the state would not be able to recruit additional soldiers. Despite the rather altruistic rationale said to underpin today's policies—that the state has an absolute obligation to care for those who served it on the battlefield—the four historical concerns of conserving the force, ensuring good morale, placating veterans, and bolstering future recruiting still underpin today's policies.

While today's military is unique in many ways, today's wars and the way we care for their casualties—both in service and as veterans—progresses along a well-established path that extends back into history. For example, while the current conflicts in Iraq and Afghanistan have resulted in fewer wounds from gun and artillery fire and more from improvised explosive devices (IEDs), such as roadside bombs, these injuries are echoes of the Germans' use of land mines in their withdrawal from Italy and retreat toward Berlin in 1945. IEDs often result in burns, traumatic brain injury (TBI), or the loss of a limb (or some combination of the three), just as land mines did during World War II. Even the changes in battlefield medical technologies that have profoundly altered the treatment wounded and injured soldiers receive are firmly built on the legacy of World War II. Today's rapid evacuation of the seriously wounded from the battlefield to military fixed-facility hospitals enables early entry into definitive care and follow-on rehabilitative services; its antecedents are in the air evacuation system developed at the end of World War II. In July 1945 alone, more than 12,000 patients were flown back to the hospitals in the United States.

In one way, however, today's soldiers are very different from those who fought in all our major wars, and the way they are being employed is also different. In World War II, soldiers served for the duration of the conflict, spending years overseas separated from their families except for the occasional letter. Today's soldiers are in frequent and intimate contact with their families. While the Vietnam conflict was brought into the living rooms of Americans through television, that contact was still largely impersonal. Since 9/11, contacts have increasingly become very personal as access to the internet has expanded and cell phones have become ubiquitous.[1] The post-9/11 conflicts are the first prolonged ones ever fought in which the Army has been made up entirely of professional soldiers. While the majority of troops in battle today are recent recruits, they are all volunteers, and today's force is made up of an extraordinary large number of career personnel who have served a number of tours in the combat theater, with the result that many soldiers have served multiple deployments. Suicides, incidents of post-traumatic stress disorder (PTSD), divorce, and postdeployment spousal violence are of great concern to today's military leaders.[2]

As previously noted, this is the second of two volumes that cover the evolution of care for the casualties of war throughout history. The first starts with the ancient world and goes through America's wars, starting with our colonial period and ending with World War II. The present volume continues to the current conflicts in the Middle East. Each volume is arranged chronologically, with a separate chapter for each of our major military conflicts. As much as possible, these chapters identify how the military mobilized for the conflict; how the military medical establishment was organized; the state of medicine at the time; the major injuries and illnesses sustained; and how soldiers were cared for on the battlefield, in the military before separation, and after the war as veterans, paying special attention to amputations and psychiatric disorders. As presented, the story unfolds chronologically, and information is presented that is relevant to the period of the chapter. As a result, statements concerning then "current"

---

[1]   An Air Force sergeant recently told me about his cell phone contact with his wife, also a serving member of the Air Force, stationed in Afghanistan. She called to talk with their daughter, who was not home, and asked to have her call later that night, when she got home. It seems that calling around the world and into a war zone has become as common as calling a family member across town.

[2]   In an interview on September 24, 2012, with Greg Barnes of the *Fayetteville Observer*, Defense Secretary Leon E. Panetta

> voiced concern over suicide rates throughout the military and acknowledged the complexity of the issue. . . . "Just like sexual assault, when it comes to suicides, we have got to make our leadership in the military aware of what this problem is about," he said. . . . The issue has to be at the top of all leaders' agendas, he said, and should be one of the things he and other leaders talk about when they meet with troops. (Lyle, 2012)

situations, policies, and problems reflect the period under discussion and not the contemporary state of affairs.

Amputees have been the focus of attention for centuries, with psychological injury only recently recognized as a significant malady of war. Throughout history, amputees have been the most visible of the war wounded. Even as the incidence of amputations has decreased, fascination with amputees can be seen today with the myriad "wounded warrior" programs that focus primarily on this most visible consequence of war.

As medicine has advanced and as physicians have learned to control disease and reduce the mortality from wounds, advances in psychiatry have made us acutely aware of how combat, even the expectation of combat, can result in what are often called *invisible wounds*: psychological wounds with debilitating mental and physical manifestations. While it is certain that such casualties have always been with us throughout history—ancient texts have vividly described psychological impairments—specific diagnoses and treatments are relatively recent. This book also highlights the development of psychiatric services, given their importance today.

The last chapter of each volume ties the evolution of care together by identifying broad domains that determine the quality of care a wounded soldier would receive. As presented in the first volume, these domains are (1) the nature of combat itself, the kind of wounds received, and the ability of physicians and surgeons to deal with disease and the consequences of wounds; (2) the ability to deliver medical services on and, later, off the battlefield; (3) the increasing role of national governments in providing care—financial, domestic, and rehabilitative—to veterans after the battle; and (4) finally, the more-recent awareness of psychological and cognitive injuries—the invisible wounds of war—that transcend the immediate battle. These domains were present in antiquity and follow throughout history to this day. The last chapter in this volume thus reprises the summary chapter of the first volume and extends the information presented from the end of World War II to the present day.

CHAPTER TWO

The Beginning of the Cold War: The Partition of Korea, U.S. Demobilization After World War II, and the Postwar Army Medical Department

When North Korean forces entered South Korea on June 25, 1950, the United States was unprepared for war in the Far East. While the United States had been engaged in a Cold War with the Soviet Union for five years—ever since the end of World War II—the focus was on Europe. Moreover, American military power was at a nadir of its World War II strength, when more than 8 million men and women were serving in the Army and millions more in the other services.

The Expansion of International Communism: Korea, a Tempting Target

In summer 1950, South Korea was a small and largely agricultural country occupying the southern half of the divided peninsula it shared with the communist Democratic People's Republic of Korea. The peninsula was partitioned as a result of agreements made during World War II among the allied powers. Japan had formally annexed Korea in 1910 and occupied the entire peninsula at the start of the war. The future of Korea was discussed at the Cairo Conference of November 1943, when the United States, Britain, and China declared their intention to see that Korea became an independent state in "due course," at some undetermined point in the future. In the meantime, once the war was over, it was agreed that Korea would be administered as a trusteeship by the wartime powers.

After the Soviet Union declared war on Japan, the United States proposed that the 38th parallel become the line of demarcation so that the Soviets could accept the surrender of Japanese troops in the northern part of the peninsula.[1] In December 1945, at a meeting of foreign ministers in Moscow, it was agreed that a joint Soviet-American

---

[1] There was never any formal wartime agreement between the United States and the Soviet Union to divide Korea. The 38th parallel north was selected only to facilitate the surrender of Japanese troops. The United States was at a disadvantage because it had no troops in the area when Soviet troops entered Korea on August 12, 1945. Almost a full month passed before U.S. troops arrived (U.S. Army Center of Military History, 1997, p. 4).

commission would set the terms for the "organization of one provisional democratic government for the whole of Korea" (U.S. Army Center of Military History, 1997, p. 5). When the commission failed to agree on how to administer Korea, the matter was submitted to the United Nations (UN) General Assembly.

In January 1948, the UN Temporary Commission on Korea arrived in country with the purpose of holding countrywide elections. The Russians, however—professing that the Korean question was beyond the scope of the UN—refused to permit the commission to enter their zone of occupation in the northern part of the peninsula. Subsequently, elections were held in the U.S.-occupied area in the South. The Republic of Korea was established in the former U.S. zone on September 9, 1948 (Lee, 2006). American occupation troops were gradually withdrawn, leaving behind a small detachment of troops to train South Korea's security forces.

The failure to reach an accord with the Soviet Union in Korea was matched by similar acrimony in Europe. So, when South Korea was invaded President Harry Truman could not tell whether the invasion was an isolated incident or the first stage of a worldwide confrontation with the proxy states of the Soviet Union. If it were the latter, the main event would be played out in Europe and not the Far East, and Truman acted accordingly because the forces he had at his disposal were a mere shadow of what had existed at the end of World War II.

The U.S. Army After World War II

While the United States emerged as the undisputed winner of World War II (with the strongest economy and the most technologically advanced military), its military was nevertheless widely troubled by 1950. The United States was not only unprepared for active conflict in Korea, it was unprepared for its commitments around the world. When the war had ended in August 1945, just five years earlier, the U.S. Army had had more than 8 million soldiers in its ranks (Sparrow, 1952, p. 139). Now, with an active conflict at hand, the Army's strength was down to 591,000 (Association of the U.S. Army, 1992), a number reminiscent of the pre–World War II level of slightly fewer than 200,000. Moreover, the problem was not only numbers but also the poor state of training and readiness of American forces.

The United States had a strong tradition of a limited standing army and had, after each past war, demobilized the vast majority of service members as soon as possible. The demobilization after World War II was no exception; looking back, the Army characterized its demobilization as "one of the cardinal mistakes" of World War II (Sparrow, 1952, p. 297).

Demobilizing an Army of Individuals

On May 10, 1945, even before the Japanese surrender, the Department of War announced that the Army's plan for a partial demobilization would not be based on unit affiliation, as had been the case in previous wars, but on each soldier's Adjusted Service Rating, which considered time in service, time overseas, combat awards, and the number of "dependent children under age 18 up to a limit of three children" (Department of War, 1944).[2] While those who took a short-term view received the plan well, some argued that the world had changed, and with it, the U.S. role had altered forever, with different views playing out on the editorial pages of American newspapers. For example, the *Washington Evening Star* saw the plan in a favorable light, commenting that

> it is doubtful that there could be a better or fairer plan for military deployment and demobilization than the one just announced by the War Department. (as quoted in Sparrow, 1952, p. 113)

On the other hand, the editorial board of the *Kansas City Star* took a more prophetic view, citing the need for American military power in the years ahead:

> [t]he part the United States is to play in the years ahead will depend upon how strong this nation maintains itself in the decade or two following final peace. If, when real V-day comes, we start letting our navy, our air force, and our army disintegrate then our voice for peace in the future will carry little weight. (as quoted in Sparrow, 1952, p. 114)

In fact, the demobilization policy—while ostensibly fair for individual soldiers—played havoc with units around the world because critical soldiers were moved with little regard for the integrity or readiness of the unit they left behind or for the needs of the Army to meet the requirements for the planned invasion of Japan and its new postwar obligations. By late winter 1945, it was clear that the point system needed to be augmented by a length-of-service policy to complete the transition to the normal peacetime method of procuring men for the Army. In October 1945, the departing Army Chief of Staff, GEN George C. Marshall told President Harry Truman that, "based on the current intake of personnel, a two-year policy will not permit the U.S. to meet overseas commitment" (Marshall, 1945, p. 2). He noted that the viability of the policy would depend on the percentage "of trained soldiers that can be obtained by voluntary enlistments and the future of inductions through the Selective Service Act" (Sparrow, 1952, p. 242). Soon after, GEN Dwight D. Eisenhower, the new Chief of Staff of the Army, concluded "that the Army was running out of replacements and that commanders would have to perform their mission with fewer troops" (Sparrow, 1952, p. 242). The Joint Staff *optimistically* estimated that our forces in Europe "could operate in an emergency for a limited period at something *less than 50% normal war-*

---

[2] The rating system, as implemented on May 10, 1945, awarded one point for each month of Army service; one for each month overseas; five for each combat award; and 12 for each dependent child, up to the limit of three children, as prescribed in Secretary of War, 1945.

time efficiency" (Sparrow, 1952, p. 266, emphasis in the original). While the change in policy in winter 1945 can be seen in Figure 2.1, the Army's strength was, by June 1946, only one-quarter of what it had been on V-E Day.

Key to the future viability of the Army was the continuation of the draft, but Congress, under pressure from the public, pressed Truman to end conscription. Truman agreed to end the draft on March 31, 1947. Within less than a year, however, the deteriorating political situation in the world—the communist coup in Czecho-slovakia in February 1946 and the confrontation with Russia over Berlin—as well as the failure of the Army to recruit sufficient volunteers (with a requirement of 30,000 recruits per month, the Army was able to attract only 12,000 volunteers), led Truman to ask that the draft be reinstated. However, by February 1949, the situation in Europe cooled, and inductions were suspended. That summer, the Associated Press reported that "unless an unfortunate emergency develops, the peacetime draft is expected to expire on June 25, 1950" ("Army Manpower Draft Expected to End in June," 1949). As it turned out, that was the day North Korean forces invaded South Korea. Three days later, Congress voted an extension of the Selective Service Act.

Figure 2.1
Strength of the Army and the Drawdown, May 1945–June 1946

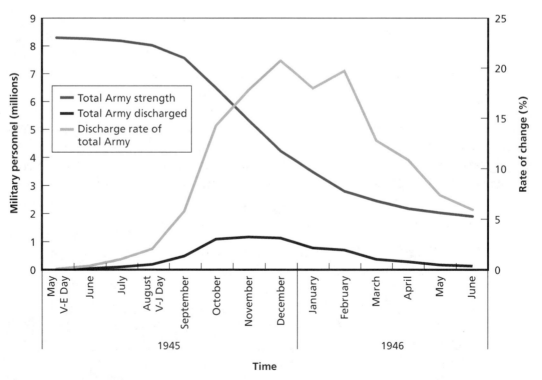

SOURCE: Data from McMinn and Levin, 1963, p. 14.

Demobilization and Transformation of the Army Medical Department

The demobilization of the Army Medical Department, including both personnel and hospitals, started even as the invasion of the Japanese home islands was pending. It was the hope of Army leaders that they could continue to meet the Army's needs while transforming the department into a modern health delivery organization incorporating what it had learned from the massive influx of civilian physicians and other health providers during World War II. Unfortunately, demobilization left the Army's medical establishment unprepared for the invasion of Japan and, later, the Korean War.

Demobilization of Personnel

The task the Army Medical Department faced immediately after V-E Day was to resize and restructure for the coming campaign against the home islands of Japan and to provide the medical support required for war-torn Europe and the American troops that remained. Accordingly, the Surgeon General started to shift personnel and restaff units in accordance with the Army's Adjusted Service Rating discharge policy. In the European and Mediterranean theaters, personnel with high scores received orders to return to the United States "to help care for the expected concentration of patients" soon to arrive from Europe and the Pacific Theater (McMinn and Levin, 1963, p. 487). Moreover, for medical units transiting through the United States on their way to the Pacific, those who had not yet served overseas replaced those with high Adjusted Service Rating scores. Figure 2.2 shows the drawdown program for the Medical Department and Medical Corps (physicians) from V-E Day to June 1946 relative to the overall size of the Army.[3] Despite the fact that medical personnel were key to a successful demobilization, the Medical Department drew down more quickly than the rest of the Army. When the war in Europe ended in May 1945, there were 80 members of the department for every 1,000 in the Army; by June 1946, that number had fallen to fewer than 60 per 1,000.[4]

To meet the demands on the Medical Department overseas and at home in Army hospitals and separation centers, physicians and surgeons were demobilized more slowly than the rest of the department; in May 1945, they constituted 7 percent of the

---

[3]   The Medical Department consists of officers and enlisted personnel in a number of corps, such as the Medical Corps and the Dental Corps. Physicians and surgeons were assigned to the Medical Corps. In May 1945, the Medical Department had a total strength of 666,710, while the Medical Corps had a total strength of 46,750, By June 1946, the Medical Corps' strength was 13,134 (McMinn and Levin, 1963, p. 14). It is interesting to note that the Surgeon General's office and the Army's Adjutant General could not agree on the size of either the Medical Department or the Medical Corps. For example, at the end of December 1945, the Adjutant General's office and the Surgeon General's office reported that the Medical Department had a strength of 330,678 and 323,085, respectively; the Adjutant General's office and the Surgeon General's office reported that the strength of the Medical Corps was 27,060 and 47,339, respectively.

[4]   It should be noted, however, that while the Medical Department lost 86 percent of its officers and 91 percent of its enlisted personnel between the end of World War II and the start of the Korean War—June 1945 to June 1950—it was still "nearly three times as great as" it was before the buildup for World War II began (Cowdrey, 1987, p. 8).

Figure 2.2
**Size of the Medical Department and Medical Corps Relative to the Overall Size of the Army,
May 1945–June 1946**

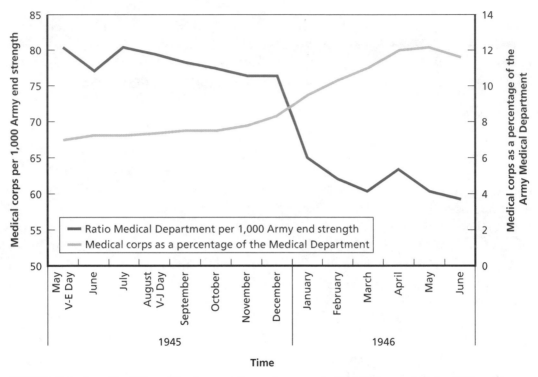

SOURCE: Data from the Office of the Surgeon General, as reported in McMinn and Levin, 1963, p. 14.

department, but in June 1946 they made up almost 12 percent. However, the lag in the demobilization of physicians did not go unnoticed by Congress, which became increasingly impatient with the pace of the drawdown. One senator charged the Surgeon General's office with "an incredible degree of incompetency, inefficiency, and general neglect . . . in dealing with the return of doctors and surgeons" (as quoted in McMinn and Levin, 1963, p. 493).

Closing of Army Hospitals

It was not only personnel that were being drawn down. At the end of June 1945, the number of beds authorized at general and convalescent hospitals was 212,949, with an authorized level at stations of 51,561, (McMinn and Levin, 1963, p. 211). A year and a half later, the Army (including the Air Forces) had only 54 station hospitals with 15,715 beds; 14 general hospitals with 34,846 beds; and only one convalescent hospital, Old Farms (McMinn and Levin, 1963, p. 314). Late in 1950, on what turned out to be the eve of the Korean War, the Army closed four large general hospitals: Murphy, Oliver, Valley Forge, and Percy Jones. These hospitals had cared for the most critical patients, particularly amputees, after V-J Day.[5] Now, "for patients requiring long-term care and expert rehabilitation the hospitals of the Veterans' Administration (VA) usually were the next step after they left the Army hospitals" (Cowdrey, 1987, p. 296).

Rebuilding the Medical Department

As the demobilization continued, a big problem for the Army Medical Department was its inability to retain or attract enough medical personnel to fill authorized positions. Table 2.1 shows the Regular Army fill rate and the ratio of reserve to regular officers in six categories of officers serving in the Army Medical Department in December 1947.[6] The Army was able to fill only 40 percent of its Regular Army positions in the Medical Corps. As a result, 84 percent of all physicians serving on active duty were reserve officers, most of whom were completing their initial period of obligated service after receiving their medical training at government expense during the war through the Army Specialist Training Program (ASTP).

The Army Specialized Training Program

ASTP provided the cushion the Surgeon General relied on to help meet the immediate postwar requirements for physicians and other health professionals. It was built on the wartime program to ensure the future supply of technicians and specialist (see Palmer, Wiley, and Keast, 1948). In December 1942, the Army and Navy each established programs that sent enlisted men to school in a variety of professions, including the

Table 2.1
Medical Department Officer Strength, December 1947

Component	Total	Reserve Officers	Regular Officers	Ratio of Reserves to Regular Officers	Regular Fill Rate
Medical Corps	7,702	6,496	1,206	5.4	0.402
Dental Corps	1,652	1,220	432	2.8	0.581
Veterinary Corps	399	201	198	1.0	1.065
Medical Service Corps	2,762	2,022	740	2.7	0.724
Army Nurse Corps	4,960	3,812	1,148	3.3	0.508
Women's Medical Specialist Corps	512	370	142	2.6	0.347

SOURCE: Cowdrey, 1987, p. 13.

---

[5] Murphy and Percy Jones were reopened within a year to handle Korean War casualties (see Cowdrey, 1987, pp. 294–298).

[6] Officers were commissioned in the Regular Army or in one of the reserve components (RCs), the Army Reserve or National Guard. The personnel rules dictating the terms of service and retirement were different for those holding regular or reserve commissions. Those holding regular commissions were basically the full-time staff; those holding reserve commissions were the temporary staff.

medical professions. At its zenith, 145,000 soldiers were enrolled, but by late 1943, the pressing need for men to fill combat units dramatically reduced the size of these programs, with only 35,000 soldiers enrolled by March 1944. That summer, the program to train future Army dentists was terminated. In 1945, Army Chief of Staff George C. Marshall proposed continuing support for these programs only to the end of the 1945–1946 academic year and only for students who were to receive their medical degrees by June 1946, who would then serve on active duty. For the students who were not scheduled to graduate, the Army's support stopped in March 1946. If an enlisted student decided to continue his medical training, presumably paid for by the VA, he could be transferred to the Enlisted Reserve Corps. Students who did not continue to study medicine were discharged from the Army.

For the Army, the more than 13,000 young physicians who graduated ASTP with a three-year obligation to serve on active duty were critical as a short-term fix (see Cowdrey, 1987, p. 12). By July 1948, ASTP graduates made up a majority of the Medical Corps, and planners noted that the Medical Department would not be able to perform its mission without them.

The Army recognized that the use of ASTP graduates was just a stopgap measure and that things had to change. New emphasis was placed on providing educational opportunities for career medical officers and on establishing Reserve Officer Training Corps (ROTC) programs at civilian medical schools. In addition, the distinguished medical consultant program that had been so important during the war in bringing state-of-the-art practices to the Medical Department was made permanent. Congress also played its part by voting additional compensation for non-ASTP doctors and dentists. However, with a large number of physicians completing their service obligations in 1948, the Army had a shortage of 12,000 medical officers by the end of 1949. By June 1950, when the war in Korea started, the Far Eastern Command had only one-half of the Medical Corps officers it was authorized.[7]

Long-Term Changes

Before World War II, the majority of Army physicians were general practitioners, with only a few specialists (mainly surgeons).[8] During the war, their ranks swelled with civilian specialists of all kinds providing direct medical care to the troops, leaving the career medical officers largely free to administer the system with the help of a new group of civilian hospital administrators. After the war, returning to the prewar arrangements was untenable both in terms of the worldwide responsibilities of the Army and the standards of medical practice. The Surgeon General clearly understood that, if Army medicine was to succeed, it would have to look a great deal more like its

---

[7]   There were 318 Medical Corps officers authorized and only 156 assigned (Cowdrey, 1987, Table 7, p. 68).

[8]   Milner, 1964, p. 14, notes that "in May 1939, the [Medical] department had on its rolls exactly 77 specialty board diplomats . . . [with none] in such important specialties as anesthesiology, . . . orthopedic surgery, and urology . . . [;] of the 37 leading medical societies in being at the time, it had no representation at all in 21."

civilian counterparts, and the Army would have to initiate a number of changes in how it procured physicians, nurses, and other health professionals.

First, with the mass of civilian doctors returning home after the war, the Army found itself critically short of highly trained professional experts. Clearly, the Army could not go back to the prewar structure of 1939, which had not been entirely adequate even then. Medical Corps officers' strength in September 1939 was 1,098—all regulars—and had reached a World War II peak of 47,990 in July 1945, with 1,261 regulars and 46,729 reserve officers (Milner, 1964, pp. 23–24). To meet its long-term need, the Army established ROTC units at medical and other health professional schools. This put thousands of students into the pipeline who would receive commissions at the end of their training. In addition, select members of the Medical Department were sent to civilian institutions for specialty training, and five Army hospitals were designated as teaching hospitals with appropriate residency programs.

Second, something had to be done to address the problem of the Nurse Corps. Reflecting the status of women in the armed forces at the time, the legal authorities for commissioning female nurses had to be addressed. Effective at the beginning of fiscal year (FY) 1948, Army nurses had to transfer their wartime commissions to the Regular Army or reserve commissions. While almost 1,600 received Regular Army commissions, the majority were given reserve commissions—nurses on extended active duty with reserve, rather than regular, commissions ended up dominating the corps. Both groups, however, were not enough to meet the needs, and civilian contract nurses were hired to fill the gap.

Third, the role of nonphysician officers was addressed with the establishment of the Medical Service Corps, which replaced the separate Medical Administrative, Pharmacy and Sanitary Corps. This not only "united medical administrators with officers in the allied sciences . . . [but helped] alleviate the shortage of doctors" (Cowdrey, 1987, pp. 20–21). Henceforth, the only doctor in an administrative post at an Army hospital would be the commander or, in large hospitals, the commander and his deputy. This one move reduced the number of medical officers the Army "required" by 7.5 percent.

Military Hospitals

The first Secretary of Defense, James Forrestal, wanted to "achieve the maximum degree of coordination, efficiency and economy" by improving utilization of hospitals and coordinating medical plans and programs (Rearden, 1984, p. 109). In December 1947, he set up the Committee on Medical and Hospital Services under the leadership of Dr. Paul Hawley, the newly retired Chief Medical Director of the VA.[9] In early 1949, the Hawley committee made a number of recommendations to eliminate obvious duplication of services, but according to Hawley, the surgeons general were "noncooperative . . . in order to safeguard their own bureaucratic turfs" (Cowdrey, 1987,

---

[9] Dr. Hawley was a retired major general in the Army Medical Corps when he joined GEN Omar Bradley at the VA in 1945. He had been the chief surgeon in the European theater during World War II.

p. 25). Nevertheless, in 1949, the new Secretary of Defense, Louis Johnson, established the Medical Services Division—later renamed the Office of Medical Services—to "set and control general policies, standards and programs for the medical services of the . . . services" (Rearden, 1984, p. 110).[10] He was determined to close 18 military hospitals (Rearden, 1984, p. 110), the Army's share of which was to be four general hospitals—a reduction of almost 5,500 beds, or 35 percent of the Army's general hospital capacity (Marble, 2008, p. 72).

Reconsidering the Roles of the Army and Veterans Administration

A critical issue in determining the need for Army hospitals was the respective roles of the Army and VA in caring for soldiers at the end of their enlistments. During World War II, the ability of the VA to receive patients was severely limited by a shortage of critical personnel and a lack of facilities.[11] This changed after the war; as early as mid-1948, Army Surgeon General Raymond Bliss was under pressure from the Assistant Secretary of the Army to make better use of VA facilities by discharging patients with chronic illnesses and little prospect of ever returning to active duty. In 1949, Congress passed the Career Compensation Act of 1949 (Pub. L. 81-351, 1949), which established the Temporary Disability Retired List (TDRL). This was followed by Executive Order (EO) 10122 in April 1950, which gave primary responsibility for "hospitalization of members or former members of the uniformed services placed on the temporary disability retired list or permanently retired for physical disability or receiving disability retirement pay who require hospitalization for chronic diseases" (EO 10122, 1950) to the VA. However, in 1952, the law was changed so that military retirees who had completed 20 years of active service could elect to receive care in a military hospital, rather than at the VA (EO 10400, 1952).

On the eve of the Korean War, the policy on the respective roles of the Army and VA was set, even if the way it would be implemented was open to interpretation. It took the Army two years to update its regulations to reflect the EO, and even then, the Army left the interpretation of "optimum hospital improvement" in the hands of the physicians treating each individual patient (Polo, 2009, p. 22). Thus, the policy was that the military health system would focus on military personnel, serving others only on a space-available basis. But in practice, policy was still ambiguous when it came to transferring severely wounded or chronically ill soldiers who had little prospect of returning to active duty from an Army to a VA facility—an ambiguity that continues to this day, particularly when it comes to the continued service of amputees.

---

[10] This office would later become the Office of the Assistant Secretary of Defense for Health Affairs.

[11] Unfortunately, the VA had a "low Federal priority rating" and could not obtain either the labor or materials it needed (Adkins, 1967, p. 167). In early 1944, the Department of War started to assign physicians and dentists to work at the VA.

The Army Medical Department on the Eve of the Korean War

The smaller, reorganized medical department was very different from what it had been before or immediately after World War II. In the five years after World War II, the Army had started to remake itself into a modern, specialty-oriented medical system. Women were more accepted as partners in the delivery of services, as were those in allied health fields. If this new system had any shortfalls, it was that its focus on specialty medicine made it less prepared to provide support for combat forces in the field. This was a system designed to care for garrison forces stationed around the world. Shortages of medical personnel persisted, but the Medical Department felt that it could make do until the current class of residents had completed its training. The low point would be June 1950 (Cowdrey, 1987, p. 35).

CHAPTER THREE

The Korean War

Invasion

On June 25, 1950, forces from the North Korean People's Army crossed the 38th parallel demarcation line that had separated the two halves of the Korean Peninsula since the end of World War II. The North Koreans engaged the ill-prepared forces not only of the Republic of Korea but also of the United States. Within hours of the invasion, the United States called for a meeting of the UN Security Council—a meeting the representatives of the Soviet Union boycotted, as they did a subsequent meeting two days later.

In retrospect, this was a colossal political blunder because, in the absence of the Soviet Union, the Security Council recognized the legitimacy of the South Korean government, called on member states to provide assistance to the South Koreans to repel the invaders, authorized the unified UN command, and asked the United States to designate the commander of the unified forces. The following day, the President named General of the Army Douglas MacArthur as Commander in Chief, UN Command.

The condition of the U.S. Army President Truman could employ in summer 1950 is legendary. Popular sentiment against a large standing military establishment and eagerness to affect economies in government had forced drastic reductions in defense expenditures, making this Army a shadow of what it had been just five years earlier, at the end of World War II. Not only had authorized strength been reduced to 630,000, but actual strength was almost 39,000 below that level (Stillwaugh, undated, p. 3). Only one of the 12 American combat divisions, including two U.S. Marine Corps divisions, was up to authorized strength. The one exception was the 1st Infantry Division, half a world away in Europe.

As a result, there were no U.S. combat units in Korea in early summer 1950. The nearest forces were the four divisions of the Eighth Army in Japan, and given that their primary mission was the occupation of Japan, "[n]o serious effort" had been made "to maintain combat efficiency at battalion or higher level" (Glass and Jones, 2005, Ch. 5,

p. 3).[1] Moreover, many of the soldiers were young; most had never been exposed to hostile fire—only "one in six were combat veterans" (Garrett, 1999, p. 23)—and the newly arrived replacement troops "had a high percentage of lower intelligence ratings. In April 1949, 43% of Army enlisted personnel in the [Far East Command], rated in class IV and class V (the two lowest classes) on the Army General Classification Test" (Glass and Jones, 2005, Ch. 5, p. 3). Just months earlier, the Army Inspector General judged the readiness of the Eighth Army to be low. He highlighted "the general lack of skills on the part of junior soldiers, . . . [but] reserved the bulk of his criticism for officer leadership," singling out the service units, such as medical support units, for being "blissfully ignorant of even the rudiments of military training" (Hanson, 2010, p. 29).

Mobilization

Within days of the invasion and on the recommendation of the Joint Chiefs of Staff, President Truman moved to increase the size of the armed forces, with the Army to gain 5,000 officers and 45,000 enlisted men. This limited response has been characterized as a partial or even a creeping mobilization, with the Truman administration proceeding cautiously because "there existed the possibility that Korea might be only a diversionary action to a larger Communist aggression" (Stillwaugh, undated, p. 13). Calling up the National Guard, as many suggested, was not feasible because "the real problem was not manpower, but the lack of modern equipment" (Stillwaugh, undated, pp. 15–16). As a result, the initial defense of Korea and any immediate offensive actions would have to come from existing forces, selectively augmented by individuals who possessed needed skills, such as physicians, surgeons, and nurses. Initially, this augmentation took the form of involuntary extensions of enlistments and overseas tours. Over time, however, it would also include stripping the continental armies of experienced and trained individuals; calling up units and members of the Organized Reserve Corps and National Guard; resuming conscription; and, later, drafting health professionals.

The First Engagement of American Forces in the Korean War: Task Force Smith

Even before the Security Council's actions on June 27, 1950, President Truman ordered U.S. military forces to assist in the defense of Korea. The initial American response was from air and naval forces based in Japan. The first ground troops, the 406 officers and men of Task Force Smith—approximately one-half of a battalion combat team of the 21st Infantry Regiment, 24th Division—were airlifted to the port city of Pusan on July 1. Because of the limited airlift available, the Task Force Smith did not include tanks or engineers to place mines. Also missing were contingents normally part of a

---

[1]   Hanson, 2010, p. 29, presents a contrary view, suggesting that there had been considerable improvement in U.S. combat units' readiness in the year preceding the outbreak of the war and that incapacity of commanders at battalion and above was the major problem U.S. Army units faced in the first few months of the war, not small-unit readiness and lack of cohesion.

regiment combat team, such as military police, air defenders, forward air controllers, and signal and reconnaissance platoons. However, Task Force Smith did include a medical platoon.

After disembarking from its aircraft, Task Force Smith was quickly dispatched north by truck and rail to block the approaches to Pusan. Reinforced by elements of the 52nd Field Artillery Battalion, they engaged the North Koreans on July 5 but were overwhelmed.[2] The task force lost 150 dead, wounded, or taken prisoner.[3]

The ultimate failure of Task Force Smith, often attributed to it being part of a "woefully unprepared and poorly equipped post–World War II force" (Sullivan, 1992, p. 18), must be weighed against the failure of senior commanders to fully appreciate the situation on the ground in Korea: Their certainty that the North Koreans would wither in battle as soon as they saw American troops reflected nothing more than the hubris of American commanders.

The experience of Task Force Smith does illustrate well a recurring theme in the history of military medicine: the importance of medical support to maintain the cohesion of fighting units. The Roman historian Livy noted the "demoralization of the fighting line by the misery of the wounded, when the primal duty of evacuation is neglected" (Garrison, 1922, p. 52). Some 2,500 years later, the lesson was relearned. The men of Task Force Smith "fought well, surrounded for hours, but when the breakout was attempted, and the men knew that some of the wounded were being left behind, the unit began to fail and unit cohesion broke down" (Garrett, 1999, pp. 18, 30–31). So even in the first hour of the engagement in Korea, the importance of medical support was apparent—support that would eventually become one of the success stories of the Korean War.

Medical Support

The first medical unit to arrive in Korea was an understrength medical platoon assigned to provide medical support to Task Force Smith. It was soon followed by the 8055th Mobile Army Surgical Hospital (MASH),[4] which disembarked in Pusan on July 6, 1950. The MASH, rather than a larger evacuation hospital, was the logical first unit to send. By design, it was small and self-contained and seemed best suited to meet the

---

[2] Collins, 1969, pp. 45–55, provides a compelling account of Task Force Smith and the battle.

[3] Garrett, 1999, p. 18, reports that, in the battle,

> 148 American infantrymen were killed, wounded, or missing. All five officers and ten enlisted men of the forward observer liaison, machine gun and bazooka group were lost. North Korean casualties in the battle before Osan were approximately 42 dead and 85 wounded; four tanks had been destroyed or immobilized. The enemy advance was delayed perhaps seven hours. (Tucker, 1992)

[4] Richard Hooker, author of the book and resulting television series, *M*A*S*H*, was assigned to the 8055th MASH, on which he based the fictitious 4077th MASH (Hooker, 1968).

emergency at hand.[5] Deploying a MASH provided medical Echelon III capability in an Echelon II environment (see Table 3.1).

Mobile Army Surgical Hospital

American military historian Clay Blair says of the Korean War that, "[t]o the several generations born since it was fought, the 'Korean War' is little more than a phrase in a history book" (Blair, 1987, p. ix). Blair's contention notwithstanding, millions of Americans knew the Korean War through the antics of Hawkeye Pierce and the other characters of a television series, *M*A*S*H*. It has been estimated that, on February 28, 1983, almost one-half of the total American population watched the last episode of the series about a mythical Army hospital during the Korean War.[6] While the show *M*A*S*H* was great fun, what went on at a real MASH was deadly serious—especially for the soldiers fighting the war in Korea.

On the eve of the Korean War, the Army had formally established five MASHs, but none were effectively fielded, and none were in the Far East. The first MASH to see combat, the 8055th MASH, was hastily organized on July 1, 1950, with "ten medical officers, 95 enlisted men and 12 nurses assigned" by stripping available personnel from other units in Japan (Cowdrey, 1985, p. 5). By July 10, it was at work in Taejon, Korea, alongside the clearing company of the 24th Infantry Division. It operated as designed, providing forward surgery for those who could not stand the journey to the 8054th Evacuation Hospital in Pusan or traveling by air to Japan or to a Navy hospital ship off the coast. However, the realities of war in Korea broke the very design of the MASH as MASH units grew and were "located too far to the rear (25 miles)" (Cowdrey, 1987, p. 179).

To be effective, this small, 60-bed surgical hospital was designed to fit into a medical evacuation (medevac) scheme (Table 3.1), to provide an Echelon III capability in an Echelon II environment, and to serve the so-called nontransportable close to the front. However, the lack of transportation, an inadequate road and rail network, and the volatile tactical situation soon overwhelmed the MASHs, including the later-deployed 8063rd and 8076th MASHs. In November 1950, the 8055th and the other

---

[5]   The standard for MASH operations required that it could be

> disassembled, loaded onto vehicles, and ready to depart with 6 hours' notice. After arrival at its new destination, it was operational within 4 hours. Each MASH operated five surgical tables in a shift with a highly organized system of managing shock patients. An ambulance platoon was attached to each MASH to facilitate the rapid evacuation when postoperative recovery was complete. Additionally, four helicopters were attached to each MASH. They, in turn, were utilized for resupply, rapid patient delivery to the MASH, and comfortable evacuation from the MASH. (Woodard, 2003, p. 508)

[6]   For decades, the last episode of *M*A*S*H* has been known as the most-watched TV show finale in history, with an estimated 50.1 million homes—106 million viewers—tuned in. In terms of the percentage of the population that saw the show, 46.96 percent, it remains the most widely seen TV show in history. See, for example, Nededog, 2017.

Table 3.1
Echelonment of Medical Support—Chain of Casualty Evacuation: MASH Provides an Echelon III Capability in an Echelon II Environment

Echelon	Facility	Brought By	Responsibility	Medical Protocol
I	Aid station or unit dispensary	Walking, manual transport or litter, ambulance or other vehicles	Unit medical personnel	Apply initial battle dressing
II	Collecting stations to clearing stations	Walking, manual transport or litter, ambulance or other vehicles	Medical battalions, squadrons or regiments, collecting, ambulance and clearing elements	Triage; medical aid measures
	MASH	Motor and air ambulance (helicopters)	Surgical care for patients who could not be moved	Emergency surgery to stabilize prior to transportation to Echelon III facility
III	Field or mobile hospitals; evacuation hospitals; convalescent hospitals	Ambulance, rail, airplane	Army Medical Service or Independent Corps Medical Service	Initial wound surgery; "debridement"; no suturing; rest and short-term recuperative services
IV	"Communication zone" general hospitals; hospital centers; station hospitals	Rail, water transport, airplane, ambulance	Medical service of the theater of operations	Reparative surgery
V	General or special hospitals in the Zone of the Interior	Rail, water transport, airplane, ambulance	Medical service of the General Headquarters or Zone of the Interior	Reconstructive surgery, rehabilitative surgery

SOURCE: Adapted from "Medical Treatment in World War II," undated; Rostker, 2013.

MASH units first expanded to 150 beds and, eventually, to 200 beds.[7] Moreover, without deployed field hospitals, the MASHs soon became more than surgical hospitals, also seeing nonsurgical patients. The chief surgeon of the 8076th MASH noted, "We had to improvise in our treatment. . . . The MASH units were responsible for treatment of all the wounded who were brought to its tents" (Apel and Apel, 1998, p. 63). Figure 3.1 shows a tactically deployed MASH in Korea; notice the helicopter in the lower right corner.

Transportation of the Wounded

The chain of casualty evacuation incorporates all the echelons shown in Table 3.1, extending from the battlefield to the hospitals in the United States. Transporting the wounded from the place of wounding to a medical facility is the first critical link. Historically, if the wounded could not be moved quickly enough to the rear, the capabilities of the rear had to be moved to them. Thus, the need for forward surgery and the positioning of a MASH was driven by the condition of the wounded and their inability

Figure 3.1
Deployed Mobile Army Surgical Hospital in Korea

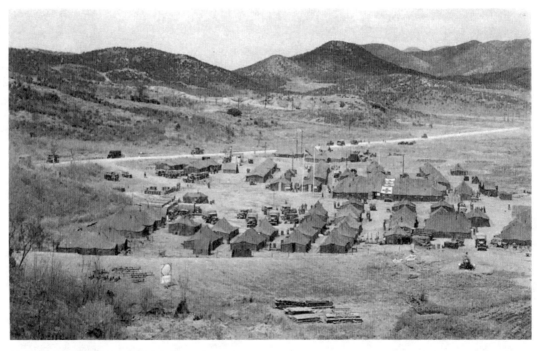

SOURCE: Ginn, 1997, p. 240.

---

[7]   It was not until February 1952 that the MASH table of organization and equipment (TO&E) was changed back to 60 beds, but MASHs continued to function as 200-bed semievacuation hospitals throughout 1952 (Lindsey, 1954, p. 84).

to withstand the journey to an Echelon III medical facility. Similarly, the conditions of postoperative patents and the rigors of transporting them to higher-echelon facilities dictated how the higher echelons were structured.

Transportation of the Wounded in Korea

In Korea, the fluid tactical situation, the limited highway net, the rough roads, and the mountainous terrain were greatly negated by the use of helicopters, enabling "hospitals . . . [to] stay longer in each location and allow four or five days of postoperative care for a patient before further evacuation" (Blumenson, 1955, p. 111). The helicopter will forever be linked with the MASH in the minds of the American people thanks to the opening of the TV show *M*A*S*H*, which depicted the types of helicopters and jeep ambulances actually used in Korea. Figure 3.2 illustrates these vehicles. The jeep ambulance, developed during World War II, was the workhorse in the mountains of Korea, as the following report from a Medical Company of the 7th Infantry attests:

> Normally, litter jeeps from our medical company collecting station pick up their patients at the battalion aid station. In this operation, however, the litter jeeps passed the aid station and came up the road to a point only fifty yards from the base of the mountain on which the battalion was fighting. . . .
>
> A man wounded on the firing line was immediately treated then he was carried down the mountain by a five-man litter team. The trip took an hour and a half.
>
> Once the patient reached the jeep evacuation point his bandages were checked and adjusted, and his general condition observed. Seriously wounded were loaded two

Figure 3.2
Helicopters and Jeep Ambulances Were Critical in Transporting the Wounded in Korea

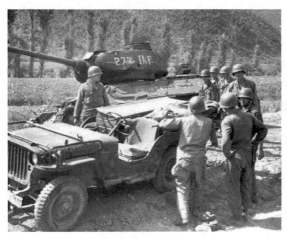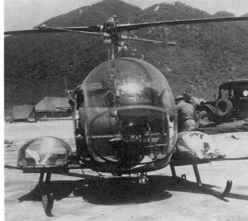

SOURCE: U.S. Army photos.

to a jeep; lightly wounded were often loaded seven to a vehicle—one in the front seat, four in the back, two on the hood.

The jeeps bypassed the battalion aid station and took the patients to the advanced clearing station. Here the seriously wounded were evacuated by helicopter. (Sarka, 1955, pp. 110–111)

For the seriously wounded, however, Korea was helicopter country:

The entire nation was marked by poor roads ruined by tank traffic, railroads with bombed-out track and bridges, mountainous terrain with ridges up to 6,000 ft. Conditions deteriorated in rainy weather, which washed out roads, and winter weather, which covered roads with snow and iced over bridges. Tactical positions in those mountains became impassable for ground vehicles. The helicopter was the only solution. (Apel and Apel, 1998, pp. 67–68)

Generally, there were enough helicopters to transport the worst cases, except during heavy combat, when the surgeons selected the worst cases. "Roughly speaking, something less than half of the true surgical [cases were] . . . moved by helicopter" (Lindsey, 1954, p. 80).

Air Evacuation from Korea to Japan and the United States

Evacuation of wounded, injured, or ill persons from Korea was governed by the theater evacuation policy,[8] which specified "number of days, the maximum period of noneffectiveness (hospitalization and convalescence) that patients may be held within the theater for treatment" (Field Manual [FM] 8-10-6, 2000, p. 1-4). A number of factors influence the specific policy, including the nature of the operation, the number and type of patients, the means of evacuation, the availability of replacements, and the in-theater medical resources. Since World War I, the number of days patients are held in theater has steadily decreased. During World War I, the Army hospitalized patients in theater for up to 150 days. During World War II, the limit was generally 60 days. "Obviously, transportation technology is the most significant reason for the evolution of shorter evacuation policy" (Rice, 1979, p. 87).

World War II

At the beginning of World War II, "it was commonly believed that air evacuation of the sick and wounded was dangerous, medically unsound, and militarily impossible . . . even when it was necessary to evacuate casualties over long distances" (Vanderburg,

---

[8]   Evacuation policy is not only a means of regulating "patient buildup and flow during wartime operations; it is equally important as a resource planning tool" (Rice, 1979, p. 86). The 1979 Defense Resources Management Study argued that shortening the time a patient spent in theater would allow "limited airlift assets to haul more combat troops and material and fewer hospitals and physicians to the front during the early critical days of a war" (Rice, 1979, p. 86) and can allow the use of "private-sector, Veterans Administration, and Public Health Service beds and physicians . . . in CONUS" (Rice, 1979, p. 88).

2003, p. 8). From the Army Air Corps prospective, according to the Surgeon of the 3rd Air Force, Lt Col Malcolm C. Grow, a major stumbling block was the Army Surgeon General, who reportedly did not "accept the airplane as a vehicle for casualty transportation" (Vanderburg, 2003, p. 8). Soon, however, the aircraft that had transported men and supplies to overseas bases were being reconfigured with removable litter supports, and patients were making the return trip back to the United States.[9] In this way, by January 1942, the Army Air Force had transported more than 10,000 casualties back to the United States from Burma, New Guinea, and Guadalcanal. One problem, however, was that there were not enough physicians to put one on every flight. Starting in early 1943, "Flight Nurses," Army nurses who had completed four weeks of training in aeromedical physiology, aircraft loading procedures, and survival skills, were assigned to the new Army Air Forces Evacuation Service. In 1943, 173,500 wounded and sick personnel were evacuated to the United States. In 1944, that number grew to 545,000 (Department of the Air Force, Office of the Surgeon General, 1976, p. 11). Despite the increased use of aircraft, medevac was still primarily done by ship, even during the last year of World War II. Even then, in August 1945, the month that saw the largest number of casualties returned to the United States by air, almost six times more patients returned home by ship than by air transport (Rostker, 2013, p. 198, Figure 8.3).

Korea

After the war, in 1949, the Joint Chiefs of Staff ordered that, in the future, air evacuation would be the primary means of returning patients to the United States.[10] However, when war started in Korea, there was no established air evacuation system.[11] As a result, most patients were evacuated by ship from Korea to Japan, even though empty cargo planes were available.[12] This changed in late August 1950 with the establishment of the Far East Air Force's Combat Cargo Command. Soon, C-54, C-46, and C-47 aircraft that offloaded personnel and cargo at forward airfields were transporting casualties further south in Korea or to Japan. In the first six months of the war, intratheater medevac—within Korea, from Korea to Japan, or within Japan—totaled 48,947

---

[9] Link and Coleman, 1955, pp. 352–418, tells the complete story of aeromedical evacuation (AE).

[10] The Joint Chiefs of Staff made the case, in *Report by the Logistics Plans Committee* (June 17, 1949), that "21 times more medical personnel are required for transportation of patients on surface vessels than required for transportation by air" (Hall and Nolan, 1950).

[11] Clingman notes that, "During the first three months the aeromedical evacuation process was not well organized because of the lack of personnel; inexperienced personnel and inadequate supplies and equipment; and the absence of a theater directive or policy on medical evacuation" (Clingman, 1989, p. 35).

[12] During the initial phase of the war, through "September 15, 1950, 13,015 wounded were evacuated from Korea, of whom only 3,855 (29.6 percent) were evacuated by air, even though 36,000 wounded could have been flown out on empty cargo planes" (Department of the Air Force, Office of the Surgeon General, 1976, pp. 12–13).

patients (Clingman, 1989, p. 38). By the end of the war, there had been more than 311,000 trips; that number was higher than the total casualties because it included multiple movements of patients (Futrell, 1983, p. 593).

Intertheater medevac from Japan to the United States was the responsibility of the Military Air Transport Service. At the beginning of the war, about 350 patients a month were being flown from Japan to the continental United States (CONUS). It was a long trip. Initially, the route from Japan was through Guam and Kwajalein, on to Wake or Midway, with a stop in Hawaii, and finally to Travis Air Force Base (AFB) in California—a 23-hour flight. Between September 2, 1950, and December 31, 1953, 38,516 Army soldiers were evacuated to CONUS—19,465 for battle injuries; 5,974 for nonbattle injuries; and 13,077 for disease—with 95.4 percent going by air transport (Clingman, 1989, p. 49).

In less than a decade after the end of World War II, the whole system of casualty evacuation had radically changed. From the use of helicopters to long-range transport aircraft, the time from wounding to definitive care in the United States had been dramatically reduced, with more to come. At the end of 1951, with air evacuation still in its infancy, Air Force Brig Gen Wilford Hall prophetically wrote that, in the future, "air evacuation, while not in itself a method of treatment, acts as a catalyst, for it sharply cuts the time needed to move a patient to the hospital for definitive care and, therefore, speeds up the initiation of the entire healing process" (Hall, 1951, p. 1028).

Medical Support on the Move

For World Wars I and II, a common picture of medical support can be drawn of medical units advancing in support of a relentless march forward. The picture does not hold for the Korean War. The medical support provided varied greatly for each of the four very distinct phases of that war: the invasion and defense of the Pusan Perimeter; the counteract and advance, including the breakout from Pusan and the Inchon landing; the Chinese assault and counterattack; and the period of stalemate. Figure 3.3 shows the buildup of American forces assigned to divisions and the corresponding buildup of medical personnel assigned to the deployed medical battalions during the four phases of the war. By summer 1951, the buildup was essentially complete, with the strength of the medical battalions being roughly 2 percent of total divisional strength.

Invasion
During the initial days of the Korean War, troops flooded into southeastern Korea to stem the tide of the advancing North Koreans and to form a defensive perimeter around the port city of Pusan.[13] By the end of July 1951, there were one evacuation hospital and three MASH units in Korea: the 8055th, the 8063rd, and the 8076th.

---

[13] Appleman, 1960, covers the initial period of the Korean War.

Figure 3.3
Buildup of American Forces: Total, Divisional, and Medical, July 1950–July 1953

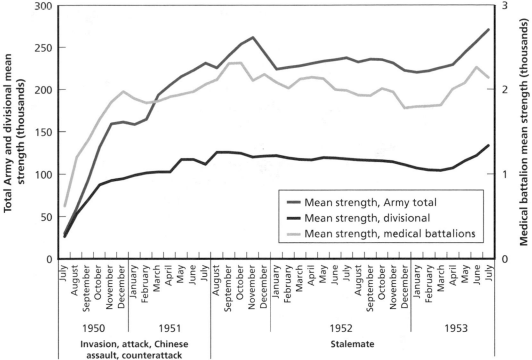

SOURCE: Data from Reister, 1973, pp. 3–4.

Originally designed to support a single division, the MASH units soon found that they had to support more than one division and more than just American forces as troops from other nations joined the fight. After intense fighting, the line held, and the medical situation stabilized,[14] but the cost was horrendous. By mid-September 1950, American casualties numbered more than 4,500 battle deaths; 12,000 wounded; 400 reported captured; and more than 2,100 reported missing in action (Webb, 2006, p. 26). The one saving grace for the wounded was that, in defending a perimeter, they could be evacuated quickly to hospital ships offshore or to airfields for a relatively quick flight to a hospital in Japan. And for the most seriously wounded, the proximity to Japan meant that "within ten to fourteen days of the time they fell in a Korean battle-field . . . [they would receive] definitive treatment . . . [in the states, well] beyond the capabilities of the Far East Command" (Cowdrey, 1987, p. 82).

---

[14] Cowdrey, 1987, pp. 82–84, discusses this further.

The Landing at Inchon, the Breakout from the Pusan Perimeter and Crossing the 38th Parallel

September 1950 saw a complete reversal of the situation on the Korean Peninsula, with the MASHs on the move. Early in the month, the three MASH units were in the south supporting the Eighth Army's defense of the Pusan Perimeter. On September 15, the newly created X Corps, comprising the 7th Infantry Division and the 1st Marine Division, landed at Inchon, the port city for the South Korean capital of Seoul, successfully cutting off the North Korean forces attacking Pusan. (The 1st MASH, 121st Evacuation Hospital, and the 4th Field Hospital were part of the invasion force.) The next day, the Eighth Army counterattacked. By September 18, UN forces started to break out of the perimeter, and "a general enemy withdrawal began . . . [which] turned rapidly into a rout" (Cowdrey, 1987, p. 105). Cowdrey provides a vivid description of the "almost bewildering . . . movements of the MASHs as they sought to maintain close support" for the advancing American troops (Cowdrey, 1987, pp. 107–112).

On October 9, 1950, troops from the 1st Cavalry Division crossed the 38th parallel, which separated the two Koreas. On October 24, the North Korean capital of Pyongyang fell; two days later, the X Corps landed on Korea's east coast. In less than six weeks, the Eighth Army had moved more than 300 miles. By the end of November, however, the advance would turn into a retreat when two new foes entered the war: the Chinese and winter.

The Chinese Communist Assault

On October 1, the Chinese Premier, Chou En-lai, warned that China would intervene if UN forces crossed the 38th parallel. The warning went unheeded. In response, nearly 300,000 Chinese Communist Forces (CCF) soldiers in 30 divisions secretly crossed into North Korea (Stewart, 2003, p. 7). They first struck Republic of Korea forces on October 25 in what was initially thought to be a "token gesture" (Gammons, 2006, p. 29). By November 1, it was clear that this was no token gesture. Through the month of November, a number of battles resulted in significant losses for the UN forces. At the battle of Ch'ongch'on (November 25–28), "the 2nd Division alone took almost 4,500 battle casualties, . . . a third of its strength" (Stewart, 2003, p. 13). The 8076th MASH was in the teeth of it:

> Rapidly the hospital was overloaded with hundreds of wounded men. Surgeons and nurses had to cope with them despite below-zero cold. Intravenous solutions froze in liter flasks. Diesel fuel for heating would not flow unless mixed with kerosene. Space heaters burned out under continuous operations, and ice forming in gasoline caused electric generators to fail. Lights in the operating room winked out, leaving surgeons to work by the glow of potbellied stoves and the unsteady beams of hand-held flashlights. Nurses boiled water on the stoves to clean surgical instruments, but ice formed in the water before they were finished washing. Surgeons' hands were so cold that they would hardly hold their instruments, much less

operate, and the bodies of the wounded steamed as the surgical knives cut them open. (Cowdrey, 1987, p. 123)

On November 27, the CCF attacked the X Corps, the 1st Marines Division, and Army 7th Infantry Division at the Chosin Reservoir, forcing them to move south in an epic withdrawal to the sea. If medical support is challenging during an advance, it is even more so during a retreat. Casualties soar and are not limited to combat troops but also include medical personnel. One medical battalion lost eight doctors, two dentists, and nine Medical Service Corps officers.

It should be noted that, for this campaign, the number of nonbattle casualties—principally from frostbite from the below zero cold but also from "digestive disorders, shock, and nonbattle injuries"—far exceeded battle casualties. The 1st Marine Division alone reported 4,395 battle casualties and 7,338 nonbattle casualties.[15]

At the port of Hungnam on Korea's east coast, the Americans established a strong defensive perimeter as the 8076th MASH leapfrogged in retreat to the beachhead and eventually to hospital ships waiting offshore. However, this was no Dunkirk. On December 24, 1950, "the X Corps completed its withdrawal from Hungnam with over 105,000 troops, . . . along with 98,100 refugees" (Stewart, 2003, p. 26). Within a month, the X Corps had been refitted and redeployed to help the Eighth Army hold the new defensive line south of Seoul. By mid-March, Seoul was retaken; by April, a new line was established just south of the 38th parallel. A series of attacks and counterattacks followed, but the UN had learned to deal with "the Chinese style of warfare—characterized by furious offensive operations, only marginally sustained, followed by withdrawal and regrouping" (McGrath, 2003, p. 26). By July 1951, the front was again north of the prewar boundary. The fluidity of the battlefield had the whole medevac system on the go; "the 8055th [and] the 8076th [MASH units] operated in nine locations between New Year's Day and the end of May . . . . During the year the 8076th would admit 21,508 patients—1,048 during the single most active week in February, of whom 741 were battle casualties" (Cowdrey, 1987, p. 168).

It was not only the MASHs that were on the move. The 121st Evacuation Hospital, for example, had landed with the rest of the X Corps at Inchon in September 1950. It moved north with advancing troops but in December 1950 was evacuated from Hungnam with the rest of the X Corps. It set up outside Pusan, but by early April 1951, it was in Seoul supporting I Corps. It moved again when the CCF counterattacked, then again when the UN forces retook Seoul. "During 1951 nearly 46,000 admissions flooded the 121st Evacuation Hospital. . . . Admissions ranged from none on some days to more than 600 on others" (Cowdrey, 1987, pp. 170–171).

---

[15] For November 27 to December 24, 1950, the 1st Marine Division reported 604 killed, 114 dead of wounds, 192 missing, and 3,485 wounded—for a total of 4,395. "The bulk of these casualties occurred between 27 November and 11 December" (Appleman, 1990, p. 345).

Stalemate

On June 1, 1951, Secretary of State Dean Acheson indicated U.S. willingness to accept a cease-fire line in the vicinity of the 38th parallel. A month later, the Chinese and North Koreans agreed to cease-fire negotiations, ushering in a period of static warfare reminiscent of the trench warfare of World War I, as shown in Figure 3.4, with continuous patrolling punctuated by intense fights for local strongpoints. As the negotiations ebbed and flowed, intense local attacks and counterattacks took countless lives and continued to tax the skills of the newly arrived surgeons, who undertook the harshest kind of on-the-job-training—learning the skills of combat medicine not taught in medical school and for which they were not prepared. Even to the end, with the cease-fire lines well in place, carnage continued. During the last two months of the war, approximately 100,000 Communist and nearly 53,000 UN soldiers were killed, captured, or wounded (Birtle, 2006, p. 34).

Medical Personnel

For the first critical months of the war, medical personnel came from those available in the Far East and those the Army could send from the United States and Europe.

Figure 3.4
An Echo of World War I: 7th Infantry Division Trenches,
July 1953

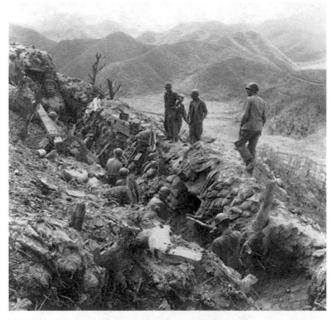

SOURCE: U.S. Army Center of Military History, 2010.

Critical shortages were partly addressed when the Navy assigned 98 physicians to help staff the Eighth Army and X Corps (Cowdrey, 1987, p. 140). Eventually, new physicians arrived from home as a result of a new draft of doctors, and a system was developed for sharing the burden—"nine months of actual service for those in forward areas" (Cowdrey, 1987, p. 231)—for all personnel. However, the interplay of these two policies—the draft and rotation of personnel—created a number of problems, not the least of which was the need to train the newcomers to fill the vacancies as medical personnel rotated home.

Doctor Draft

For the Army, the initial call-up of reserve physicians and dentists was inadequate to meet the demand. It was soon clear that extraordinary measures were needed. While the Selective Service law had been reestablished in 1948 in response to the heightened tensions in Europe, its requirement for registering men between the ages of 18 and 26 was not effective in filling the need for physicians and dentists. Since the 1948 law did not include a provision allowing the conscription of "medical professional and specialists," as earlier laws had, new legislation was necessary. By early September 1950, Pub. L. 81-779, the so-called doctor draft law, was before President Truman for his signature (Hinton, 1950; Hershey, 1953, p. 9).[16] Nevertheless, until the draft could become functional, World War II veterans—"the very group the law was designed to keep out of uniform"—were being recalled.[17] In fact, no drafted medical officer reached Korea until January 1951 (Cowdrey, 1987, p. 230).

The new law authorized drafting physicians and dentists as privates into the Army, but the real objective was to "coerce professionals into accepting reserve commissions in the medical [and dental] corps" (Flynn, 1993, p. 154). To do this, the new law established a priority system for induction as a way of putting pressure on those next in line to be drafted to apply for a reserve commission (Hershey, 1953, pp. 36–37). Dr. Howard A. Rusk, Chairman of the Health Resources Advisory Committee of the National Security Resources Board, reported that

> there was almost unanimous agreement in all circles that those physicians and dentists who received their professional training at Government expense or who were deferred from military service to continue their medical education had a moral obligation to serve the country during this emergency. (Rusk, 1952)

---

[16] For more on Pub. L. 81-779, see Hershey, 1953, pp. 118–120; on the regulations, see Hershey, 1953, pp. 137–140).

[17] During the first year of the war, 43,000 Army officers and 125,000 Army enlisted men were (individually) recalled to active duty, many before those in the reserve units. In the face of public outcry, the Army explained that "active reservists, because they were better prepared, had to be husbanded for any greater national emergency that might arise" (Gough, 1987, p. 30).

Those to be taken first were men who had trained at government expense during World War II or who had been given a deferment to attend a preprofessional program and had served less than 90 days. Next to be called would be those in the same category who had served more than 90 days but less than 21 months. The third priority group was made up of those who had not served. In the fourth group were veterans who had trained at government expense or had been deferred during World War II but had served more than 21 months.

On October 16, 1950, more than 16,000 doctors and dentists who had been previously deferred or trained by the government registered and were assigned to Priority Groups 1 and 2. In January 1951, 100,000 more doctors and dentists registered and were assigned to Priority Groups 3 and 4. By June 30, 1951, more than 131,000 doctors and dentists had registered (see Table 3.2). With a draft call of about 300 a month, just the threat of being drafted as a private into the Army was enough to get the required number to voluntarily take commissions.[18]

By 1952, the first two priority categories were exhausted. Moving into Priority Groups 3 and 4, however, created problems: "[A]n extremely high percentage of the men in Priority 3 are above the age of 40, whereas the military services primarily need younger men for field and sea duty" (Rusk, 1952). In addition, "physicians released from active duty complained about not being properly utilized," and there was "great dissatisfaction on the part of a large number of medical officers who thought they were not being treated fairly" (Berry, 1976, p. 279). Those in Priority Groups 1 and 2 thought that the doctors who had not served in World War II should be forced to serve. As the draft reached deeper into Priority Group 3, younger doctors and dentists were being drafted, impacting the internship and residency programs of many hospitals. Despite these problems, the law was extended with minor changes, eventually to

Table 3.2
Special Registrants—Physicians and Dentists—by Priority and Profession, June 30, 1951

Priority	Total	Physicians	Dentists
1	14,399	10,549	3,850
2	3,238	2,505	733
3	45,678	31,138	14,540
4	61,459	46,632	14,827
Total	123,774	90,824	33,950

SOURCE: Hershey, 1953, p. 37.

---

[18] The Surgeon General of the Army "advised physicians to take a commission as soon as they got a draft notice" (Flynn, 1993, p. 157).

be replaced by the Berry Plan (Berry, 1976), which focused on new medical and dental school graduates.

By the end of the war, in 1953, 13,000 physicians and 6,500 dentists were on active duty, which was "8 percent of all the physicians and dentists in practice in the United States" (Flynn, 1993, p. 156), a number substantially smaller than the 30 percent of all physicians and dentists who had served during World War II (Flynn, 1993, p. 154). About one-half of these were the result of the draft. Unlike World War II, in which soldiers served for the duration, Korean War draftees and the physicians and dentists who took reserve commissions served for only one year.

Rotation System

One of the most controversial programs during the Korean War was the personnel rotation system. As the war settled into a stalemate in September 1951, the Army introduced a system of points to determine when a soldier could "rotate home." When fully implemented, those with as little as nine months in the forward areas were eligible to rotate home.

This system was designed to improve morale by giving "every soldier a definite goal in an otherwise indefinite and seemingly goalless war" (Birtle, 2006, p. 27). Overall lower manpower quality, less-well-trained soldiers, and less-experienced leaders had deleterious effects on military efficiency; the system, by one account, "did nothing to improve military medical services. Like their nonmedical counterparts, medical personnel were rotated out at about the time that they were beginning to know their jobs well" (Sandler, 1999, p. 221). As a result, "there were very few, if any, individuals on duty in 1952 Korean hospitals who had ever seen the [MASH] unit move" (Woodard, 2003, p. 510). The high turnover translated into inadequate care for some of the wounded, as this account by Cowdrey illustrates:

> In October and November 1952 a large number of men with infected wounds reached the hospitals in Japan. The reason was not only the increased combat during October but also the arrival in the Eighth Army . . . of a large number of surgical replacements with hardly any experience in the treatment of massive traumas in a septic environment. (Cowdrey, 1987, p. 254)

The rotation system introduced during the Korean War was unique in military history. In previous wars, soldiers joined for the duration. In a few cases, soldiers might be sent home after some extended period of combat. For example, during World War II, Marines were rotated back to the states if they survived three campaigns. Many old hands were already back in the states before Iwo Jima and Okinawa, and many of the men in those campaigns were on their third operation (Frank and Shaw, 1968). The Army Air Corps also sent aircrews home after they completed a specified number of combat missions (Little, 1968, pp. 1–2). However, nothing had ever been tried on such a large scale before the Korean War. The twin rationalizations were fairness and combat fatigue, but what enabled this policy was a seemingly inexhaustible number of replacements fed by a draft and a manpower pool that was larger than what was needed just to replace combat losses. While some argued the policy had deleterious effects on the efficiency and proficiency of the Army (for example, Marshall, 1956, p. 14), others saw in it an emotional anchor, arguing that it limited the negative psychological impact of combat, especially at a time when the "the troops derived scant satisfaction either from enthusiastic popular support back home or from identification with those whose freedom they were fighting to save."[19] The rotation system used in Korea would be used again during the Vietnam War and was the subject of a "searing . . . brutal critique" that invoked the issues of fairness and combat fatigue that remain the underpinnings of the decision on whether or not to rotate troops (Towell, 2004, p. 44).

Field Medical Training

The draft and the rotational system exacerbated the problem of the lack of physicians trained to operate under battlefield conditions. Well-trained physicians and outstanding hospital care do not automatically translate into lifesaving care for the casualties of war. No civilian analogies prepared Army physicians for what they experienced in Korea, as a young surgical resident from Ohio explained, recalling his experience on arriving in Korea in spring 1951:

> No one had ever shown any of us the first military manual on how to do things militarily. We just had to figure out the best way to do it and get it done. Then we taught the next guy who came to our units, and they taught the next guy. That's the way the MASH operated. We did that with medical things also. The first doctor figured out the best way to do it, then taught the next doctors how it should be done. (Apel and Apel, 1998, p. 35)

By 1951, with the draft swelling the ranks and the rotation policy replacing experienced doctors with new ones fresh from civilian life, the problem became acute as "young physicians, some with only a year or 2 of training, were called to active duty and often sent directly to the combat theater. These doctors with limited surgical training and often no military training provided most of the battlefield care" (Baker, 2016, p. 259). Accordingly, Secretary of Defense George Marshall ordered the secretaries of the military departments "to appoint a board of officers in [each] department to prepare and implement plans for bringing field medical services for the combatant forces up to the level of competence already existing in the hospitals" (Cowdrey, 1987, p. 192). The problem of training medical personnel for combat would not be solved

---

[19] Towell, 2004, p. 38, which also notes that the

> decisions to limit soldiers' time in the combat theater during the Korean and Vietnam wars were based on the Army's analysis in the late 1940s of the incidence of psychiatric casualties in World War II. Service leaders concluded that, in future conflicts, the duration of any soldier's exposure to combat should be limited in order to reduce the number of troops who broke down emotionally under the stress of combat.

until the Army stopped relying on drafted physicians to care for those wounded in combat and until the field of trauma medicine was ultimately established.

Casualties

Battle Casualties

Battle casualties fall and rise according to a number of factors, including the weapons used, combat tactics, terrain, and weather. In Korea, as in World War II, the mortality-morbidity ratio of one killed to four-plus wounded seemed to hold. Moreover, the "anatomic region frequency of wounding has been almost the same in the Civil War, World War I, World War II and the Korean action . . . [with] infantry comprising only 20 percent of total army strength, yet it suffers about 70% of the total casualties" (Holmes, 1952, p. 74). In general, shell fragments cause the greatest number of wounds, but small arms bullets cause the greatest number of deaths, by a ratio of two to one.[20]

Killed in Action

The two Korean Wars—the one of intense combat and the other of stalemate, as depicted in Figure 3.4—are also reflected in the casualty figures. Figure 3.5 shows the killed-in-action (KIA) rates for the U.S. Army Divisional and regimental combat teams. The initial KIA rate from July 1950 declined sharply with the stabilization of the Pusan Perimeter in August, only to rise again with the landing at Inchon in September 1950. It fell again as the North Koreans retreated in October, then increased with the Chinese attacks in November 1950. By mid-January, the situation had stabilized, as reflected in low KIA rates in December and January, only to rise again as the UN counterattacked in February. As Figure 3.6 shows, the rate remained relatively low for the rest of the war, punctuated by sharp rises for relatively short periods as both sides mounted local attacks to gain tactical advantage along what would become the final cease-fire line.

Wounded in Action

Statistics reflecting the wounded-in-action (WIA) rate show a similar but more volatile pattern (see Figure 3.7). As expected, the WIA rate exceeds the KIA rate in every month, and the two series are highly correlated, with a correlation coefficient of 0.807.[21] On average, during the 37 months of the war, the monthly annualized WIA rate was 4.5 times the KIA rate. In one notable exception, the two rates were almost equal.

---

[20] Holmes, 1952, presents a comprehensive description of relative morbidity and mortality of wounding agents, the nature of wounds, wounding agents, the relationship between combat tactics and wound incidence, and anatomic regions of wounds.

[21] Correlation based on data presented in Reister, 1973, pp. 110–111.

Figure 3.5
Killed-in-Action Rates, July 1950–February 1951: U.S. Army Divisions and Regimental Combat Teams

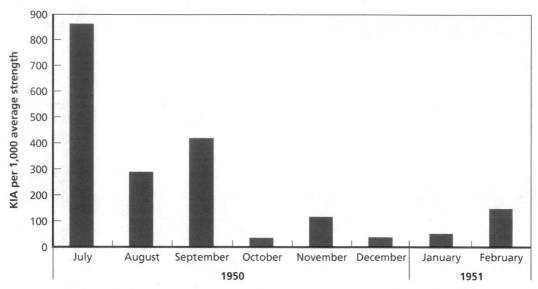

SOURCE: Data from Reister, 1973, pp. 110–111.

During the first month of the war (July 1950), when units were being thrown into the breach to stem the North Korean advance and when the medical infrastructure was struggling to take hold, there were almost as many KIAs as there were WIAs: 1,858 KIAs and 2,097 WIAs. The following month, 1,259 American soldiers were KIA and 3,502 were WIA—a WIA/KIA ratio of 2.78. During the stalemate, the average monthly ratio was 4.71.[22]

Comparing World War II and Korea

Causative Agent

Compared with World War II, fewer casualties in the Korean War were caused by explosive projectile shells (artillery, mortar, and bazooka), rockets and bombs, and booby-traps. Accordingly, more casualties were from small arms, grenades, land mines, and other fragments and explosions. "In Korea, 27 percent of the nonfatal wounds were from small arms [bullets] compared to 20 percent for all of World War II. The

---

[22] Reister makes a slightly different calculation in his "index of combat mortality," which he describes as the ratio of the number KIA to the number WIA, including those who died of wounds (DOW). He notes that, in World War II, the ratio was 3.9, excluding the Air Corps. In comparison, the ratio in Korea was 4.1 wounded to one killed (Reister, 1973, p. 15).

Figure 3.6
Killed-in-Action Rates, July 1950–July 1953: U.S. Army Divisions and Regimental Combat Teams

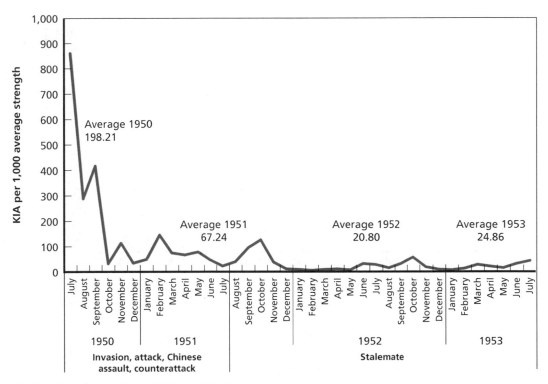

SOURCE: Data from Reister, 1973, pp. 110–111.

proportion from explosive projectiles (51 percent) was lower in Korea than the 58 percent for World War II" (Reister, 1973, p. 36).[23]

Location of Wounds and Body Armor

While steel helmets to protect the head were considered an essential part of battle dress in World War II, little was done to protect the thorax and abdominal areas, where most wounds occurred (see Table 3.3). The Army Air Corps developed flak jackets to protect bomber crews, and the Navy had similar armored jackets to protect personnel on the decks of aircraft carriers, but such jackets generally proved heavy and bulky, especially for ground combat soldiers. In 1943, the Dow Chemical Company laminated layers of

---

[23] According to Holmes, Enos, and Beyer, 1954, p. 218,

> about 75 [percent] of wounds are caused by shell fragments; not shrapnel, as they are erroneously called. The mean size of these fragments is less than 50 grains and about 1 cm. in greatest dimension. Distance from the shell explosion is usually from 1 to 25 meters for the wounded-in-action, and probably much closer for the killed-in-action. . . . [a]bout 70 percent of all missile wounds were of a penetrating type, that is, having a wound of entrance but no wound of exit, rather than a perforating type or "thru and thru" wound.

Figure 3.7
Killed-in-Action and Wounded-in-Action Rates, July 1950–July 1953: U.S. Army Divisions and Regimental Combat Teams

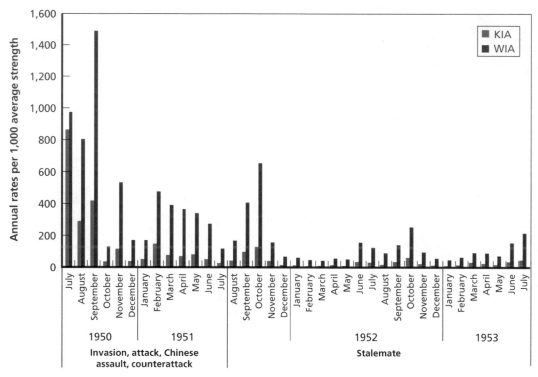

SOURCE: Data from Reister, 1973, pp. 110–111.

Table 3.3
Distribution of Anatomical Location of Wounds, World War II and Korean War

Anatomical Location	World War II (%)			Korean War (%)		
	KIA	DOW	Nonfatal Wounds	KIA	DOW	Nonfatal Wounds
Head	35.6	19.7	7.4	37.9	25.4	6.8
Trunk	36.4	52.1	15.2	36.8	50.2	15.4
Thorax	21.2	21.0	8.3	22.6	20.2	8.1
Abdomen	15.2	31.1	6.9	14.2	30.0	7.3

SOURCE: Data from Reister, 1973, p. 43.

fabric made from fibrous glass filaments into what came to be known as Doron armor plates. These were "sewn into standard utility jackets and first used in the last stages of the Okinawa battles of 1944" (Baker, 2012, p. 427).

The widespread use of modern ballistic body armor came during the Korean War. By one account, it was "the premier innovation from the viewpoint of medics and front-line soldiers alike" (Cowdrey, 1987, p. 210) and provided both a medical and psychological boost to the troops.[24] At the start of the war, the Army did not have protective body armor. Tests during World War II showed that it was too heavy and restricted movement. In the November 1950, a wound ballistics team was sent to the Far East Command to study casualties.[25] On its return to Washington in May 1951, the team recommended that the Surgeon General field a trial of an armored vest. Laboratory tests already completed showed that, while it would not be possible to defeat most bullets with any reasonable weight of body armor material then available, most of missile fragments that were causing perforating wounds or extensive tissue damage were lower-velocity, lower-energy fragments that could be defeated. For example, the "armored vests developed by the U.S. military services are designed primarily to stop fragments of mortar shells, hand grenades and other types of low-velocity missiles—the type which cause the majority of battlefield wounds" (Army Quartermaster Museum, 1952).

It was clear that steel could not be used because of its lack of flexibility and excessive weight, but layers of nylon cloth by itself and Doron molded to conform to the contours of the body with nylon shoulder supports might prove effective.[26] The Marine Corps preferred a Doron vest,[27] while the Army preferred an all-nylon vest. Eventually, 31,000 of the Marine Corps Doron vests and 20,000 of the Army all-nylon vests were ordered.

Test results showed why body armor gained such widespread acceptance among soldiers despite its added weight and bulkiness. A survey of those who used the armor found that "over 85 percent of the men stated that they felt safer and more confident when wearing body armor" (Herget, Coe, and Beyer, 1962). The combat field trials found that the Army's all-nylon T-52 armored vest (see Figure 3.8) deflected "approximately 65 percent of all types of missiles, 75 percent of all fragments, and 25 percent of all small-arms fire. . . . The armor has reduced torso wounds by 60 to 70 percent, while those inflicted in spite of the armor's protection were reduced in severity by 25 to

---

[24] There were negative consequences; Herget, Coe, and Beyer, 1962, p. 743, recounts that "soldiers who had previously used body armor expressed a reluctance to their unit leaders to go out on patrols when body armor was not available."

[25] The finds of the wound ballistics team are from Herget, Coe, and Beyer, 1962.

[26] The fibers of nylon trap jagged fragments of the low-velocity missiles that cause the majority of combat wounds. Ballistic tests reveal that nylon, weight for weight, is superior even to steel in stopping fragments from exploding missiles (Army Quartermaster Museum, 1952).

[27] In spring 1951 the Marine Corps combat-tested 40 vests with curved Doron panels. On November 16, 1951, they ordered 2,000 Doron vests, with the first 500 arriving on January 30, 1952, and first used in combat on February 21, 1952 (King, 1953).

Figure 3.8
Army T-52-2 Armored Vest

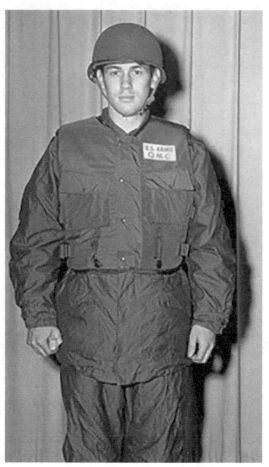

SOURCE: Army Quartermaster Museum, 1952.

35 percent" (Army Quartermaster Museum, 1952; see also Herget, Coe, and Beyer, 1962, pp. 741–742).[28]

The effects of body armor may possibly be reflected in the overall reduction in casualties between Word War II and the Korean War.[29] After the war, it was noted that

---

[28] The T-52-2 weighed approximately 8 pounds and consisted of "12 layer[s] of flexible, spot-laminated Nylon-duck, enclosed in a heat-sealed water-repellent vinyl envelope. The T-52-2 Model (the 5,000 shipped to Korea late in 1952) is designed to be worn as an outside garment and has an outer cover of 6 ounce, nylon fabric. It has adjustable side straps to assure a snug fit. . . . [They were] made in three sizes—small, medium, and large" (Army Quartermaster Museum, 1952). The vest would eventually be issued as the M-1951 and, later, the M-1952 Fragmentation Protective Body Armor vests.

[29] Cowdrey, 1987, p. 255, observes that, "[f]or all wounded who reached a medical installation, the mortality rate declined from World War II's 4.5 percent to 2.1 percent in 1951 and again 1.8 percent in 1952."

"the body armor in current use has been designed primarily for the reduction of battle KIA. Any reduction of WIA is a gratuitous and natural expectancy" (Herget, Coe, and Beyer, 1962, p. 221).

Overall Measures of Survival

Overall measures of survival that reflect the performance of military medicine during the Korean War mask the great volatility of the conflict. The hot battles and rapid maneuver that marked the first months of the war were followed by what one observer has called the "peculiarly favorable circumstances that existed in the latter 2 years of the war" (Lindsey, 1954, p. 71). That said, Reister, in the Army's official accounting of medical statistics for World War II, provides a number of measures that suggests that a Korean War soldier was more likely to survive than his World War II counterpart (Reister, 1975, p. 15).

Battle Deaths

Battle deaths include those KIA but also those who later DOW, those declared dead from missing-in-action reports, and those who died from nonbattle causes when they were prisoners of war (POWs). The ratio for the Korean War (43.2 per 1,000 average annual strength) was lower than that for the European Theater of Operations from June 1944 to May 1945 (51.9 per 1,000 average annual strength) (Reister, 1973, p. 15).

Ratio of Battle Deaths to "Hit" as a Measure of Lethality

One measure of lethality is the number of deaths compared to the number of soldiers hit. In Korea, 21.8 percent of those hit died, compared to 25.1 for those hit in the European theater and 28.8 percent for all of World War II (Reister, 1973, p. 15).

The Combat Mortality Rate

An index of combat mortality is the ratio of the number KIA to the number of WIA, including DOWs. In World War II, the ratio for Army ground forces was 3.9 wounded to one KIA for all theaters; in Korea, the ratio was 4.1 wounded to one killed. So, slightly more were wounded than killed in Korea than in World War II.

The Case Fatality Rate

During the Korean War, 77,788 wounded soldiers were admitted to medical treatment facilities. Of these, 1,957 died of their wounds, for "a case fatality rate of 2.5 percent. This rate is markedly lower than the 4.5 percent recorded for all of World War II" (Reister, 1973, p. 16).

Nonbattle Casualties
Disease

The scourge of an army in the field throughout history has been disease. By World War II, however, deaths from disease had ceased to be a major case of deaths. As shown in Table 3.4, this was also true during the Korean War, although the disease death rates

Table 3.4
Deaths from Disease, by Major U.S. Conflicts

	Deaths from Disease (%)	Per Year per 1,000 Average Strength
Mexican War	85.0	103.90
Civil War, Union	65.0	71.20
Spanish American War	87.9	34.00
World War I[a]	48.1	16.50
World War II		
Total outside CONUS	1.8	0.65
European theater	1.5	0.55
Mediterranean theater	1.9	0.41
Southwest Pacific area[b]	12.6	1.03
Pacific Ocean area[c]	3.9	0.64
Korean War	2.4	0.67

SOURCES: Beebe and DeBakey, 1952, p. 21; Reister, 1975, pp. 70–71; Reister, 1973, p. 17.

[a] The World War I numbers would have been considerably lower if not for the influenza outbreak at the end of the war.

[b] Includes the Admiralty Islands, Australia, Borneo, Celebes, New Britain, New Guinea, and the Philippines.

[c] Includes Bora-Bora, Fiji, Gilbert, the Hawaiian Islands, Iwo Jima, Japan, the Marianas and Marshall Islands, Ryukyus, New Hebrides, New Zealand, Palau Islands, Samoa, the Solomon Islands, and Tongatabu.

were somewhat higher than they had been in either the European or Mediterranean theaters. The higher overall rates during World War II are attributable to higher rates in Africa, the Middle East, China, and Alaska.

The single greatest cause of deaths from disease—40 percent—was "infective and parasitic disease. . . . Acute respiratory disease, largely pneumonias, contributed over 6 percent of the deaths from disease" (Reister, 1973, p. 17). The fact that only 33 soldiers died from respiratory disease is a tribute to the advances made in medical science during the first half of the 20th century. Diseases of the digestive system, particularly dysentery and diarrhea, caused more than 37,000 deaths during the Civil War.[30] A century later, during the Korean War, despite the horrendous conditions during the first months, only 25 soldiers died from diseases of the digestive system (Reister, 1973, Table 16, p. 17).

---

[30] Derived from Woodward, 1870, Table C, p. 637.

Cold Injuries—The Forces of General Winter

In November 1950, the fortunes of war changed for the UN troops. The Chinese Communist troops coming from the north were accompanied by an icy wind that drove the thermometer below zero. Cowdrey called it the "Forces of General Winter," telling us that,

> [i]n the Chosin reservoir area, temperature dropped 40 degrees over the night of 10–11 November, from 32° to −8°F. More than 200 Marines had to be hospitalized by Navy medics. Water-soluble medicines froze: plasma had to be warmed for an hour or more to be usable. The Eighth Army also suffered. On the 13th extremely cold weather struck the 2d Division. Here, too, aid stations complained that plasma was freezing. (Cowdrey, 1987, p. 116)

The situation was made worse by the lack of adequate cold-weather supplies. In the advanced north, units outran their supply lines. Those who received their cold-weather gear found their feet got wet from perspiration when they put on their snowpacs—winterized boots worn over heavy socks and a felt insole—resulting in frequent cases of frostbite. Table 3.5 illustrates the impact that the cold had on the Army, showing that, during December 1950 and January 1951, more soldiers were taken off the line because of cold-weather injuries than were wounded. By the following year, new cold-weather gear arrived. Replacing snowpacs with "Mickey Mouse boots" clearly had an impact, but the tactical situation had also changed.[31]

The Changing Nature of War Casualties

Throughout history, the most lingering and visible impression of the casualties of war has been the amputee. Arguably, those who become psychologically disabled by the invisible wounds of war can now claim that distinction. Looking at how these two types of casualties have evolved over the past 150 years, since the Civil War, provides a broader view of how war has evolved for the individual soldier. As the physical calamity of war has been reduced, we have become more aware of the psychological tolls our soldiers pay. The war in Korea is a case in point.

---

[31] A further note on the Mickey Mouse boot:

> The new boot was issued first to the Marine Corps then to the Army. The boot was designed with two layers of rubber with a layer of wool pile insulating material in between. They were referred to as thermos boots because of a sealed air layer within the insulating material. Neither air nor moisture could be exchanged with that layer due to the sealed rubber, preventing heat from escaping the foot, protecting the wearer from frostbite down to −20° F. By mid-November 1951, all Army and Marine Corps troops in Korea had the new boots. ("Mickey Mouse Boots," undated)

Table 3.5
Comparison of Wounded-in-Action and Cold-Weather Injuries,
Korea, 1950–1953

	WIA	Cold Injuries	Ratio of Cold Injuries to WIA
Winter 1950–1951			
November	4,079	840	0.21
December	1,330	1,980	1.49
January	1,390	1,825	1.31
February	3,995	1,195	0.30
March	3,312	615	0.19
Winter 1951–1952			
November	1,561	330	0.21
December	673	150	0.22
January	599	230	0.38
February	454	295	0.65
March	399	30	0.08
Winter 1952–1953			
November	901	30	0.03
December	494	80	0.16
January	408	90	0.22
February	540	45	0.08
March	788	0	0.00

SOURCE: Data from Reister, 1973, pp. 114–115.

Loss of a Limb

Over the past century and a half, not only have amputations become less common and survival rates increased, but new programs for the rehabilitation of amputees mean that those who do lose a limb can regain most of the mobility and dexterity they have lost. In fact, starting in 1950, the Army not only allowed amputees who could be gainfully employed to remain on active duty but also allowed amputees from World War II to return. Their time away from the Army was treated as a normal "broken service." By the end of 1951, more than 1,500 handicapped soldiers were on active duty (Office of the Surgeon General, 1951).

Amputations

For the individual soldier, the possibility of losing a limb has always been the starkest reality of war. The statistics on amputations for the Civil War are appalling. On the Union side, the official account—reported in *The Medical and Surgical History of the War of the Rebellion*—is that 17.4 percent of all wounds resulted in an amputation, with 26.3 percent of the amputees dying after the amputation.[32] As Table 3.6 shows, 12.1 percent of those who survived their wounds were amputees, and almost 21,000 veterans of the Union Army were amputees. At the end of the war, a report by the Sanitary Commission noted that most disabled veterans were amputees because the "sick either get well, die, or as invalids, find light employment, while limbless men take much longer to accommodate themselves to their condition" (Bellows, 1865, p. 13).

World War I

In World War I, with advances in medicine, the number of amputations was reduced sharply; for instance, "only 25 percent of the cases of compound fractures are now fatal instead of 66 percent" (Keen, 1918, p. 15). In total, 2.9 percent of those WIA who survived the war were amputees (Beebe and DeBakey, 1952, p. 194). In World War II, the corresponding number was 2.5 percent. In total, almost 15,000 returning veterans of

Table 3.6
Amputation Survivors—Civil War, World Wars I and II, and the Korean War

Conflict	Extremities Wounded	Individuals Wounded	Surviving Amputees	
			Number	As a Percentage of Surviving Wounded
Civil War	Upper[a]	83,536	12,860	15.4
	Lower[b]	89,528	8,002	8.9
	Total	173,064	20,862	12.1
World War I	Upper	55,000	2,359	4.3
	Lower	69,000	2,044	3.0
	Total	154,000	4,378	2.8
World War II[c]	Upper	167,000	3,152	1.9
	Lower	248,000	11,760	4.7
	Total	599,000	14,912	2.5
Korea[c]	Upper	21,002	454	2.2
	Lower	26,270	1,023	3.9
	Total	47,272	1,477	3.1

SOURCES: Beebe and DeBakey, 1952, p. 194; Reister, 1975, p. 400; Otis and Huntington, 1883, p. 877; Reister, 1973, pp. 48, 160.

[a] Shoulder, arm, forearm, wrist, and hand.

[b] Hip, thigh, leg, ankle, and foot.

[c] The World War II and Korea numbers include nonbattle amputations, which are not included in the World War I numbers. In Korea, there were also 1,120 traumatic amputations (Reznick, Gambel, and Hawk, 2009, p. 33).

---

[32] The most prevalent amputations were of a hand or finger, which most, 97 percent, survived. The next largest groups were amputations of the thigh, leg, and upper arm. The survival rates for these groups were 46 percent, 77 percent, and 76 percent, respectively (Otis and Huntington, 1883, p. 877).

World War II were amputees (Beebe and DeBakey, 1952, p. 194). In Korea, the amputation rate was essentially the same, with almost 1,500 returning veteran amputees.

World War II

During and after World War II, the Army's approach to amputations was extremely conservative "because of the tremendous possibilities of modern reconstructive surgery. The operation was almost never performed unless the extremity was damaged beyond salvage or . . . conditions developed which endangered life or made further efforts to save the limb futile" (Hampton, 1957, p. 245). That said, amputations as a result of acute injuries of major arteries remained a problem, as one landmark study noted: "There was little unanimity of opinion concerning either concepts of management or procedures of choice" (DeBakey and Simeone, 1946, p. 534).

DeBakey and Simeone's review of World War II data from the Mediterranean and European theaters shows that almost 20 percent of major amputations were the result of major arterial injuries.[33] The review also showed the importance of immediate treatment to reestablish circulation to the damaged limb, noting that incidents of amputation correlated with the time lag between wounding and operations. There was a 63-percent amputation rate when arterial wounds were not addressed—circulation restored—within the first 20 hours after the wounding. The corresponding rate when circulation was restored within 10 hours of the wounding was 37 percent (DeBakey and Simeone, 1946, p. 541).[34]

Korean War

The policy of the Army Medical Department at the start of the Korean War was basically to ligate all vascular wounds, a procedure that had not changed much since the time Roman Legions held the field. Ligation—the tying off of a damaged blood vessel—had been described in ancient texts by Hippocrates and Galen. During World War II, ligation still accounted for 92 percent of all treatments of arterial wounds, with a corresponding amputation rate of 48.9 percent. A somewhat lower amputation rate, 35.0 percent, when arteries were repaired with sutures appears in DeBakey and Simeone, 1946, p. 557, but this procedure was "time-consuming and required a great deal of specialized technical skill" (Jahke and Seeley, 1953, p. 159).

In the interwar period, advances in arterial surgery were moving forward in civilian hospitals (Howard, 1998, p. 717), so that newly inducted surgeons assigned to MASH units started to take advantage of new tools and techniques for arterial surgery

---

[33] DeBakey and Simeone, 1946, p. 539, reports amputations caused by vascular injuries as 14.5 percent for the Mediterranean theater and 23.1 percent for the European theater.

[34] After about six to eight hours, the wounded limb had been deprived of oxygen and nutrition too long for the limb to be saved. DeBakey and Simeone, 1946, pp. 541–542, also notes that "infection is probably not an important factor . . . [in operations done within ten hours of wounding], though it plays an increasingly important role after the ten-hour period and undoubtedly accounts for at least a portion of the unhappy results in the group observed 20 hours or more after wounding."

that had been developed in civilian hospitals, despite the threat of disciplinary action (see Apel and Apel, 1998, pp. 149–177).[35] Apel and Apel explained that the

> methods under experimentation in the research hospitals and the methods we used in MASH 8076 were vein grafting [removing a portion of a vein from elsewhere in the patient's body and inserting it into the injured artery] or anastomosis [removing the injured portion of the artery and suturing the artery end to end]. (Apel and Apel, 1998, p. 153)

Late in 1952, a surgical team from the Army Medical Service Graduate School at Walter Reed brought to Korea a new tool for working on damaged arteries, the Potts' clamp.[36] Despite a shortage of such devices in civilian hospitals in the United States, each MASH eventually received one clamp, and the "amputation rate . . . [fell] from 49% during World War II to approximately 7% to 13%" (Howard, 1998, p. 718).

Cowdrey called these new procedures "the most outstanding forward-area clinical innovation" of the war (Cowdrey, 1987, pp. 206–207). Soon, arterial segments taken from corpses were being preserved in antibiotic solutions to be used as grafts, and "[l]imbs that would have become gangrenous only a few years earlier were saved from the knife" (Cowdrey, 1987, p. 207). Hughes, 1958, p. 558, provides support for Cowdrey's conclusion, noting that, in a group of patients with arterial wounds, the amputation rate following ligation was 51.4 percent, and the rates following anastomosis, vein graft, and artery grafts were 9 percent, 11.8 percent, and 33.3 percent, respectively, with an overall amputation rate of 13 percent for all methods of repair (see also Hughes, 1954a, and Hughes, 1954b). But Hughes also notes that the

> amputation rate following vascular repair could have been further reduced except for the . . . prolonged time interval between injury and arterial repair . . . . The average time from injury to operation was 9.2 hours, . . . and . . . results were generally better in those vessels repaired with ten hours after injury. (Hughes, 1958, p. 560)

Time Lag for Surgical Treatment: World War II and Korean War

At the end of World War II, DeBakey and Simeone wrote that "time-lag in military surgery is a military matter . . . [;] from a military standpoint, it is doubtful that the time-lag can be greatly reduced" (DeBakey and Simeone, 1946, p. 542). It

---

[35] According to Apel and Apel, 1998, p. 152, "it was brand new in the civilian hospitals, and the army did not allow it. . . . The art of vascular surgery was in the developmental stage." The order to ligate was also standard procedure for the Navy (Spencer, 2006, p. 907).

[36] A Potts' clamp is "a fine-toothed, multiple-point, vascular fixation [clamp] that imparts limited trauma to the vessel while holding it securely" ("Clamp: Potts' c.," 1995). These clamps were used in the "blue baby" operations pioneered by Drs. Alfred Blalock and Helen Taussig at Johns Hopkins.

appears, however, that the time lag was, in fact, reduced during the Korean War. The average of 9.2 hours Hughes reported between wounding and "surgical treatment" to repair seriously damaged arteries is considerably better than the average of 15.2 hours DeBakey and Simeone reported. Unfortunately, this was still longer than the goal of surgically repairing damaged arteries within six to eight hours of wounding. However, the 9.2 hours Hughes reported might overstate the time lag because there was a general increase in the proportion of the wounded reaching surgical and evacuation hospitals on first day after being wounded over the course of the war (see Figure 3.9).

Rehabilitation of the Amputee

To say the least, the Army was ill prepared for the influx of casualties from Korea. Given the uncertainty of how long the conflict would last, the U.S. Department of Defense (DoD) was reluctant to authorize any permanent increase in the size of the Army's medical establishment. With the change in fortunes after the Inchon landing and the breakout from Pusan, it seemed for a while that the flow of casualties would soon stop. However, by spring 1951, it was clear that it would not.

In the months after the invasion, the Army took a number of measures to care for the wounded returning from Korea. Some patients were sent to Navy hospitals;

Figure 3.9
Army Wounded-in-Action Evacuees, by Month of Wounding, July 1950–August 1953

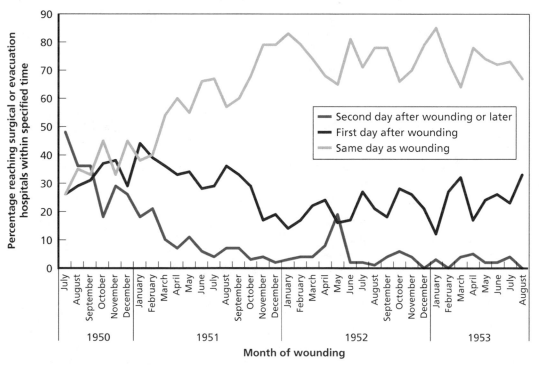

SOURCE: Data from Reister, 1973, p. 81.

reserve medical personnel were called up; three general hospitals were reactivated; and Pub. L. 81-779 was passed to allow the drafting of physicians.[37] Under orders from the Secretary of Defense, the Army suspended admissions of VA patients into military hospitals and expedited the transfer of patients deemed unlikely to return to duty to the VA, including amputees. The Navy and Army were allowed to retain amputees needed for "research" and "less severe" amputees who might return to duty (Marble, 2008, p. 74). The decision did not go down well with the Army, whose leadership questioned the quality of care at VA hospitals and even the financial disparity between service pay and VA benefits. Finally, it took both the personal intervention of the Assistant Secretary of Defense for Health Affairs and the retirement of the Army Surgeon General in May 1951 for the Army to start sending patients to the VA.

The Psychologically Impaired

Psychiatric care received during the Korean War was firmly built on the system originally developed during World War I and "rediscovered" during World War II. The focus was on the immediate impact of combat and not on its long-term impact, which was not fully recognized until after the Vietnam War.[38]

Army Psychiatry Prior to the Korean War: World War I and World War II

World War I

Neuropsychiatric casualties were not recognized until the Civil War and then were not effectively addressed until World War I.[39] Before the United States entered World War I, the Army tried to learn as much as it could from the allies' experience with neuropsychiatric cases. In 1916, it sent Dr. Thomas Salmon to England to observe and

---

[37] It was not only the Army that found itself short of physicians; the shortage extended to the Central Intelligence Agency (CIA), which entered into an agreement with DoD to defer physicians subject to being drafted willing to sign on for duty with the agency (CIA, Historical Staff, 1973, p. 15).

[38] Today, combat stress reaction (CSR), also known as *combat fatigue*, in the field is clearly differentiated from delayed-onset and long-term PTSD. The discussion here is about the former, consistent with the focus on theater medicine.

[39] This book follows the Army's common use of the term *neuropsychiatric*, although there is an important distinction between neurology and psychiatry. The former is concerned with organic diseases and disorders of the nervous system, while the latter is concerned with functional disorders (Menninger, 1948, p. 3). Glass, 1966, pp. 3–4, notes that, in

> the Russo-Japanese War (1904–6), an organized program was developed, for the first time, in which mental illnesses of military personnel were treated by specialists in psychiatry. Because the increased mental cases overtaxed the capability of the Russian Army Medical Service, the problem was turned over to the Red Cross Society of Russia which established psychiatric treatment facilities in cities near the front as well as in rear home areas.

The services received and their outcomes are illustrated by the experience of the Central Harbin Hospital opened in early 1904. Special ambulances were provided with a psychiatrist in attendance to quickly move casualties to the clinic. While "a key ingredient for success was prompt psychiatric treatment close to the battlefield," 85 percent of patients were transferred to Moscow for "a ticket home" (Wanke, 2005, p. 22).

"contribute information which might aid in formulating plans for dealing with mental and nervous diseases among our . . . forces when they are exposed to the terrific stress of modern war" (Salmon, 1917, p. 7).[40] In England, he found there was no common vocabulary that would enable psychiatry to classify behaviors in a readily understood manner, provide a diagnosis, and offer a preferred course of treatment for what they would see on the battlefields of Europe. Nevertheless, Salmon fundamentally accepted the neuropsychiatric view that had taken hold by the time of his visit and drew some important lessons concerning the organizational and treatment modalities of the British. The system the Americans put into place as a result took full advantage of what the British and French had learned:

> Patients with war neuroses improved more rapidly when treated in permanent hospitals near the front than at the base, better in casualty clearing stations . . . than even at advanced base hospitals, and better still when encouragement, rest, persuasion, and suggestion could be given in a combat organization itself. (Salmon and Fenton, 1929, p. 303)

Following the British model, a psychiatrist with the rank of major was assigned to each division, along with supporting staff. He was central to the implementation of the Army's policy of caring for mental patients in field hospitals close to the front and returning as many as possible to their own organizations within two to five days. Even the majority of the more-severe cases that were evacuated to special psychiatric hospitals were eventually returned to duty, since "the primary function of the hospital was to return as many cases as possible to duty with their divisions, and in as short a time as possible" (Salmon and Fenton, 1929, p. 332). For example, at Army Neurological Hospital No. 1, more than 60 percent of those admitted were "restored" within an average of 10 to 14 days to a "state of apparent stability" (Salmon and Fenton, 1929, p. 331).

Salmon recognized the question of returning the psychologically impaired to their units was central to the design of the American military psychiatry system, even without consideration for the long-term mental health of the soldier. Reflecting on the experience during World War I, Salmon and Fenton later wrote:

> The question before the hospital staff with nearly half of the hysteria and fear cases was: Which is wiser from the standpoint of army efficiency, to send these men back to the front line on the chance that they will carry on or to send them to Base Hospital No. 117 to be reclassified as labor troops? One's first impulse was to carry out the former alternative, especially if one were dealing with a plain case of fear. There was another point of view to consider, however, and that was the line officer's. Even if the hysterical and fear cases were not contagious in the front line, the

---

[40] Salmon held a commission as a major in the Medical Officers' Reserve Corps; in civilian life, he was medical director of the National Committee for Mental Hygiene. After the war, from 1923 to 1924, he served as the president of the American Psychiatric Association.

chances were that they would not be individually dependable. There were exceptions, of course. Furthermore, at a time when every available bit of transportation was needed for wounded men, a seat in an ambulance for a relapsed nervous case seemed rather superfluous. (Salmon and Fenton, 1929, p. 333)

As finally developed, the American system incorporated the concepts of *echelons of care* (many layers of treatment) and employed the principals of *proximity* (forward treatment), *immediacy* (early treatment in forward settings), *expectancy* (with the expectation that the soldier will return to his unit), *simplicity* (no involved or lengthy treatment, lest the soldier believe himself really very ill), *effective labeling* (the casualty tag of "not yet diagnosed" left the soldier with nothing to reinforce his notion that he was really sick, not just tired or a "little nervous"), and *centrality* (a central clearing point to evaluate casualties to ensure that those who might be returned to their units were not sent home) (Jones, 2000, pp. 3–5). After a rocky start, these concepts eventually were rediscovered in World War II's system of psychiatric care.

World War II

After World War I, the writings of Sigmund Freud and the advent of psychoanalysis captured the popular imagination, but the vast majority of the 2,295 members of the American Psychiatric Association (Grob, 1991, p. 427) did not share that enthusiasm. They were predominantly concerned about the treatment of psychotic patients in large state mental hospitals. As a result, the very language of psychiatrists, as captured in the *Standard Classified Nomenclature of Disease*,[41] updated in 1942, was judged to be "totally inadequate" for the "special problems encountered in the practice of psychiatry in the military setting" (Menninger, 1948, p. 258). The much-used diagnosis of *psychoneurosis* reinforced the notions that the soldier's impairment was not related to battle conditions but to a failure to screen out those predisposed to such reactions and that such soldiers should immediately be discharged. During the war, the Army would gradually develop a nonspecific diagnosis of "exhaustion" and a new classification scheme of "transient personality reactions to acute or special stress."[42] It would take the experience of the war and the successful treatment of neurotic symptoms in noninstitutional settings to "reinforce the growing importance of psychodynamics and [the] psychoanalytic model that ultimately became the basis for postwar transformation of the specialty" (Grob, 1991, p. 427).

---

[41] Grob, 1991, p. 427, notes that "the classification system incorporated in the *Statistical Manual* was only of marginal concern to psychiatrists and their patients. Its categories were quite general. For the goal was to facilitate the collection of institutional data rather than to provide definitive diagnoses that in turn were related to specific therapies."

[42] According to Office of the Surgeon General, Army Service Forces, [1946] 2000, p. 925, a "normal personality may utilize, under conditions of great or unusual stress, established patterns of reaction to express overwhelming fear or flight reaction. The clinical picture of such reactions differs from that of neuroses and psychoses chiefly in points of direct relationship to external precipitation and reversibility."

On the eve of World War II, the Army was convinced that it would avoid such problems by screening out those predisposed to neuropsychiatric problems before such individuals ever joined the Army. Accordingly, "there was no effective plan or real preparation for the utilization of psychiatry" (Glass, 1966, p. 17).[43] In a move to cut costs in 1940, the position of division psychiatrist, the centerpiece of the British and American psychiatric program of World War I, was eliminated. The position was not reauthorized until November 1943, once the lessons about treating neuropsychiatric casualties on the battlefield had been learned all over again.

In retrospect, screening during World War II did not achieve its goal.[44] The number of neuropsychiatric disorders was reported to be "two to three times that of World War I despite the fact that rejections for psychiatric reasons were five to six times greater than those of World War I" (Glass, 1966, p. 7). Not only did screening fail to eliminate neuropsychiatric casualties, it also meant that the Army did not focus on factors it *could* control and allowed the views of some commanders to persist that those who had psychiatric combat breakdowns were merely cowards.[45] It was only after separating a large number of soldiers that the Army gave serious attention to preventing "psychological" discharges by improving leadership, changing personnel policy,

---

[43] This emphasis on screening had a profound impact on the nation's mobilization program; 1,250,000 men were rejected in 1942 and 1943 because of mental and emotional abnormalities. This was about 12 percent of those examined and was higher than any other cause of rejection. During the last six months of 1943, 20 percent of the men examined were rejected for neuropsychiatric reasons (Menninger, 1944, p. 807). It appears, however, that the vast majority of men rejected could have made "good soldiers."

[44] After the war, a number of studies

> led to a general recognition that the psychiatric standards and procedures of World War II were obviously overcautious and, hence, caused a considerable and unnecessary loss of potential military manpower. They also indicated that psychiatric and psychological criteria at the time of examination for military service generally have not proved a reliable index for efficiently predicting future behavior and, furthermore, that greater proficiency can be accomplished by observing individuals with psychiatric difficulties under military conditions, rather than by psychiatric screening, at the time of their examination. (Berlien and Waggoner, 1966, p. 191)

By the time of the Korean War, the chief of the Army's Psychiatry and Neurology Consultants Division and his coauthor would write:

> Lists of completely or partly disqualifying diagnoses have been prepared on the assumption that the use of such a screening device would result in the selection of men who would function creditably. We are all too aware that this method is grossly inadequate, that many men inducted under our standards were worthless, while many men that fall far short of the written standard function extremely well. The potential functioning of the individual soldier depends so much on his future motivation, associations with others, unit identification, exposure to privation and dangers, and a host of other things that by their very nature cannot be known at the time of the screening examination. (Peterson and Chambers, 1952, pp. 250–251)

[45] Weinstein, 1973, pp. 133–136, describes the range of breakdowns. Drayer and Glass, 1973, p. 27, describes the famous "slapping" episode involving GEN George Patton. Rather than an isolated incident, "it symbolized in concrete fashion the attitudes of many line and medical officers. In essence, men who broke down in combat were cowards and derelict in their responsibilities to their country and fellow soldiers. General Patton later said he sought to shame the man and help him regain his self-respect" (Weinstein, 1973, p. 130).

and addressing motivation and developed a classification scheme that recognized the transitory nature of "exhaustion."

Army Psychiatry on the Eve of the Korean War

In spring 1950, the Far East Command was the largest overseas Army command, with 108,500 soldiers; it was larger than the Army in Europe, which had strength of 103,800 (Glass and Jones, 2005, Ch. 5, p. 2). At the time, there were nine psychiatrists in the Far East, eight of whom were residents with less than two years training serving a three-month rotation from Letterman and Fitzsimons Army Hospitals. Needless to say, their stay in the Far East was extended with the invasion of South Korea, and they provided the backbone of an emerging system of care that took root in Korea, Japan, and Okinawa. They had two other things going for them: First, they were able to tap the experience of World War II colleagues, and second, there was now an accepted working definition of "combat exhaustion," which recognized "combat-induced psychiatric disorders" (Glass and Jones, 2005, Ch. 5, p. 6).[46]

The experience of World War II came in two ways: First, in the late 1940s the Medical Department set out to capture the lessons that had been learned during World War II. *Combat Psychiatry: Experiences in the North African and Mediterranean Theaters of Operation, American Ground Forces, World War II* (ed. Hanson, 1949) was published just in time for it to become "the textbook for the orientation of neuropsychiatric personnel in the Far East Command" (Glass and Jones, 2005, Ch. 5, p. 5). Second, one of the authors, COL Albert J. Glass, arrived in Japan in late September 1950 to take up the duties of Theater Consultant in Neuropsychology.[47]

Colonel Glass quickly reinstituted the tenets of PIES—a mnemonic for *proximity*, *immediacy*, *expectancy*, and *simplicity*—as the organizing paradigm around which psychiatric services would be delivered. Later, the notion of *centrality* would be added, that is, "having a casualty evaluated prior to departing from the combat zone" (Jones, 2000, p. 15). The goal, as it had been in World War II, was to keep as many fighting men on the line as possible.

---

[46] In a 1952 article, Peterson and Chambers referred to *combat exhaustion* as an "observation diagnosis, designed to take into consideration the factors of fatigue, combat, and exhaustion." They explained that the term *exhaustion* "implies a potential automatic recuperation, . . . [and using the term] relieves the doctor of the necessity of making a premature, perhaps ill-considered diagnosis, eliminating an almost inevitable cross-sectional diagnosis of mental mechanisms, rather than of disease of personality process" (Peterson and Chambers, 1952, p. 251).

[47] Menninger, Farrell, and Brosin, 1966, p. 67, calls "the development of the consultant system in the Medical Department . . . one of the most important progressive steps made during" World War II, noting that

> as representatives of the Surgeon General, the professional consultants are concerned essentially with the maintenance of the highest standards of medical practice. It is their function to evaluate, promote, and improve further the quality of medical care by every possible means, and to advise in the formulation of the professional policies of the Surgeon General and to aid in their implementation. (Menninger, Farrell, and Brosin 1966, p. 76)

Psychological Casualties During the Korean War

The neuropsychiatric casualties and psychiatric services mirrored the operational situation as it developed in Korea. From a state of unpreparedness and after the initial overwhelming North Korean attack, casualties ebbed and flowed as the battle line advanced, retreated, advanced again, and then stabilized. As with other medical support, psychiatric care improved as old lessons were relearned and new lessons incorporated.

Phase 1: Invasion

During the initial onslaught of North Korean troops, as South Korean and UN forces attempted to stem the tide and establish a defensive perimeter around the harbor city of Pusan, there were no dedicated psychiatric services or the "possibility of holding any patients for interdivisional treatment" (Glass and Jones, 2005, Ch. 6, p. 1). All medical personnel were needed at forward clearing platoons, and the physically wounded were evacuated to Japan. During this period, psychiatric casualties were

> low in view of the high battle casualty rate, the terror spread by enemy atrocities on the captured and wounded, the series of apparent defeats. . . . Men were forced to fight for survival. It was far safer to remain with the group than to become a straggler. Evacuation of psychiatric casualties was best accomplished in combat units rather than through vulnerable medical facilities. (Glass, 1952, p. 1388)

By mid-August, as the defense stiffened, divisional psychiatrists were assigned to the four American divisions on the line, and psychiatric treatment units were established in or near division clearing stations. Applying the principles that "combat fatigue should be treated as near the scene of combat, and as quickly as possible" (Peterson and Chambers, 1952, p. 252), recovery rates of between 50 and 90 percent were reported, with less than 10 percent repeat cases. Nevertheless, during this phase of the war, some 1,800 psychiatric casualties were evacuated to Japan where "only 50 percent . . . were salvaged for even noncombat duty" (Glass, 1954, p. 359). Glass attributed the low salvage rate to the fact that the "comfort and safety" of a hospital or hospital ship "mitigated against the motivation of psychiatric patients to face again the rigors of combat" (Glass, 1954, p. 361).

Phase 2: The Landing at Inchon, the Breakout from the Pusan Perimeter, and Crossing the 38th Parallel

As noted earlier, September 1950 saw a complete reversal of the situation on the Korean Peninsula. On September 15, the U.S. X Corps landed at Inchon, well behind the North Korean lines. The next day, the Eighth Army counterattacked, and by September 18, UN forces started to break out of the Pusan Perimeter. On October 9, 1950, the 1st Cavalry Division crossed the 38th parallel, and on October 24, the North Korean capital of Pyongyang fell. Two days later, the X Corps landed on Korea's east coast.

During the initial fighting near Pusan, psychiatric casualties were "elevated," in concert with the tempo of battle. However, as the breakout turned into a rout of the North Korean forces, cases fortunately "dropped precipitously, as . . . expected when victorious troops are rapidly advancing with few battle casualties," since the division psychiatric centers were too far to the rear of the rapidly advancing troops to operate effectively (Glass and Jones, 2005, Ch. 7, p. 2). In addition, the newly assigned division psychiatrists limited their activities to the treatment and evacuation of soldiers, rather than taking on the unfamiliar responsibilities of working with commanders to prevent such casualties.

As the front moved north, arrangements were made to provide second-echelon psychiatric care in the Inchon-Seoul area for patients who could not be treated and returned to duty within a few days. Meanwhile, the practice of concentrating most psychiatric casualties evacuated to Japan at the 361st Station Hospital near Tokyo was proving to be a problem, which led to a program to decentralize services. After the war, Glass explained the problem this way:

> Many psychiatric patients were adversely affected by the environment of this hospital either to maintain a stubborn persistence of symptoms or develop more severe manifestations than were previously noted. This resistance to improvement and return to any type of duty is not surprising when the comfortable atmosphere of a fixed hospital situated in the midst of peaceful and pleasurable Tokyo is compared with the monotonous, primitive, and hazardous existence of Korea. In addition, they could readily observe and envy the frequent evacuations to the Zone of Interior of other psychiatric patients, who were seemingly being rewarded for persistence of severe mental symptoms by being sent home. (Glass, 1954, p. 363)

In December, the Army established two hospitals in Tokyo and Osaka. As Glass saw it,

> Convalescent hospitals provided a realistic environment for psychiatric treatment. Here patients, in fatigue uniform, instead of hospital garb, participated in an active daily program of calisthenics, supervised athletics, marches, and other training activities. Under this regime, there was less benefit from clinging to symptoms and no suggested evidence of possible evacuation to the Zone of Interior. . . . The far better results attained by psychiatry in convalescent hospitals over those of fixed hospitals argues strongly for its similar use in [the] future. (Glass, 1954, p. 364)

Phase 3: The Chinese Communists' Assault

From late October to the end of November, UN forces faced what was believed to be a "token" presence of CCF backing their North Korean allies. This all changed during the night of November 25, when the communist forces counterattacked. In the ensuing battle, the 2nd Division alone took almost 4,500 battle casualties—almost one-third of them in late November and December. One might have expected to see a precipitous rise in psychiatric casualties, but that was not the case. According to one report,

> this relative low incidence of psychiatric casualties to battle casualties during rapid withdrawal . . . was indicating lessened contact with the enemy, moving away from danger, and inability of division medical services during such times to detect or diagnose psychiatric problems. . . . [D]ivisional psychiatric centers were dislocated and on the move. Intradivisional psychiatric treatment did not become operative until . . . stabilized defensive positions were established along the 38th Parallel. (Glass and Jones, 2005, Ch. 8, p. 2)

After a lull in fighting along the 38th parallel in December 1950, the attack on UN forces resumed, pushing them south of Seoul. By mid-January 1951, however, the North Korean and Chinese attack had run its course. With improved analysis of intelligence and new offensive tactics that employed armor supported by infantry, air, and artillery, all designed to "inflict a maximum of enemy casualties with minimum self-losses" (Glass and Jones, 2005, Ch. 7, p. 1), Seoul was retaken by mid-March.[48] By April, a new line just south of the 38th parallel was established; by July 1951, the front was again north of the prewar boundary.

Initially, there was a marked drop in morale as "the expectation of an early victory in November had turned to bitter defeat in December" (Glass and Jones, 2005, Ch. 8, p. 5). Unexpectedly, the official rate of psychiatric casualties remained low. What did increase, however, were the disabilities from disease and noncombat injuries, including frostbite and self-inflicted wounds, which Glass and Jones believed was a different manifestation of the missing psychiatric casualty reports, e.g., the true number was "canceled among the numerous evacuees for subjective complaints and non-disability conditions" (Glass and Jones, 2005, Ch. 8, p. 5).

The late winter offensive increased battle casualties and generated a commensurate, but less than expected, increase in the number of psychiatric casualties. Glass and Jones attributed this to an increase in morale; the positive effects of new tactics on reducing fear from the human-wave attacks; and the introduction of a rotation policy, which saw the first troops taken off the line in mid-April 1951. In a later account, Glass and Jones also highlighted "improved medical discipline," that "now experienced divisional medical officers had learned to realistically appraise subjective complaints and firmly close the door of medical evacuation except for those disabled from mental or physical causes" (Glass and Jones, 2005, Ch. 9, p. 2). Starting in March 1951, it became theater policy that division psychologists controlled the decisions about returning psychiatric casualties to combat, even for soldiers sent to higher echelons for care. The initials DSB, standing for *Don't Send Back*, were added to the diagnosis of combat exhaustion on the emergency medical tag. For casualties retained within the divi-

---

[48] Hayes, 1999, pp. 196–199, discusses the improved analysis.

sion, division psychiatrists were often able to obtain reassignments to less-strenuous positions.

As the situation stabilized and as the administrative procedures of the Eighth Army morphed from supporting a peacetime occupation force to a combat army, new ways were developed to handle soldiers and officers with personality or behavior disorders. Because regular procedures for administrative discharge of enlisted personnel were time consuming and because a general discharge under honorable conditions— the normal action taken—would have been seen as an easy way out of combat, "it was agreed that divisional psychiatrists . . . [could] medically evacuate mild personality problems . . . [who would be given] a rear area assignment" (Glass and Jones, 2005, Ch. 9, p. 9). Ineffective officers, on the other hand, were removed from their units, and a permanent discharge board at Eight Army Headquarters in Tokyo expedited their cases, with final determination made at the Department of the Army in Washington.

Phase 4: Stalemate

The advent of peace talks in summer 1951 changed the military objective but not the intensity of combat action. The goal now was not to occupy North Korea but to improve the UN's position to establish a short and more defensible battle line. Despite the increase in battle casualties, the rate of psychiatric casualties hardly changed. Glass later wrote that "perhaps the principal reason for the continued relatively low incidence of psychiatric admissions was the influence of rotation" (Glass and Jones, 2005, Ch. 11, p. 2). The rotation system changed the whole personnel dynamic along the front. Not only did it break group cohesion, it also played on the mind of the individual soldier. Those nearing rotation became known as "short timers," and many tried not to "tempt fate," exhibiting what one psychiatrist called the "short timer's attitude." Such behavior was readily understood, and units would often send short timers to a safe position in the rear.[49]

Phase 5: Armistice and the Return of Prisoners of War

In World War II, there were approximately 130,000 American POWs, of whom Japan held about 27,000. By one account, the death toll among these prisoners was more than 40 percent, a number comparable to the 38 percent often cited for the Korean War. These rates are sharply different from the death rate of a little over 1 percent for prisoners held by Germany.[50] Cowdrey suggests that

---

[49] The prophetic stories of short timers being killed on their last day in Korea was brought home by the final scene of the third season of *M*A*S*H*: It was reported that, on his way home, Colonel Henry Blake's plane had been shot down and that he had been killed.

[50] Charles A. Stenger developed these figures for the Department of Veterans Affairs Advisory Committee on Former Prisoners of War. The Center for Internee Rights, an internee advocacy group, has somewhat higher figures for POWs interned by Japan. The center reported that Japan had held 36,260 American POWs and that 13,851 of the POWs had died in captivity, resulting in a slightly lower percentage of POW deaths, 38.2 percent. See Reynolds, 2002, p. 21. Ritchie, 2002, p. 901, presents the death rate among Korean War POWs.

the experience of many former Korean POWs resembled those of World War II survivors of Japanese prison camps. In some respects they were worse . . . . Complicating a difficult homecoming for POWs were attacks by their own countrymen . . . [with] energetic charlatans . . . spread[ing] the legend that American prisoners during the Korean War had been uniquely spiritless, dying without cause and yielding without reason to enemy pressures. (Cowdrey, 1987, pp. 354–355)

On April 20, 1953, the first exchange of POWs took place at Panmunjom. For most, the process went as expected, but soon the "curiously 'flattened' personalities of those imprisoned for an extended period were noted; these men answered when spoken to, volunteered nothing, and showed little emotion" (Cowdrey, 1987, p. 349). Based on interviews with the POWs during their return to the United States, reports started to circulate that some POWs had collaborated with their North Korean and Chinese captors.[51] What followed were charges that American POWs had been "brainwashed" (Mayer, 1956), which resonated well with the anticommunist themes of the McCarthy era.[52] A more dispassionate account found that the behavior shown immediately after repatriation "did not last very long" and that the behavior that seemed so alarming was a normal reaction to the stress of being a POW: "One of the most prevalent reactions of POWs to severe and chronic physical and psychological stress is a withdrawal from involvement with the environment and constriction of overt behavior and emotional responses" (Strassman, Thaler, and Schein, 1956, p. 1001). This POW "apathy syndrome serves to maintain personality integration in the face of severe reality and psychological stresses" (Strassman, Thaler, and Schein, 1956, p. 1003). Nevertheless, the returning POWs soon found themselves embroiled in the anticommunist hysteria of the day, which saw them not as returning heroes but as untrustworthy dupes of an international communist conspiracy.

Accounts of improper behavior filled the press and were used to portray not only the evils of Communism but also the growing decadence of American society, and the POWs themselves were vilified. In 1962, *Harvard Business Review* published a statement by a group "familiar with the first-hand evidence" to "set the record straight"

---

[51] Dr. William Mayer conducted these interviews, as noted in Jones, 2005, Ch. 12, pp. 3–4. His views were widely disseminated as a series of recorded lectures, now available in Mayer, 2014. The argument that many POWs collaborated was carried through in Kinkead, 1959, and refuted in Biderman, 1963.

[52] In 1962, Dr. Mayer told a congressional committee that, during his time in the military, he "became concerned deeply over the preparation which was being given to our troops from a psychological standpoint, for their role." He went on to say:

> I became concerned deeply with the methods used by the Communists to control people. I became concerned . . . because it appeared to me that we Americans had no built-in, God-given immunity to the personnel management methods and corruption of human control that Communists have applied to millions of the freedom-loving people elsewhere in the world. I believe that we need to take stock and respond to this new challenge of Communist domination of human beings, appraise it realistically, and attempt to create the proper counter measures, not just for prisoners of war in the future, but for our whole people. (Mayer, 1962, p. 1152)

(reproduced in Biderman, 1962, pp. 94–95). The authors concluded that "[t]he behavior of the Korean War prisoners did not compare unfavorably with that of their countrymen or with the behavior of people of other nations who have faced similar trials in the past" (Biderman, 1962, p. 94). It also pointed out that, while 21 Americans refused repatriation and chose to stay in North Korea, more than one-half of North Korean and Chinese POWs—some 88,000—refused repatriation. Nevertheless, as late as 2006, half a century after the POWs returned from Korea, stories continued to circulate that many POWs showed signs of "hopelessness," and "give-it-upitis," proving our soldiers "lacked religious faith" (Wilson, 2006; Ritchie, 2002).

One result of the Korean POW situation was EO 10631, signed August 17, 1955, which prescribed the Code of Conduct for Members of the Armed Forces of the United States (see Box 3.1). President Eisenhower's declaration accompanying the promulgation of the code clearly saw it in terms of standards concerning behavior in captivity:

> Every member of the Armed Forces of the United States is expected to measure up to the standards embodied in this Code of Conduct while he is in combat or in captivity. To ensure achievement of these standards, each member of the armed forces liable to capture shall be provided with specific training and instruction designed to better equip him to counter and withstand all enemy efforts against

---

Box 3.1
Code of Conduct for Members of the Armed Forces of the United States, 1955

I
I am an American fighting man. I serve in the forces which guard my country and our way of life. I am prepared to give my life in their defense.

II
I will never surrender of my own free will. If in command, I will never surrender my men while they still have the means to resist.

III
If I am captured I will continue to resist by all means available. I will make every effort to escape and aid others to escape. I will accept neither parole nor special favors from the enemy.

IV
If I become a prisoner of war, I will keep faith with my fellow prisoners. I will give no information or take part in any action which might be harmful to my comrades. If I am senior, I will take command. If not, I will obey the lawful orders of those appointed over me and will back them up in every way.

V
When questioned, should I become a prisoner of war, I am bound to give only name, rank, service number, and date of birth. I will evade answering further questions to the utmost of my ability. I will make no oral or written statements disloyal to my country and its allies or harmful to their cause.

VI
I will never forget that I am an American fighting man, responsible for my actions, and dedicated to the principles which made my country free. I will trust in my God and in the United States of America.

SOURCE: Quoted from EO 10631, 1955.

him, and shall be fully instructed as to the behavior and obligations expected of him during combat or captivity. (EO 10631, 1955).

For Dr. William Mayer, the Army psychiatrist who conducted many of the original interviews of POWs and who most forcefully raised the specter of communist brainwashing and moral weakness, the code fell short of what was needed. As he saw it, "when the code was first announced, it was emphasized by the President that this was not a formula for being a prisoner-of-war, that the principles of this code were first principles of the American society. . . . Now the code has not been taught in those terms" (Mayer, 1962, p. 1166).

Nonbattle Psychiatric Casualties

In the initial months of the war, most American troops were assigned to combat units, but as the war matured, increasing numbers of support troops arrived in Korea. Moreover, as the war settled into a dulling sameness for these rear-area troops, military psychiatrists began to see a rise in psychiatric problems:

> The terrors of battle are obvious in their potentialities for producing psychic trauma, but troops removed from the rigors and stress of actual combat . . . continued to have psychiatric disabilities, sometimes approximating the rate sustained in combat, as in psychoses. Other stresses relegated to the background or ignored in combat are reinforced . . . when time for meditation, rumination, and fantasy increases the cathexis caused by such stresses, thereby producing symptoms. . . . [B]oredom, segregation from the opposite sex, monotony, apparently meaningless activity, lack of purpose, lessened chances for promotion, fear of a renewal of combat . . . are psychological stresses that tend to recrudesce and receive inappropriate emphasis. (Marren, 1956, p. 719)

For Franklin Jones, a leading military psychiatrist, this "situation resembled that of nostalgic soldiers of prior centuries. In these circumstances, the soldier sought relief in alcohol abuse and, in coastal areas, in drug abuse . . . and sexual stimulation" (Jones, 2000, p. 14). While he noted that "these problems were scarcely noticed at the time," they foreshadow more prevalent problems in Vietnam. These so-called "garrison casualties" would become the "predominant psychiatric casualties of the Vietnam War" (Jones, 2000, p. 14).

Legacy

In the minds of the American public, the two most enduring stories to come out of the Korean War were those of Task Force Smith, reflecting the unpreparedness of the American military after the World War II, and the epic adventures portrayed in the TV series *M*A*S*H*. The Korean conflict also had a lasting influence on military medicine.[53]

The Legacy of Task Force Smith

The story of Task Force Smith dominates the historical accounts of the first days of the war and has become a useful mantra for the Army in pressing its claim for resources in the face of pending budget cuts. Besides being useful for bureaucratic purposes, can we blame the initial defeats in Korea of the "ill-trained, ill-equipped [and] ill-led" American troops, as suggested by Clay Blair (1987, p. 115) and others? Even Blair recognized that our efforts constituted a "piecemeal and disorganized waste of precious lives and equipment" and that we left on the battlefield "enough weapons, equipment and ammo" to "fit out one or two North Korean regiments."

The real lesson to be learned from Task Force Smith was the importance of good intelligence and a concept of operations that included an appropriate appreciation of the enemy and a realistic assessment of our own capability. To paraphrase a familiar quotation from Shakespeare's *Julius Caesar*: The fault, dear Brutus, lies not in our readiness, but in our arrogance and contempt. Richard Wiersema contended that "MacArthur's strategy in effect doomed the 24th Division to a piecemeal employment in front of the North Koreans" (Wiersema, 1997, p. 42), quoting Blair, 1987, p. 78: "MacArthur did not hold the [North Korean Army] in high regard; on the contrary, he was contemptuous of it." Wiersema went on to say that the assumption was "that the North Koreans would not fight once they encountered American soldiers" (Wiersema, 1997, p. 42). He then made a case that our forces were in no

> way ideally trained, equipped, or manned, or that the Eighth Army in 1950 presents an acceptable standard of readiness for the American Army. The point is simply that those shortcomings did not lie behind the ignominious retreat to the Pusan Perimeter and that no amount of extravagance in funding, rigor in training or zealousness in the pursuit of discipline would have reversed the outcome. It was not the North Korean Army that shattered the admittedly brittle 24th Division; MacArthur, and Dean, executing MacArthur's concept, accomplished that for them at least twenty-four hours before Task Force Smith began its forty year march into the Army's institutional memory as a metaphor for unreadiness. (Wiersema, 1997, p. 44)

The Task Force Smith myth of defeat because of excessive budget cuts in the post–World War II period may not only be a poor reading of history; it also ignores the fact that the American military that so many have derided as having been unprepared

---

[53] Possibly the most important legacy of the Korean War had nothing to do with casualties or medical care: the full and final racial integration of the U.S. armed forces. While proclaimed in 1948 by President Truman, integration was not actually accomplished until the Korean War. See Pash, 2012, pp. 168–181.

and unready was able to occupy the North Korean capital of Pyongyang just three months later, in September 1950. While a second failure of intelligence—the Chinese Communist Army was massively entering the war, with 300,000 troops—resulted in an epic and orderly retreat, the Army remained a potent fighting force and soon was again north of the line that divided the two Koreas. All this was accomplished with basically the same Army that had been in place when the Korean War started in June 1950 because it would take months before new troops were trained and new equipment procured.

Lessons Learned by the Army Medical Department

Despite the fact that the war took place only five years after World War II, many things in the world had changed. The Army Medical Department considers eight notable advances in combat care to have emerged from the Korean War (see Box 3.2).

"Choppers" and the MASHs they supported became the prototypes for today's trauma care and influenced the development of the emergency medical system in the United States.[54] New surgical techniques, despite large numbers of battle casualties, reduced the number of related amputations in the "first deviation from the practice of ligation started by Pare more than a century earlier" (Rasmussen and Cherry, 2009). The policy of rotating surgeons to front-line units helped train a new generation of surgeons in the advanced repair of arteries. The body armor first introduced in Korea would become standard issue in the next war.

The Korean War fortified the principles of PIES for the treatment of combat psychiatric casualties, returning up to 90 percent of combat psychiatric casualties to battle. That success notwithstanding, military psychiatry, as practiced during the Korean War, failed to address two issues that would challenge the very foundations of military psychiatry in the years ahead: the emergence of nonbattle psychiatric casual-

---

Box 3.2
Army Medical Department Advances in Combat Care from the Korean Conflict

Fluid resuscitation adequate to correct shock and prevent organ failure
Availability of board-certified surgical specialists
Forward availability of definitive surgery
Use of helicopters for patient transport
Primary repair and vascular grafts for injured vessels
Use of hemodialysis in theater of operations
Identification of high output renal failure
Recognition of seasonal variation in bacteria recovered from battle wounds

SOURCES: Murray, Hitter, and Jones, 2016, p. 2; Pruitt, 2008, p. S7.

---

[54] As Ravage, 2006, p. 16, notes, "[m]odeled after the mobile army surgical hospital (M.A.S.H.) units, the nation's first hospital-based civilian trauma units were established in 1966 at San Francisco General Hospital and Chicago's Cook County hospitals."

ties and the lingering effects of combat, in what came to be known as PTSD—both issues that would become critical in Vietnam.

CHAPTER FOUR

From Korea to Vietnam—1954 to 1964

The stalemate in Korea finally came to an end in summer 1953. Two events are generally credited with bringing the conflict to a close. First, the new Eisenhower administration upped the ante by "hinting at Panmunjom . . . and elsewhere to the effect that if the deadlock in the peace talks were not soon broken, Washington might not confine the war to Korea and might employ atomic bombs in Asia" (Blair, 1987, p. 971). Second, the death of the Soviet leader Joseph Stalin on March 5, 1953, brought new leaders to the Kremlin. Within a month of Stalin's death, the communists accepted the UN proposal for a limited exchange of POWs. Finally, on July 27, 1953, at 10:00 p.m., hostilities ceased along an armistice line that exists to this day. The Cold War, however, did not end. In retrospect, the Korean War was only the first military battle and was soon to be followed by another conflict in Asia: Vietnam. In the meantime, the United States turned its attention to caring for its newest veterans and creating a military and security order better prepared than the one that had existed in 1950 to face the threat from international communism.

The Veterans of the Korean War: America's Invisible Veterans

Mention of V-E or V-J Day immediately brings to mind World War II and the image of a jubilant crowd in Times Square, New York. Americans have no such mental images about the announcement that the Korean War had ended. In fact, for most of the time American forces were fighting in Korea, the engagement was not even called a war. It was initially referred to as a "police action" or a conflict, but not a war. The military sociologist, Charles Moskos summed it up this way:

> Unlike World War II, the war in Korea never resulted in total mobilization. At the height of the Korean buildup in 1952, less than 3,700,000 Americans were in uniform. . . . Military service in the Korean War did not become the modal generational experience of young men in the early 1950s. . . . The American public was never to feel the effects of the war in Korea in any way resembling their involvement in World War II. (Moskos, 1970, pp. 9–10)

Those drafted for World War II served for the duration of the war, but for those who served in Korea, being drafted was more like being on a conveyer belt that took them from their home, to Korea, and back home in short order. During the Korean War, combat troops served between nine and 12 months and, even then, rotated on and off the line. Rear-echelon troops served 18 months (Kolb, 1997, p. 25). As the war ended, one unflattering account published in the *New York Times* characterized them as being "adrift, . . . thoroughly indifferent," attributing much of their attitude to being a "product of the impersonalized pipeline system" (Barrett, 1953, p. 24). But the cause of detachment may have gone deeper than that. For one thing, those who served in Korea were considerably younger than their World War II counterparts: The age group was "narrower, without the wide age variation found among World War II veterans. . . . Thus, among Korean veterans there were more problems that are adolescent and postadolescent in type and concerned with early adult adjustment" (Tompkins, 1955, p. 35).

The veterans of the Korean War also carried a burden unknown by the veterans of any other war, the charge that they were morally weak, with many of them collaborating with the enemy. Military sociologist Charles Moskos reminded us that,

> when the repatriation of American prisoners of war began 1953, the American public was suddenly exposed to new and disquieting terms—collaboration, brainwashing, "give-up-itis." These ominous words portended a strictly negative image of American behavior in Communist prison camps. (Moskos, 1970, p. 11). . . . [And] contributed to an inverted placement of blame for the war's unsatisfactory outcome. The American soldier himself was held up to question. (Moskos, 1970, p. 33)

Today, the Korean War is often referred to as "the forgotten war," and one might extend that to refer to veterans of that war as the forgotten veterans.[1] In fact, their story is the precursor to that of the troubled return of veterans from the Vietnam War a decade or so later.

The Veterans Administration in 1950

If the veterans of the Korean War were different from the veterans of World War II, so was the VA that treated them. Arguably, in the five years between the end of World War II and the start of the Korean War, no other American institution had changed more than the VA. The change can be seen by looking at the VA before and during World War II and the VA of 1950, at the start of the Korean War.

---

[1] In January 1953, an editorial in the *Army Times* said, "Certainly—in many respects—it [Korea] is the most 'forgotten war,' and the men who fight it are lonesome symbols of a nation too busy or too economy-minded to say thanks in a proper manner" (as quoted in Kolb, 1997, p. 27).

The VA Before World War II

In 1940, on the eve of World War II, the recently formed VA could only be called a backwater of American medicine. Created in 1930 through the amalgamation of the Veterans' Bureau, the National Homes for Disabled Volunteer Soldiers, and the Bureau of Pensions, the new agency had largely become a warehouse for neuropsychiatric veterans, many of whom were indigent and whose disabilities were not connected to their prior military service. This came about as the result of the World War Veterans Act of 1924 (Pub. L. 68-242), which substantially expanded veterans' access to the hospitals of the Veterans' Bureau. It was originally thought that "not too many veterans would take advantage of this" expanded benefit (Adkins, 1967, pp. 131–132), but by 1940, 84.5 percent of all admissions to VA hospitals or domiciliary facilities were veterans with non–service-connected problems (Administrator of Veterans Affairs, 1941, Table 6, p. 53).[2]

The Veterans Administration During World War II

The limited capabilities of the VA notwithstanding, as the United States prepared for war, President Franklin Roosevelt approved a Federal Board of Hospitalization recommendation that the VA should care for members of the armed forces who were injured or who incurred disabilities in line of duty and whose physical rehabilitation the Army or Navy could not feasibly undertake.[3] When the war started, it soon became clear, that the VA was incapable of handling the casualties that were returning from overseas battlefields. Within the first year of the war, about 15 percent of the VA's physicians, dentists, nurses, and administrators were called to or had volunteered for military service. By June 1942, the staffing situation had become so critical that the Department of War agreed not to call up VA doctors who held reserve commissions; by December 1943, the Selective Service stopped drafting VA physicians and dentists. In early 1944, the Department of War started to assign physicians and dentists to work at the VA.[4] The problem was not only the lack of personnel; it was also the lack of adequate facilities. The VA's 91 hospitals were designed to handle about 62,000 patients, which was not even enough for the pre–World War II veterans' population (Adkins, 1967, p. 149).

The inability of the VA to provide care for World War II casualties became a national scandal. Newspaper stories appeared with such headlines as "Veterans Hospitals Called Backwaters of Medicine" and "Third-Rate Medicine for First-Rate Men" (Maisel, 1945). Most notable were an 11-part series by Albert Deutsch in the New York newspaper *PM* and Albert Q. Maisel's two-part series in *Cosmopolitan*, which

---

[2] A decade earlier, in 1930, the percentage of non–service-connected admissions stood at 69.1 percent (Director U.S. Veterans' Bureau, 1930, Table 13, p. 48).

[3] To be clear, the policy was to maximize the use of the VA. Neither the Army nor the Navy was prepared to undertake rehabilitation programs that were not focused on returning service members to combat units.

[4] GEN Omar Bradley noted that, when he took over the VA on August 15, 1945, "there were then 2,300 full-time doctors in VA, of whom 1,700 were on 'loan' from the Army and Navy" (Bradley and Blair, 1983, p. 457).

was later reprised in the more widely read *Reader's Digest*.[5] On December 4, 1944, President Roosevelt took steps to limit the flow of casualties to the VA. He ordered the Secretary of War to ensure that no overseas casualty was discharged from the service until he or she had received "the maximum benefits of hospitalization and convalescent facilities," including "physical and psychological rehabilitation, vocational guidance, prevocational training and resocialization" (Roosevelt, 1944). On June 30, 1945, there were 20,774 World War II veterans in VA hospitals, compared with 58,345 in Army convalescent hospitals and 152,971 in Army general hospitals.[6] Thus, as the war was ending, the VA was caring for less than 10 percent of Army's most serious casualties.

The Veterans Administration After World War II

In the months following the end of the war in Europe, the VA underwent significant changes. Within days of the fall of Nazi Germany, GEN Omar N. Bradley, the second highest-ranking Army officer in Europe, was reassigned as the new head of the VA.[7] Almost immediately, Bradley made major changes at the VA that he would later characterize as "radical and revolutionary" (Bradley and Blair, 1983, p. 458). Even before he officially took over the VA, Bradley recruited former members of his old European staff to join him in Washington. He appointed MG Paul Hawley, the former chief surgeon of the European theater, to be the VA's new chief medical director. And one month after he was sworn in as administrator, Bradley announced "a sweeping reorganization" (Adkins, 1967, p. 195) by decentralizing operations. He created 13 branch offices, each a small-scale version of the VA, led by a deputy administrator with broad decisionmaking powers. He implemented Hawley's plan to revitalize the VA's medical staff by creating a professional medical corps independent of Civil Service regulations. He also set up a new advisory board to help guide the VA, established VA hospital affiliations with medical schools, organized physician training programs at VA hos-

---

[5] In 1941, Deutsch began to write a daily column for *PM*. In 1945, his 11-part series criticizing the maltreatment of psychiatric patients in veterans' hospitals led the House Committee on Veterans Affairs to demand the names of his news sources. He refused and was voted in contempt of Congress. Later, the committee rescinded its action, and the VA adopted many of Deutsch's suggestions for improving treatment. The American Newspaper Guild gave him its Heywood Broun Award in 1945 and 1946 for this series. See Beard, 1963.

[6] Another 50,078 patients were at regional hospitals and 51,561 at station hospitals (Smith, 1956, p. 211).

[7] Bradley wrote that he was devastated when he received the news and that he was

> reluctant to go to any desk job in Washington before the war with Japan was over, especially one outside the Army and one that seemed on first blush so inconsequential and demeaning. . . . The only job in Washington I wanted was Chief of Staff of the Army. And yet I could not refuse the assignment. . . . [Eisenhower] assured me that he would do everything within his power to see that sooner or later I was named Chief of Staff. (Bradley and Blair, 1983, p. 440)

Bradley eventually made his peace with the new job, telling one reporter,

> I don't think there's any job in the county I'd sooner not have nor any job in the world I'd like to do better. For even though it is burdened with problems, it gives me the chance to do something for the men who did so much for us. (Bradley and Blair, 1983, p. 446)

pitals, and put a new emphasis on rehabilitation. During his stewardship of the VA, the agency grew precipitously. Between 1945 and 1947, the budget increased from $177.6 million to more than $500 million; employment at the VA was up from 65,000 to 200,000; and funding for hospital and domiciliary facilities grew from $17.9 million to $242.8 million (Gambone, 2005, p. 52).

As noteworthy as the growth of the new VA was, so were the cutbacks that were put in place after Bradley left the VA to become Chief of Staff of the Army in 1948.[8] As early as February 1947, the VA was forced to institute a hiring freeze and to curtail all but essential travel. By 1949, it had also cut back on the ambitious hospital construction program Bradley and Hawley had put in place. Predictably, physicians, usually the best, began to resign.

By one account, on the eve of the Korean War, "more than four thousand authorized beds, the equivalent of sixteen average-sized hospitals, . . . [were empty] because the staffs needed to maintain them were unavailable" (Gambone, 2005, p. 468). The staff shortage was aggravated by the loss of VA personnel to the Korean War effort as reserve personnel were called to active duty and medical personnel were drafted.

The VA at the Start of the Korean War: The Rusk Committee Report

Two weeks before the outbreak of hostilities in Korea, President Truman appointed a special committee to review the veterans' hospitalization program and needs of disabled veterans, paying special attention to the problem of paraplegics and amputees. The committee was headed by Dr. Howard A. Rusk, considered by many to be the founder of rehabilitation medicine in the United States. Since the Korean War broke out shortly after the committee started work, it paid particular attention to the "Korean situation in its review and recommendations" (Dennison, Abramson, and Rusk, 1950, p. i). The committee's September 22, 1950, report provides a unique picture of the state of the VA at the start of the Korean conflict.

The committee was concerned about the "[r]ecent precipitate cuts in personnel . . . [that] have brought about a number of resignations, and have caused many of the young doctors in training to decide against a career in the Veterans' Administration." The report stated that "[s]uch actions in the future must be avoided at all costs" (Dennison, Abramson, and Rusk, 1950, p. 1). The committee argued that medical personnel employed by the VA should not be mobilized, e.g., reservists employed by the VA should not be called up; the current medical staff should be exempt from being

---

[8] Bradley's replacement was Carl R. Gray, Jr. Bradley thought him a "poor choice" (Bradley and Blair, 1983, p. 468). Gray turned the clock back. He

> restored the centralized VA bureaucracy . . . priority for hospital construction and facilities purchase again passed to the congressional pork barrel. Gray himself was forced out as VA administrator after a Senate investigation . . . revealed a familiar story of politicization and bureaucratic incompetence. (Gambone, 2005, p. 55)

drafted;[9] and, in the future, VA staff should not be allowed to join military reserve units. Their recommendations notwithstanding, "as a result of the Korean situation, VA hospitals lost a large number of employees to the military" (Gray, 1953, p. 23).[10]

Problems

The Rusk committee highlighted a number of concerns about the VA program in 1950 that resonate today. It found that interdepartmental coordination of medical services was a "primary problem," as was the administration organization of the VA, which the committee called "cumbersome and unwieldy" (Dennison, Abramson, and Rusk, 1950, pp. 1, 3). The committee focused on four problems: the inability of the VA to appropriately staff its facilities, waiting times to gain access to VA hospitals, the transfer of disabled soldiers from DoD to the VA, and the care of veterans whose medical needs were not related to their military service.

Staffing

Despite the fact that more than 2,000 staff were lost to the armed forces during the Korean War and with 915 unfilled positions in June 1954 (Administrator of Veterans Affairs, 1954, p. 25), the overall staffing remained relatively constant throughout the Korean War (see Table 4.1). The largest numbers of vacant medical positions were in psychiatry and neurology, medical residents, and nurses.

Waiting for Admission to VA Hospitals

At the heart of the VA's problems in 1950 were, first, the "unavailability of qualified medical personnel, particularly in such specialties as tuberculosis and psychiatry; second, the difficulty of attracting competent medical personnel to service in remote areas" (Dennison, Abramson, and Rusk, 1950, p. 14).[11] For veterans, particularly those with neuropsychiatric problems, for whom the bed occupancy rate was over 95 per-

---

[9] At the time, 19 percent of VA residents and 50 percent of regular physicians—38 percent of the entire medical staff—held reserve commissions, constituting 8 percent of the Armed Forces medical reserve (Dennison, Abramson, and Rusk, 1950, p. 24).

[10] The VA reported that, at

> the end of fiscal year 1952, shortages of medical personnel still existed at many VA stations. Between the approximate date of the outbreak of the Korean situation and the end of fiscal year 1952, 682 physicians (including 478 residents), 78 dentists, 750 nurses, and 1,995 other medical personnel had been separated from the Veterans Administration to enter on extended active duty with the Armed Forces. Nearly one-third of the losses of physicians occurred during fiscal year 1952. (Gray, 1953, p. 24)

[11] The Rusk committee reported that,

> [a]s of June 30, 1950, 87.4 percent of all operating Veterans' Administration beds were occupied (tuberculosis hospitals, 86.0 percent; neuropsychiatric hospitals, 95.1 percent; general medical and surgical hospitals, 79.7 percent). This, however, does not represent the true picture, as, while some hospitals near metropolitan areas are overcrowded even to the extent of using emergency beds, many hospitals in remote areas are not fully utilized. (Dennison, Abramson, and Rusk, 1950, p. 16)

Table 4.1
**Veterans' Administration Medical Personnel During the Korean War,
June 1950–June 1953**

	FY				
	1950	**1951**	**1952**	**1953**	**1954**
Physicians					
Full-time	3,991	4,014	4,160	4,160	4,384
Regular part-time	990	988	1,003	936	N/A
Residents and interns	2,251	2,011	1,895	1,937	N/A
Dentists					
Full-time	929	903	901	904	894
Regular part-time	9	5	5	6	N/A
Residents and interns	0	0	5	12	N/A
Nurses					
Full-time	13,258	13,734	14,304	13,799	14,754
Regular part-time	78	69	62	131	N/A

SOURCES: Administrator of Veterans Affairs, 1952, p. 25; Gray, 1953, p. 25; Administrator of Veterans Affairs, 1954, p. 26; Administrator of Veterans Affairs, 1955.

cent, these problems manifested in long waits for care.[12] Table 4.2 shows the waiting periods for each type of hospital. While the average time waiting was not reported, the Rusk committee found that about three-quarters of those waiting admission were on the list more than 40 days. It should be noted, however, almost all those on the waiting list were veterans with non–service-connected disabilities. The waiting lists would have been longer had not the VA initiated an outpatient program built around the so-called mental hygiene clinics, which reduced the demand for psychiatric beds by a reported 25 percent (Dennison, Abramson, and Rusk, 1950, p. 22). At the time, 1950, the demand for such outpatient services was expected to rise 20 percent per year.

Transfer of Military Patients to the VA

Despite the fact that EO 10122 gave primary responsibility for physically disabled soldiers and veterans to the VA, the Rusk committee felt that there was a need to clarify policy for the care of soldiers "whose disabilities are such that it is obvious they will be unable to return to active duty, should be transferred *on military status* to Veterans' Administration specialized facilities" (Dennison, Abramson, and Rusk, 1950, p. 4; emphasis added). The Rusk committee thought that VA centers should care for

---

[12] The committee noted that the VA was "having difficulty staffing the number of neuropsychiatric beds . . . . The residency training program is barely keeping pace with the attrition rate of qualified psychiatric personnel. The greatest part of the staffing difficulty arises from the relatively remote locations of some Veterans' Administration neuropsychiatric hospitals" (Dennison, Abramson, and Rusk, 1950, p. 21).

Table 4.2
Waiting Lists for Admission to Veterans' Administration Hospitals, as of June 15, 1950

Length of Waiting Period	Type of Hospital to Which Veteran Is Awaiting Admission			
	Neuropsychiatric	General Medical and Surgical	Tuberculosis	Total
1 to 20 days	513	2,225	115	2,853
21 to 40 days	628	1,956	100	2,684
>40 days	8,218	9,636	1,211	19,065
Total	9,359	13,817	1,426	24,602

SOURCE: Dennison, Abramson, and Rusk, 1950, p. 19.

the rehabilitation of the blind, the hard of hearing, paraplegics, amputees, the tuberculous and other groups . . . [those requiring] plastic surgery, chest surgery, and other types of specialized medical care. . . . [because the VA centers had] well-trained, experienced . . . personnel as well as the services of outstanding civilian consultants. (Dennison, Abramson, and Rusk, 1950, p. 4)

Care for Veterans with Non–Service-Connected Disabilities

Of particular concern to the Rusk committee were veterans receiving care unrelated to their military service. This issue would be a central theme throughout the 1950s. Some even argued that programs to care for veterans had created a special class of citizens who were receiving "free hospitalization for disabilities which occurred after their military service, and . . . drawing veterans' pensions in addition to social security, despite the fact that they had no injuries in service" (Booth, 1958, p. 19).

The data the Rusk committee reported showed that, on January 31, 1950, 51.2 percent of the 109,618 patients being cared for in a VA hospital were receiving care for service-connected disabilities, and an additional 16.4 percent were receiving care as "service-connected cases being treated for non–service-connected disabilities" (Dennison, Abramson, and Rusk, 1950, p. 54). The committee saw this as an open-ended commitment and argued that, until Congress clarified its policy on how veterans "should be cared for by the Veterans' Administration regardless of the origin of the disability, and in what numbers, . . . there can be no way to establish requirements upon which an adequate and appropriate . . . hospital program could be developed" (Dennison, Abramson, and Rusk, 1950, p. 12).

Serving the Veterans of the Korean War

As noted, during both World War I and World War II, soldiers were recruited and drafted for the duration of the conflict, but this was not the case for the Korean War. As a result, despite the fact that the number of American combat troops on the line in

Korea at any point in time was generally less than 250,000, some 6.8 million service men and women served during the Korean War and were therefore entitled to VA benefits and services after the war ended.[13]

Initially, those in the armed forces fighting in Korea did not receive the same benefits as those in World War II because "military service in Korea was technically peace-time service, and veterans of peacetime never have received the same measure of benefits as those who served in time of war" (Adkins, 1967, p. 231). After an unfortunate and embarrassing incident in which a disabled Korean War casualty was denied services at a local VA hospital, Congress passed Pub. L. 82-28 on May 11, 1951, providing the same benefits as those available for World War II veterans. Other legislation followed (see Fisher, 1975, p. 117). The Combat Duty Act of 1952 (Pub. L. 82-488, Title VII, 1952) gave Korean War service members retroactive combat pay from the start of the war. The Veterans Readjustment Assistance Act of 1952 (Pub. L. 82-550, 1952) provided assistance for schooling, as had the World War II G.I. Bill, and 2.3 million—43 percent of Korean War veterans—had enrolled in the program by 1960.[14] Despite having to pay tuition out of a monthly stipend, rather than having it paid separately, Korean War veterans were more likely than World War II veterans to enroll at institutions of higher education (see Table 4.3).

By the end of the Korean War, 2.897 million Korean War veterans had returned to civilian life, as the VA reported for FY 1954 (Administrator of Veterans Affairs, 1955, p. 12). By the end of the decade, that number had grown to 5.482 million (Administrator of Veterans Affairs, 1961, p. 7), including the 18 percent who had also served

Table 4.3
Enrollment as of June 30, 1960 in Veterans Training Program by Type of Program: World War II and Korean War Programs

	Korean War Veterans (%)	World War II Veterans (%)
Institution of higher learning	51	29
School below college level	36	44
On-the-job training	9	18
On-the-farm training	4	9
Total	100	100

SOURCE: Administrator of Veterans Affairs, 1961, p. 71.

---

[13] For the purpose of receiving VA benefits, the Korean War era extended from June 27, 1950, to January 31, 1955 (Administrator of Veterans Affairs, 1957, p. 1).

[14] The VA reported in 1957 that 7.8 million of the 15.37 million World War II veterans were trained under the Servicemen's Readjustment Act of 1944 (Pub. L. 78-346, 1944), or 50.1 percent of those eligible (Administrator of Veterans Affairs, 1957, pp. 15, 103).

in World War II (see Table 4.4). As of June 30, 1960, there were 120,073 beds in VA hospitals, the majority of which were for psychiatric patents—54,034 for psychotic patents and 4,380 for other psychiatric patients (Administrator of Veterans Affairs, 1961, p. 15). Korean War patients, however, never made up more than 10 percent of the total patient load at VA hospitals.

Psychiatric Services

On the average day in FY 1960, there were by far more psychiatric patients in VA hospitals than any other type of patient.[15] Moreover, many of these were long-term patients: Only 8.5 percent of those with a diagnosis of "psychoses" were hospitalized for less than 90 days, and the remaining 91.5 percent—of a total of 55,545 patients—had a reported "length of stay of more than 90 days" (Administrator of Veterans Affairs, 1961, p. 190).[16] In addition, the VA ran 67 outpatient mental hygiene clinics, with an enrolled veteran population of 31,000. An additional 14,400 veterans also received

Table 4.4
Korean War Veterans, as of June 30, 1960

Year	Total Living Veterans (000)	Korean War Veterans (000)	Hospitalized Korean War Veterans	
			Total	As a Percentage of All Hospitalized Veterans
1951	18,813	Not reported	Not reported	Not reported
1952	19,288	921	3,000	2.9
1953	20,138	1,963	4,930	4.7
1954	20,850	2,897	7,746	7.0
1955	21,878	4,015	9,740	8.7
1956	22,381	4,682	10,916	9.5
1957	22,633	5,105	11,064	9.7
1958	22,727	5,353	Not reported	Not reported
1959	22,666	5,448	Not reported	Not reported
1960	22,534	5,482	Not reported	Not reported

SOURCES: Veterans' Administration annual reports (Administrator of Veterans Affairs, 1952–1961).

---

[15] The VA reported "average daily patient load by type" as 56,728 for psychiatric; 9,037 for tuberculosis; 4,708 for neurological; and 40,935 for general medical and surgical patients (Administrator of Veterans Affairs, 1961, p. 169).

[16] The pattern is somewhat different for those admitted in 1959:

> 51 percent of the 24,800 psychotic patients admitted during 1959 were discharged within 90 days after their admission, leaving 49 percent who required care for 90 days or more. An additional 15 percent of the psychotic

"treatment from fee-basis physicians and contract clinics" (Administrator of Veterans Affairs, 1961, p. 36). These programs were staffed with psychiatrists, as well as 500 clinical psychologists and 1,400 social workers.[17]

The substantial psychiatric services available to veterans in 1960 masked the unmet demand for these services. With 95 percent of the beds in the 39 psychiatric hospitals filled (Administrator of Veterans Affairs, 1961, p. 18), almost 14,000 veterans were on waiting lists for psychiatric beds to open up.[18] As it had since the end of World War II, the VA was aggressively trying to grow its own mental health professionals. At the end of 1959, the VA had 349 psychiatric residents, with 775 clinical and counseling psychologists and 410 social workers in training (Administrator of Veterans Affairs, 1961, pp. 45–46). Nevertheless, there were 130 unfilled positions in psychiatry,[19] 73 for clinical psychologists, and 73 for social workers (Administrator of Veterans Affairs, 1961, p. 31).

A Fresh Look at Veterans' Program: The Bradley Commission and the Pension Act of 1959

By the mid-20th century, almost one-half of the American population was made up of veterans and their families, about 81 million in total.[20] In January 1955, President Eisenhower appointed a commission "to carry out a comprehensive study of the laws and policies pertaining to pension, compensation, and related nonmedical benefits for our veterans and their dependents (Eisenhower, 1955; see also EO 10588, 1955), chaired by his old military colleague, GEN Omar Bradley, who had also served as the

---

patients admitted were released after 3 to 6 months of treatment, so that 34 percent were still under treatment 6 months after their admission. (Administrator of Veterans Affairs, 1961, p. 24)

[17] The VA did not report the number of psychiatrists on staff, but noted in 1955 that there were

more vacancies for physicians in psychiatry and neurology than in any other specialty—98 out of 257, in reality the shortage was greater since requests by hospitals for psychiatrists are related to the maximum number recruitable rather than to the number necessary for a definitive therapy program. In 14 of the 38 neuropsychiatric hospitals there was a total of only 74 full-time psychiatrists to care for a total of more than 15,000 patients. (Administrator of Veterans Affairs, 1955, p. 28)

[18] According to VA, at

the end of fiscal year 1960, there were 21,677 (208 tuberculosis, 7,612 medical, surgical, and neurological, and 13,857 psychiatric) veterans on the waiting list. None of these were waiting for treatment of a service-connected disability. . . . Forty-five percent of the eligible veterans on the waiting list were already in hospitals at no expense to the Veterans Administration. Most of these veterans had psychiatric disabilities. (Administrator of Veterans Affairs, 1961, p. 25)

[19] On June 30, 1958, the number of unfilled positions in psychiatry and neurology was reported as 128 positions, and the number in psychology and social work as 46 and 80, respectively (Administrator of Veterans Affairs, 1959, p. 25). For 1959 and 1960, the VA did not report the number of vacant positions for psychiatry and neurology but did report the numbers for psychology for the two years as 75 and 73 and for social workers as 97 and 73 (Administrator of Veterans Affairs, 1961, p. 31).

[20] As noted in Bradley Commission, 1956a, p. 23, the actual count of veterans at the time was 25 million.

VA administrator immediately after World War II. Given that veterans' programs had grown up over time from a patchwork of legislation, President Eisenhower wanted Bradley to provide a set of "fundamental principles, which I can use as the basis for making recommendations to the Congress for modernization of these benefits and clarification of their relationship to our broader Government social insurance and family protection programs" (Eisenhower, 1955). Eisenhower was acutely aware that, in the years since the Veteran's Bureau, the predecessor to the VA, had been created after World War I, the nation had undergone sweeping changes. In particular, the nation had

> instituted policies to maintain high and stable employment and developed the broad social security programs to provide economic assistance to the aged and the needy. These developments reflect[ed] the growth of the Government's obligations and a more adequate recognition of its responsibilities, and they have also had an important effect on its fiscal situation. (Eisenhower, 1955)

Now he wanted a systematic assessment of

> the structure, scope, philosophy, and administration of pension, compensation, and related nonmedical benefits furnished under Federal legislation to our veterans and their families, together with the relationships between these benefits and others which are provided our citizens without regard to their status as veterans. (Eisenhower, 1955)

A year later, in a report that resonates today, the President's Commission on Veterans' Pensions reported its findings and recommendations (Bradley Commission, 1956a).[21] General Bradley summed it up in the commission's transmittal letter to President Eisenhower:

> Existing veterans' benefit programs on the whole are working well and are being soundly administered. Veterans as a group are better off economically than nonveterans. The Commission was especially impressed with the recent trend away from the old backward-looking pension philosophy. The present practice of assisting the veteran in his immediate readjustment to civil life is much more effective. A veteran now receives help when he needs it most.

> While the general situation is good, the Commission's studies did reveal some important weaknesses and inequities that can and should be corrected. One of the most serious is that under some of the programs benefits are not being channeled sufficiently to those who have sacrificed the most or whose needs are great-

---

[21] The 2004–2007 Veterans' Disability Benefits Commission found the work of the Bradley Commission "particularly compelling" (Veterans' Disability Benefits Commission, 2007, p. 23) and was "mindful of the . . . Bradley Commission principles, which have provided a valuable and historic baseline" (Veterans' Disability Benefits Commission, 2007, p. 2).

est. There is also a decided need for long-range programing and for coordination between related programs, especially between the veterans' non-service-connected pension program and the general social security programs. (Bradley et al., 1956)

The Status of Veterans at the Midpoint of the 20th Century

At the midpoint of the 20th century, the veteran population, largely made up of the aging World War I veterans and younger men and women who served in World War II, were doing substantially better than their nonveteran counterparts in terms of incomes, occupational status, job mobility, marital status, home ownership, and liquid assets" (Bradley Commission, 1956c, p. 118).[22] Using figures from 1952, the commission reported an education level—median years completed—for World War II veterans of 12.2 years, compared with 9.1 for nonveterans. The impact of the GI bill was clear. Twice as many veterans as nonveterans had been to and completed college, and the high school graduation rate itself was almost double.[23] The advantage that veterans had over their nonveteran counterparts was reflected in their incomes, which grew relative to nonveterans after World War II (see Figure 4.1). At first, veterans lagged behind, but within a year they were at parity and soon outpaced their nonveteran contemporaries.

Veterans Benefits Programs

The Bradley Commission highlighted the three forms of benefits veterans were receiving and the issues surrounding each:

- *Readjustment assistance*, designed to help those leaving service transition back to civilian life, was a revolutionary new program at the end of World War I that was greatly expanded by the GI Bill of 1944 for World War II veterans and subsequently extended to the veterans of the Korean War. These benefits included education and training assistance, unemployment allowances, loan guarantees, and reemployment preferences.
- *Service-connected benefits* were received by "veterans who are disabled as a result of military service or for the dependents of veterans who die as a result of service, . . . [including] medical and hospital care for injuries resulting from service, vocational rehabilitation for the disabled" (Bradley Commission, 1956a, p. 33).
- *Non–service-connected benefits* were provided, "not by virtue of any needs arising directly from military service, but on the ground that the Government owes

---

[22] The report noted that one explanation for the status of veterans was that, "[f]actually, veterans were by and large the physical and perhaps mental superiors of the contemporary male population. Through the exacting processes of military requirement and selection they were, so to speak, the 'Nation's best'" (Bradley Commission, 1956c, p. 118). See also Bradley Commission, 1956a, pp. 92–97.

[23] The "some college" (1 to 3 years) and graduation rates for veterans were 11.0 percent and 12.4 percent respectively, compared with 6.6 and 6.7 percent for nonveterans. The high school graduation rate for veterans was 32 percent, compared with 18 percent for nonveterans (Bradley Commission, 1956c, Table 5, p. 106).

Figure 4.1
Ratios of Median Annual Income of Male Veterans and Nonveterans of World War II, 25 to 44 Years Old, 1947–1954

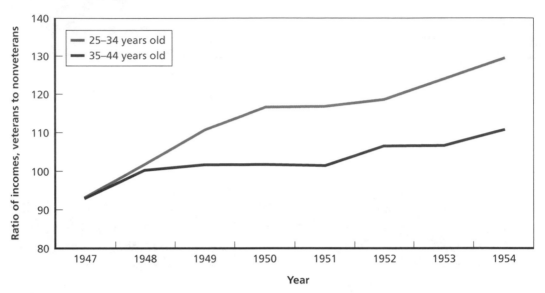

SOURCE: President's Commission on Veterans' Pensions, 1956c, p. 101.

an obligation to those who were in military service during wartime periods" (Bradley Commission, 1956a, p. 34). Besides cash awards in the form of pensions and bonuses, medical and hospital care has been included since 1924.[24]

As the Bradley Commission saw it, "[s]ervice-connected benefits should be accorded the highest priority among the special programs for veterans. Service-connected compensation and related benefits should be liberal, even generous" (Bradley Commission, 1956a, p. 138).[25] Readjustment benefits were temporary and were an "effective alternative to the backward-looking and less constructive 'old soldiers' pensions" (Bradley Commission, 1956a, p. 138).[26] They thought, however, that the non–service-connected benefits were problematic (Bradley Commission, 1956a, pp. 348–392; Bradley Commission, 1956f). According to the commission, their

justification is weak and their basic philosophy is backward looking rather than constructive. Our society has developed more equitable means of meeting most of the same needs and big strides are being made in closing remaining gaps. The non-

---

[24] Appendix A of Bradley Commission, 1956b, provides a short history of the veterans' pension through the Korean War.

[25] Bradley Commission, 1956a, pp. 146–196, provides an extensive discussion.

[26] See also Chs. VIII and IX in Bradley Commission, 1956a, pp. 231–319.

service-connected benefits should be limited to a minimum level and retained only as a reserve line of honorable protection for veterans whose means are shown to be inadequate and who fail to qualify for basic protection under the general Old-Age and Survivors Insurance system. (Bradley Commission, 1956a, p. 138)

Caring for Veterans with Service-Connected Disabilities

The Bradley Commission undertook a comprehensive review of the benefits received by those with service-connected disabilities (see Bradley Commission, 1956a, pp. 146–230; Bradley Commission, 1956e; and Bradley Commission, 1956d). As noted, such benefits dated back to colonial times and were at the heart of the nation's commitment to provide for those who served and their families. After 1949, this obligation was met through either the VA's disability compensation system or the disability retirement system of the armed forces.[27] The Bradley Commission reported in 1955 that 2.1 million veterans were receiving disability compensation, and another 800,000 were on the disability retirement rolls.

The VA administered two types of monetary awards for service-connected disabilities. The first, focusing on anatomical disablement, reflected a historical approach codified in the Civil War Era's General Law of 1862, which by 1955 provided specific payments for specific disabilities, including loss or loss of use of limbs or creative organs; blindness; deafness; and, at the time, tuberculosis. The second type of award, reflecting the concept of workers' comprehensive insurance from World War I, was to ensure that the disabled veteran and his family would have the essential means to achieve economic security (Bradley Commission, 1956a, p. 147).[28] The former benefit was rather clear cut, while the latter, focusing on some measure of impairment, introduced a high degree of judgment, which created a great many problems in practice. The Bradley Commission concluded that

> the present Veterans' Administration Schedule for Rating Disabilities is in many respects not in conformity with up-to-date standards. Some ratings are unrealistic in view of the current level of medical and other scientific knowledge. In many areas, the standards embodied in the schedule show evidence of looseness in application, which produces inequities in the granting of some awards. (Bradley Commission, 1956a, p. 158)

---

[27] In keeping with the Career Compensation Act of 1949 (Pub. L. 81-351, 1949) and EO 10122, 1950.

[28] The Bradley Commission explained that

Among other special veterans' benefits for service-connected disabilities are: continuing medical and hospital care, special life insurance, prosthetic appliances, special aids for the blind, a one-time award of $1,600 toward purchase of an automobile or other conveyance for loss, or loss of use, of one or both hands or feet or both eyes (incurred in World War II or the Korean conflict); and a single grant of up to $10,000 to cover not more than one-half the purchase price of a special house for veterans who have suffered the loss, or loss of use, of lower extremities. (Bradley Commission, 1956a, p. 147)

The Veterans' Pension Act of 1959

The Bradley Commission found that

> A practically universal social-security system protects veterans and nonveterans alike against the ordinary risk of life. Consequently, the veterans' pension program needs reorientation in its scope and direction. . . .

> The Commission recommends that the veterans' pension benefits be coordinated with those payable under OASI [Old-Age and Survivors Insurance], which now covers 9 out of 10 veterans and nonveterans. It is proposed that this be done by maintaining a separate veterans' pension program, but changing the present eligibility standards to take account of all income, including OASI but not public-assistance payments, as resources in determining need for a pension. Accordingly, veterans' pensions would supplement the income of the eligible beneficiaries from OASI and other sources up to a guaranteed minimum. (Bradley Commission, 1956a, p. 18)

Despite the recommendation of the Bradley Commission, Congress reaffirmed its commitment to the 22 million veterans and 2.5 million widows and surviving children of deceased veterans with non–service-connected disabilities via the Veterans Pension Act of 1959 (Pub. L. 86-211, 1959; see Karter, 1959, p. 18). As Congress saw it, the system should "provide a liberalized and new pension . . . based on the general principle of need and giving the greatest amount of pension to those in the greatest need" (Byrd, 1959, p. 1). Accordingly, the 1959 pension system provided that veterans with a service-connected disability would qualify for a pension based on the degree of the disability and the age of the veteran but with little consideration of other income maintenance programs. While the new pension would be tied to both disability rating and the income of the veteran and his spouse, the minimum disability rating needed to qualify for a pension would decrease with age, so that, at age 65, a disability rating of only 10 percent would be all that was needed to qualify for a pension (Byrd, 1959, p. 3).

For the first time, the VA could recognize more than the veterans' own income; the law provided that

> the wife's income in excess of $1,200 will be considered as the income of the veteran . . . ; the Administrator of Veterans Affairs [has] the authority to deny or discontinue a pension when the net worth of the veteran, widow, or child is sufficiently large that it is reasonable for a part of the assets to be used for maintenance. (Karter, 1959, p. 19)

Congress also required that the pension be means tested:

> A needs test must be met before pension can be paid. A reasonable rule should relate the amount of pension paid to the extent of the pensioner's need. Pension is not and never has been intended to support those who receive it on a standard above similarly situated persons who work and pay taxes. Pension is intended as an

honorable means of providing a measure of security . . . [for] those who are in need. (U.S. Senate Committee on Finance, 1959, p. 8)

The new law, however, was only loosely connected to other social security programs. It excluded from the calculation of net income a number of sources of income, particularly public assistance and welfare payments and pension payments from private retirement plans. Social Security—also known as OASI—was excluded up to an amount equal to the veteran's contributions; for example, "[a]fter the veteran has recouped his original dollar outlay in these plans, all future benefits will be counted" (Karter, 1959, p. 19). The VA Administrator summed up the new pension program this way:

Disability pensions are now available to these veterans if they are seriously disabled for causes not related to service. The basic pension rate is $66.15 monthly and is raised to $78.75 when the disabled veteran is 65 years of age or has been on the pension rolls for 10 consecutive years. Those who require aid and attendance are paid $135.45 per month. No pension, however, is paid to a single veteran whose annual income exceeds $1,400 or to a married veteran with an annual income in excess of $2,700.[29]

The ultimate outcome of the Bradley Commission and the Veterans Pension Act of 1959 was to leave little changed.

"Pay Any Price, Bear Any Burden" . . . The Advent of Vietnam

On January 20, 1961, President John Kennedy told the world that "that the torch has been passed to a new generation of Americans." He pledged that, in the new postcolonial states, such as South Vietnam, "one form of colonial control shall not have passed away merely to be replaced by a far more iron tyranny" (Kennedy, 1961)—referring, of course, to a communist form of government. What may not have been perceived at the time was that this lofty statement soon would be translated into young Americans fighting in the jungles of Vietnam—a fight that was years in the making.

A Line in the Sand—Picking Up the Pieces Left by France in Indochina

By 1893, Indochina was a largely pacified French colony. In September 1940, Japan invaded Indochina, and the Vichy French colonial authorities, backed by the force of the Japanese Army, ran Indochina for the next five years. With the support of the United States, an indigenous independence movement, the Viet Minh, led by Ho Chi Minh, opposed both the French and Japanese occupiers. By late 1945, the surrender

---

[29] Letter from VA Administrator Sumner G. Whittier to Senator Harry Byrd, Chairman, U.S. Senate Committee on Finance, dated July 24, 1959 (Byrd, 1959, p. 17).

of the Japanese had left a power vacuum the Viet Minh exploited. On September 2, 1945, as the Japanese formally surrendered on the USS *Missouri* in Tokyo Bay, the Viet Minh declared the Democratic Republic of Vietnam in Hanoi. That declaration notwithstanding, under the terms of the Potsdam Agreement, all of Indochina—Vietnam, Laos, and Cambodia—was to be returned to France, and the *status quo ante* was to prevail, with a transitional force of solders from Nationalist China replacing the Japanese in North Vietnam and the British occupying South Vietnam until the French could take over. French rule in South Vietnam was restored in October 1945. During 1946, Chinese troops withdrew from the north, and there was open warfare between the Viet Minh and the French. The French nominally controlled the cities, and the Viet Minh retreated to the jungle.

Over the next eight years, the French, increasingly backed by the United States, fought the Viet Minh. Between 1950 and 1954, the United States spent "$3 billion on the French war and by 1954 was providing 80 percent of all war supplies used by the French" ("The Vietnam War: Seeds of Conflict, 1945–1960," 1999). The first American aid to the French, a mere $15 million, was authorized by President Truman just days after the North Koreans invaded South Korea; two months later, on September 27, 1950, the United States established the Military Assistance Advisory Group in Saigon. In the mind of American policymakers, Korea and Vietnam were both part of vast communist expansion that had to be contained. Later during the Eisenhower administration, this was given a name: the Domino Theory. The idea was that a Communist victory in Vietnam would result in surrounding countries falling one after another, like a falling row of dominoes, a rationale a succession of Presidents used to justify ever-deepening U.S. involvement in Vietnam.[30]

The end of French colonial rule in Vietnam effectively came at 5:30 p.m. on May 7, 1954, when 10,000 French soldiers surrendered to the Viet Minh at Dien Bien Phu, a besieged military base in northwest Vietnam. By the end of July 1954, the Geneva Accords on Indochina divided Vietnam along the 17th parallel, formally creating the two countries of North and South Vietnam but providing for a plebiscite to be held within two years to reunite the country. A massive relocation program followed, with populations moving from north to south and vice versa, as nearly 1 million members of the Roman Catholic minority moved south.

---

[30] At the presidential press conference on April 7, 1954, Robert Richards of Copley Press asked President Eisenhower: "Mr. President, would you mind commenting on the strategic importance of Indochina to the free world?" The President responded:

> you have the possibility that many human beings pass under a dictatorship that is inimical to the free world. . . . [Y]ou have broader considerations that might follow what you would call the "falling domino" principle. You have a row of dominoes set up, you knock over the first one, and what will happen to the last one is the certainty that it will go over very quickly. So, you could have a beginning of a disintegration that would have the most profound influences. . . . Asia after all, has already lost some 450 million of its peoples to the Communist dictatorship, and we simply can't afford greater losses. (Eisenhower, 1971)

With the French withdrawal from Vietnam, it now fell to the United States to bolster the noncommunist government in South Vietnam, particularly by training and arming its army. The first direct shipment of military aid arrived in January 1955. On October 26, 1955, the Republic of South Vietnam was proclaimed, with former Prime Mister Ngo Dinh Diem, as its president. In January 1957, the Soviet Union proposed permanent division of Vietnam into North and South, with the two nations admitted separately to the UN. The United States rejected the proposal, unwilling to recognize communist North Vietnam. Later that year, Viet Minh guerrillas began a widespread campaign of terror in South Vietnam, including bombings and assassinations. But North Vietnam did not make the critical decision to press the fight in South Vietnam until May 1959. The following year, the National Front for the Liberation of South Vietnam (Viet Cong) was established. At this point, the American military involvement in Vietnam and the rest of Indochina was still minimal—the Eisenhower administration had sent 700 American military advisors to South Vietnam—but that would soon change.

On January 19, 1961, the last full day of the Eisenhower administration, the President-elect, the outgoing President, and their senior staffs met to discuss the transition of foreign policy that was to take place the following day. There were four sets of notes from the meeting and as many interpretations of what was said and what was meant.[31] It is clear, however, that the immediate focus of concern at the meeting for the situation in Southeast Asia was not Vietnam but neighboring Laos. That Eisenhower saw Laos as the linchpin for all of Indochina was clear, but there was a substantial difference of opinion among the note takers as to his recommended course of action, particularly his views on committing American troops beyond the level already engaged. However, within months, President Kennedy moved to strengthen the U.S. military commitment to South Vietnam.

During his inaugural address, President Kennedy said: "Let us never negotiate out of fear. But let us never fear to negotiate. Let both sides explore what problems unite us instead of belaboring those problems which divide us" (Kennedy, 1961). Kennedy got the chance to test that proposition with Nikita Khrushchev in Vienna the following June. James Reston of the *New York Times* described what happened:

> Kennedy went there shortly after his spectacular blunders at the Bay of Pigs, and was savaged by Khrushchev.
>
> I had an hour alone with President Kennedy immediately after his last meeting with Khrushchev in Vienna at that time. Khrushchev had assumed, Kennedy said, that any American President who invaded Cuba without adequate preparation was inexperienced, and any President who then didn't use force to see the invasions through was weak. Kennedy admitted Khrushchev's logic on both points.

---

[31] Greenstein and Immerman, 1992, covers the controversy about what was said and what was meant.

> But now, Kennedy added, we have a problem. We have to demonstrate to the Russians that we have the will and the power to defend our national interests. Shortly thereafter, he increased the defense budget, sent another division to Europe and increased our small contingent of observers and advisors in Vietnam to over 16,000. (Reston, 1979)

Kennedy's War in Vietnam: 1961–1963

America's involvement in Vietnam grew steadily during President Kennedy's tenure in office but was unable to check the growing strength of the Viet Cong. During the years Kennedy was in office, the strength of the Viet Cong grew from approximately 5,000 to 100,000.[32] Starting in Laos and the Central Highlands, the CIA and a Special Forces (SF) military command organized the Civilian Irregular Defense Group to check the infiltration of men and equipment from the north and counter the growing strength of the Viet Cong.

Not only did the United States provide SF, it provided military advisors and highly mobile transportation in the form of helicopters manned and maintained by American troops.[33] By 1964,

> each of South Vietnam's divisions and corps was supported by Army helicopters. . . . In addition to transporting men and supplies, helicopters were used to reconnoiter, to evacuate wounded, and to provide command and control. The Vietnam conflict became the crucible in which Army airmobile and air-assault tactics evolved. (Stewart, 2005, p. 296)

In addition, military advisers were placed at the sector (provincial) level and were permanently assigned to infantry battalions and certain lower-echelon combat units, and with the expansion came demands for better support, including medical support.

Medical Support

By the end of the first year of the new Kennedy administration—1961—there were more than 4,000 American military personnel on the ground in South Vietnam. To provide medical care for the troops, a field hospital was deployed and operational at

---

[32] Stewart noted,

> The number of infiltrators alone during that period was estimated at 41,000. The growth of the insurgency reflected not only North Vietnam's skill in infiltrating men and weapons but also South Vietnam's inability to control its porous borders, Diem's failure to develop a credible pacification program to reduce Viet Cong influence in the countryside, and the South Vietnamese Army's difficulties in reducing long-standing Viet Cong bases and secret zones. (Stewart, 2005, p. 293)

[33] On December 11, 1961, 82 U.S. Army H-21 helicopters and 400 men arrived in South Vietnam. Twelve days later, these helicopters were committed to the first air-mobile combat action in Vietnam, lifting approximately 1,000 Vietnamese paratroopers into battle with the Viet Cong about ten miles west of the Saigon. See Tolson, 1989, p. 4.

Nha Trang, along the central coast by early April 1962.[34] This 100-bed hospital was the only U.S. Army hospital in Vietnam, and given its limited capacity, a 15- to 30-day evacuation policy was enforced.

The hospital was not only responsible for supporting the growing number of medical detachments scattered throughout the country, it also become the focal point of all medical matters in Vietnam. Its commander had an additional assignment—was dual hatted—as the medical advisor to the commander of U.S. Army Support Group, Vietnam, an arrangement that was judged by those involved to be totally unsatisfactory.[35] The situation would not change until June 1965, when the Department of the Army authorized a full-time surgeon–administrative officer to the U.S. Army Support Command, Vietnam (USASCV) medical section. As the American presence in Vietnam grew, the USASCV medical section was renamed the Office of the Surgeon, Headquarters, U.S. Army, Vietnam (USARV), with responsibility for the health services of the entire Army medical structure in Vietnam, including unit-, division-, and Army-level medical service (Neel, 1991, pp. 10–12).

Vietnam at the Time of President Kennedy's Assassination

Weeks before his assassination, President Kennedy sought to clarify his policy toward South Vietnam. He said, "[t]he security of South Viet-Nam is a major interest of the United States," and that while "the political situation in South Viet-Nam remains deeply serious," "the military program in South Viet-Nam has made progress and is sound in principle, though improvements are being energetically sought" (Office of the Press Secretary, 1963). He even thought that "by the end of this year, the U.S. program for training Vietnamese should have progressed to the point where 1,000 U.S. military personnel assigned to South Viet-Nam can be withdrawn" (Office of the Press Secretary, 1963). Just days after assuming the presidency, Lyndon Johnson expressed similar sentiments but seemed less sanguine about the progress being made. He ordered the cancellation of the planned reduction of American military personnel.[36]

---

[34] This was not the first medical unit sent to Vietnam. To meet the immediate medical needs during the buildup, three medical detachments were sent to Vietnam in January and February 1962, each as part of a transportation company (Neel, 1991, p. 4). The April 1962 deployment also included the 57th Medical Detachment (Helicopter Ambulance) with five UH-1, "Huey," aircraft (Dorland and Nanney, 1982, p. 24).

[35] At the end of 1962, the hospital commander reported that "one of the major problems he faced as hospital commander was that of insufficient personnel in his headquarters section, leading to the absence of a 'cohesive, balanced organization to accomplish the administrative and logistics burdens of attached units'" (Neel, 1991, p. 5).

[36] On November 26, 1963, the National Security Advisor, McGeorge Bundy, told his colleagues that the new president had new guidance: "Programs of military and economic assistance should be maintained at such levels that their magnitude and effectiveness in the eyes of the Vietnamese Government do not fall below the levels sustained by the United States in the [recent past]" (Bundy, 1963). The planned reduction of American military personnel was off the table, at least for the foreseeable future.

CHAPTER FIVE

The American War in Vietnam

As Lyndon Johnson assumed the Presidency in November 1963, the situation in South Vietnam was growing steadily worse. The new leader of South Vietnam told Johnson that he did not think his forces could withstand a full-scale attack by the Viet Cong without more American support. With his own election coming the following fall, Johnson did not want to face the electorate after sending American troops to fight in the jungles of Southeast Asia. So, he decided to increase pressure on North Vietnam by sending Asian mercenaries to carry out acts of sabotage. As part of the program, the USS *Maddox* was sent to the Gulf of Tonkin to examine North Vietnamese naval defenses. The North Vietnamese responded by sending three torpedo boats to "attack" the *Maddox*. In retaliation, Johnson ordered the bombing of four North Vietnamese torpedo-boat bases and an oil storage depot. Johnson's decision to bomb military targets in North Vietnam received overwhelming backing from Congress with the passage of the so-called Gulf of Tonkin Resolution. In the House, 416 supported the president with no dissenters. In the Senate, 88 supported Johnson and only two dissented. The resolution authorized Johnson "to take all necessary measures to repel any armed attack against the forces of the United States, . . . [and] to assist any member or protocol state of the Southeast Asia Collective Defense Treaty requesting assistance in defense of its freedom" (Pub. L. 88-408, 1964). The terms of the resolution were open ended.

What followed was a steady escalation of the conflict. Regular North Vietnamese Army units began moving south, with increased American air raids on the North. Facing a deteriorating military situation in the South, Johnson ordered U.S. Marines into South Vietnam to protect the large airfield at Da Nang in March 1965. Soon, their mission expanded to allow them to conduct offensive operations close to their bases. A few weeks later, to protect American bases in the vicinity of Saigon, Johnson approved sending the first Army combat unit, the 173rd Airborne Brigade, to South Vietnam, and American military strength in South Vietnam soon passed 50,000. On July 28, 1965, President Johnson announced an escalation of American military strength in South Vietnam, with a goal of 175,000 by the end of the year.

Initially, American forces were employed defensively, but U.S. ground units were soon seeking out and engaging main-force enemy units in an attempt to halt their infiltration into South Vietnam. While a full account of the military conflict in Vietnam is well beyond the scope of this book, suffice it to say that the American advantages of firepower and mobility never proved decisive and were matched by the Viet Cong's ability to infiltrate troops from North Vietnam. Although the Americans had some success, it could best be measured in terms of the inability of the North Vietnamese to achieve their goals. Likewise, the North Vietnamese and Viet Cong goal of defeating the Americans was thwarted. What resulted, prior to 1968, was a stalemate with neither side able to achieve a strategic advantage over the other.

The whole tenor of the war changed in the aftermath of the Viet Cong's Tet offensive, which started on January 30, 1968, and lasted for months in various parts of the country. Tet was a well-coordinated series of surprise attacks against military and civilian command-and-control centers throughout South Vietnam. While Tet was a military defeat for the Viet Cong, in that they lost a great many troops and were unable to permanently take control of any population centers, it changed the political landscape in the United States. Just months before, the American commander in Vietnam, GEN William Westmoreland, had assured the American public that the North Vietnamese were "unable to mount a major offensive . . . I am absolutely certain that whereas in 1965 the enemy was winning, today he is certainly losing . . . We have reached an important point when the end begins to come into view" (Dougan and Weiss, 1983, p. 66). Despite the devastating losses that the North Vietnamese and the Viet Cong suffered during Tet,[1] American strategy thereafter was one of negotiations, Vietnamization (Dougan and Weiss, 1983, pp. 152, 176), and withdrawal. It would take another seven years before Saigon would finally fall, but in retrospect, after Tet, it was just a matter of time. When it came, the offensive was not in the form of a popular uprising or a victorious Viet Cong defeating the South Vietnam Army but as an across-the-board invasion of the South by conventional forces from North Vietnam.

The American Soldier of the Vietnam War

Generally, countries mobilize to go to war by calling up reserve units, putting industry on a wartime footing, curtailing domestic production to make resources available for the war effort, rationing critical goods, increasing taxes, and imposing conscription. None of this happened when the United States started to send ground troops to Vietnam. In general, reserves were not called up;[2] industrial production was not commandeered; goods were not rationed; and taxes were not raised until 1968, when a 10-percent surcharge was imposed on individual and corporate income taxes. Most

---

[1]   Dougan and Weiss, 1983, vividly presents the details of the Tet Offensive and the other traumatic events of 1968. Willbanks, 2009, and "Tet Offensive: Turning Point in Vietnam War," 1988, discuss the impact of Tet.

[2]   DeVries, 2009, covers the contribution of select National Guard and Reserve units.

important, conscription did not have to be imposed because it was already in place. All that was needed was for the Army to ask the Director of Selective Service to increase the draft calls and for Congress to appropriate the money to pay, train, and equip the troops. The county did not mobilize for the war in Vietnam but simply grew into it.

The Vietnam War was the last war America fought with largely a conscripted (drafted or draft-motivated recruits and enlistees) Army.[3] As in the previous war, in Korea, the manpower resources of the country were largely untapped. Unlike World War I and World War II, the men drafted for military service did not serve for the duration of the conflict but for a specific time, and those sent to Vietnam generally spent less than a year in country. Of the 26.8 million men who came of draft age during the Vietnam era—between August 1965, when retaliatory strikes began and when the Tonkin Gulf Resolution was passed, and March 28, 1973, when the last American troops departed South Vietnam—only one in four (10.9 million) served in the military. Of these, fewer than one in five (1.6 million) saw combat in Vietnam, with another 550,000 serving in Vietnam but not in combat units. (See Baskir and Strauss, 1978.) Figure 5.1 shows the troop levels in Vietnam from 1959 to 1973, when the last American troops were withdrawn.

On average, Vietnam-era soldiers were 19 years old, which was substantially younger than the 26 years of the World War II soldiers (Camp, 2011, p. 13). While there are no definitive studies on the socioeconomic backgrounds of those who saw combat in Vietnam, it appears that not all shared the likelihood of such service equally. Initially, blacks were disproportionally represented among combat deaths, but after concerted efforts to bring this number down, battle deaths of blacks were proportional to their share of the population by the end of the war.[4] By one account, combat soldiers were twice as likely to have come from low-income than from more affluent families. In general, high school graduates, and even high school dropouts, were almost twice as likely to be in the military during the Vietnam era than college graduates and considerably more likely to be sent to Vietnam and serve in a combat unit (Baskir and Strauss,

---

[3] The impact of the draft was both direct and indirect. Of the approximately 26.8 million men of the Vietnam generation, 16 million never served; 2.2 million were drafted; and 8.7 million enlisted. A previous report employed a constructed draft pressure variable using the variation in actual draft calls to estimate that 28 percent of those who volunteered from 1967 through 1999 were motivated to join to avoid being drafted and thus gained more flexibility in their ultimate assignment (Rostker, 2007, p. 245). As noted in that report, however, this might well underestimate the true effect of the draft because of the unmeasured impact of the uncertainty of being drafted independent of the relative effect of the actual size of the draft call. A better measure of the effect of the draft came from the 1970 lottery. When draft-eligible young men had unambiguous information concerning the likelihood of being drafted, an estimated 77 percent of non–prior-service accessions were draft motivated.

[4] Baskir and Strauss note:

> At the end of World War II, blacks comprised 12 percent of all combat troops; by the start of the Vietnam war, their share had grown to 31 percent. In 1965, blacks accounted for 24 percent of all Army combat deaths. The Defense Department undertook a concerted campaign to reduce the minorities' share of the fighting. That share was reduced to 16 percent in 1966, and 13 percent in 1968. (Baskir and Strauss, 1978, p. 8)

Figure 5.1
Troop Levels in Vietnam

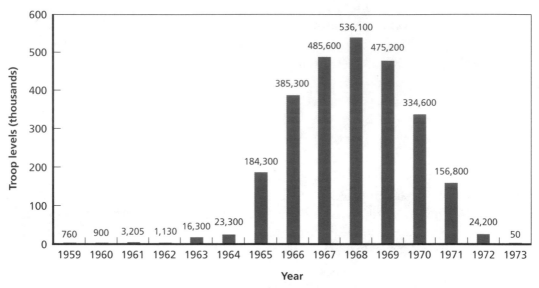

SOURCE: Data from "Allied Troop Levels—Vietnam, 1960 to 1973," 2008.

1978, p. 9). It should be noted, however, that young men were not entirely helpless to affect their chances of serving in a combat unit in Vietnam. Given that reserve units were not being sent to Vietnam, many young men signed up for service in the National Guard and Army, Navy, Air Force, and Marine reserve programs.[5] Many more volunteered for service in the military, including enlisting in the Army, to get their choice of jobs in the hope of avoiding being sent to Vietnam. Between July 1969 and June 1970, two-year draftees made up 68 percent of Army enlisted combat arms jobs, with three-year volunteers, who exercised an option to choose a job, making up only 4.1 percent. Two-year volunteers and those who did not elect to choose a job filled the remaining combat arms jobs.[6] The impact of such a disparity was impressive. In 1969, "Army draftees were being killed in Vietnam . . . at nearly double the rate of non-draftee enlisted men" (Glass, 1970, p. 1747).[7]

---

[5]   Given that National Guard and Army Reserve units were generally not called up during the Vietnam War, young men flocked to sign up for such units, and the units had long waiting lists. For example, in 1970, the Air National Guard and Air Force Reserve took in more than 20,000 new airmen from civilian life. The same year, the regular Air Force separated 105,000 trained airmen, of whom fewer than 300 joined Air Reserve Force units. See Rostker, 1973, p. 37.

[6]   See "How Army Fills Combat Jobs" in Glass, 1970, p. 1753.

[7]   Glass, 1970, p. 1747, reports the following statistics for 1969:

During 1969, Army draftees were being killed in action or wounded at the rate of 234 per 1,000. Draftee deaths were 31 per 1,000. By contrast, Army enlisted volunteers were killed or wounded at a rate of 137 per 1,000, and 17 per 1,000 died. Both draftees and volunteers served 12-month tours of duty in Vietnam.

The All-Volunteer Force

The draft—military conscription—not only provided the manpower to prosecute the Vietnam war, it was the catalyst that turned the American people against the war and ushered in a revolution in the way manpower would be procured for military service in the future, as an all-volunteer force.[8] While the new all-volunteer force was "to a large extent a political child of the draft card burning, campus riots, and violent protest demonstrations of the late 1960s and early 1970s" (U.S. Senate, Armed Services Subcommittee on Manpower and Personnel, 1978, p. 50), it came too late to have much of an impact on the way manpower was procured for most of the war.

The path to the volunteer force was rather direct.[9] It began in fall 1968, when the Republican candidate for President, Richard Nixon, announced his opposition to the draft (Nixon, 1968). It continued with the recommendation of the commission he set up that "the nation's interests will be better served by an all-volunteer force, supported by an effective stand-by draft, than by a mixed force of volunteers and conscripts" (Gates et al., 1970, p. iii). It culminated in his signing, on September 28, 1971, the law that extended the draft for only two years and committed the country to an all-volunteer force (Pub. L. 92-129, 1971; Lee and Parker, 1977, pp. 138–147). As the American war came to an end on January 27, 1973, the Secretary of Defense, Melvin Laird, announced that "with the signing of the peace agreement in Paris today, . . . the Armed Forces henceforth will depend exclusively on volunteer[s]. Use of the draft has ended" (Office of the Assistant Secretary of Defense for Public Affairs, 1973). For all practical purposes, however, the impact of the draft was substantially reduced after pay was raised to implement an all-volunteer force. Table 5.1 illustrates the trend in non–prior-service accessions and the role the draft played.

Casualties

Battle Casualties

Vietnam was a "dirty" war. It was dirty because of the types of wounds and the environment in which the battles took place. Fighting along waterways and rice patties, where human and animal excreta were common, meant that wounds were frequently contaminated. Only the rapidity of evacuation and the "ready availability of whole blood, well-established forward hospitals, advanced surgical techniques, and improved medical management" (Neel, 1991, p. 49), such as the widespread use of antibiotics,

---

[8]   In 1973, shortly after becoming a U.S. Senator, Sam Nunn (D-Georgia) told the Georgia General Assembly, "the concept [of the All Volunteer Force] is a clear result of the Vietnam war because it caused the President and Congress to yield to the tremendous pressure to end the draft at almost any price" (Nunn, 1973). See also Vandiver, 2014.

[9]   A detailed account can be found in Rostker, 2007.

Table 5.1
Non–Prior-Service Accessions, Total DoD and Army, with Draftees, by
Year, 1964–1973

Year	Draftees (000)	Non–Prior-Service Accessions		Draftees as a Percentage of DoD Accessions
		Total DoD (000)	Army (000)	
Period of draft-motivated volunteers				
1964	112	486	268	23.0
1965	231	414	205	55.8
1966	382	903	488	42.3
1967	228	770	489	29.6
1968	296	843	533	35.1
1969	284	821	455	34.6
1970	163	632	376	25.8
Transition to an all-volunteer force				
1971	94	544	314	17.3
1972	50	418	187	12.0
1973	<1	455	215	0.1

SOURCES: For draftees, Selective Service System, undated; for non–prior-service accessions, Office of the Assistant Secretary of Defense for Manpower, Reserve Affairs, and Logistics, 1978, p. 193.

held infections to a minimum.[10] By one estimate, "in Vietnam more than 30,000 lives were saved than would have been the case if the medical care had been only as good as the highly efficient care given the wounded in the Korean conflict" (Hardaway, 1999, p. 392).[11]

---

[10] Of wounded soldiers admitted to hospitals between March 1966 and July 1967, 70.2 percent received antibiotics. The most common antibiotic was penicillin, which was administered almost 92 percent of the time. Other antibiotics were frequently given, such as streptomycin, which was given to one-half the patients who received an antibiotic. (See Hardaway, 1988, p. 39.) Experimental delivery systems were also tested in Vietnam. One of these was an antibiotic packaged as an aerosol, which was distributed to various tactical units and produced good results (Neel, 1991, p. 57).

[11] Note that the casualties of the Vietnam War included those who were injured or became ill while serving and those whose injuries and illnesses had delayed onset and were not recognized for some time after the war ended. The latter, importantly, included PTSD and a list of medical conditions linked at some level to exposure to Agent Orange. The different types of casualties are discussed separately in this chapter, first the immediate casualties in their own section and then the delayed casualties as part of a larger section on veteran care.

Causative Agent

Vietnam was very different from the three other major conflicts fought in the 20th century. While there were important large-scale battles between American and regular North Vietnam Army units,[12] combat was best categorized as guerrilla warfare throughout most of the war and in most places.[13] In that regard, the only conflict remotely similar was the Philippine insurrection at the turn of the 20th century, some 65 years before. For American soldiers on the ground, however, "evidence suggests rather strongly that the insurgents controlled the timing and scope of battle."[14] Throughout the country, American soldiers were under constant psychological pressure as patrol routes were booby trapped with the punji traps or trip wires attached to grenades or mines—the infamous "Bouncing Betty." As a result, compared with previous wars, more casualties were caused by small arms fire, booby traps, and mines, and many fewer were caused by artillery and other explosive projectile fragments (see Table 5.2).[15]

The increase in the mortality rate from small arms in Vietnam is attributable to the tendency for the rounds from such weapons as the American M18 and North Vietnamese and Viet Cong AK-47 to shatter when entering a body, resulting in severe tissue damage.[16] Both sides made extensive use of mines, particular the claymore mine, which sprayed high-velocity fragments forward, resulting in deep wounds. The blast usually forced tremendous amounts of dirt and debris into the wound, resulting in massive contamination, as reflected by the much higher rate of infection. The Viet Cong's use of crude punji-stick booby traps seldom resulted in death but frequently resulted in infected wounds.

---

[12] One example is the battle for Khe Sanh (Dougan and Weiss, 1983, pp. 40–63).

[13] The nature of the war has been heavily debated. Some argue that it was a conventional war, finally won by the conventional forces of North Vietnam overwhelming the conventional forces of South Vietnam. Others see it as a revolutionary war fought with guerrilla tactics. For the soldiers on the ground, it could be either. (See Krepinevich, 1986, p. 269.)

[14] Vickers, 1993, p. 119, tells us that "88 percent of all engagements in early 1967 were initiated by the insurgents. The monthly average battalion sized attacks dropped from 9.7 per month during to last quarter of 1965 to 1.3 per month in the last quarter of 1966. During the same period, small-scale attacks increased by 150 percent."

[15] The data presented averages over the whole period. Neel, 1991, p. 53, notes that, by 1968,

> troops were usually engaging the enemy in his defensive positions. Wounding from small arms fire decreased from 42.7 percent in June 1966 to 16 percent in June 1970, while the percentage from fragments (including mines and booby-traps) rose from 49.6 percent in 1966 to 80 percent in 1970.

[16] Fackler, undated, p. 6, makes the point that

> The erroneous assumption that the amount of kinetic energy "deposited" by a projectile is a measure of the damage it produces continues to mislead. Wounds that result from the same amount of "kinetic energy deposit" can differ widely, depending on the predominant tissue disruption mechanism (crush or stretch), and the anatomic location of the disruption.

See also Cubano and Lenhart, 2013, pp. 1–16.

Table 5.2
Agents of U.S. Army Deaths and Wounds in World War II, Korea, and Vietnam, January 1965–June 1970

Agent	Deaths (%)			Wounds (%)		
	World War II	Korea	Vietnam	World War II	Korea	Vietnam
Small arms	32	33	51	20	27	16
Fragments	53	59	36	62	61	65
Booby traps and mines	3	4	11	4	4	15
Punji sticks	—	—	—	—	—	2
Other	12	4	2	14	8	2

SOURCE: Neel, 1991, p. 54.

While the data from Neel in the Army's official medical history of Vietnam show a comparison between wars, Hardaway's data from sample of the wounded during a 15-month period (March 1966 to July 1967) are more robust (Neel, 1991; Hardaway, 1988; Hardaway, 1978).[17] The lethality of small arms and mines and the high rate of infections for punji-stick wounds are consistent with Neel's data presented in Table 5.2. The hospital mortality rate of 1.8 percent is much better than comparable rates for World War II (3.3 percent) and the Korean War (2.4 percent) (Hardaway, 1988, p. 42).

As low as hospital mortality rate was, it may well overstate the true hospital mortality rate because so many critically wounded soldiers were brought to military hospitals within minutes of being wounded who, in previous wars, would have died on the battlefield. The priority air ambulance crews gave to the critically wounded and the rapidity of evacuation led to a mortality rate for those arriving within one hour of being wounded that was half that for those arriving 18 hours after being wounded.[18]

Location of Wounds

The wound location is critical in determining the chance of survival and the long-term prospects for recovery. In stark terms, a senior medical officer told a Senate committee that,

---

[17] Hardaway's sample was of 17,726 injured soldiers of the approximately 30,000 admitted to Army hospitals. An additional 27,000 had lesser wounds and were not admitted to a hospital but are counted in the official statistics of wounded (Hardaway, 1978, p. 635).

[18] Of those who died from wounds after being admitted to a military hospital, "34 percent died very soon after admission, 57 percent of deaths occurring by the end of the first day of hospitalization. Only 10 percent of deaths occurred after 14 days" (Hardaway, 1988, p. 58).

if the patient does not die, only the head injury cases, of the severe wounds, represent long-term cases. The chest and belly cases, although severe and life threatening, do not usually cause long-term rehabilitation problems. Lesser wounds of the extremities, although not life threatening in most cases, on the other hand, may require extensive and long-term rehabilitation and treatment. (Whelan, 1969)

Neel reported the distribution of wounds presented in Table 5.3. Hardaway presents similar data for March 1966 through July 1967 but, importantly, includes mortality rates (see Table 5.4). The mortality rate for wounds of the abdomen of 3.94 percent is most noteworthy because a similar rate was 21 percent for World War II and 12 percent for the Korean War.[19]

Overall Measures of Survival and Battle Casualties

During the Vietnam conflict, the number of American deaths reflected the phases of the Americanization and subsequent Vietnamization of the war (see Figure 5.2). The number of service members who died in Vietnam increased sharply as American troops entered the battle, peaking in 1968. After the Tet Offensive, the numbers dropped almost as sharply as they had risen.[20]

Table 5.3
Locations of Wounds in Hospitalized U.S. Army Casualties in
World War II, Korea, and Vietnam

Anatomical Location	World War II (%)	Korea (%)	Vietnam (%)
Head and neck	17	17	14
Thorax	7	7	7
Abdomen	8	7	5
Upper extremities	25	30	18
Lower extremities	40	37	36
Other	3	2	20

SOURCE: Neel, 1991, p. 54.

---

[19] The reductions in the mortality rates for wounds of the pancreas and ureter were most notable. The mortality rate for a wound of the pancreas was 58 percent during World War II, 22 percent during the Korean War, and just 5.7 percent during the period studied in Vietnam. For wounds of the ureter, the mortality rate was 41 percent for World War II, 50 percent for the Korean War, and 10.5 percent for the Vietnam sample (Hardaway, 1988, p. 42).

[20] Battle casualties associated with the Tet Offensive are hard to estimate because the initial assault was followed by three other offensives stretching into June 1968 (U.S. Department of State, 2015). By one account, "the bitter fighting took a heavy toll on allied forces; U.S. losses were 3,895 dead and the South Vietnamese suffered 4,954 killed in action" (Willbanks, 2009). Smith, 2000, places the total KIAs for all of 1968 at about 14,600; Smith's overall numbers generally track with the official numbers presented in National Archives, 2013.

Table 5.4
Analysis of Traumatic Wounds Among Patients Admitted to U.S. Army Hospitals in Vietnam, March 1966–July 1967

	Number Admitted	Admitted (%)	Died in Hospital (%)	Infection Rate (%)
All wounds	17,726	100.00	1.81	3.90
Result of hostile action	13,896	86.77	1.86	4.32
Nonbattle injury	2,119	13.23	1.39	2.45
Location of wound				
Head and neck	4,180	23.58	2.98	2.87
Thorax	3,490	19.69	7.06	3.84
Abdomen	2,454	13.84	3.94	6.89
Upper extremities	7,106	40.01	1.14	3.69
Lower extremities	8,838	49.86	1.09	5.04

SOURCE: Data from Hardaway, 1978, p. 636.

Figure 5.2
Vietnam Conflict Deaths

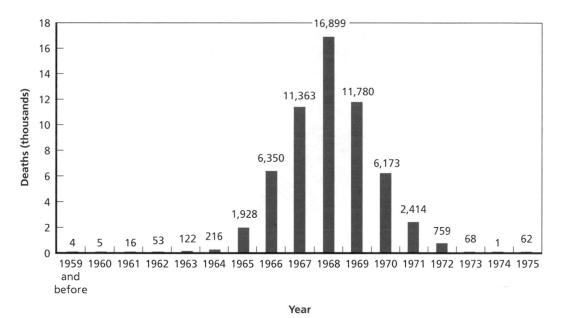

SOURCE: National Archives, 2013.

Officially, 58,220 American service men and women died as a result of the Vietnam conflict. The vast majority, almost 81.5 percent, were battle casualties. The rate of battle deaths was much lower than in either Korea or World War II. During the critical period between June 1965 and June 1969, the battle death rate for Vietnam was

21.9 per thousand average troop strength, as compared with 43.2 for Korea and 51.9 for the European theater between D-Day and the end of the war (Whelan, 1969).[21] Measures that show the "more immediate realities of combat engagements germane to physicians" (Carey, 1987, p. 6) consider the numbers KIA, WIA, and DOW. Where *hit* includes all KIA, WIA, and DOW, 27 men died for each 100 seriously hit in World War II, 22 per 100 hit in Korea, and 23 U.S. soldiers died per 100 hit in Vietnam. If one considers the percentage of the wounded who died, the experience in Vietnam was actually worse than that in Korea. During the Vietnam War, 3.6 percent DOW, compared to 2.5 percent during Korea and 4.5 percent during World War II (Carey, 1987, p. 9, Table 3). The relative consistency of these numbers suggested to some at the time that a limit may have been reached and that many of the improvements in battlefield medicine since World War II chronicled here have had no significant influence on the overall survival rate of seriously wounded soldiers.[22] Nevertheless, improvement was reported in the post-9/11 conflicts, as discussed in Chapter Seven.

Nonbattle Casualties

As a sign of how the nature of war has changed, fatalities from accidents were ten times more common than deaths from illnesses, the historic scourge of armies. Given that more than 2.6 million men and women served in South Vietnam, it is remarkable that fewer than 1,000 died from illnesses (National Archives, 2013; "Vietnam War Statistics," 2015). By comparison, during World War I, just half a century before, more died of disease (55,868) than were KIA (36,693).[23]

While modern medicine had largely eliminated disease as a major cause of death among soldiers in combat in Vietnam, "disease accounted for approximately 70 percent of all hospital and quarters admissions" (U.S. Army Medical Service Historical Unit, 1966, p. 20). However, this was "over 25 percent lower than the corresponding rate for Korea and less than half the rate for European theater of operations in World War II from D-Day to V-E Day" (Whelan, 1969).

Given the tropical location of Vietnam, it was not surprising that malaria was a "hazard of major proportions" (U.S. Army Medical Service Historical Unit, 1966, p. 18). During the buildup in 1965, incident rates reached a high during November of 109.8 cases per 1,000 average strength per year, and "it was not uncommon for malaria patients to be absent from their usual duties for 6 to 8 weeks" (U.S. Army Medical

---

[21] Carey, 1987, p. 6, reports the rate for the period July 1965 to December 1970 as 18 per 1,000 average strength per year.

[22] Carey, 1987, p. 9, argues that "these parameters have remained so intransigent that any deviation in the future will demand great scrutiny to ascertain the true cause."

[23] See Rostker, 2013, pp. 127, 132.

Service Historical Unit, 1966, p. 18).[24] Given that drug-resistant malaria was "recognized as the greatest disease threat in overseas operations" (U.S. Army Medical Service Historical Unit, 1966, p. 42), research was focused on the development of new drugs that would be effective against drug-resistant strains of malaria. Diarrhea, the perennial scourge of military camps, was a constant problem but less of a concern.

The Changing Nature of War Casualties

As noted in Chapter Three, the amputee has, throughout history, been the most visible and lingering reminder of war and its casualties. Today, that distinction may well belong to those who suffer the psychological wounds of war. But when the war in Vietnam started, medical authorities did not recognize that term. Vietnam plays an important role in how these two casualties are perceived today.

Amputations

The Civil War produced the largest number of military amputees for the United States. The medical records of the Union Army show that 21,000 amputees survived the war (Rostker, 2013, pp. 92–96).[25] While the overall size of the Union Army during the Civil War and the number of soldiers that served in Vietnam were not very different, the numbers of amputations were distinctly different (see Table 5.5).

The reduction in absolute numbers notwithstanding, the high prevalence of amputations in Vietnam compared with previous wars in the 20th century, even as arterial surgery became more common, reflected extensive wounding from rifle and machine gun fire, mines, and booby traps.[26] These mechanisms have "inherently greater destructive potential than shell fragments and made the proportion of limb-threatening wounds greater" (Mayfield, 1994, p. 131).[27] While rapid evacuation by air

---

[24] The Army Surgeon General's Annual Report noted that the "vast majority of the infections occurred among tactical units' personnel while in areas removed from base camps and under circumstances which thwarted efforts to apply effective individual protective measures against mosquitoes" (U.S. Army Medical Service Historical Unit, 1966, p. 18).

[25] Congress provided Union amputees with artificial limbs, and by the end of the first three years of the program, in 1865, the Army had issued more than 6,000 artificial arms and legs. Amputees who fought for the Confederacy were not eligible, but the individual Southern states provided some assistance (Rostker, 2013, p. 105).

[26] Whelan reported to the Senate in 1969 that

> only 81 attempts to repair an artery were made . . . in Western Europe during World War II. About 300 such repairs were done during the Korean War. In Vietnam, several thousand artery repairs have been done. This has become standard procedure at every hospital and is performed by almost all surgeons. The result is salvage of limbs that would otherwise require amputation. (Whelan, 1969)

[27] Mayfield also notes that "mines and booby traps, weapons that exploded at very close range, caused the greatest trauma and accounted for approximately 55 percent of all amputations in one series. On the other hand, gunshot wounds caused only 8 percent of the amputations in the same series" (Mayfield, 1994, p. 131).

Table 5.5
Prevalence of Amputations

Conflict	Wounds of the Extremities	Amputations	Prevalence of Amputations[a]
Civil War	173,064	20,862	12.1
World War I	154,000	4,378	2.8
World War II	599,000	14,912	2.5
Korean War	47,272	1,477	3.1
Vietnam War	99,000	5,283	5.3

SOURCES: Beebe and DeBakey, 1952, p. 194; Reister, 1975, p. 400; Otis and Huntington, 1883, p. 877; Reister, 1973, pp. 48, 160; "Vietnam War Statistics," 2015.

[a] Amputations as a percentage of wounds of extremities.

ambulance saved many lives, the proportion of those surviving multiple amputations rose sharply. Mayfield put the number at 2 percent for World War I and 5 percent for World War II. While comprehensive figures are not available for Vietnam, Mayfield further noted that, in two studies, the prevalence of multiple extremity amputations rose to 19 percent and 18 percent, respectively (Mayfield, 1994, p. 131).

Amputees were usually evacuated from Vietnam to a hospital in Japan within a few days of their operations and then on to hospitals in CONUS, usually within two weeks. Given the quality of medevac services, these patients were generally in better shape than those who arrived more quickly, within days of wounding. A common problem along the evacuation chain, however, was that traction was not maintained on the skin of the open stump, so that patients arrived at a CONUS hospital with bones protruding.[28] Moreover, the delay in getting the amputee from Vietnam to CONUS meant that the healing process and rehabilitation were separated, a growing concern among those engaged in the rehabilitation process.[29]

---

[28] Mayfield, 1994, p. 133, discusses the problems with maintaining proper skin tension. The author also suggested that, if "future wars require evacuation of amputees, a uniform inter-service education program should be designed that includes established guidelines and specific directives concerning maintenance of continued skin traction to the stump by self-contained methods" (Mayfield, 1994, p. 151). See also Dougherty, 1993, p. 762.

[29] Brown explained:

The growing conviction that rehabilitation could not be separated from treatment increased concern about evacuation policies that moved the patient from facility to facility, undermining the continuity of care that was increasingly seen as vital to prompt, successful rehabilitation. Furthermore, a transient commitment to the patient, the normal consequence of a lack of continuity of care, quite naturally fostered a depersonalization of the patient-doctor contact, a situation that frustrated the physician intellectually and sometimes, because of his compassionate concern, emotionally. The patient, however, experienced more than mere frustration; he inevitably felt afraid and abandoned. With each move to a new hospital scene, he became more reluctant to commit himself fully to a new doctor-patient relationship. No sooner was he familiar with a team of physicians and

The care received in Army CONUS hospitals, moreover, was quite inconsistent, with some amputees being transferred to the VA even before their wounds had closed. Apparently, patients often gained "financial benefit by becoming medically retired as soon as their general condition was stabilized. Therefore, many of these amputees were not fitted with prostheses, but were discharged from Army Hospitals to Veterans Administration Hospitals" (Mayfield, 1994, p. 136). Such transfers were not strictly necessary because those medically retired could still be treated in Army hospitals. Moreover, even those who did not receive medical retirements might be transferred to the VA. At certain times of the war, when large numbers of casualties flooded the system, patients were quickly medically boarded out, and amputees were transferred from the Army to the VA.[30]

Amputees who remained in the care of the Army were generally treated as ordinary orthopedic patients. Several Army hospitals eventually approached the level of an amputee rehabilitation center, such as Army's Valley Forge General Hospital, which in 1968 accounted for about 10 percent of all amputees. Data from Valley Forge, including a detailed 1971 review of 410 cases and a ten-year follow up study (LaNoue, 1971), provide important insights. The follow-up study contained information on 205 cases. Blasts accounted for 86 percent of the cases; missiles and crushing accounted for 8.3 percent and 4.8 percent of the cases, respectively. Of the 48 percent of the cases followed for ten years, 96 percent had been fitted with prostheses, and 88 percent of those were wearing their artificial limbs ten years later (Dougherty, 1993, p. 762).

Another center for the care of amputees was at the Fitzsimons Army Hospital in Denver. The orthopedic program there grew rapidly with an influx of amputees after Tet, tripling the program within a year to more than 900 patients. Given its proximity to the Rocky Mountains, the hospital pioneered an innovative sports rehabilitation program that eventually trained 400 amputees to ski. The program was motivated by "reports of Austrian skiers who had returned to skiing after World War II in spite of amputations" (Brown, 1994, p. 198). Such approaches to rehabilitation, however, were still controversial. The orthopedic consultant for the Surgeon General's Office, who was also the chief of orthopedics at Walter Reed General Hospital, felt that the program was "inappropriate to the mission of an Army hospital" (Brown, 1994, p. 201).

---

nurses and a hospital environment than the whole scene and all the characters in it (save the principal one—the patient) were changed to another. (Brown, 1994, p. 191)

[30] In 1969, a Senate committee was told it was Army policy to retain wounded patients until it was "determined that they have received optimum hospital improvement." They further explained that "optimum improvement" meant that the patient had reached the point at which his "medical fitness for further active military service can be determined, and it is considered probable that further treatment after a reasonable period in a military hospital will not result in material change in the patient's condition, which would alter his ultimate type of disposition or amount of separation benefits." In the event of separation, the Army would take "immediate action to secure a bed . . . in a Veterans Administration hospital" (Whelan, 1969).

Quandary for the Rehabilitation of the Amputee: The Handoff from the Army to the Veterans Administration

In theory, the roles of the Army and the VA were clear once the amputee was returned to the United States. The Army was responsible for initial treatment of the seriously wounded, but the norm was to transfer those whose continuing service was unlikely, such as amputees, to a VA hospital. In practice, the length of time spent in an Army hospital fluctuated "according to administrative policy, whim, physical considerations, staffing patterns, and bed availability" (Brown, 1994, p. 193). For patients, however, the policy meant, in practice, that "both continuity and quality of care usually suffered. Some felt expendable, abandoned, or culled, probably with reason" (Brown, 1994, p. 193).

In its history of the Vietnam War, the Army acknowledges that

> An arbitrary period of time rather than the degree of recovery was the determining factor in the decision to discharge or transfer a patient. This approach, which reserved military hospital beds for more acute rather than protracted care, was, from the administrative viewpoint, both useful and practical. But it could adversely affect rehabilitation, and its effectiveness from an overall medical point of view was debatable. (Brown, 1994, p. 189)

> [To make matters worse,] the Veterans Administration hospital chosen for the casualty was often the one closest to his home, which was not necessarily the facility best equipped to care for him. Ironically, many wounded soldiers were sent to veterans' hospitals with no capability for managing their particular treatment or rehabilitative needs. (Brown, 1994, p. 193)

The handoff and issues of continuity of care were even more problematic because standards of rehabilitation medicine were changing. In the years prior to Vietnam, the approach to wartime amputee care was essentially "heal the stump, fit it with a prosthesis, train the patient in its use, and discharge him to civilian life" (Brown, 1994, p. 197). Moreover, patient care was fragmented, with physical medicine focusing on kinesiology, gait patterns, and occupational therapy, which excluded ward surgeons and nurses from the rehabilitation process. By the time of Vietnam, there was a growing realization that "treatment and rehabilitation were indistinguishable parts of one another and should not be considered separately. In other words, rehabilitation should start immediately as a part of the therapeutic endeavor" (Brown, 1994, p. 190). The medevac process that moved patients from Vietnam to Japan and other military medical centers in the Far East, then on to CONUS weeks later, frustrated this emerging model of continuity of care. By one account, this made "patients more passive in their own rehabilitation. Moreover, shifting around often created an attitude of skepticism and cynicism about their government's concern for them, since multiple transfers were obviously for the benefit not of the patient but of the administrative process" (Brown, 1994, p. 191). Ironically, the increase in casualties in the wake of the Tet Offensive had a positive effect on the continuity of care for some because more wounded were being sent directly from Vietnam to a military hospital in CONUS.[31] While there were problems with early evacuation, as already noted, the ability to provide early treatment and continuity of care resulted in "the impression that their rehabilitation progressed both more smoothly and more rapidly than that of evacuees retained longer in Southeast Asia. . . . [But even then, the] patient was not assured of continuity of care" (Brown, 1994, pp. 192–193). It would not be until the wars in Iraq and Afghanistan that the quality of medevac would reach the point that patients could be evacuated without compromising their care and transported directly to specialized military medical centers, where treatment and rehabilitation could be truly united under a policy that retained amputees through the rehabilitation. In 1968, that was at best a dream, one not to be realized for a half century, as the case of former U.S. Senator Max Cleland attests.

A Tale of Two Senators: Senators Robert Dole, 1945, and Max Cleland, 1968

Bob Dole served in the U.S. Senate from 1969 to 1996. Max Cleland served in the U.S. Senate from 1997 to 2003. They shared more than their service in the Senate. Both were soldiers who had suffered major debilitating injuries in combat, and both wrote books describing the care they received after their injuries (Dole, 2005; Cleland, 2000). They were different, however, in that one was a World War II veteran, the other a Vietnam veteran. They were also different in the care they received, a difference that reflected how the Army generally cared for combat casualties from Vietnam. The consequences of the different treatment these two veterans received influenced the way care is given today.

On April 14, 1945, 2LT Bob Dole was severely wounded in Italy. He passed through the five-echelon medevac system, finally arriving at Winter Army General Hospital in Topeka, Kansas on June 12, 1945. The selection of this particular hospital was in keeping with the Army's policy of sending patients to hospitals near their hometowns. Dole received extensive physical rehabilitation at Winter and stayed there until November 10, 1945, when he was transferred to Percy Jones General Hospital in Battle Creek, Michigan. Given that Winter was near his home in Russell, Kansas; that the war was over; and that the Army was demobilizing, Dole might have expected to remain at Winter when the hospital was turned over to the VA on November 30, 1945. But the Army was not yet ready to release him.

Percy Jones General Hospital was one of the Army's largest major medical centers, including a general hospital, a convalescent hospital, and a number of annexes.

---

[31] Brown, 1994, pp. 191–192, notes that

> The sudden influx of large numbers of casualties forced the abandonment of the policy that had permitted casualties from Vietnam to spend weeks to months in hospitals in Vietnam, in the Philippines, or in Japan before their evacuation to the United States. Hospitals in Southeast Asia and Japan were quickly filled, making it necessary to send patients directly from Vietnam to the United States, where a much higher proportion of patients with open wounds, open stumps, and fresh, unhealed fractures were being received.

While its authorized capacity was 3,414 beds, it had a population of more than 16,500 by April 1945, including both patients and operating personnel (Smith, 1956, pp. 198, 276).[32] When Dole arrived, it was "the army's main center for paraplegics and amputees. . . . The hospital was also well known for its rehabilitative work in assisting disabled soldiers in reclaiming their lives" (Dole-Shalala Commission, 2007a, p. 193). Dole was assigned to Percy Jones for the next two years and eight months, until he was medically retired.

By spring 1947, both Dole and the doctors at Percy Jones concluded, as noted in his official record, that "[n]o further treatment is indicated for this patient" (Dole, 2005, p. 249). While he had physical therapy at Percy Jones and private care from a surgeon in Chicago,[33] he had not regained use of his arm. He had his last physical examination on May 14, 1948, and went before the Army Retirement Board on May 26, 1948. He was officially retired at the rank of captain on July 29, 1948 (Dole-Shalala Commission, 2007a, p. 254). While Dole later received services from the VA (e.g., the use of a Sound Scriber, a precursor of a portable tape recorder, which he used in law school), his medical retirement from the Army gave him options that soldiers who were simply medically discharged did not have.

On April 8, 1968, a little over two months after the Tet offensive had begun, CPT Max Cleland of the First Air Cavalry Division, taking part in an operation to break the siege of Khe Sanh, was wounded by an exploding grenade. He was immediately medevaced to the 38th Surgical Field Hospital at Quang Tri, some 24 minutes by air ambulance, where he was rushed into surgery. Treatment started well within the golden hour after wounding, but not even immediate care could alter the fact that he had lost his lower right arm and both legs. His wounds were so extensive that if they had occurred during any previous war, Cleland would have died on the battlefield. But this was Vietnam. A week after being wounded he was in surgery again at the 106th General Army Hospital near Yokohama, Japan; ten days later, he was on an Air Force C-141 for a 16-hour flight to Washington, D.C. A total of 18 days had passed from when he was first wounded to when he arrived at Walter Reed Army Hospital, in the late evening of April 26, 1968. This was, all in all, a more rapid evacuation than the one Bob Dole had taken 23 years before.

Unlike World War II, when the Army built out its hospital infrastructure to provide care, this time little was done to expand capacity. The conditions Cleland found at Walter Reed were far from ideal, especially with the influx of casualties after Tet:

---

[32] Dole-Shalala Commission, 2007a, pp. 192–193, reports that, by the time he arrived in November 1945, the hospital center housed more than 11,000 wounded soldiers; it peaked at 11,427.

[33] While a patient at Percy Jones, Dole sought care from a private surgeon who performed a number of operations trying to restore the use of his arm. While the Army did not pay for these private operations, the surgeon waived his fee, and his neighbors in Russell, Kansas, paid for the hospital costs. The Army did grant him "sick leave" to go to Chicago and then provided the rehabilitation services he needed at Percy Jones.

> The wounded arriving daily from Vietnam were straining the hospital facilities. Men on litter beds waited on each side of me. Less critically wounded men, along with other casualties from accidents and illness, filled the hallway in a long line. (Cleland, 2000, p. 60)

The initial examination confirmed his condition and set him on a course of treatment. He had a traumatic amputation of the right arm below the elbow and surgical amputation of the right and left legs above the knees. He was told, "your right leg is coming along fine, . . . but your left leg and right arm will probably need skin grafts. . . . After that [the skin grafts] we'll send you to physical therapy. We will see how your stumps heal before we decide what to do about fitting you with limbs" (Cleland, 2000, p. 61).

By mid-June 1968, wheelchair-bound Cleland had recovered enough strength to take a weekend pass away from the hospital. The skin graft on his arm was a success, and he was fitted with an artificial arm. Physical therapy soon expanded to occupational therapy as he learned practical skills. After four months at Walter Reed, Cleland's case was evaluated. He had hoped that he would be fitted for limbs but was told that he needed more physical therapy. In October, he was fitted with "stubbies." For the first time since he entered Walter Reed, he was excited about his progress. His excitement was quickly dashed when he was told that he was being discharged from Walter Reed and the Army and being sent to a VA hospital. He recalled:

> Back in those groggy days when I first entered Walter Reed, I had indeed said I was willing to go to a VA hospital if it meant my getting home sooner. My future was sealed. Even while I had been learning to walk on my stubbies, preparation was under way to send me to the Veterans Administration. . . . A triple-amputee was not regarded as a "normal" amputee. My rehab program was seen as "long term." Such cases were to be sent to the VA. (Cleland, 2000, pp. 102–103)

The VA was an unwelcome surprise. He wrote that "within two and a half hours of leaving Walter Reed, I had been stripped of rank, denied the amenities to which I had been allowed at another government hospital just up the street, and given no identification except a [claim] number" (Cleland, 2000, p. 114). A new fellow patient, sensing Cleland's frustration, told him, "the trouble with us . . . is that you and I are combat casualties. The VA doesn't know what to do with us" (Cleland, 2000, p. 116). It was older veterans from previous wars that populated the hospital.

Soon, Cleland was out of the VA hospital and in his own apartment, taking physical and occupational theory as an outpatient. He finally forced a showdown, insisting on being fitted for the full set of legs that, to date, the Army and the VA would not provide. However, because the prospects of him ever truly walking were not good, the VA would authorize only old-fashioned wooden limbs, not the new plastic limbs with hydraulics:

My hopes for a quick and simple fitting of artificial limbs were gone. The drama of being a battlefield casualty and the careful attention one received at Walter Reed was in the past. I felt like I was now a discarded warrior and an expense to my government. (Cleland, 2000, p. 126)

Against all odds, the following June (1969), 14 months after being wounded, Max Cleland "walked across the front lawn of his home in Georgia" (Cleland, 2000, p. 131). His journey was markedly different from that of Bob Dole. While both eventually received medical retirement, the Army kept Dole on active duty much longer than it did Cleland. In neither case was there any expectation that these wounded officers would return to their previous jobs. However, in Dole's case, the standard for discharge was "no further treatment is indicated for this patient." In Cleland's case, he was retired and sent to the VA, even though further treatment was clearly indicated.

Max Cleland's time with the VA was not over after he learned to walk. Later, a friend told him about the VA Prosthetics Center in New York, where he was fitted with the latest plastic legs with hydraulic knees that fitted him "perfectly" (Cleland, 2000, p. 136). In December 1969, he testified before the Senate Veterans Affairs Committee on the way the VA was handling returning Vietnam veterans. He later became a staff member of that committee, then a state senator in Georgia. In 1977, he became the VA administrator, appointed by the former governor of Georgia, President Jimmy Carter.

Psychiatric Casualties in Vietnam

Psychiatrists were engaged in Vietnam from the very beginning.[34] During the peak years of 1967 to 1970, 23 Army psychiatrists provided psychiatric care in Vietnam: One was assigned to each of the seven combat divisions,[35] and one was assigned to each of the evacuation surgical or field hospitals or to one of the two neuropsychiatry

---

[34] Norman Camp has provided the most comprehensive account of the Army's psychiatric program during Vietnam (Camp, 2011; Camp, 2015). He captured the Army's psychiatric community's ambivalence about Vietnam:

> Following the war, the Army Medical Department did not commit to developing a historical summary of psychiatry in Vietnam or study these problems for "lessons learned." Furthermore, the Army evidently lost, abandoned, or destroyed documentation at the conclusion of hostilities that could serve as primary source material. (Camp, 2011, p. 10)

The first psychiatrist to serve in Vietnam was MAJ Estes Copen, from October 1962 to February 1963, when there were only 8,000 military advisors in Vietnam (Jones and Johnson, 1975, p. 49).

[35] Division psychiatrists had two roles: serving as advisors to the division commander on the morale and seeing to the mental health of the troops and the treatment of psychiatric casualties with the "aid of ancillary personnel." This included a division social worker and two enlisted social work specialists assigned to each of the three medical companies of the medical battalion (Jones and Johnson, 1975, p. 50). In the field, much of the work was done by "psychiatric technicians, usually college educated young men who had been given a very intensive Army course in mental health. They proved to be very talented and ingenious fellows who were more easily able to identify with the enlisted men" (Colbach, 1985, p. 258).

specialty detachments (Camp, 2015, p. 74).[36] A senior psychologist, who acted as the neuropsychiatric consultant to the commanding general, served in Saigon. Over the course of the war, approximately 140 psychiatrists were deployed to Vietnam. One-third received their training at one of the two Army training programs, at Walter Reed Army General Hospital or Letterman Army General Hospital, San Francisco, California. The remainder were trained in civilian institutions and introduced to military psychiatry through an introductory course at the Army's Medical Field Service School at Fort Sam Houston, Texas. The Army training stressed the prevention and treatment of combat breakdown. Assignments within Vietnam were based on the expectation that combat stress would be their main concern and that the application of the traditional paradigm on "proximity, immediacy, and expectancy" would prevail.

The story of the psychiatric casualties of the Vietnam War is a tale of three wars: the one that ended with the start of the Tet Offensive in January 1968; the one of the initial post-Tet period, from late 1968 to 1970; and the one that covered the final withdrawal of American troops, ending in 1973.

Psychiatric Casualties from 1965–1968: Casualties Before Tet

Before the Tet Offensive, there were remarkably few incidents of psychiatric impairment; in fact, the number was much lower than that reported for World War II. During the first two years of the war, only 5 percent of all evacuations were for psychiatric or neurological reasons, compared with 23 percent for World War II and 6 percent for Korea. Officially, during this period, there were only three reported psychiatric cases per 1,000 men per year, lower than for any previous wars and only slightly higher than the early psychosis-only rate in the entire Army (Tiffany and Allerton, 1967, pp. 812–813). As late as 1970, psychiatrists were complimenting themselves on the fact that "the most significant psychiatric finding of the conflict has been that the number of casualties has remained surprisingly low. The incidence of psychiatric problems requiring hospitalization has remained about the same [as for] a comparable stateside force" (Bourne, 1970, p. 482).[37] Credit was given to a wide array of things: the rotation policy

---

[36] Jones and Johnson notes that the psychiatric teams consisted of

> three psychiatrists, one neurologist, one nurse, one psychologist, two social workers, and approximately one dozen enlisted nursing, social work, and psychology specialists. . . . Psychiatric patients who could not be expected to be returned to useful duty within two to four weeks were ordinarily evacuated out of country. (Jones and Johnson, 1975, p. 51)

See also Camp, 2015, pp. 109–117.

[37] The treatment for the small number of psychiatric casualties followed the Army's well-established principles of PIES to the extent possible, given the unique situation that was war in Vietnam. Given the terrain and the extensive use of evacuation helicopters, soldiers who might have previously been initially cared for on or near the battlefield were immediately evacuated to rear-area hospitals, rather than being helped at an aid station or clearing company. Once at a hospital, however, psychiatric casualties were separated from the general population to deemphasize "the hospital atmosphere and install the attitude of expecting to return to duty" (Tiffany and

of 12 months in theater;[38] the type of combat—"brief, intensive, and sporadic episodes, with periods of relative calm and safety interspersed" (Tiffany and Allerton, 1967, p. 813); hot meals being provided by helicopter to troops in the field; the availability of rest-and-recreation centers inside and outside the combat zone; and, finally, a wide variety of local distractions, some sanctioned and others not. Collectively, it was noted that "these policies have exerted a profound although unmeasured effect in reducing the incidence of psychiatric casualties" (Bourne, 1970, p. 483). Among all the self-congratulations, however, COL William J. Tiffany, Jr., the Chief of Psychiatry and Neurology Consultant in the Army Surgeon General's office, provided a prophetic warning: "[T]he absence of combat exhaustion may have to do with seasoned and motivated troops: if this is true, we might expect a change if 'greener' and less motivated troops replaced those who have completed their tours" (Tiffany and Allerton, 1967, p. 813). As it turned out, Colonel Tiffany did not have long to wait for the change he thought might come. Leaving aside the "greenness" of the troops before and after 1968—junior enlisted soldiers sent to Vietnam in 1965 and 1966 were, like their successors, mostly draftees—troops arriving in Vietnam in late 1969 and thereafter were decidedly less motivated.

Psychiatric Casualties from 1968–1970: Casualties After Tet

The American Army after the Tet Offensive was a far cry from the American Army that had taken the field in 1965. Troops that started to arrive in late 1968 reflected the tumultuous times that had developed in the winter, spring, and summer of 1968 across America—increased opposition to the war, social and racial upheaval, and an epidemic of illicit drugs—and not the idyllic Army of the 1950s and early 1960s.[39] The General Counsel of the postwar Presidential Clemency Board reported that "twelve thousand individuals either deserted during a Vietnam tour or deserted when they received orders to report to the war zone" (Baskir and Strauss, 1978, p. 114). By any measure, the behavior of the troops serving in Vietnam worsened, with absent without leave (AWOL) incidents, less-than-honorable discharges, drug abuse incidents, and disciplinary actions all increasing. And some things were new to the Army: not only widespread refusals to take orders but actual killing of superior noncommissioned officers (NCOs) and officers by their men, in what came to be known as *fragging*.

Allerton, 1967, p. 812). For example, in January 1966, 86 psychiatric patients were hospitalized, but only 29 of these were evacuated.

[38] It would later be argued that the 1-year rotation policy, rather than being a way to control combat stress, actually added to it. Camp, 2011, p. 16, argues that, "over time the resulting churning and ultimate depletion of experienced military personnel in theater . . . had a hugely negative effect on commitment and cohesion and consequently morale." Nevertheless, the alternative, unit rotation, had its own problems and would have required a massive mobilization of Reserve and National Guard units, which is exactly what was done 30 years later to support operations in Afghanistan and Iraq.

[39] Shephard, 2001, pp. 343–344, describes the "generational conflict" that was "coming to the boil." See also Baskir and Strauss, 1978, for an account of who actually did the fighting.

The mental health of the Army as a whole was deteriorating, and this can be seen in the statistics on the incidence rates of psychiatric conditions across the Army, but especially in Vietnam (see Figure 5.3). In the official Army medical history of the war, General Neel recounted the situation as follows:

> Until 1968, the neuropsychiatric disease rate in Vietnam remained roughly stable and parallel with that for the rest of the Army. In that year, however, Army-wide rates began to increase, and rates in Vietnam increased more precipitously than in any other location where substantial numbers of American troops were serving. . . . Rising rates showed increases in all areas of psychiatric illness: psychosis, psychoneurosis, character and behavior disorders, for example.
>
> The extent of the problem is evident from several statistical indices. Rates for admission to hospital and quarters for neuropsychiatric cases in Vietnam more than doubled between 1965 (11.7 per 1,000 per year) and 1970 (25.1 per 1,000 per year). . . . In terms of estimated man-days lost, neuropsychiatric conditions were the second leading disease problem in the theater in 1970; the 175,510 figure for that year is more than twice as high as the estimate for 1967 (70,000), reflecting a steady increase over the 1967–70 period. (Neel, 1991, p. 45)

Of particular concern was the use of illicit drugs. While no comprehensive statistics on the prevalence of drug abuse in Vietnam are available, surveys of soldiers indicate that illegal drug use was widespread; one 1969 study, from Cam Ranh Bay, reported that 53.2 percent of departing enlisted men had tried marijuana, one-half of

Figure 5.3
Incidence Rates of Psychiatric Conditions, Army-Wide, 1965–1970

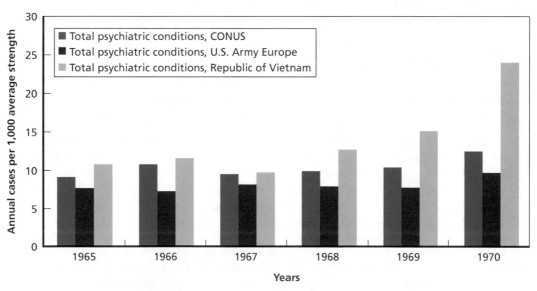

whom used had it for the first time in Vietnam. The reported use of opium among this sample nearly tripled during their time in Vietnam, rising from 6.3 percent to 17.4 percent (Neel, 1991, p. 47).

It should be noted that the data Neel presented covers only the period through the first nine months of 1970. American troops were engaged in combat in Vietnam several years longer, as forces were drawn down and finally withdrawn in 1973. While the numbers are significantly lower than before Tet, these were the years of the greatest psychiatric and behavioral problems. Given the tempo of operations, these were years that should have shown a reduction in psychiatric casualties, which unfortunately did not decline but increased. While the Army was ready to deal with traditional combat stress, which, as Camp pointed out, "did not materialize in the numbers expected" (Camp, 2011, p. 10), it was less equipped to deal with the "unprecedented flood of psychosocial casualties. . . . [that] consisted of disciplinary problems, racial disturbance, attacks on superiors, drug abuse, and the rising prevalence of soldiers diagnosed with character disorders." These problems were on the rise even as troop numbers were being reduced. While some prominent senior medical officers saw the emerging trends of the changing mental health picture, the Army did not adjust accordingly, as Camp's retrospective makes clear: "[D]espite this warning, there were no structural changes in the organization of mental health assets in Vietnam nor modifications in the selection, preparation, or deployment of mental health personnel sent as replacements to the theater" (Camp, 2011, p. 20).

Psychiatric Casualties from 1970–1973: Casualties During the Withdrawal from Vietnam

Camp referred to the drawdown years after 1970 as the years of "the severe breakdown in soldiers' morale and discipline" (Camp, 2011, p. 10) with "an unprecedented flood of psychosocial casualties . . . [and] the rising prevalence of soldiers diagnosed with character disorders" (Camp, 2011, p. 10). To be more specific, he highlighted the driving factors of the drawdown phase of the war from 1970 to 1973:

> Unrelenting public opposition to the war may have accelerated the American pullout, but the process severely demoralized those who were sent there during the drawdown years. Many soldiers interpreted antiwar sentiment as criticism of them personally—not the war more generally. In addition to accelerating rates for psychiatric conditions and behavior problems, two new and very alarming behavior problems emerged in 1970, primarily among lower-ranking enlisted troops: (1) widespread heroin use and (2) soldier assaults on military leaders with explosives ("fragging")—symptoms unmistakably indicating that the US Army in Vietnam was becoming seriously compromised. (Camp, 2015, p. 52)

Jones and Johnson, 1975, provides a statistical account of these years (see Figure 5.4). The authors attribute the jump in evacuations to the widespread illicit use

Figure 5.4
Rate of Evacuation of Psychiatric Patients from Vietnam and as a Percentage of Total Evacuations

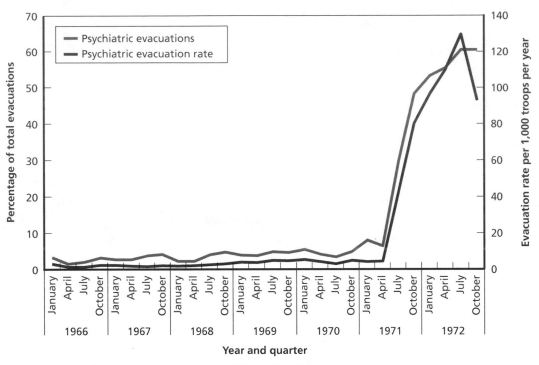

SOURCE: Adapted from Jones and Johnson, 1975, pp. 61–62.

of drugs and the initiation of a urine analysis drug screening program, with those who tested positive being evacuated as psychiatric casualties. The rise in the psychiatric casualties goes hand in hand with the rise in other measures of an increasingly dysfunctional Army, such as AWOL and desertion rates (see Figure 5.5).

The effects of the illicit use of drugs on the Army, and the other services, are also suggested by results from Datel's military psychiatric epidemiological study at Walter Reed Army Institute of Research. He found that the worldwide psychiatric incidence rate for active-duty Army personnel in mid-1973, after troops had been withdrawn from Vietnam, approached that seen at the height of the Korean conflict:

> The psychosis rate for worldwide active duty Army has never been higher than it was at the time of the last observation point, mid-1973. The same assertion can be made with respect to character and behavior disorder and with respect to character and behavior disorder combined with mental illness diagnoses relegated to "other." Similar incidence trends are apparent in the Navy and Air Force as well.

> Active duty Army neuropsychiatric outpatient visits consumed almost twice the proportion of active duty Army out-patient visits for all causes in 1972 that they

Figure 5.5
AWOL/Desertion Rates per 1,000 Troops Worldwide During the Vietnam Era

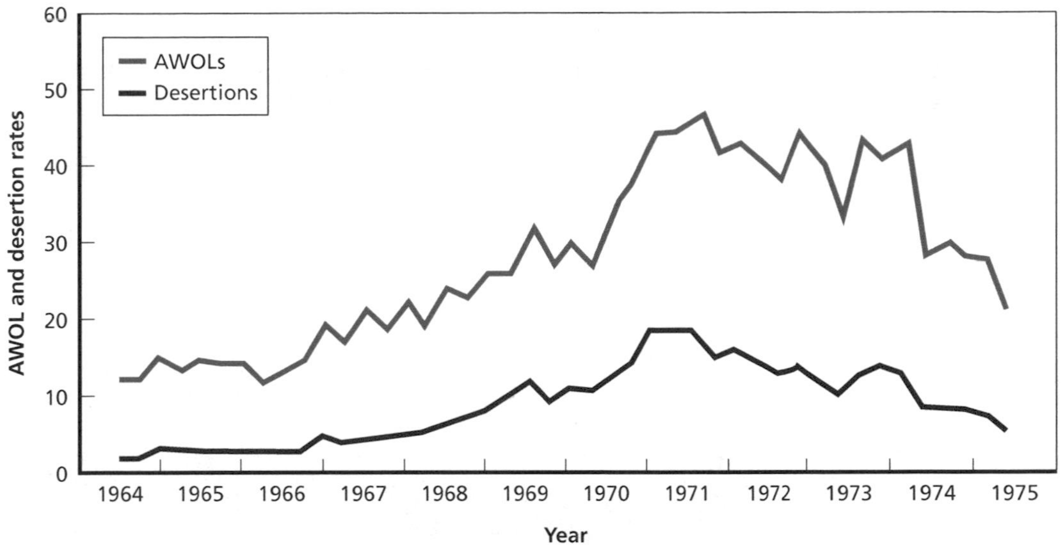

SOURCE: Camp, 2015, p. 26.

did in 1962. The proportion of Army hospital beds in continental United States occupied by neuropsychiatric patients compared with beds occupied by patients for all causes was greater in mid-1973 than it has ever been—including the "psychiatric disaster" period of World War II. For better or for worse neuropsychiatric patients remain in CONUS Army hospitals for longer periods than they did in World War II. (Datel, 1975, p. 15)

Datel did not make any direct observations on the actual use of illicit drugs. However, after considering and rejecting what he refers to as "time-worn hypotheses"—that these trends might be caused by a change in the personnel composition of the force or by wartime activity—he was left with one: that "the rising psychiatric incidence is drug-related" (Datel, 1975, p. 16).

A New Tool for Psychiatrists

Illicit drugs were not the only kind widely used in Vietnam. Before Vietnam, the treatment of combat-generated psychiatric casualties was generally limited to sedatives. During World War II, psychiatrists used sodium amobarbital and pentobarbital for nighttime relief. As part of a therapeutic program, sodium pentothal was used to facilitate the emotional release of repressed traumatic combat experiences in what was labeled "therapy under sedation" (Menninger, 1948, p. 311). During Vietnam, new tranquilizers were "commonly prescribed by psychiatrists and primary care physicians and had displaced the sedatives from the Korean War era in the treatment of a wide variety of conditions, including those affecting combat-exposed troops" (Camp, 2015,

p. 236). The effects of these new medications were never rigorously studied, but at least one psychiatrist working in Vietnam in the early days of the war—before Tet—thought "use of tranquilizing medications is one of the most important factors in keeping the psychiatric rates in Vietnam at a low level" (Camp, 2015, p. 237).[40]

The wide use of psychotropic medications is reflected in responses to a retrospective survey of Army psychiatrists who had served in Vietnam that the Walter Reed Army Institute of Research conducted in 1982:

> [P]sychiatrists who acknowledged some exposure to combat reaction cases indicate that they extensively used and highly valued these medications (neuroleptics and anxiolytics) in the treatment and management of soldiers suffering from a wide variety of combat-generated symptoms. (Camp, 2011, p. 31)

Figure 5.6 depicts the extent to which various drugs were prescribed for soldiers returning to duty following treatment for CSR.

Therapy was not, however, the only use for these drugs. There is a long history of using drugs to enhance performance on the battlefield.[41] Reportedly, performance-enhancing drugs proved useful in Vietnam but not without consequences:

> During the Vietnam conflict, methylphenidate (Ritalin) and sometimes dextro-amphetamine (Dexedrine) were standard issue drugs carried by long-range reconnaissance patrol . . . soldiers. The[se soldiers] found the most efficacious use to be upon completion of a mission when fatigue had developed and rapid return to the base camp was desirable. *Other than mild rebound depression and fatigue after the drug was discontinued, no adverse effects were reported.* (Jones, 1995b, p. 125, emphasis added)

Given the drug problem in Vietnam, Jones asked: "If the United States has declared war on drugs, how can it possibly justify prescribing similar drugs to American soldiers for use in combat?" (Jones, 1995b, p. 124; see also Howe and Jones, 1994, pp. 121–122). His answer was that, during war, "it is necessary to give American soldiers every safe, feasible, and competitive advantage" (Jones, 1995b, p. 124). But he then asked, "Will the parents and spouses of America tolerate soldiers being given drugs to induce them to risk their lives and possibly die?" (Jones, 1995b, p. 125). He suggested that administering such drugs constitutes a risk, and if there are adverse reactions, "the uniformed services owe it to them to provide long-term follow-up,

---

[40] See also Datel and Johnson, 1978.

[41] According to Schneider,

> The ancient Assyrians, Egyptians, and Greeks reportedly used opiates before and during battles to sustain or enhance bravery and courage. . . . The most extensive modern use of performance-enhancing drugs occurred during World War II by German, Japanese, and English soldiers. Amphetamines were noted to be useful not only to stave off fatigue and drowsiness but also to improve memory, concentration, physical strength, and endurance. (Schneider et al., 2011, p. 152)

Figure 5.6
Recollections of Patterns for Psychotropic Medications "Routinely Prescribed" for Soldiers Returned to Duty Following Treatment for Combat Stress Reactions

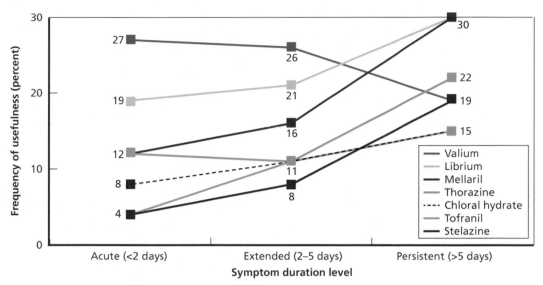

SOURCE: Camp, 2015, p. 250
NOTE: Represents percentage of combat psychiatrist participants endorsing use, by symptom duration. N = 47.

and treatment or compensation for any complications of the therapy that may arise" (Jones, 1995b, p. 125). While there is no way to definitively attribute addiction, drug abuse, or the psychiatric problems Vietnam veterans reported to the use of these drugs, Dr. Harry Holloway, the former director of neuropsychiatry at Walter Reed Army Institute of Research and former chairman of the Department of Psychiatry at Uniformed Services University of the Health Sciences (USUHS) suggested that "the use of chlorpromazine (Thorazine) and similar medications in Vietnam rendered some soldiers more susceptible to . . . chronic post-traumatic stress disorder" (as reported in Howe and Jones, 1994, p. 122).[42]

From Psychiatric Casualty to PTSD

Just as the war in Vietnam is no longer remembered for the low psychiatric casualties that characterized its early years and better remembered for psychological problems during the drawdown, e.g., the breakdown in discipline and drug abuse, so is it remembered for the postwar psychological difficulties so many of its veterans encountered. Vietnam brought into question the very singular explanation of the lingering effects of combat. Numerous books and journal articles have been written on the subject (e.g.,

---

[42] Moreover, Colbach recounted that "many soldiers went into the field with Thorazine or Mellaril in their pockets" (Colbach, 1985, p. 261).

Jones and Wessely, 2005), and a complete treatment of the subject is beyond the scope of this enterprise. However, Camp provides a cogent summation:

> Over the years since the war, disputes have arisen as to the relative weight to give various etiologic influences (e.g., predisposition and personality, traumatic extent of combat theater circumstances, and post-Vietnam experience [particularly social dynamics]). These disputes have complicated the diagnosis and treatment of PTSD and related adjustment difficulties. Many behavioral science observers have commented on the considerable potential for postwar adjustment difficulties to be powerfully affected by psychological and social dynamics that are not the direct consequence of combat zone "trauma." (Camp, 2011, p. 30)

An Unexpected Casualty of Vietnam: Military Psychiatry

How did the legitimacy of military psychiatry itself became a casualty of the Vietnam War? Until Vietnam, the unquestioned obligation of the military psychiatrist was to the Army and not to the patient.[43] The paradigm for care of the psychiatric combat casualty was operationalized in a mnemonic, PIES, which was thought to be an effective way to conserve manpower and return psychiatric casualties to the fight. Dr. William Menninger, the Chief Consultant in Neuropsychiatry to the Surgeon General of the Army during World War II and later president of the American Psychiatric Association said that

> [t]he daily responsibility of every psychiatrist who worked with troops in action was to aid the psychiatric casualty sufficiently to justify sending him back into the line. In other words, the medical officer treated the casual soldier only until he was able to return to combat, *even though after so doing he would probably again become worse.* (Menninger, 1948, p. 37; emphasis added)

In World War II, the whole psychiatric community mobilized for the fight. The Vietnam War fractured that same community. In March 1971, an overwhelming majority of the American Psychological Association's members indicated that they favored termination of the war. At its annual convention that year, the American Psychological Association withdrew recognition of the military psychiatry section. The following year, the association declared: "We find it morally repugnant for any government to extract such a heavy cost in human suffering for the sake of abstract conceptions of national pride or honor" ("Psychologists, MH Groups Attack Vietnam War," 1972, p. 1). The fracture not only reflected the antiwar conviction of the majority of

---

[43] Howe and Jones highlight the debate this way:

> In conjunction with the controversial Vietnam conflict, a frank and impassioned debate erupted within psychiatry concerning the proper role for psychiatrists in time of war, especially military psychiatrists. Underlying this debate was the critical moral or ethical question for whom does the military psychiatrist work—the individual patient or the military organization? (Howe and Jones, 1994, p. 116)

the members of both the American Psychiatric Association and the American Psychological Association, but the very ethical foundation on which military psychiatry had been built: Was the psychiatrist's first obligation to the Army or to the longer run mental health of his patient?[44] Is it ethical to employ "a treatment regimen designed to induce symptomatic soldiers to believe that facing further combat risks would be in their best interest or that of the nation" (Camp, 1993, p. 1000)? Similarly, is it ethical to administer drugs that could negatively affect the long-term health of soldiers to improve their performance on the battlefield? These questions are as fundamental as questions about the morality of war itself. They are ones that the psychiatric profession and the military still struggle to answer (Weisfeld, Weisfeld, and Liverman, 2009).[45]

Medical Support

Following well-established doctrinal lines, the originally planned medical support for combat troops in Vietnam was to be provided by the medical units assigned to the various divisions and separate brigades deployed to Vietnam backed up by a central medical establishment. The realities of Vietnam—in terms of the deployment of forces, the changing technology, and the fluidity of combat operations—resulted in what have been described as "far-reaching modifications" (Neel, 1991, p. 87) to the traditional linear, five-level medical support model from both world wars and even the MASH model of the Korean conflict.

Division and Brigade Medical Support

Each division sent to Vietnam included a medical battalion with four medical companies. Each separate brigade included one medical company. Each medical company had three platoons, each with three sections, which provided medical support to infantry and tank battalions or armored cavalry squadrons. When President Johnson announced a significant increase in deployments to Vietnam in July 1965, one of the first units to be deployed was the 1st Cavalry Division (Airmobile), a new kind of formation built around helicopters—the UH-1 (Huey) troop carrier helicopter, the AH-1

---

[44] An Army psychiatrist who shared his personal struggle with these central issues for military psychiatry brings these questions home. He wrote that, having

> acquiesced to my role as a military psychiatrist, I then had to accept that my obligation to my individual patient was far superseded by my obligation to the military and, eventually, to my country. This focus is the main ethic of military psychiatry. . . . I'm sure I would sound more positive if I were writing about World War Two or even Korea. Those of us who served in Vietnam went to the wrong war. (Colbach, 1985, p. 265)

[45] In 2015, 40 years after the fall of Saigon, Camp lamented that, as far as the Army was concerned, "there [still] was no acknowledgment of the critical—and evidently latent—ethical dilemmas associated with the combat psychiatry forward treatment doctrine" and that "leaders in military and civilian psychiatry [still need] to reconcile the dilemmas that became so torturous to practitioners . . . during the Vietnam War" (Camp, 2015, pp. 407–408).

attack helicopter, the CH-47 Chinook cargo helicopter, and the CH-54 Skycrane cargo helicopter—rather than ground vehicles. The new organization was well suited for the kind of war being waged in Vietnam. In the absence of a network of roads and with an enemy with no effective antiair capability, helicopters were ideal. Eventually, all Army units in Vietnam made extensive use of helicopters, following the paths the 1st Cavalry Division had pioneered. This included the extensive use of helicopters as air ambulances.

The medical battalion of the 1st Cavalry Division included an air ambulance platoon of 12 helicopters and an aircraft maintenance section. These helicopters transported the wounded from the battlefield to a division clearing station. In addition to the helicopter units that were part of the division, a separate group of air evacuation helicopter units, known as Dust Off helicopters, belonged to the echelons above division—to the corps or logistic command or to the Army medical brigade or medical command—and transported the wounded outside the division's area of operations. In practice, however, these helicopters could play many roles, depending on exigent conditions.

Given its own extensive air ambulance assets, the 1st Cavalry Division adhered to the traditional evacuation model. By one account, 95 percent of the division's casualties were first evacuated to one of its clearing stations and then, if warranted, went on to a surgical hospital (Neel, 1991, p. 88). There were times, of course, when wounded patients could not tolerate this two-stage process, and the most severely wounded were evacuated directly from the battle to a surgical, evacuation, or field hospital.

The divisions that did not have their own air ambulances units, such as the 25th Division, followed a different model and evacuated their wounded directly to surgical hospitals using helicopters assigned to and operating from the hospital. To augment the receiving hospital and because the new process freed up medical personnel in the echelons of care that were being bypassed, divisional medical companies were sometimes set up adjacent to the receiving hospitals. This provided additional beds for the less severely wounded and a facility to hold patients not ready to return to duty. In these cases, the traditional functions of a division clearing station and those of the hospital merged. The extent to which the divisions relied on the Dust Off helicopters, which they did not formally own, is shown in the following account:

> In 1968, the 25th Medical Battalion [of the 25th Division] operated facilities at three locations and treated 75,184 patients. Dust-off helicopters flew 8,159 missions and evacuated more than 20,000 patients. In 1969, the 25th Medical Battalion treated more than 58,000 patients. That same year, Dust-off aircraft flew approximately 7,000 missions and evacuated about 14,000 patients. (Neel, 1991, p. 89)

The experience of the 25th Division was duplicated throughout Vietnam. By midsummer 1967, it was apparent that the formal doctrine and organization of field medical services had to change. In practice, the critical role the chain of evacuation from battalion aid station to division clearing station had played in past wars gave way to the direct evacuation of the wounded to a surgical, evacuation, or field hospital well to the rear of the division's area of operations. As a result, and after extensive study, decisions were made to reduce the number of physicians in the division from 34 to 12 and to eliminate one-half of the divisional wheeled ambulances and their crews. In a radical departure from the past, "by the end of 1970, all were operating under the general concept that physicians should not be assigned to combat and combat support units" but could best be utilized in rear areas (Neel, 1991, p. 98). In effect, the paradigm of care had shifted from one that emphasized bringing the surgeons to the wounded to one of bringing the wounded to the surgeons and giving immediate care in a more pristine facility.

Nondivisional Medical Support

As noted, the first Army hospital deployed to Vietnam arrived in April 1962. Between then and April 1965, this single, 100-bed army hospital was the only hospital facility in country. As troop levels increased, however, so did the Army's capacity to provide hospital beds. By the end of 1965, there were two surgical hospitals, two evacuation hospitals, and several field hospitals, with a total of more than 1,600 beds. Over the next three years, five surgical hospitals, nine evacuation hospitals, and two field hospitals were deployed, and a convalescent center was established at Cam Ranh Bay. By December 1968, there were more than 5,000 Army hospital beds in Vietnam (Neel, 1991, pp. 60–61). Figure 5.7 shows the locations of these hospitals.

Modular, Self-Contained, and Transportable Medical Units

Vietnam was a different kind of war. The battlefront was fluid, but the helicopter allowed transport of critically wounded and ill patients to hospitals far from the combat zone. The MASH units of the Korean War, which had brought the skills of the surgeon up to the front line, were no longer needed. Helicopters now transported the wounded to physicians working in modern facilities, where teams of medical specialists could deliver outstanding care. The modular Medical Unit, Self-Contained, Transportable (MUST) replaced the 60-bed Korean-era MASH unit (see Figure 5.8).[46] But in reality, MUSTs were hardly mobile. They were semipermanent, air-conditioned, fully equipped hospi-

---

[46] Neel, 1991, p. 65, notes that

> MUST-equipped surgical hospitals were operated for several years in Vietnam with mixed success. These units consisted of three basic elements, each of which could be airlifted and dispatched by truck or helicopter. The expandable surgical element was a self-contained, rigid-panel shelter with accordion sides. The air-inflatable ward element was a double-walled fabric shelter providing a free-space area for ward facilities. The utility element or power package contained a multifuel gas turbine engine which supplied electric power for air-conditioning, refrigeration, air heating and circulation, water heating and pumping, air pressure for the inflatable elements, and compressed air or suction. In addition, other expandables were used for central materiel supply, laboratory, X-ray, pharmacy, dental, and kitchen facilities.

Figure 5.7
U.S. Army Hospitals in Vietnam, as of December 31, 1968

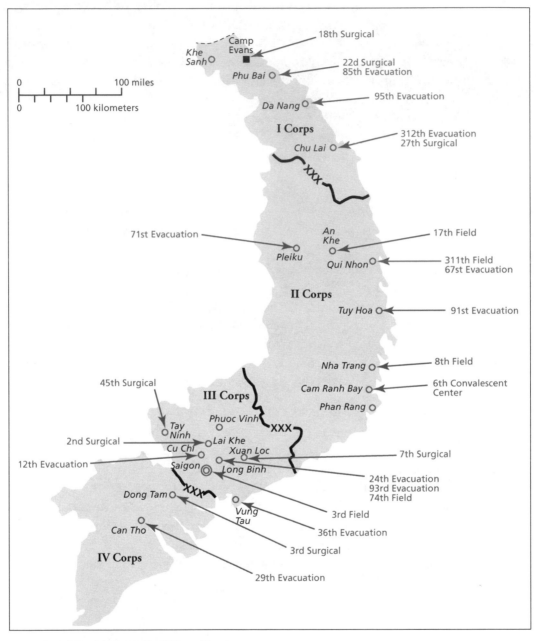

SOURCE: Adapted from Neel, 1991, p. 62.

tals. Expandable, mobile shelters with inflatable double-walled fabric walls replaced the tentage of previous wars. Turbine-powered utility packs provided electrical power and air-conditioning and maintained the internal pressure of the shelters. Sections could be

Figure 5.8
The Medical Unit, Self-Contained, Transportable

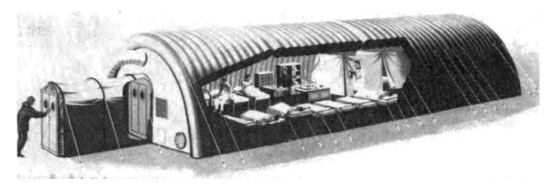

SOURCE: U.S. Army Medical Service Historical Unit, 1964, p. 115.
NOTE: The MUST, shown here configured as a ward, was 20 ft. wide and 52 ft. long. It could be erected by six men in about 30 minutes.

configured as wards or X-ray facilities, laboratories, pharmacies, dental clinics, or kitchens. Additional modules could easily be added.

6th Convalescent Center

Given the limited number of hospital beds available and the need to be able to surge during an emergency, the patient evacuation policy for Vietnam was established as a 15-day minimum or a 30-day optimum. Generally, the policy worked well, with nearly 40 percent of those injured through hostile action and 70 percent of other surgical patients returning to duty (Neel, 1991, p. 69).[47] However, in one area, the policy was not working: Large numbers of malaria and hepatitis patients were evacuated. There was a clear need for a convalescent facility in country, which was met with the establishment in 1966, of the 6th Convalescent Center at Cam Ranh Bay, adjacent to the South China Sea. During its first year of operation, some 7,500 patients were admitted, with an average patient load of about 1,000. Between 50 and 65 percent of all admissions were malaria patients, but hepatitis patients and some postoperative patients were also admitted. Overall, almost all were returned to duty within a month (Neel, 1991, p. 68).

Organization of Nondivisional Medical Support

Just as the chain of evacuation changed in Vietnam, so did the command and control of nondivisional medical assets, which evolved into the independent Medical Com-

---

[47] Medical evacuation policy identified who would be kept in theater with the goal of returning to duty and who would be evacuated from the theater. A 15-day policy meant that a soldier who was expected to recover and return to duty within 15 days was kept, and a soldier who was not expected to do this was sent home. When those sent home were actually evacuated out of theater depended on when they could fly and on evacuation assets. It could be less than or more than 15 days (e.g., those with injuries affecting an ear stayed longer, until they could handle the change in air pressure during flight).

mand (see Figures 5.9–5.13). In 1965, as troop levels increased, the medical structure matured into two medical groups reporting to the commander of the 1st Logistical Command. In December 1965, the Surgeon General and the commander of USARV, General Westmoreland, decided to deploy a medical brigade. In March 1966, the 44th Medical Brigade became operational as a subordinate unit of the 1st Logistical Command.

By 1967, and after a number of staff studies, it was decided that the 44th Medical Brigade should report directly to the USARV commander to facilitate

> medical planning and medical statistical reporting, and in implementing the rec-
> ommendations of professional consultants; and the greater ease in the management
> of medical personnel to be realized by assigning the brigade directly to USARV
> headquarters. (Neel, 1991, p. 23)

On August 10, 1967, the change was made, with the commander of the 44th Medical Brigade also assuming the position of USARV command surgeon. Finally, to eliminate duplication and overlap of staff functions, the command surgeon's office and the 44th Medical Brigade were eliminated, and the staffs merged into the U.S. Army Medical Command, Vietnam in 1970.

Looking back on his experience in Vietnam, MG Spurgeon Neel, the most experienced medical officer to have served in Vietnam and the author of the Army's official medical history of the war, summarized the lessons learned about how to organize medical support for a military campaign:

> The commander of the medical command, regardless of echelon, should function
> as the staff surgeon to the responsible supported commander. Medical capability

Figure 5.9
U.S. Army Medical Command
Staff Structure in Vietnam,
February 24, 1962–April 1, 1965

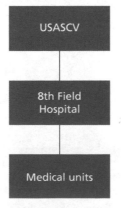

SOURCE: Neel, 1991, p. 6.

Figure 5.10
U.S. Army Medical Command Staff Structure in Vietnam, November 1, 1965–
February 17, 1966

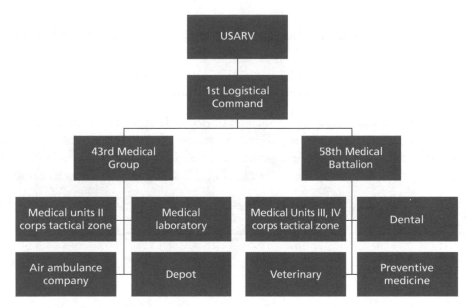

SOURCE: Neel, 1991, p. 14.

Figure 5.11
U.S. Army Medical Command Staff Structure in Vietnam, May 1, 1966–
August 10, 1967

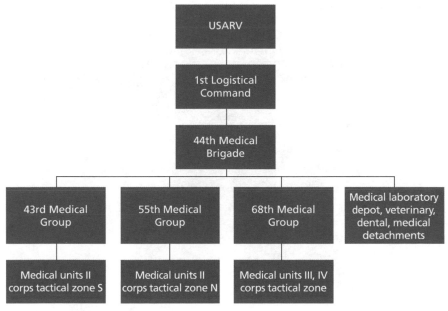

SOURCE: Neel, 1991, p. 20.

Figure 5.12
U.S. Army Medical Command Staff Structure in Vietnam, August 10, 1967–March 1, 1970

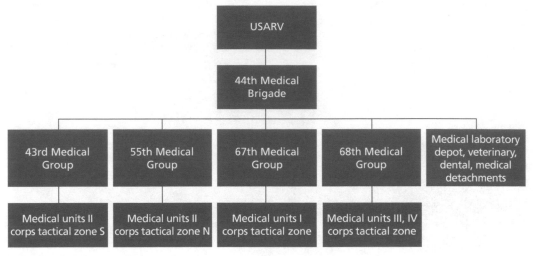

SOURCE: Neel, 1991, p. 24.

Figure 5.13
U.S. Army Medical Command Staff Structure in Vietnam, March 1, 1970

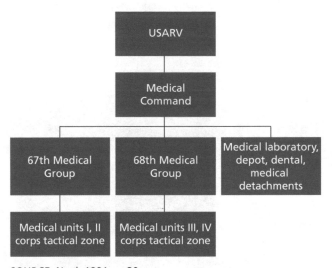

SOURCE: Neel, 1991, p. 29.

must not be fragmented among subordinate elements but rather centrally directed and controlled by the senior medical commander. No nonmedical commanders should be interposed between the medical commander and the line commander actually responsible for the health of the command. Specifically, logistical commanders, with their broad materiel-related functions, should not be made responsible for a task so critical and so uniquely professional as the provision of health services. The well-being and care of the individual soldier must not be submerged in, or subordinated to, the system responsible for the supply and maintenance of his equipment. The issues involved are too great to risk failure or marginal accomplishment. (Neel, 1991, p. 169)[48]

The Evolution of Medical Support in Vietnam

It is often said that battle plans work until the first shot is fired (Greer, 2005, p. 75). That was the case with medical support in Vietnam. Most critical to how medical support evolved in Vietnam was the use of helicopters for medevac, which complemented the changes in the skills of a new generation of surgeons. Helicopters made it possible to transport the wounded directly from the battlefield to modern, well-equipped hospitals, where specialists trained to provide the specific care needed were waiting. The convergence of these two developments was a long time in the making, and so was the realization that winning the war also entailed winning the "hearts and minds" of the Vietnamese people.[49]

Helicopters and Intratheater Medical Evacuation in Vietnam
The use of helicopters in Vietnam for medevac not only reduced the time from injury to treatment but also allowed more efficient organization of medical support. For centuries, the goal was to bring medical care as far forward as possible, close to the casualty; now the goal was to bring the casualty, as quickly as possible, to the right medical support in the rear. Interestingly, not the Americans but the French were the first to

---

[48] General Neel's observation stands in stark contrast to the arrangements that were common in militaries less than a century before. In Great Britain, the regimental hospital was abolished, and a modern organization of battlefield care was established only in 1873. The last of the great powers to establish an autonomous military medical service was the French in 1889. In the United States, the permanent Army Medical Department was established in 1818, but medical officers were not given the same military rank, pay, and privileges as other officers until 1857. During World War II, the Army Surgeon General retained decisions about only professional standards of care; operational control of medical units was left to the theater commanders and their chief medical officers. It was basically this organizational structure that operated in Vietnam.

[49] In his 1966 annual report, the Army Surgeon General elaborated on the latter point:

> The Vietnamese conflict has been described as two wars—the military effort against the enemy and the day-to-day struggle to win the minds and hearts of the people. In addition to medical support for the military effort, the Army Medical Service has been deeply engaged in this second effort. Medical personnel have served ably and with dedication in the Military Advisory Assistance, the Medical Civic Action, and the Military Provincial Hospital Assistance Programs. They have shared their medical knowledge and instructed their Vietnamese military and civilian counterparts in the most recent medical advances. In their spare time, Army Medical Service personnel have also worked voluntarily with the Vietnamese orphanages and sought out opportunities for expanding their help to such agencies. (U.S. Army Medical Service Historical Unit, 1966, p. iv)

use helicopters to transport casualties in Vietnam, evacuating some 5,000 by helicopter during the French Indo-China War.[50]

Medevac by helicopter started with the arrival of the first medical detachments in April 1962. The 57th Medical Detachment (Helicopter Ambulance) had five UH-1/Hueys and provided support throughout the country. As American operations expanded, so did the range and missions of the 57th, even as old problems resurfaced. Dedicated ambulances, whether wheeled or rotary winged, are relatively new on the battlefield. During the initial days of the Civil War, responsibility for ambulances lay with the Quartermaster Corps, and it was not unusual to see ambulances commandeered as baggage carts for Union officers. It was not until ambulances were given to the Medical Department that anything like a dedicated ambulance corps was sustained. It would finally take a general order issued by the commander of the Army of the Potomac that threatened placing officers who commandeered ambulances for other purposes under "arrest for trial for disobedience of orders" (McClellan, 1862). During the early days in Vietnam, the same scenario played out. The aircraft of the 57th were sometimes cannibalized to provide spare parts not only for their own aircraft but also those of other units, to the extent that, at one point, only one medevac helicopter was operational. A proposal to transfer the 57th from the Medical Service to the Army Transportation Corps, which controlled all other Army helicopters in Vietnam, was actively considered and narrowly rejected. Several times, commanders tried to commandeer standby evacuation aircraft, often for routine administrative tasks, and asked that the 57th aircraft use removable red crosses so that the aircraft could be used for general-purpose missions. Eventually, none of these proposals took hold; by the end of the first year, air evacuation had matured to the point that these missions had an official designation, *Dust Off* (see Figure 5.14).

During this initial period, most Dust Off missions flown by the 57th were in support of the Army of (South) Vietnam and its American advisors. As American involvement increased in fall 1964, so did the need for more helicopter ambulances, and the 82nd Medical Detachment became operational on November 7, 1964. It was assigned to the 44th Medical Brigade to fly Dust Off missions.

One of the first Army units to deploy as part of the Americanization of the war was the 1st Cavalry Division (Airmobile), which included an air ambulance platoon of 12 helicopters and an aircraft maintenance section as part of its medical battalion. Unlike the medical helicopters that were part of the 44th Medical Brigade, these helicopters used the call sign "MEDEVAC." Initially, medevac flights evacuated the wounded only to the division rear battalion aid stations and division clearing stations. The Dust Off helicopters, however, provided transportation to hospitals. Eventually,

---

[50] While this number was less than one-third of what the United States evacuated during the Korean War, it was dwarfed by the almost 900,000 sick and wounded casualties evacuated during the American war in Vietnam (Dorland and Nanney, 1982, p. 4).

Figure 5.14
Dust Off Medevac Helicopter in Operation in Vietnam

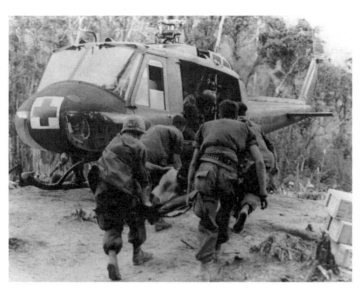

SOURCE: U.S. Army Photo.

the medevac helicopters also began to transport the critically wounded directly to hospitals.

Vietnam, if nothing else, was a laboratory to discover the best way to use helicopters for medevac. In September 1965, a medical company (air ambulance) was deployed to Vietnam. Assigned to the company were 24 UH-1D helicopters, 28 officers, and a large number of enlisted personnel. The unit was broken up and dispersed to three locations, each in a different operational area. While this arrangement provided the needed support for the tactical units on the ground, it proved to be a coordination headache for the company commander, with maintenance being carried out at three locations. Figure 5.15 shows the deployment of Dust Off units in Vietnam in 1969.

In a March 1967 report to the Commander in Chief, U.S. Army, Pacific, General Westmoreland attested to the overall success of the AE program. He stated that he had only one-half of the air ambulances he needed and that he had taken steps to alleviate the shortage, including giving the existing air ambulance companies "more nonmedical aircraft, giving basic medical training to those assault and transport crewmen who might find themselves evacuating the wounded, and even designating certain aircraft in the airmobile assault units to carry a medical corpsman during attacks" (Dorland and Nanney, 1982, p. 55).

Just as the organization for AE matured in the crucible of war, so did the equipment, tactics, and techniques of AE. The original air ambulances sent to Vietnam in 1965 were standard—the UH-1A and B, the basic Army utility aircraft. These were far better than the medevac helicopters used in Korea but left a lot to be desired. While

Figure 5.15
Dust Off Aeromedical Evacuation Units in South Vietnam, December 1969

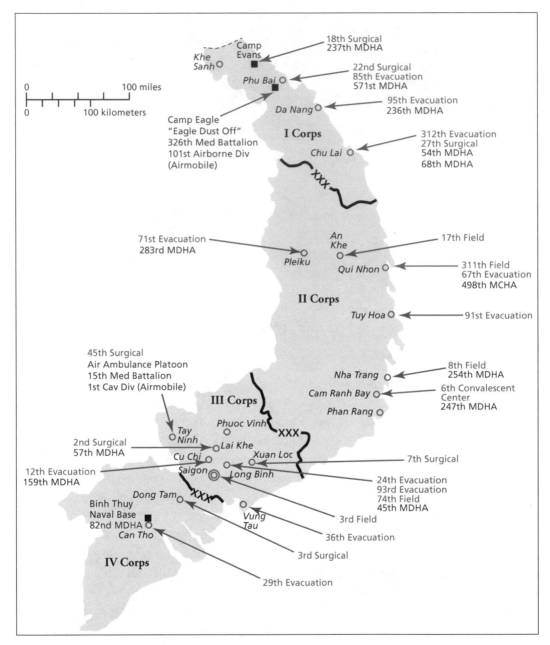

SOURCE: Adapted from Neel, 1991, p. 62.

they did allow patients to be carried inside the main cabin, with a corpsman providing in-flight care, they were so underpowered that their utility was limited. The aircraft were configured to carry three litter patients against the back wall of the cabin. However, given the standard four-man crew—pilot, aircraft commander-pilot, crew chief, and corpsman—the aircraft were often limited to one to two patients. The lack of power proved a particular problem in the heat and mountains of Vietnam.

The next version, the UH-1D, was not much better. The new UH-1Ds had a longer body and greater capacity—six litters or nine ambulatory patients—but even with longer rotor blades providing additional lift, the lack of engine power limited the aircraft's potential. This lack finally began to be overcome in July 1967 as the new L-13 engine was introduced for the UH-1H.[51] The Huey's propulsion problem had been solved (Dorland and Nanney, 1982, p. 69). The fact that the UH-1H was fully instrumented for night flight and poor weather was an added bonus.

The added power and instrumentation of the UH-1H came at the right time to meet the additional stress on aircraft and crew from the introduction of the hoist. Given Vietnam's terrain, it soon became clear that there was a need to lift the wounded into a helicopter hovering above ground obstacles that made a landing impossible. What was finally developed was a winch mounted on supports on the right-side door of the aircraft. This winch could be swung outside the cabin and used to lower something to the ground—a variety of litters, harnesses, baskets, and even a jungle penetrator that could cut through the dense jungle to extract ambulatory wounded (see Figure 5.16). Hoist missions, however, were particularly dangerous. An aircraft was ten times more likely to take an enemy hit during a hoist mission than during a standard mission. Nevertheless, more than 8,000 hoist missions were flown during the war.

As the war progressed, it settled into a deadly routine for the Dust Off and medevac crews. Most missions were classified as area-support missions. Aircraft were dispersed and responded to calls to evacuate the wounded as they came in. In some cases, particularly for the medevac helicopters that belonged to divisions, aircraft were assigned to support specific operations. Missions were prioritized according to the criticality of the wounded as determined by commanders on the ground, who also indicated the security of the pickup zone. Unfortunately, the information provided was not always accurate, and the realities on the ground did not always reflect what was communicated. This was particularly unfortunate, given the storied willingness of Dust Off and medevac pilots and crews to fly into harm's way to retrieve a critically wounded soldier. Air ambulances flew single-aircraft missions, usually without armed escorts; despite the prominent red cross painted on their sides, these aircraft suffered about 3.3 times as many losses as the rest of the Army's helicopter fleet.[52] Overall,

---

[51] A comparison of the lifting power of the D and H models makes the point. The new engine had 27 percent more horsepower than the previous engine but consumed 9 percent less fuel. Test results were even more impressive. In a fly-off of aircraft on a normal 95-degree day in the Western Highlands, each aircraft hovered 20 ft above the ground, and the maximum load for each aircraft was computed. Under these conditions, the maximum load for the UH-1D was 184 pounds. The corresponding maximum load for the UH-1H was 1,068 pounds.

[52] The losses were even 1.5 times greater than those of nonmedical helicopters on combat missions (Dorland and Nanney, 1982, p. 117).

Figure 5.16
Jungle Penetrator Being Deployed
on the Hoist

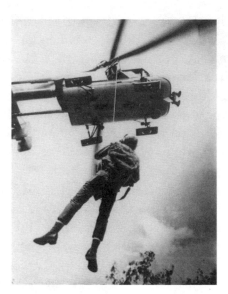

SOURCE: U.S. Air Force.

slightly more than one-third of the 1,400 air ambulance pilots themselves became casualties, being either killed or wounded.[53]

Over the course of the war, air ambulances amassed an admirable record. Between May 1962 and March 1973, when the last American ground units were withdrawn, these aircraft transported between 850,000 and 900,000 patients, about 45 percent of whom were American soldiers. Air ambulances gave first priority to patients in immediate danger, and it is estimated that "the percentage of wounded among air ambulance patients was . . . between 30 and 35 percent" (Dorland and Nanney, 1982, p. 116). Of the approximately 120,000 Army WIA who were admitted to medical facilities, something like 90 percent arrived by air ambulance. Shortening the time from wounding to definitive treatment in a rear medical facility was certainly a factor in reducing the number of soldiers dying from wounds to 19 percent. The corresponding statistic was 29.3 percent for World War II and 26.3 percent for the Korean War.[54]

---

[53] Dorland presents the figures as 40 killed by hostile fire or in crashes as a result of hostile fire; 180 wounded; and 48 killed and 200 injured from nonhostile crashes, many at night and in bad weather (Dorland and Nanney, 1982, p. 117).

[54] The hospital mortality rate during Vietnam was actually higher, at 2.6 percent of admissions, than during Korea, at 2.5 percent. This reflected the fact that so many more of the wounded who would have died in the field in previous wars now made it to hospitals before dying. The improved survival rate for those who were wounded paints a more accurate picture of how things improved in Korea (Dorland and Nanney, 1982, p. 116).

In-Country Medical Regulation

The aeromedical helicopters were ubiquitous in Vietnam. By 1969, there were 116 field-army-level air ambulances assigned to two companies and 11 separate detachments. But this was only half the story of improved medical support for the wounded. The other half was a dedicated medical radio network,[55] an effective real-time system regulating the flow of wounded to appropriate medical facilities, and the availability of surgical subspecialists with the skills to care for specific traumas.

As the number of hospitals and the number of casualties increased,[56] so also did the need for a system to control the flow of patients to proper medical facilities. During the buildup of American troops, the newly arrived 44th Medical Brigade became responsible for regulating all patients. Here is how it worked:

> Medical regulating started on the battlefield. Medical groups placed regulators (senior noncommissioned officers) in areas of troop concentration or at the site of a combat operation. In co-operation with the local medical unit, the regulator radioed requests for evacuation to the supporting Dust-off unit. . . .
>
> The patient was flown directly to the medical treatment facility best able to give the care required. This might or might not be the one nearest the site of injury. The decision as to the proper destination hospital was based on several factors. Distance was less important than time; the objective was to reduce the time between injury and definitive treatment to the minimum. Information based on the preliminary in-flight evaluation of the injury and the condition of the patient, knowledge of existing surgical backlogs, and the over-all casualty situation were other considerations. If the aircraft commander questioned the destination selected by the medical regulator because of his knowledge of the patient's condition, a physician was consulted by radio while the patient was still in transit before the decision became final. The inbound medical aircraft commander informed the receiving hospital by radio of his estimated time of arrival, the nature of the casualties on board, and any special reception arrangements that might be required. Thus, the receiving hospital was able to have everything in order to receive casualties and begin definitive surgical care. (Neel, 1991, p. 74)

The effectiveness of this AE system in Vietnam is seen in these statistics: During World War II, the average time from wounding to definitive treatment was 10.5 hours;

---

[55] Prior to the war, in 1957, the best thought was that "there is no real requirement for a separate communications net for the control of aeromedical evacuation" (Page and Neel, 1957, p. 1199).

[56] At the peak in 1968, there were 11 evacuation, five field, and seven surgical hospitals in Vietnam, as well as a convalescent center at Cam Ranh Bay. In total, 5,283 hospital beds were available (Camp, 2011, p. 14).

during the Korean War, it dropped to 6.3 hours; and in Vietnam, it was 2.8 hours, with many patients arriving within 20 minutes of their wounding (Arnold, 2015, p. 222).[57]

Intertheater Medical Evacuation

The movement of patients out of Vietnam was challenging. The nearest offshore U.S. hospital was almost 1,000 miles away, at Clark AFB in the Philippines; the nearest complete hospital was in Japan, 2,700 miles away. Casualties destined for CONUS had to fly more than 7,800 miles to reach Travis AFB, California, and almost 9,000 miles to reach Andrews AFB, near Washington, D.C. (Howard, 2003, p. 38).

Over the course of the war, a number of evacuation routes were used. Initially, evacuations were to Thailand or Clark AFB in the Philippines; from there, evacuees were routed either to CONUS or to Tripler General Hospital in Hawaii; the U.S. Army Hospital, Ryukyu Islands (Okinawa); or to a military hospital in Japan. (In summer 1966, hospital capacity in Japan was greatly expanded to care for patients who could be returned to duty within 60 days.) In June 1967, flights were initiated from Da Nang to the United States through the Philippines, Guam, and Hawaii. By December 1967, there was regular service between Tan Son Nhut, Cam Ranh Bay, and Da Nang Air Bases in Vietnam to Japan. While the Vietnam-to-Japan flight lasted only six hours, the next leg back to the United States took much longer; those bound for the eastern half of United States flew 18 hours via Elmendorf AFB, Alaska, to Andrews AFB, outside Washington, D.C. Those bound for the western part of the country had a 10-hour direct flight to Travis AFB, California. The long trip took its toll, and starting in August 1968, patients were held in Japan or sent to the Philippines or Okinawa for additional care and stabilization before being sent on to the United States.

While initially, in 1965, transportation was provided by propeller-driven aircraft, patients were soon being carried out by jet-powered C-141s and C-9s. The C-141 Starlifter was the workhorse of the fleet. Used to transport troops to Vietnam, C-141s were quickly reconfigured to carry 80 litter patients, 121 ambulatory patients, or a combination of 36 litter and 54 ambulatory patients (Neel, 1991, p. 77).[58] The standard medevac crew consisted of two flight nurses and three medical technicians (Mabry, Munson, and Richardson, 1993, p. 942). In 1968, the C-9A Nightingale, a modified version of the McDonnell Douglas DC-9, went into service, mainly within CONUS. It could

---

[57] These data are somewhat different from those presented in Chapter Three, which reported on the time lag for wounds involving "seriously damaged arteries." There is no doubt that the time lag was very much shorter in Vietnam.

[58] Clingman noted that C-141s could be reconfigured in as little as 25 minutes, but these "unscheduled flights posed the most problems. . . . The efficient use of the unscheduled missions required a lot of coordination between the aeromedical evacuation control centers, airlift operations or airlift control centers, transport squadrons, the individual aircraft crews, and the medical facilities involved" (Clingman, 1989, p. 101).

carry 40 ambulatory patients, 40 litter patients, or a combination of both (Vanderburg, 2003, p. 10).[59] The record of AE during the Vietnam War was impressive:

> During the 1968 Tet Offensive, 688 patients were processed within the Pacific Aeromedical Evacuation System on a single day. In May 1968, 12,138 casualties were evacuated from Vietnam on 154 AE missions. By 1969, the Military Airlift Command AE system evacuated an average of 11,000 casualties per month. An all-time single-day high of 711 patients were moved out of Vietnam on March 7, 1969. In the closing months of 1969, patient movements began to decline to less than 7500 per month. (Vanderburg, 2003, pp. 10–11)

Wound Shock Trauma Care

Extensive helicopter use was not the only medical innovation in Vietnam. Mortality from traumatic wounds caused by shock is as old as warfare itself. Not until the American Civil War was shock thought to be a separate problem from the physical wound, requiring attention apart from direct treatment of the wound. Even with this insight, progress was slow in coming. During World War I it was "recognized that shock and resuscitation were important and that intravenous fluids and blood were required and should be given in large amounts" (Hardaway, 2004, p. 267). However, as late as 1930, scholarly articles appeared that blamed shock on "damaged and dying tissues" (Hardaway, 2004, p. 266). During the early years of World War II, the Army refused to send blood overseas, citing the use of blood plasma, logistics, and shipping-space priorities. Eventually, the heightened mortality rates forced a change in policy, and whole blood was shipped to overseas theaters. During the Korean War, as the military situation stabilized, whole blood was generally available and extensively used. During Vietnam, there was a marked increase in the utilization of whole blood. The use of whole blood, occasionally even before the arrival of an air ambulance, contributed to the low mortality rate in Vietnam by better preparing the wounded for evacuation.

Building on the experience of Korea, the Division of Surgery of the Walter Reed Army Institute of Research constructed the first shock trauma center in 1963. In 1965, such a center was deployed to Vietnam and became the focal point for care, training, and continued research. In 1966, the National Research Council recognized the care wounded soldiers were receiving in Vietnam, noting that, "if seriously wounded, their chances of survival would be better in the zone of combat than on the average city street" of the United States. In particular, the

> [e]xcellence of initial first aid, efficiency of transportation, and energetic treatment of military casualties have proved to be major factors in the progressive decrease in death rates of battle casualties reaching medical facilities, from 8 percent in World

---

[59] The work of the medevac crews is highlighted in Clingman, 1989, pp. 105–106.

War I, to 4.5 percent in World War II, to 2.5 percent in Korea, and to less than 2 percent in Vietnam. (Committee on Trauma and Committee on Shock, 1966, p. 12)

Specialized Casualty Care

Superb specialized surgical care was also a hallmark of the Vietnam War. In marked contrast with the generation of physicians and surgeons who fought in World War II, the Medical Corps officers who served in Vietnam had extensive graduate training.[60] Given the explosion of medical knowledge during and after World War II, the response was threefold: The period of formal training was extended; the practice of medicine became more specialized;[61] and medical care was no longer organized around a single independent practitioner. In 1966, the Council on Medical Education of the American Medical Association noted a trend in civilian practice that was no less applicable to the way care was provided in Vietnam:

Institutionalized practice, in a hospital [or] a clinic . . . permits a higher quality of total service than the relatively independent practitioner can offer. A variety of skills, specialized knowledge in different areas, a more competent corps of para-medical aides, and expensive equipment that the solo practitioner can rarely afford *are all brought together for the benefit of the patient who takes his medical problems to physicians based in a hospital or a group practice clinic.* (Citizens Commission on Graduate Medical Education, 1966, p. 25; emphasis added)

The individual skills of the highly trained surgeons who served in Vietnam is illustrated by the frequency of vascular surgeries. During World War II, only 81 such surgeries were attempted. The number grew during the Korean War, to about 300. In Vietnam, such surgeries were relatively common, and not only thoracic but also gen-

---

[60] In 1966, the Millis Report noted:

The medical student's first four years are spent in medical school, an institution that has education as its primary goal. Successful completion results in receipt of the M.D. This degree used to mark the end of formal medical education, but now it comes about halfway along the road. Following its receipt, the typical young physician now spends a year as an intern, three, four, or even more years as a resident, and perhaps a year or two in sponsored practice before his colleagues, particularly of the specialty boards, consider his medical education to be complete. (Citizens Commission on Graduate Medical Education, 1966, p. 9)

[61] In 1931, 84 percent of all private-practice physicians reported themselves to be general practitioners. By 1960, that number had declined to 45 percent; just five years later, the reported number was 37 percent. In 1966, only 15 percent of recent medical school graduates reported that they were planning on entering general practice (Citizens Commission on Graduate Medical Education, 1966, p. 34; see also Ludmerer, 1999, pp. 180–190). Since Vietnam, and consistent with this shift, family medicine was recognized as a specialty in 1969, and the numbers of physician assistants and nurse practitioners have increased. In 2015, 13 percent of active physicians were in family practice, and 21 percent were primary-care physicians. Including physician assistants and nurse practitioners, just over 50 percent of clinicians in the United States are in primary care.

eral and orthopedic surgeons routinely performed repairs.[62] Ultimately, however, given the nature of the wounds and that multiple wounds were common, it was the ability to work in teams that saved lives. For example, a team including a "neurosurgeon, ophthalmologist, oral surgeon, otolaryngologist, and plastic surgeon" [might treat a head wound.] If the casualty had multiple injuries, more than one surgical team operated simultaneously" (Neel, 1991, p. 50).

Personnel by the Numbers

In 1953, at the end of the Korean War, the Army Medical Corps had 5,714 officers. By 1960, that number had dwindled to 3,676 physicians and surgeons but, after that, grew steadily. At the height of the Vietnam War, 7,154 medical officers were on active duty (Greenwood and Berry, 2005, p. 135). During the most critical period, however, many fewer Medical Corps officers were available (see Table 5.6).

During the buildup of forces in Vietnam, there were critical shortages of some surgical specialties, as the Army Surgeon General noted in his 1966 annual report.[63] Relief came with the institution of the so-called doctors' draft and realignment of the Berry Plan that saw more physicians coming to active duty after completing their specialty training.

The Berry Plan

The Berry Plan was the way male medical school graduates could be certain that they would not be drafted into the Army when they completed their basic medical education. The Berry Plan allowed graduating male medical students, who would normally be subject to being drafted, to continue their education with the understanding that, at

---

[62] Neel, 1991, p. 50, notes that the "high level of skill was maintained despite the turnover of medical officers. Since surgeons arriving in Vietnam were not adequately prepared by their background in civil trauma to treat combat casualties, they were attached to experienced teams for orientation and learned technique in the operating room."

[63] According to the Army Surgeon General's 1966 annual report, the

> requirements for surgical specialty support in Southeast Asia reached a peak during the first half of fiscal year 1966 and continued at a high level during the latter part of the year. Until the doctor draft began in April, the major source of surgical specialists for Southeast Asia was from class I hospitals. The chief shortages, as noted last year, occurred in the specialties of anesthesiology, general surgery, and orthopedic surgery. Lesser publicized, but equally important shortages of operating-room nurses, nurse anesthetists, and enlisted operating-room technicians also occurred. As a result, surgical service was curtailed to some degree at nearly all class I hospitals. Every effort was made to maintain the integrity of the class II teaching hospital system, but in a few instances, reassignment of class II staff members to Southeast Asia without replacement was required. Also, it became necessary to curtail tours of duty for certain surgical specialists in Europe, with later replacement of vacancies projected as civilian physician procurement was implemented and Southeast Asia tours of duty were completed. The shortage of anesthesiologists became most critical, and vacancies could only be filled by use of on-the-job trainees. Notwithstanding these shortages, many of which were temporary, surgical service in both class I and class II hospitals continued in a highly competent and professionally satisfying manner. With few exceptions, it is anticipated that increased physician procurement will alleviate surgical specialty shortages as fiscal year 1967 begins. (U.S. Army Medical Service Historical Unit, 1966, pp. 12–13)

Table 5.6
Strength of the Army Medical Department, by Corps

Corps	1964	1965	1966	1967	1968	1969	1970	1971	1972	1973
						End of FY				
Medical	4,759	4,662	5,549	6,303	6,251	7,154	7,000	6,025	5,667	5,055
Dental	2,493	2,149	2,617	2,656	2,748	2,810	2,761	2,520	2,524	2,245
Veterinary	556	562	608	637	635	636	610	537	503	501
Medical Service	4,236	4,305	4,864	5,639	5,890	6,033	5,606	5,466	5,060	5,325
Nurse	2,971	3,071	3,725	4,531	4,734	4,817	4,781	4,752	4,173	3,769
Medical Specialist	450	456	460	502	584	627	682	601	507	475
Total officers	15,465	15,205	17,820	20,268	20,842	22,077	21,440	19,923	18,434	17,370
Enlisted	43,659	44,301	44,644	54,853	52,812	48,472	47,865	49,259	N/A	N/A

SOURCES: U.S. Army Medical Service and Historical Unit, 1964, p. 70; U.S. Army Medical Service and Historical Unit, 1965, p. 66; U.S. Army Medical Service and Historical Unit, 1966, p. 84; U.S. Army Medical Service and Historical Unit, 1967, p. 67; U.S. Army Medical Service and Historical Unit, 1968, p. 71; U.S. Army Medical Service and Historical Unit, 1969, p. 67; U.S. Army Medical Service and Historical Unit, 1970, p. 71; U.S. Army Medical Service and Historical Unit, 1971, p. 70; U.S. Army Medical Service and Historical Unit, 1972, p. 74; U.S. Army Medical Service and Historical Unit, 1973, p. 29.

the end of their postgraduate training, they might be required to serve on active duty. (Those who were not called to active service were required to join the Ready Reserve for three years after completing training, from which they could only be activated in time of war or a national emergency declared by Congress or the President.) Here is how it worked: During 1964, the Army was allocated 785 medical school Berry Plan graduates, of whom 194 were to report for active duty after completing internships and the rest after residency training. As shown in Table 5.7, the size of the program grew during the war, even as the percentage of participating physicians deferring active service so they could take specialty training declined. Even with the reduction in the numbers continuing past their internships, the Berry Plan and the military's own residency training program could not fill the need. As a result, all the services turned to the Selective Service System to conscript trained health professionals. The Army Surgeon General explained that

> Special Calls were necessary because the number of qualified physicians who had volunteered for active duty was insufficient to meet the buildup requirements of the Armed Forces in connection with Southeast Asia. Some of the physicians called will serve as general duty medical officers and some will serve as specialists. Before the buildup, most of the need for specialists in the Armed Forces medical services was filled by volunteers who were deferred for specialty training in the Berry plan and by physicians completing their military residency training. However, the increased need for specialists has exceeded the numbers normally produced by the Berry plan and military residency training program. (U.S. Army Medical Service Historical Unit, 1966, p. 86)

As a result, the vast majority of the physicians who served in the Army during the Vietnam War were drafted.

Table 5.7
Berry Plan During Vietnam

	1964	1965	1966	1967	1968	1969	1970
Total medical school graduates participating in the Berry Plan	2,987	3,330	3,811	4,842	5,299	5,781	5,583
Allocated to the Army, accepted commissions	785	1,068	1,096	1,228	1,625	2,260	NC
Active duty after internship	194	211	328	451	695	1,583	NC
Deferred for residency training	591	857	768	777	930	677	NC
Deferred as a percentage of those accepting commissions	75.3	80.2	70.1	63.3	57.7	30.0	NC

SOURCE: Data from U.S. Army Medical Service Historical Unit, 1964–1970.

NOTE: NC = The program changed, and reported data were not comparable with those from previous years.

The Draft

On January 17, 1964, the Director of Selective Service System was ordered to draft 1,050 physicians, with 650 assigned to the Army (U.S. Army Medical Service Historical Unit, 1964, pp. 70–73). The following year, almost 600 additional physicians were drafted into the Army (U.S. Army Medical Service Historical Unit, 1965, p. 69). In 1966, there were three separate special draft calls; in total, 3,400 physicians were drafted into the Army. Additional draft calls in 1967 and 1968 provided more than 2,000 more physicians. In total, the Selective Service drafted almost 8,300 physicians for the Army; similar numbers were drafted for the other services.[64]

Nurses in Vietnam

Standing near the Vietnam Memorial on the Mall in the nation's capital is the Vietnam War Women's Memorial (Figure 5.17). It depicts three uniformed nurses and a wounded soldier. Most of the nurses who served in Vietnam were women, almost 80 percent, and almost all the women were nurses. They were largely volunteers,[65] young, and inexperienced.[66] They averaged less than 24 years old—not much older than the majority of the soldiers they cared for—and the majority, 65 percent, were new to the profession, with less than two years of experience (West, undated, p. 1). They were idealistic, as the words of one nurse suggest: "My reason for going was that there were American troops there that needed help, they needed the things that I could give them in my nursing profession" (as quoted in West, undated, p. 2).[67] They generally served for a single, one-year tour. In total, more than 5,000 Army nurses served.

The first contingent of ten Army nurses arrived in the Republic of Vietnam in spring 1962. They were assigned to the 8th Field Hospital, Nha Trang. The number steadily grew, especially after the deployment of troops in 1965. By the end of 1965, 215

---

[64] The numbers were extracted from the various reports of the Army Surgeon General for 1964 through 1972. The draft program ended with the advent of the all-volunteer force, which was announced in 1970 and went fully into effect in 1973. After 1970, however, the program was dramatically cut back. Nevertheless, physicians who had previously enrolled in the Berry Plan were still called to active service at the end of their training. The Berry Plan provided specialists to the Army well into the 1980s (Rostker, 2007, p. 287).

[65] Female nurses were almost always volunteers. However, some male nurses were drafted. In April 1966, there was a special draft call (number 38) to provide 700 male nurses for the Army. Eventually, this produced 27 warrant officers and 124 commissioned officers for the Army Nurse Corps (Feller and Moore, 1995, p. 39). Female nurses serving in the reserve medical units were ordered to active duty in April 1968. All the U.S. Army Reserve medical units returned to reserve status in January 1970 (Feller and Moore, 1995, p. 42).

[66] As Neel, 1991, p. 144, notes: "Assigning nurses was further complicated by the fact that 60 percent of the nurses assigned had less than 6 months' active duty and lacked experience in combat nursing. . . . This problem was solved by the institution of intensive training programs in each unit and continuous counseling and guidance by more experienced nurses."

[67] The exploits of Army nurses were dramatized for television from 1988 through 1991 in a show called *China Beach*, much as *M*A*S*H* had told the story of a medical unit in Korea. The show was based on a book called *Home Before Morning: The Story of an Army Nurse in Vietnam* (see Van Devanter, 1983).

Figure 5.17
Vietnam War Memorial: Women's Memorial

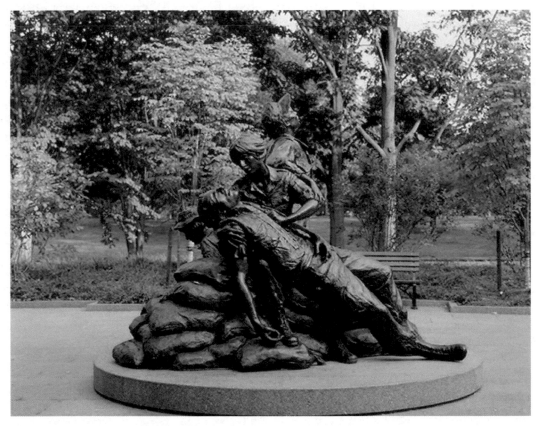

SOURCE: Photograph in the Carol M. Highsmith Archive, Library of Congress, Prints and Photographs Division.
CREDIT: Glenna Goodacre designed the monument, which was unveiled on Veterans Day, November 11, 1993. It depicts three women, one caring for a soldier.

Army nurses were serving in Vietnam (Feller and Moore, 1995, p. 39).[68] The number of assigned nurses peaked at 900 in January 1969. By July 1970, with the drawdown of forces, 650 were assigned (Neel, 1991, p. 142). The last Army nurse left Vietnam on March 29, 1970. During the war, roughly 6 percent of military nurses were wounded; nine Army nurses were killed, seven of whom were women (Steinman, 2000, p. 20). The only nurse to die as a result of hostile fire was 1st Lt. Sharon A. Lane.

---

[68] The Medical Command in Japan also cared for the sick and wounded from Southeast Asia. There was only one hospital in Japan in 1965, which had 100 available beds. By 1966 there were four hospitals, with a total bed capacity in excess of 3,200. There were 280 nurses assigned to the command during 1968 (Feller and Moore, 1995, p. 41).

Medical Support to the Vietnamese

When the first air ambulance detachments arrived in Vietnam in 1962, the U.S. Military Assistance Advisory Group gave them strict orders not to evacuate Vietnamese soldiers or civilians. This all changed the following year with the advent of the Army's Medical Civic Action Program (MEDCAP) and, in 1965, the development of Military Provincial Health Assistance Program, jointly sponsored by U.S. Agency for International Development and the U.S. Military Advisory Command, Vietnam (Neel, 1991, pp. 162–168).

There were actually two MEDCAP programs in Vietnam. The original program (MEDCAP I) provided U.S. military advisory teams and SF personnel to care for the sick and injured and train Vietnamese medical personnel. MEDCAP II teams were integrated into the Vietnamese hospital staffs and provided direct treatment to civilians. By the end of June 1968, a total of 22 teams were deployed: eight from the Army and seven each from the Navy and Air Force (U.S. Army Medical Service Historical Unit, 1968, pp. 38–39).

A very visible indication of the medical support that both the Vietnamese military and civilians received was the service U.S. air ambulances provided. Before 1965, 90 percent of all patients moved were Vietnamese. That number dropped to 21 percent during the Americanization of the war after 1965 and was about 62 percent during the Vietnamization program from 1968 to 1970 (Dorland and Nanney, 1982, p. 116).

Care for the Vietnam Veteran

The Veterans Administration of the Eve of the Vietnam War

On the eve of the Vietnam War, the VA reported that there were slightly fewer than 22 million "war veterans" (see Figure 5.18). In addition, the VA count of total veterans included 147,000 Regular Establishment exservicemen and -women who were receiving VA compensation for service-connected disabilities. Not counted as veterans, and not shown in Figure 5.18, were the estimated 3 million veterans who had served only during peacetime. The average age of the veterans was 45 years; Figure 5.19 gives the distribution of veterans by age.

As American combat units deployed to Vietnam, the VA health care system was the largest in the United States, with 168 hospitals, 214 outpatient clinics, 18 domiciliary centers, and two restoration centers. Where VA facilities were not available, the system also used non-VA hospitals, state homes, and private facilities. At any given time, VA hospitals had an average daily patient load of 110,000. Slightly over one-half were psychiatric patients; about one-third were medical patients; and the remainder were surgical patients. During the FY ending June 30, 1964, more than 609,000 veterans were admitted to VA hospitals—about 56,000 with psychiatric problems; 313,000 for medical conditions; and 240,000 for surgeries. Outpatient visits numbered 6.1 mil-

Figure 5.18
Veteran Population in Civilian Life, as of June 30, 1964

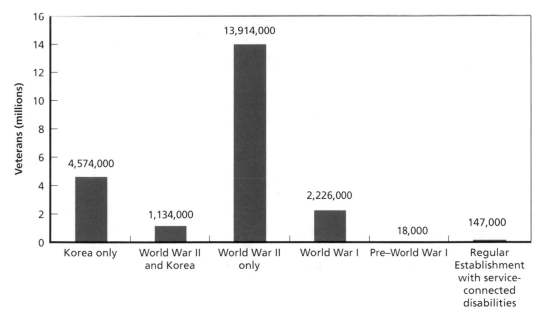

SOURCE: Data from Administrator of Veterans Affairs, 1965, p. 6.

Figure 5.19
Estimated Age of Veterans in Civilian Life, as of June 30, 1964

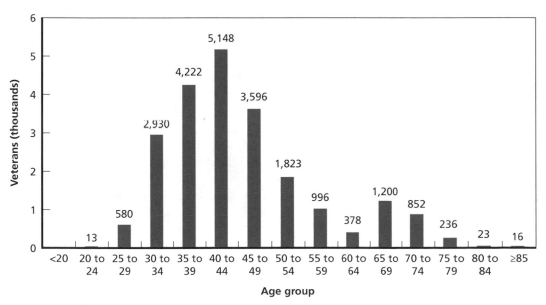

SOURCE: Data from Administrator of Veterans Affairs, 1965, p. 191.

lion. Almost 2 million veterans were receiving some compensation for service-connected disabilities, with 5.5 percent being totally disabled.[69] Most disability payments were for general medical and surgical conditions, but a significant number, about 19.1 percent, were for psychiatric and neurological diseases.[70] The VA had 172,171 full- and part-time employees; the majority, 89 percent, were in the Department of Medicine and Surgery. The VA's expenditures for FY 1964 totaled $7.052 billion (Administrator of Veterans Affairs, 1965, Table 97, p. 305).

The VA maintained a waiting list of those who were medically and legally eligible for VA inpatient care but not yet scheduled for hospital admission. In FY 1958, the list had topped out with 25,418 awaiting VA hospitalization.[71] At the end of June 1964, only 16,873 eligible veterans were on the waiting list, 10,048 requiring hospitalization for psychiatric conditions. None of the applicants on the waiting list required hospital care for a service-connected condition.

Psychiatric care was a significant part of the VA program. Care was provided in special psychiatric hospitals, in general hospitals, and at outpatient mental hygiene clinics. On average, at VA hospitals, 56,023 beds were occupied by psychiatric patients, with 50,546 being provided at one of the 42 psychiatric hospitals (Administrator of Veterans Affairs, 1965, Table 5, p. 195).

The Tsunami That Was Vietnam

By the end of 1965, almost 200,000 American troops were in Vietnam. On January 3, 1966, four months after the Marine Corps landed at Da Nang, the annual report to Congress covering the activities through June 30, 1965, did not mention Vietnam or anything that would indicate that the VA was anticipating the tidal wave that was about to engulf it (Administrator of Veterans Affairs, 1966a). Figure 5.20 shows the change in the veteran population in civilian life from 1965, the year American combat units were first deployed to Vietnam, to 1981, when most of those who had served in

---

[69] The above data are from various places in Administrator of Veterans Affairs, 1965; see also, specifically, Administrator of Veterans Affairs, 1965, Table 36.

[70] The number receiving compensation for a psychiatric or neurological disability differed by conflict. On June 30, 1964, 20.2 percent were receiving disability payments for World War II, 19.0 percent for World War I, 14.0 percent for the Regular Establishment, 14.5 percent for the Korean conflict, and 12.1 percent for the Spanish-American War (Administrator of Veterans Affairs, 1965, Tables 30–35).

[71] According to Administrator of Veterans Affairs, 1959, p. 18, the "waiting list on June 30 was as follows: 16,851 were diagnosed as neuropsychiatric cases (13,555 psychotic, 2,654 other psychiatric, and 642 neurological cases), 8,468 as general medical or surgical, and only 99 as tuberculous" cases. Forty-six percent of those on the waiting list were already hospitalized in non-VA facilities; of these, most, almost 80 percent, were psychiatric or neurological patients. The administrator noted:

> Over most of the past 11 years the neuropsychiatric portion of the waiting list has increased, although it has been fairly stable since 1955. The general medical and surgical component, which constitute the largest part of the total waiting list after World War II, is now smaller than the neuropsychiatric. (Administrator of Veterans Affairs, 1959, p. 18)

Figure 5.20
Veteran Population in Civilian Life, by Period of Service

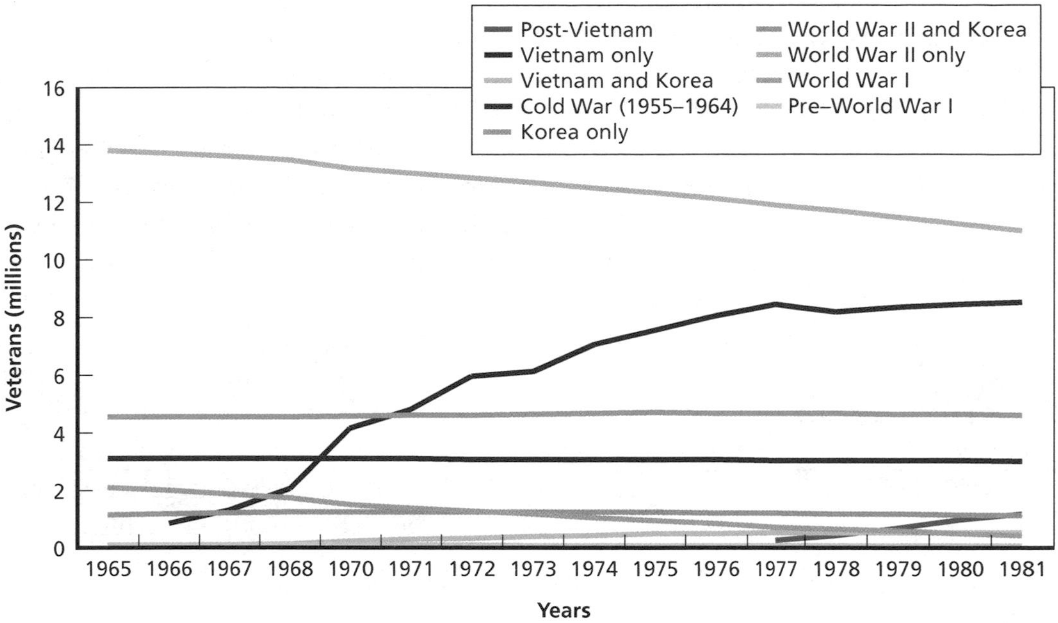

SOURCES: VA annual reports FYs 1965–1981 (Administrator of Veterans Affairs, 1966a–1982). Data not available for 1969

Vietnam had left the service. At its peak in 1977, 34 percent of all living war veterans had served during the Vietnam era, one-quarter of whom had actually been deployed to Vietnam.

Initial VA Response Vietnam

The VA administrator hardly acknowledged the sharp rise in the number of Vietnam veterans starting in 1966 in the annual report he sent to Congress on January 3, 1966, which covered the year ending on June 30, 1965. The following year, the only references the FY 1966 Annual Report made to Vietnam were about the VA's response to a request from President Johnson to provide medical treatment for 57 paralyzed Vietnamese soldiers and support the VA gave to the "cadre of 14 Vietnamese military personnel (2 physicians, 4 nurses and 8 corpsmen) [who] accompanied the patients for training in the treatment of these severe disabilities" (Administrator of Veterans Affairs, 1966b, p. 43). The administrator was, however, concerned about an increase in the veteran population that came about as a result of enactment of Pub. L. 89–358, the Veterans' Readjustment Benefits Act of 1966, in March 1966, which retroactively provided benefits for veterans who served in the Cold War after January 31, 1955. The VA estimated that some 3.911 million new veterans would qualify under this law (Administrator of Veterans Affairs, 1966b, p. 6).[72] Accordingly, the Veterans Benefits Bureau increased staffing by 4.1 percent in anticipation of "increased workload stemming from the enactment of the 'Cold War GI Bill'" (Administrator of Veterans Affairs, 1966b, p. 157). Employment at the VA's Department of Medicine and Surgery also increased by 1.6 percent, but this was attributed neither to Vietnam nor to the new law but to accommodating the "opening of new and replacement hospitals, and further implementation of the long-range plan for improved medical care staffing to maintain quality and to further effective patient turnover" (Administrator of Veterans Affairs, 1966b, p. 157).

Was Vietnam to Be a Replay of World War II?

Hindsight is always clearer than foresight, and looking back, one can clearly see the increasing number of Vietnam veterans who would soon be demanding services from the VA. However, at the time, the way the war was unfolding seemed to have clouded not only the VA's picture of the future but also of the country. The Army itself was not investing in increased infrastructure to support a large or long conflict, even as the total numbers of military personnel increased from 2.687 million to 3.547 million, or by one-third, between June 1964 and June 1968 (Defense Manpower Data Center [DMDC], 2015). Given this change, was Vietnam to be a replay of the VA's response to World War II?

The VA had been late in responding to World War II, despite a stated policy of transferring patients no longer fit for military duty to the VA for treatment and discharge. As the country mobilized after Pearl Harbor, it soon became apparent that the VA lacked the facilities and personnel to handle the large number of war casualties that might be discharged during the conflict. Yet nothing was done to prepare for the millions of veterans who would demand services once the war was over. Rather than build up the VA to handle the flow of wounded service members who were already returning to the United States, the policy was changed in late 1943 to build up the medical infrastructure of the Army and the Navy and to keep patients under military control until they "reached maximum improvement" (Peterson, 1962, p. 51). As a result, on June 30, 1945, just two months before the end of World War II, only 21,000 World War II veterans were patients in VA hospitals, compared with 58,000 soldiers in Army convalescent hospitals and 152,971 in Army general hospitals. An additional 50,078 patients were in Army regional hospitals and 51,561 at station hospitals (Smith, 1956, p. 211). So, as World War II was ending, the VA was caring for less than 10 percent of the Army's most serious casualties. Another sign of how irrelevant the VA had become was the fact that, in 1945, World War I hospital patients outnumbered World War II hospital patents in VA hospitals by more than two to one (Bradley, 1946, Table 8, p. 53). It would take the leadership of GEN Omar Bradley, the wholesale transfer of

---

[72] Some 161,000 post-Korean conflict veterans were already receiving compensation for service-connected disabilities, even before the passage of Pub. L. 89-358 (Administrator of Veterans Affairs, 1966a, p. 8).

military medical facilities to the VA, and a great deal of money before the VA could cope with the World War II veterans. But this time around, for Vietnam, there was no such safety valve. The services had not expanded their medical infrastructures, and the wounded were not being kept on active duty until they achieved maximum improvement. This time, the VA had to step up to caring for the veterans returning from war.

The VA Takes Notice of Vietnam

Finally, in its FY 1967 Annual Report to Congress, the VA acknowledged its "new role . . . of providing benefit information and assistance to servicemen in Vietnam" (Administrator of Veterans Affairs, 1966b, p. 1). To address this "new role," the VA stationed contact assistants at military hospitals in October 1966 to identify the casualties scheduled for discharge who might benefit from rehabilitation services when they arrived at a VA hospital.[73] By June 1967, the age profile of veterans in civilian life (see Figure 5.21) clearly shows the emerging Vietnam bulge of young veterans. However,

Figure 5.21
Estimated Age of Veterans in Civilian Life, as of June 30, 1964, and June 30, 1967

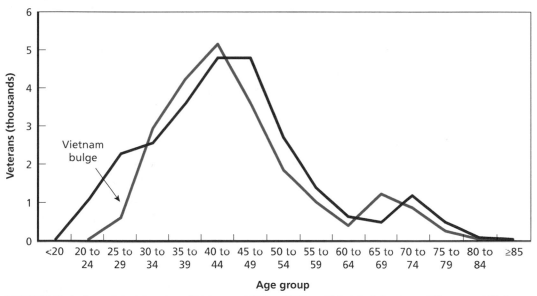

SOURCES: Data from Administrator of Veterans Affairs, 1965, p. 191; Administrator of Veterans Affairs, 1968, p. 307.
NOTE: Blue line is 1964; red line is 1967.

---

[73] The VA reported that, during FY 1967, its representatives at military hospitals had "made over 1,820 visits to some 100 military hospitals during which over 14,000 patient interviews and over 4,600 applications for vocational rehabilitation were completed" (Administrator of Veterans Affairs, 1968, p. 119). In addition, in January 1967, the VA sent two additional contact representatives to Vietnam to provide benefit assistance to men awaiting transportation home. In March, the program was expanded to five contact representatives; by the end of June 1967, they had made group presentations to 70,000 servicemen.

the average daily patient load was 6 percent lower than it had been the previous year, even as hospital admissions were up by 2 percent.

The Impact of Vietnam Veterans on the VA

The first real impact on the VA of the Vietnam War was reported in FY 1968. While this was just the beginning for the VA, it was the high-water mark of America's involvement in Vietnam; the Tet Offensive had begun in January 1968, and the long drawdown had begun. For the first time, the VA reported the number of Vietnam-era veterans in civilian life as a distinct group apart from the veterans of other wars; on June 30, 1968, there were more than 2 million Vietnam-era veterans, a number equal to over 9 percent of all war veterans (Administrator of Veterans Affairs, 1969, p. 79).[74] Their average age was 24.3 years, which made them some 15 years younger than the Korean War cohort and 23 years younger than the World War II veterans (Administrator of Veterans Affairs, 1969, Table 77, p. 318). Moreover, this new group of younger veterans was just the vanguard of the eventual 8.5 million Vietnam-era veterans that would change the face of the VA.

The impact the influx of Vietnam-era veterans had on the VA is hard to discern because it took place just as the VA was changing the way it was delivering services. Figure 5.22 shows the percentage change between FYs 1964 and 1976 in a number of factors that characterize the VA.

Over this period, the number of veterans grew by 20 percent; as one might expect, the increase in new veterans led to an increase in overall employment at the VA of 29 percent, primarily in the Department of Medicine and Surgery.[75] In real terms, VA expenditures, adjusted for inflation, also increased but by 62 percent, a number substantially larger than the percentage increase in the veterans' population. Most striking, however, was the change in the way the VA delivered services over this period, which is reflected in the sharp rise in both the total numbers of veterans admitted to VA hospitals and outpatient visits.[76] This came at the same time as decreases in the average daily patient load at VA hospitals, which reflected the amount of time patients stayed in hospitals. In FY 1976, the VA reported that 97 percent of veterans who asked to be admitted to a psychiatric or general hospital received care (National Research Council, 1977, p. 21).[77] Of these, the vast majority—70 percent—received care for

---

[74] Pub. L. 90-77, 1967, defined Vietnam-era veterans as those whose service began after August 5, 1964.

[75] The VA also used "fee-basis" physicians to provide outpatient services. In FY 1964, there were 4.9 million visits to VA medical facilities and more than 1.2 million visits to fee-basis physicians (Administrator of Veterans Affairs, 1965, p. 29).

[76] A visit is "the presence of an outpatient on 1 day in a VA medical facility or in the office of a fee-basis physician for medical services" (Administrator of Veterans Affairs, 1965, p. 2).

[77] In 1977, the National Research Council found that,

> despite the complex set of eligibility regulations governing the use of VA health care, only a very small proportion of the veterans who apply for care at VA facilities are being denied care or are dissatisfied with the amount

Figure 5.22
Change in VA from FY 1964 to FY 1976

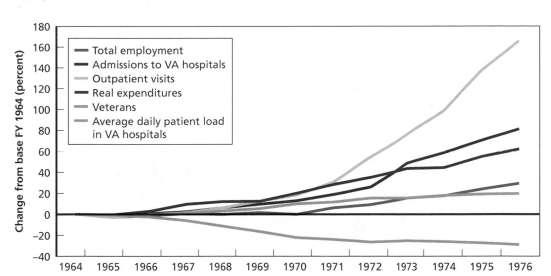

SOURCES: VA annual reports FYs 1964–1976 (Administrator of Veterans Affairs, 1966a–1977); budget deflator (Office of Management and Budget, 2015).

conditions not associated with their military service (National Research Council, 1977, p. 25, Table 2-1).

In general, the time patients spend in the hospital is related to the nature of the illness requiring treatment; the treatments and procedures followed; the age of the patient; and, to some extent, the availability of outpatient options.[78] The reduction in hospital stay time was the result of a concerted effort by the VA that was in line with similar reductions in the civilian health sector.[79] While the VA attributed much

---

of care they receive. Although some veterans may be denied the use of some VA services (especially dental care), inpatient and outpatient medical care appears to be available to almost all applicants, regardless of their eligibility status. (National Research Council, 1977, p. 22)

[78] The VA reported that, "the younger Vietnam era veteran was not staying in the hospital as long as his older counterpart since his problems tend to be less of a chronic-degenerative variety" (Administrator of Veterans Affairs, 1971, p. 8). There was also a relative decline in the number of older veterans being admitted to VA hospitals. The VA attributed this to the fact that "Medicare provides veterans with an additional source through which medical care may be obtained, . . . [and] the number of living veterans 65 years of age or older is decreasing" (Administrator of Veterans Affairs, 1969, p. 10).

[79] For example, the average length of a short hospital stay for Medicare enrollees age 65 years and over dropped from 13.8 days in 1967 to 10.9 days in 1977, as noted in Gornick, 1982, p. 50. The Department of Health and Human Services reported similar reductions were reported in 1984: "The average number of days spent by patients in hospitals fell 22 percent over a recent five-year period." The department

attributed the decline to several factors. These included advances in technology, growing acceptance of outpatient treatment, greater scrutiny of the need to hospitalize patients by government and insurers, changes in

of the decrease to changes that introduced preadmission workup and posthospitalization medical care on an outpatient basis,[80] others saw it differently. In a comprehensive report to Congress on the state of the VA, the National Science Foundation noted:

> In the last decade, an influx of patients resulting from the Vietnam War drew public attention to some of the VA's problems. The controversy over their treatment sharpened the debate between the Congress and the Executive Branch on the resource requirements of the VA hospital system. Congressional committees responsible for veterans' affairs and for VA appropriations were repeatedly told by veterans' groups and medical schools that shortages of hospital staff and equipment were jeopardizing the quality of patient care in VA hospitals and forcing some VA hospitals to deny admission or outpatient services to veterans who needed care. Congressional hearings emphasized the disparity in staff-to-patient ratios between VA hospitals and community hospitals: VA hospitals were said to be greatly understaffed. These problems were said to persist despite the rapid growth of the VA's medical-care budget in recent years, growth that roughly paralleled the general increase in costs in the health industry. (National Research Council, 1977, p. 2)

The New Paradigm for the Treatment of Psychiatric Patients for the Nation and at the VA

A substantial part of the reduction in average daily patient load at the VA came from the way psychiatric patients received care. On October 31, 1963, the VA's hospital census day for FY 1964, 87 percent of long-term patients (those hospitalized for more than 90 days) were for psychiatric conditions. By 1976, that number had dropped to 70 percent, driving down the overall percentage of long-term hospital patients, from 56.0 percent to 35.1. Between FYs 1964 and 1976 (see Figure 5.23), there was not only a significant overall reduction in the number of psychiatric patients but also a drop in the number of long-term psychiatric patients hospitalized for more than one year and a sharp rise in the proportion of psychiatric patients hospitalized for less than 90 days.

The VA attributed the reduction in hospitalized psychiatric patients to the "many changes in treatment [that] have taken place within hospitals which permit more rapid evaluation and shortened intensive treatment"[81] (Administrator of Veterans Affairs, 1971, p. 16). The VA also noted that the increased importance of outpatient psychiatric services was consistent with "efforts to reduce the institutionalization of psychotic

---

reimbursement systems, price competition among hospitals and the growth of health maintenance organizations, which have incentives to reduce the use of hospital services. (Tolchin, 1988, p. 1)

[80] Pub. L. 86–639, July 12, 1960, authorized pre- and posthospital care for a large part of the veteran population.

[81] Specifically mentioned were treatment techniques involving the establishment of simulated societies with token economies, which the VA saw as a means of bringing many institutionalized veterans with chronic psychiatric disorders "new hope" and which "permitted them to leave institutionalized settings" (Administrator of Veterans Affairs, 1971, p. 16).

Figure 5.23
Trends in the Care of Psychiatric Patients, FYs 1964–1976

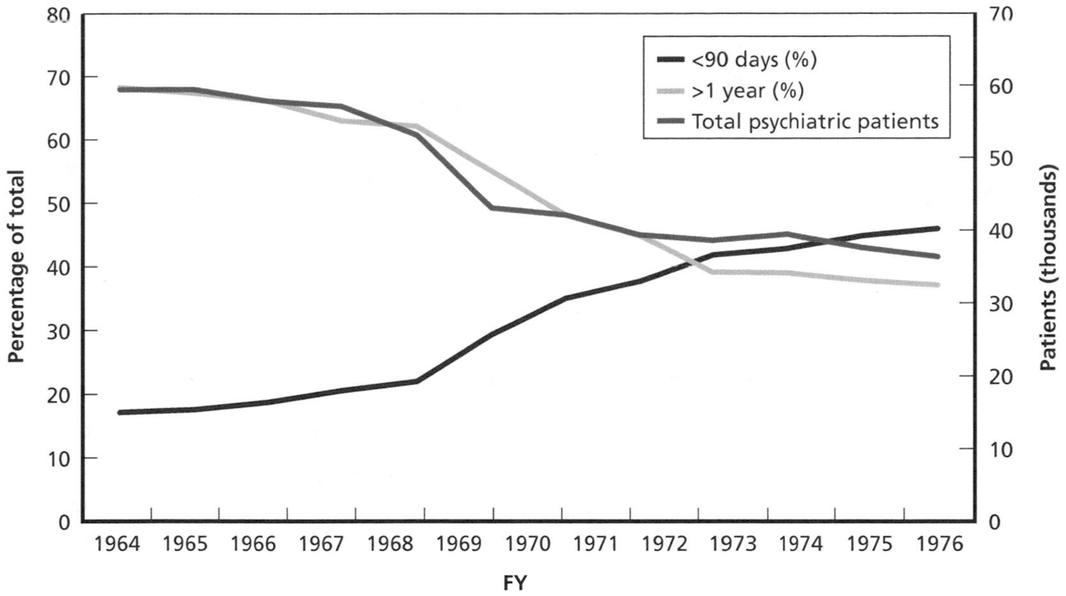

SOURCES: VA annual reports FYs 1964–1976 (Administrator of Veterans Affairs, 1966a–1977).

patients, . . . [that] dominated recent treatment regimen philosophy in both community and VA facilities" (Administrator of Veterans Affairs, 1973, p. 14). Going forward, the VA would emphasize

> the importance of early short-term treatment on an ambulatory basis as the treatment of choice . . . [and would provide] a broad array of comprehensive psychiatric services so that quality treatment can be given without undue separation of the veteran from his family, job and community. (Administrator of Veterans Affairs, 1973, p. 20)

The Joint Commission on Mental Illness and Health

At the heart of the change in the VA paradigm for care was a new way of treating mental health. Observing (1) that 47 percent of hospital beds in the United States were occupied by mental patients with an "outmoded reliance on simple custodial care in mental hospitals as the chief method of dealing with mental illness" and (2) that "experience with certain out-patient clinics and rehabilitation centers would seem to indicate that many mental patients could be better treated on an out-patient basis at much lower cost than by a hospital," Congress passed a joint resolution in 1955 calling for an "objective, thorough, and nationwide analysis and reevaluation of the human and economic problems of mental illness" (Pub. L. 84-182, 1955). The Joint Commission on Mental Illness and Health carried out the congressionally mandated study. In its final report, released at the end of 1960, the commission took a strong stand against large psychiatric hospitals in favor of small, community-based, intensive outpatient treatment centers:

> The objective of modern treatment of persons with major mental illness is to enable the patient to maintain himself in the community in a normal manner. To do so, it is necessary (1) to save the patient from the debilitating effects of institutionalization as much as possible, (2) if the patient requires hospitalization, to return him to home and community life as soon as possible, and (3) thereafter to maintain him in the community as long as possible. (Joint Commission on Mental Illness and Health, 1961, p. xvii)

States throughout the country, as well as the VA, reacted swiftly to adopt the new paradigm.[82] Over time, it became clear, however, that the expected changes had not come to pass. In 1984, the *New York Times* reported that the

> policy that led to the release of most of the nation's mentally ill patients from the hospital to the community is now widely regarded as a major failure. Sweeping critiques of the policy, notably the recent report of the American Psychiatric Association, have spread the blame everywhere, faulting politicians, civil libertarian lawyers and psychiatrists. (Lyons, 1984, p. 1)

There had been notable improvement in overcoming the debilitating effects of schizophrenia—in 1963, the average stay in a state institution for someone with schizophrenia was 11 years; by 2013, many patients with schizophrenia were to live normal, productive lives with jobs and families. However, the loss of about 90 percent of the beds in state hospitals and the facts that only one-half of the proposed community outpatient centers were ever built and that those that had been built were not fully funded had mental health professionals lamenting that there was "nowhere for the sickest people to turn, so they end up homeless, abusing substances or in prison" ("Kennedy's Vision for Mental Health Never Realized," 2013).

VA's Emphasis on Outpatient Psychiatric Treatment

The VA, however, never went as far in reducing the number of psychiatric beds in its hospitals and provided more outpatient services. Nevertheless, such issues as homeless veterans would mark the VA's future.[83] Consistent with the recommendations of the joint commission, the emphasis on outpatient mental health program was clear by FY 1976. Table 5.8 shows the relative growth and decline of outpatient and inpatient

---

[82] As Lyons, 1984, p. 1, reports: "In California, for example, the number of patients in state mental hospitals reached a peak of 37,500 in 1959 when Edmund G. Brown, Sr., was governor, and fell to 22,000 when Ronald Reagan attained that office in 1967."

[83] In 2010, veterans accounted for 10 percent of the total adult population and 16 percent of the homeless adult population. However, veterans comprised 13 percent of sheltered homeless adults in 2010 and 16 percent of homeless adults at any given time (National Center for Veterans Analysis and Statistics, 2012).

Table 5.8
Percentage Change in Psychiatric Inpatient and Outpatient VA Programs Between FYs 1967 and 1976

	FY 1976	FY 1967	Change (%)
Psychiatric hospitals			
Operating beds at end of year	11,650	17,112	−31.9
Average daily census	10,062	14,156	−28.9
Admissions	44,622	117,347	−62.0
Turnover rate	39	9	327.2
Patients treated	58,913	106,245	−44.5
Psychiatric outpatient visits			
Mental hygiene clinics	943,000	507,347	85.9
Day treatment center	502,933	239,989	109.6
Day hospital programs	167,561	6,217	2,595.2
Psychiatric outpatient caseload			
Mental hygiene clinics	170,020	82,232	106.8
Day treatment center	8,546	2,791	206.2
Day hospital programs	5,550	92	5,932.6

SOURCE: Administrator of Veterans Affairs, 1977, p. 20.

programs between FYs 1967 and 1976. Soon, the separate designation of "psychiatric hospital" would be gone from the VA's lexicon. The FY 1977 VA Annual Report was the last to highlight the VA's separate psychiatric hospitals, reporting "129 VA hospitals with services, including 22 in predominantly psychiatric hospitals and 107 in general hospitals" (Administrator of Veterans Affairs, 1978, p. 20). Thereafter, the VA reported "medical centers." The following year's annual report (FY 1978) was the last to report data separately for general and psychiatric hospitals (Administrator of Veterans Affairs, 1979, p. 127).

Quality of Care at VA Psychiatric Facilities

Even before the large number of psychiatric patients flooded the VA, the quality of care psychiatric patients were receiving was brought into question. Dr. Norman Q. Brill, the distinguished psychiatrist who had done pioneering work during and following World War II,[84] testified in 1970 to the deteriorating quality of care the VA provided,

---

[84] Today, what is known about the neuropsychiatric casualties of World War II largely comes from two studies, both led by Dr. Brill. The first was done during the war, under the auspices of the Neuropsychiatry Consultants Division of the Army Surgeon General's Office (Brill, Tate, and Menninger, 1945). The second was done after the war, under the auspices of the National Research Council and the VA (Brill and Beebe, 1955). See also Brill and Kupper, 1966b; Brill and Kupper, 1966a; and Brill, 1966.

especially with "excessive reliance on drugs in the treatment of patients" (Brill, 1970, p. 393). Brill noted that a

> physician . . . can hardly do more than prescribe medication, keep an eye on the patients' physical condition and the grossest manifestation of their mental health, and keep up with the paperwork. There is no time to do research, and little or no time to provide any intensive treatment, even when it's indicated. . . . The VA is not able to compete with State, community, private, or other facilities in recruiting outstanding people. (Brill, 1970, p. 393)

Highlighting his long-standing and growing concerns for the unsatisfactory conditions at the VA's Brentwood Neuropsychiatric Hospital in Los Angeles, where he was the consultant in psychiatry, he reported that 1,595 patients were being cared for by only ten full-time psychiatrists. He went on to tell a Senate committee that

> [e]ven this might be manageable if the patients stayed for a long time and there was not any significant turnover, but the turnover of patients is another factor that needs to be taken into consideration. There were over 3,400 admissions to the Brentwood NP [Neuropsychiatric] hospital in 1969. That's twice as many as there were in 1964 who are being taken care of by less staff—about half of what they had before—and who are responsible for examining them, diagnosing, and treating all of these patients at the same time they are taking care of the large number of patients who remain as a residual. (Brill, 1970, p. 393)

> There is a policy consistent with what is going on in many public mental hospitals of getting patients out of the hospital as rapidly as possible. From 1964 to the present time [1970], the average daily patient load has been reduced from 1,910 patients to 861 despite the . . . increased numbers of admissions—which were 1,752 in 1964 and double that amount in 1969. (Brill, 1970, p. 396)

> Adequate and continuing rehabilitation services after discharge could not be provided to the increasing numbers of patients who were being admitted and discharged. Unfortunately, in many instances, the rehabilitation consists of continuing medication and an occasional visit from the social worker and sometimes a brief visit with the doctor. (Brill, 1970, p. 399)

> I think that one of the problems that has been created by the excessive reliance on drugs[, which in part] stems from the tremendous deficiency in staff and shortage of staff[,] is that there is little opportunity to get to the causes of the patient's illness. (Brill, 1970, p. 400)

Finally, Brill suggested that, "rather than expose veterans to inadequate psychiatric treatment," state, some county, and even some private hospitals could "probably do a better job than is now being done and probably for not any more money" and suggested that "we need to reexamine the concept of having hospitals just for veterans" (Brill, 1970, p. 402).

A New Kind of Veteran and a New Kind of VA

In 1969, the VA prophetically noted it faced a "spectrum" of problems, with one end "providing benefit information and assistance to servicemen in Vietnam; at the other end, the extension and refinement of care and assistance to the needy 'older' veteran" (Administrator of Veterans Affairs, 1970, p. 1). By 1976, the spectrum was clear (see Figure 5.24). In 1976, Vietnam veterans made up 26 percent of all veterans. On average, they were almost half the age of the World War II veterans. Sandwiched between the two were the smaller groups of Korean War and Cold War veterans. The VA was now dealing with two very large veteran populations that, as far as age was concerned, were entirely distinct. However, it was not just age that marked the difference, as the VA reported in 1971:

> The Vietnam era veteran . . . [is] viewed as a major challenge by VA psychologists. Several important factors contribute to this challenge: the general psychosocial characteristics of this generation of veterans; the accelerated pace of technological and social changes in the American society; the prolonged and inconclusive nature of the Vietnam conflict; and the fact that a greater portion have sustained, and survived serious physical disabilities and emotional trauma from combat experience. (Administrator of Veterans Affairs, 1971, p. 16)

The new generation of veterans was also coming as the VA's new approach to caring for psychiatric patients was taking hold. The impressive growth of the mental

Figure 5.24
Age Profile of Living Veterans on June 30, 1976

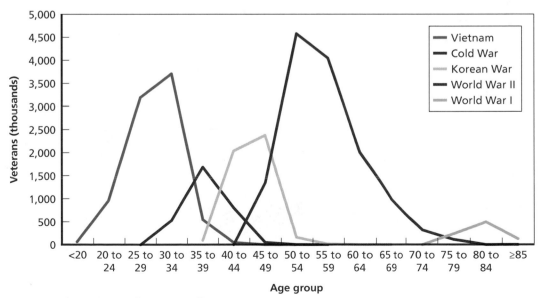

SOURCE: Administrator of Veterans Affairs, 1977, p. 125.

health program notwithstanding, the VA expressed concerns that serving this group of veterans was going to be a problem as early as 1970:

> Experience has shown that the Vietnam Era veteran is more apt to be critical of organization and tends to act impulsively, increasing the frequency of interruption of treatment before completion. To best meet the needs of this veteran, programs have been created using younger staff members as therapists, thereby improving communication. The complicated factor of drug misuse has been increasingly identified and newer approaches developed to deal with it. (Administrator of Veterans Affairs, 1971, p. 16)

Not only did the VA seem frustrated with the Vietnam veterans; those who were receiving services from the VA also seemed frustrated. A large number were asking for "age segregated wards" and with "somewhere between 30–40 percent . . . expressing dissatisfaction with VA programs or conveying feelings of isolation and powerlessness" (Administrator of Veterans Affairs, 1972, pp. 13–14). And there was more. Vietnam veterans were also different in another way. Just as the misuse of drugs was a major problem for the Army in Vietnam, particularly after 1970, it became a similar problem for the VA after 1972. In FY 1969, about 3,000 veterans were treated in a VA drug treatment program, as measured by veterans discharged from the program. In FY 1971, the number had grown to 6,800 veterans; the following year, it was 22,000 veterans (Administrator of Veterans Affairs, 1973, p. 14). Most were treated as outpatients.[85]

It was not only inside the VA that Vietnam veterans were different. In 1976, the overall unemployment rate for all male veterans was 5.4 percent, significantly less than the 9.0 percent unemployed for nonveterans. However, among Vietnam veterans, the employment rate was 8.8 percent, and "among the youngest Vietnam era veterans (20 to 24 years old) the unemployment rate was 19.6 percent in June 1976, nearly double the corresponding nonveteran rate of 10.5 percent" (Administrator of Veterans Affairs, 1977, p. 5).

Vietnam veterans were also different in that, after 1970, they were in open conflict with the government, the VA, and even the old-line veterans' service organizations, such as the American Legion, the Veterans of Foreign Wars, and the Disabled Veterans of America.[86] Vietnam Veterans Against the War, first formed in 1967, was

---

[85] A comparison of data for June 30, 1971, and June 30, 1972, indicates that inpatients in the drug dependence program increased from 574 to 1,292 patients (125 percent) and outpatients in the drug dependence program increased from 600 to 5,360 (793 percent) (Administrator of Veterans Affairs, 1973, p. 22).

[86] According to Boulton, 2014, the

> old established veterans' organizations, in particular the American Legion and the Veterans of Foreign Wars, tended to have the interests of World War II veterans at heart and were often slow to throw the full weight of their lobbying machine behind the Vietnam generation's causes. Because of this relative vacuum, the Vietnam-era bills tended to gain their form and function from the initiatives of individual politicians . . . . Bills had to negotiate a tortured path through successive obstructionists and White House administrations influenced by

organizing numerous antiwar demonstrations by 1970 and would eventually claim to have some 30,000 members (Vietnam Veterans Against the War, 2015).[87] In a more traditional vein, many more Vietnam veterans joined the Vietnam Veterans of America, which was founded in 1978 as an "advocacy organization devoted exclusively to the needs of Vietnam veterans" (Vietnam Veterans of America, 2015). Grassroots advocacy by Vietnam veterans would press the VA hard on what was first called *Vietnam syndrome* and later became known as *PTSD*, the need for special outreach programs to help with readjustment, and the treatment for the illnesses the organization argued were caused by exposure to the herbicide Agent Orange.

Posttraumatic Shock Disorder

In 1970, the *American Journal of Psychiatry* published a paper by Dr. Peter Bourne. Reflecting on his experience as the chief of the neuropsychiatric section, U.S. Army Medical Research Team–Viet Nam, Walter Reed Army Institute of Research, Dr. Bourne flatly stated that the

> Viet Nam experience has shown that we have now successfully identified most of the major correlates of psychiatric attrition in the combat zone. . . . As a result there is reason to be optimistic that psychiatric casualties need never again become a major cause of attrition in the United States military in a combat zone. (Bourne, 1970, p. 487)

Not long after, however, Bourne acknowledged that this assessment might have been too rosy. He now argued that there was

> no doubt that the rate of psychiatric attrition during the one year spent in Viet Nam by U.S. servicemen is lower than in previous wars. It is becoming increasingly apparent, however, that this represents only a part of the overall picture of the psychological effects of this war on the men who serve. The psychological and social problems of the Viet Nam veteran probably exceed those of any previous conflict. (Bourne, 1972, p. 23)

> His self-image is blighted by an alien society, which does not regard him as a hero. A sense of loneliness may foster depression. . . . Today's psychiatric facility must gear themselves to the need for treatment of the large number of emotional prob-

---

fiscal conservative budget agencies and a less-than-munificent Veterans Administration. . . . [As a result,] benefits offered by the Vietnam-era bills were lower than those offered by the 1944 G.I. Bill, not only in terms of dollar amount but also in terms of the quality of education they provided.

[87] After 1973, when the last American troops left Vietnam, Vietnam Veterans Against the War lost its *raison d'être* and, with it, membership. The group's march on Washington in July 1974, Operation Dewey Canyon IV, turned into an anti-Nixon demonstration and further alienated Vietnam veterans from the Nixon administration and the VA. "For Nixon, the long-haired and disheveled interlopers sporadically invading DC served as an unwelcome and public reminder of how the war had gone so terribly wrong" (Boulton, 2014, pp. 159–160).

lems, ignored or postponed in active duty, but often thrust into prominence upon return. (Bourne, 1972, p. 23, abstract)

That the incidence of emotional problems, even the level of hospitalization, is so high among today's veterans, makes depressingly hollow the claim that we have cut combat psychiatric attrition to a minimum. To merely delay the time at which the peak incidence of psychiatric breakdown occurs is not a notable accomplishment. (Bourne, 1972, p. 26)

Sarah Haley Challenges the Traditional Approach to Treating War Neurosis

For Sarah Haley, a young and freshly minted psychiatric social worker newly assigned to screening and triage at the Boston VA outpatient clinic, Bourne's new assessment was no revelation. In early 1969, despite the admonitions of her colleagues that the veterans they were seeing were "delusional [and] obviously in full-blown psychosis" (Scott, 1993, p. 5), Haley could not disregard the stories she was hearing. She thought that what her colleagues, mainly World War II veterans themselves, failed to see was that these patients were traumatized by what they had experienced in Vietnam. There were two problems, as Haley would later recall, that "clouded her fellow professionals' view" of the veterans coming into the Boston VA. First, as she saw it, there was a general bias against Vietnam veterans. "It was so much easier," she said, for her colleagues "to blame the . . . [Vietnam] veteran . . . [and] to romanticize . . . World War II veterans [as being] cut from sterner stuff" (Scott, 1993, p. 5). Particularly after the revelations of the My Lai massacre, many of her colleagues did not want to deal with the Vietnam veterans, thinking of them as "baby killers who should have known better" (Scott, 1993, p. 5). Second, she was repeatedly told that there was no basis for thinking that returning soldiers, now months removed from combat, were reacting to what they had experienced earlier in Vietnam, since "mental health professionals across the country assessed disturbed Vietnam veterans using a diagnostic nomenclature which contained no specific entries for war-related trauma" (Scott, 1993, p. 5).

In 1974, she recounted her experience at the VA in a groundbreaking article, "When the Patient Reports Atrocities: Specific Treatment Considerations of the Vietnam Veteran," arguing that

[p]sychotherapy with veterans who have committed atrocious acts does not follow the traditional treatment model of the "traumatic war neurosis." . . . The therapist must "be with" and tolerate the existential reality of the patient's overt or covert view of himself as a murderer. (Haley, 1974, p. 191)[88]

---

[88] On traumatic war neurosis and its treatment, Haley goes on to say that

[t]he traumatic war neurosis, as described in the literature following World War II and the Korean Conflict, involved feelings of guilt, depression, anxiety, and/or suppressive symptoms that appeared related to combat experiences but were thought to be essentially "neurotic." That is, the combat experiences, traumatic as they may have been, were in the line of duty, and persistent symptoms of guilt or depression were thought to be related to the stirring up of unacceptable, unconscious wishes and fantasies. The standard way to treat combat-

Lifton, Cleland, and Shatan Define Post-Vietnam Syndrome

Haley, however, was not the only one who thought that there were problems with the veterans returning from Vietnam. In late 1969, Max Cleland, the triplegic from Georgia, provided a Senate committee with a firsthand account of the difficulties a returning soldier had in dealing with the physical and psychological consequences of Vietnam. He described the

> inevitable psychological depression after injury, coupled with doubts that it may not have been worth it, comes months later like a series of secondary explosions long after the excitement of the battlefield is behind, the reinforcement of your comrades-in-arms a thing of the past, and the individual is left alone with his injury and his self-doubts. Anyone who deals with a Vietnam returnee, wounded or not, must understand this delayed, severe psychological symptom. And, in my opinion, more effort has to be made, especially by the VA, to insure that the small but select minority of Vietnam returnees in VA hospitals have adequate help . . . in readjusting to American life. (Cleland, 1970, p. 274)

On January 27, 1969, a noted Yale psychiatrist, Dr. Robert Jay Lifton,[89] explained to the Senate committee why Vietnam was unique—there were no battle lines[90]—and why the traditional emphasis on the trauma of combat needed to be expanded. He put Cleland's observation about having "doubts that it may not have been worth it" into a broader observation: "[W]e cannot separate the larger historical contradictions

---

related guilt and the depression of the traumatic war neurosis, therefore, was to alleviate the guilt and thereby aid repression by taking the responsibility from the individual and placing it on a higher authority (one was following orders). In addition, treatment consisted of exploring the unconscious wishes and fantasies if necessary, and to treat the consecutive depressions of the surviving soldier—the depression of leaving his family, friends, and the life he would have had if not for military service; and finally the depression caused by separating from his fellow soldiers either by their deaths or his discharge. The inappropriateness of this model for the veteran whose chief complaint involves responsibility for war atrocities is best illustrated by my first encounter with such a veteran. . . .

The therapist's ability to acknowledge and tolerate both the veteran's objective responsibility and his varying views of himself is of crucial importance in the therapist's sense of "being with" the veteran as they work toward understanding and resolution of conflict. (Haley, 1974, p. 192)

[89] For a more complete discussion of Lifton's engagement, see Nicosia, 2001, pp. 158–169.

[90] Lifton explained why the battlefield in Vietnam was so different from that in Korea, of which he had firsthand knowledge:

In Korea, there were established battlelines. The relations between Americans and South Koreans, while not without antagonisms and some expressions of racial prejudice, were nonetheless on the whole reasonably friendly. . . .

[In Vietnam,] there are no battlelines. Everything shifts, nothing is stable, just because of the nature of that war, because it is a guerrilla war and the guerrillas are so close to the people.

None of this was true in Korea, and the stresses were different. The ordinary psychological outlets of war were more available in Korea. (Lifton, 1970, p. IV-36)

surrounding the American involvement in Vietnam from the individual psychological response of our soldiers" (Lifton, 1970, p. IV-32). His frame of reference was the general psychology of the survivor. Lifton explained:

> For veterans of any war there is a difficult transition from the "extreme situation" of the war environment to the more ordinary civilian world. . . . He survives the general war environment, within which he was taught that killing was not only legitimate but proper and necessary. . . .
>
> He must . . . struggle with feelings of guilt and shame resulting directly from the war experience. . . .
>
> His overall adjustment is greatly influenced by the extent to which he can become inwardly convinced that his war, and his participation in that war, had purpose and significance. . . . (Lifton, 1970, p. IV-29)
>
> [The] inability to find significance or meaning in their extreme experience leaves many Vietnam veterans with a terrible burden or survivor guilt. And this sense of guilt can become associated with deep distrust of the society that sent them to their ordeal in Vietnam. They then retain a strong and deeply disturbing feeling of having been victimized and betrayed by their own country. . . .
>
> [T]hese men are also affected by the deep ambivalence of the American population about the war in general, an ambivalence which extends to those who have fought it. . . . (Lifton, 1970, p. IV-31)
>
> [They are reacting to] an unspoken feeling on the part of many Americans that returning veterans carry some of the taint of that dirty and unsuccessful war. (Lifton, 1970, p. IV-32)

In April 1972, the codirector of the Postdoctoral Psychoanalytic Training Program at New York University, Dr. Chaim F. Shatan, challenged the psychiatric orthodoxy with a paper presented at that the annual meeting of the American Orthopsychiatric Association meeting. Shatan wrote:

> While the government has claimed few "psychiatric casualties" among Vietnam war veterans, most symptoms are delayed in onset, due to emotional anesthesia brought on by a combination of combat trauma and the military's counter-guerrilla training, which discourages grief and intimacy. . . . [T]he symptoms reported by veterans, and their efforts in launching a self-help movement of group sessions and other activities, outside the auspices of a Veterans Administration that they find unresponsive to their needs, . . . [reflect] the inadequacy of the traditional therapist-patient relationship. (Shatan, 1973, p. 640)

In what has been described as "a landmark in the literature of post-Vietnam syndrome, and later post-traumatic stress disorder" (Nicosia, 2001, p. 170), the *New York Times* printed an op-ed on May 6, 1972, in which Shatan identified six feelings that the veterans he was working with seemed to share: (1) of guilt; (2) of being scapegoated, of being "victimized . . . by inadequate V.A. treatment . . . [and by] society at large"; (3) of rage, stemming "from the awareness of being duped and manipulated"; (4) of combat brutalization, having been given a "dehumanized image of the 'enemy'"; (5) of alienation, finding "it difficult and painful to experience compassion for others"; and (6) of doubt, "an agonizing doubt about their continued ability to love others, and to accept affection" (Shatan, 1972, p. 35). Finally, in an ironic twist, Shatan invoked Sigmund Freud, who many had used to make the case against the central role that the combat in Vietnam was playing in the psychiatric difficulties of returning veterans:[91]

> During World War I, Freud elucidated the role grief plays in helping the mourner let go of a missing part of life, and acknowledging that it exists only in the memory. The post-Vietnam syndrome confronts us with the unconsummated grief of soldiers—"impacted grief" in which an encapsulated never-ending past deprives the present of meaning. (Shatan, 1972, p. 35)

About the same time the Shatan op-ed appeared, Lifton, brought the plight of Vietnam veterans to the attention of the American public. In an article in the *Atlantic Monthly*, he wrote:

> There is something special about Vietnam veterans. Everyone who has contact with them seems to agree that they are different from veterans of other wars. A favorite word to describe them is "alienated." . . .

> [They] avoid contact with the Veterans Administration—because they associate it with the war-military-government establishment, with the forces responsible for a hated ordeal, or because of their suspicion (whether on the basis of hearsay or personal experience) that VA doctors are likely to interpret their rage at everything connected with the war as no more than their own individual "problem." . . . (Lifton, 1972, p. 56)

> [T]hey have taken on a very special survivor mission, one of extraordinary historical and psychological significance. They are flying in the face of the traditional pattern of coping with survivor emotions, which was to join organizations of veterans that not only justify their particular war but embrace war making and militarism in general. . . . [They] are turning that pattern on its head, and finding

---

[91] At the time there was a reluctance to accept the trauma of Vietnam by the branch of psychiatry that is influenced by psychoanalysis. Boulanger explains "the dogma of the childhood etiology of neuroses":

> The question of trauma is at the root of psychoanalysis, but the timing of the trauma is also significant, and it is this that has historically proved a stumbling block to the acceptance and appropriate treatment of traumatic neuroses. For it is commonly believed that the etiology of pathology ties not in adult but in childhood traumas. To argue that trauma in adult life can have a profound and long-lasting psychological consequence even among individuals who were previously normal is to contradict this developmental theory. (Boulanger, 1985, pp. 16–17)

significance in their survival by exposing precisely the meaninglessness—and the evil—of their war. . . .

[For many,] political activities become inseparable from psychological need. Telling their story to American society has been both a political act and a means of confronting psychologically an inauthentic experience and moving beyond it toward authenticity. (Lifton, 1972, p. 62)

Central to the work of both Lifton and Shatan was the thesis that the legitimacy of the Vietnam War and the way it was being prosecuted were important factors in the psychiatric functioning of veterans once removed from Vietnam. This moved the psychiatric theory from being apolitical, dealing with the soldiers themselves and what they had individually experienced, to the political realm of antiwar activism and the social issues of how returning soldiers were being treated by their fellow citizens. The therapeutic effects of veterans' "rap" groups being reported by Haley, Shatan, Lifton, and others—the healing power of political and social activism—were hard for many to reconcile with a more neutral expectation of what psychiatric treatment was all about.[92] Soon, the psychiatric and clinical psychological professions would struggle with how to deal with what was now being termed *post-Vietnam syndrome* as they worked to revise the definitive *Diagnostic and Statistical Manual of Mental Disorders* (DSM).[93]

The Battle over the DSM's Inclusion of PTSD

By 1972, it became apparent to those working with Vietnam veterans that, to make progress, something had to be done to formally recognize and legitimize a diagnosis to account for what would eventually be called *PTSD*. But that progress was not to be easy or fast.

The importance of recognition of delayed-stress disorder in the DSM cannot be overstressed. The manual was the authoritative underpinning for VA claims and legal cases that ranged from seeking compensation for the impact of negligent actions in civil cases to demands for reparations for Nazi concentration camp survivors. It was the bible against which most psychologists or psychiatrists dared not preach. DSM-I reflected the combat experience of World War II and Korea and did recognize *gross stress reaction*, reserving this diagnosis for "situations in which the individual has been exposed to severe physical demands or extreme emotional stress, such as in combat or in civilian catastrophe" (as cited in Jones, 1995a, p. 411). It did not, however, deal with delayed-onset stress reactions and even suggested that, if ongoing symptoms lasted more than a year, "another explanation should be found" (Nicosia, 2001, p. 179).

The second edition of the manual was published in 1968, soon after the start of the war in Vietnam. DSM-II renamed the category to *adjustment reaction to adult*

---

[92] On rap groups, see Smith, 1985, pp. 167–191.

[93] The American Psychiatric Association published its first edition of DSM (DSM-I) in 1952 and publishes periodic updates; as of this writing, the latest edition was DSM-V, published in 2013.

life and broke all links to combat. In retrospect, Jones suggests that this change was "unfortunate," since it suggested that "therapy should be aimed at removing the individual from the stressful environment" and is "dependent only on the individual's innate adaptive capacity rather than requiring therapeutic intervention" and that delayed onset, being removed in time from the stressful situation itself, was not possible (Jones, 1995a, p. 413).

The next opportunity to change the diagnosis in the DSM came in 1974, with the announcement in the *Psychiatric News* that a revision was in the works, with the plan of publishing DSM-III in 1980.[94] Shatan and Lifton knew "they would have to drum up support for the change" (Scott, 1993, p. 59). They enlisted the help of John Talbott, the director of the Manhattan State Hospital and a former head of the New York City chapter of the American Psychiatric Association. He arranged for a presentation at the chapter's monthly meeting on the topic of "Post-Vietnam Syndrome" and would eventually lead to an informal organization, the Vietnam Veterans Working Group (VVWG),[95] a member of which was Vietnam veteran Jack Smith.

At the 1975 annual American Psychiatric Association convention, Shatan pressed Spitzer to include a diagnosis of delayed onset stress disorder linked to combat. Spitzer said that other psychiatrists working with Vietnam veterans—several of whom who were on his task force—had come to a different conclusion, that no new diagnostic category was needed. Shatan would therefore have to "prove" that a new category was needed. Spitzer did, however, allow Shatan's group to have a seat on the Reactive Disorder Subcommittee of the DSM-III Task Force, chaired by Nancy Andreasen from the University of Iowa. In a highly unusual move, Spitzer agreed that Vietnam veteran Jack Smith, who at the time had not even graduated college, could join the subcommittee.

From a vantage point of more than 40 years later, what might seem strange today but was no laughing matter even in 1975 was that some members of the task force charged to deal with the issue of delayed onset stress adhered to the so-called "predisposition theory,"[96] thinking that

> these guys [veterans] are all character disorders. They came from rotten backgrounds. They were going to be malcontents and dysfunctional anyway. Vietnam just probably made them worse, but Vietnam is not the cause of their problems.

---

[94] The American Psychiatric Association appointed noted Columbia University professor Dr. Robert Spitzer to head the team making the revisions.

[95] Chaim Shatan organized the VVWG, which "brought together the most progressive people treating stress disorders in Vietnam veterans from around the country—forty-five professionals from New York, Massachusetts, Michigan, California, and elsewhere" (Nicosia, 2001). The group gathered data on delayed stress to submit to the American Psychiatric Association's convention.

[96] This was one of seven reasons that, prior to 1979, those "experiencing PTSD and various dislocations were in general unable to obtain effective therapeutic assistance, either from the Veterans Administration or within the private sector" (Blank, 1985, p. 230).

They're alcoholics and drug addicts. . . . Depression doesn't usually occur in people unless they've already been predisposed to it. . . . Vietnam veterans must have gone to war with a predisposition to depression. (as described in Nicosia, 2001, p. 205)

For the VVWG, the key was Nancy Andreasen. The group invited her to the next meeting of the American Orthopsychiatry Association, in March 1976, where they presented new data on the extent of postcombat disorders. This was followed in May 1976 by the annual American Psychiatric Association convention, where, to the great surprise of the VVWG, Andreasen told them to keep pressing their case. Haley later recounted:

> The unbelievable had happened. Andreasen had begun to observe delayed-stress symptoms in the burn victims she was treating, and the symptoms of her burn victims greatly resembled the problems she had been hearing of in Vietnam veterans. Though still not completely won over, a turning point had been reached in her thoughts. (as described in Nicosia, 2001, p. 207)

At the 1977 annual meeting of the American Psychiatric Association, with the support of Andreasen, the VVWG presented a major paper, and in January 1978, Spitzer and Andreasen agreed that DSM-III would contain the diagnosis for PTSD.[97] Shatan told the members of the VVWG

> The latest draft version of *DSM-III* [January 1978] incorporates most of our formulations on stress disorders, not only for combat veterans but also for Holocaust survivors and victims of other disasters, both man-made and otherwise . . . . We are happy to have reached agreement on it. (Shatan, 1978)[98]

In retrospect, it is hard to see how the American Psychiatric Association could have come to any other conclusion than to recognize PTSD. The times they were a-changing. The year before (1977), the new VA administrator, Max Cleland, had told

---

[97] The definition that was incorporated into DSM-III was revised in DSM-III-R in 1987 and again in DSM-IV (1994) and DSM-IV-TR (2000). In addition, DSM-V (2013)

> made a number of notable evidence based revisions to PTSD diagnostic criteria, with both important conceptual and clinical implications. First, because it has become apparent that PTSD is not just a fear-based anxiety disorder (as explicated in both DSM-III and DSM-IV), . . . [and] PTSD is no longer categorized as an Anxiety Disorder. PTSD is now classified in a new category, Trauma- and Stressor-Related Disorders, in which the onset of every disorder has been preceded by exposure to a traumatic or otherwise adverse environmental event. (Friedman, 2014b)

In the mid-1980s, Spitzer again headed the American Psychiatric Association's working group on the revision of DSM-III, including the revisions to the definition of PTSD, incorporating emerging results from the National Vietnam Veterans Readjustment Study (NVVRS) (Kulka et al., 1990, p. xiv). In fact, the NVVRS used the 1987 DSM-III-R definition of PTSD.

[98] The inclusion of a diagnostic category for PTSD in DSM-III was, of course, not the last word. For example see Friedman, 2014a.

the Senate that readjustment counseling would be his top priority. And the congressional logjam was about to break. In the GI Improvement Act of 1977, Congress had directed the Center for Policy Research to conduct a study documenting the status of Vietnam veterans. Preliminary reports indicated that the study had concluded that "combat veterans continue to have significantly more psychological and behavioral difficulties than Vietnam era veterans . . . not exposed to combat, or non-veterans" (Egendorf et al., 1981, p. 43). The solid wall of opposition that the American Legion, the Veterans of Foreign Wars, and the Disabled Veterans of America had built that had, on four previous occasions, thwarted the efforts of Senator Alan Cranston (D-California) to provide adjustment assistance for Vietnam veterans was cracking. Fearful that the size of the veterans' budgetary pot was only so big, the old-line veterans' organizations were even willing to pit a service-connected program for these new veterans against non–service-connected programs for the older veterans who dominated these organizations. Now, with a VA itself headed by a disabled veteran, the Disabled Veterans of America broke the united opposition to support new legislation. The final deal involved what Cleland called old-fashioned "horse trading." The Senate got Vietnam veterans readjustment centers, and the House got to have a say in choosing the locations of future VA hospitals. On June 13, 1979, as if in coordination with the change being included in the new edition, DSM-III, President Carter signed Pub. L. 96-22, which established the Vietnam Veterans' Outreach Program and the vet centers. However, as one historian noted, "the fight over the outreach program . . . [also] heightened the sense of neglect from the government and estrangement from the World War II generation felt by many Vietnam veterans" (Boulton, 2014, p. 136).

Vet Centers and the National Center for PTSD

What was officially known as the Readjustment Counseling program produced a network of community-based vet centers, detached from VA medical centers, that were designed to assist veterans and their family members by providing a broad range of counseling, outreach, and referral services to eligible veterans to help them make a satisfying postwar readjustment to civilian life. Importantly, veterans did not need a formal determination of service-connected disability to receive counseling or psychotherapy at these centers. As designed, each vet center was to be staffed by a four- or five-member team consisting of a team leader, two or three counselors with appropriate academic and experience backgrounds, and a clerical staff member.[99] Nationally,

---

[99] In 1987, the General Accounting Office (GAO; the name changed to U.S. Government Accountability Office in 2004) reported that the "majority of team leaders and counselors had master's or doctoral degrees in social work, counseling, or counseling psychology, with more than 4 years of related professional experience" (Fogel, 1987, p. 4). In a questionnaire, team leaders reported

> that half of them had over 8 years of professional experience in counseling, mental health, social work, or other social service employment; 85 percent of them had over 4 years of experience. Seventy-seven percent of satellite coordinators and 60 percent of the counselors had more than 4 years of such experience. (Fogel, 1987, p. 44)

approximately 60 percent of team members had actually served in Vietnam; 20 percent were Vietnam-era veterans; and the rest were veterans of other wars or nonveterans (Blank, 1985, p. 233). While vet centers provided as wide a range of services as possible, given their small size, most "provided group therapy for veterans and some groups for significant others as well. . . . Psychotropic medication [was] not viewed as a central modality of treatment. However, in certain cases clients [were] referred for medication as a useful adjunct to counseling services" (Blank, 1985, pp. 235–236).

Originally set up to serve only those who served in Vietnam, the centers expanded their mission in 1991 to other combat veterans who fought in Lebanon, Grenada, Panama, the Persian Gulf, Somalia, and Kosovo and Bosnia. By 1996, when Congress extended the eligibility to include World War II and Korean Combat Veterans, there were 205 such centers (Baine, 1996a, p. 1). The vet centers were further opened in 2003 to veterans of Operation Enduring Freedom (OEF), Operation Iraqi Freedom (OIF), and subsequent operations within the Global War on Terrorism. While the original focus was on PTSD, services now include individual and group counseling and assistance not only for PTSD but also for sexual trauma, alcohol and drug assessment, and suicide prevention. The centers also furnish bereavement counseling services to surviving parents, spouses, children, and siblings of service members who die of any cause while on active duty, including federally activated Reserve and National Guard personnel. Today, there are also mobile vet centers and an around-the-clock confidential center that combat veterans and their families can call to talk about their military experience or any other issue they are facing in readjusting to civilian life. The staff comprises combat veterans from several eras, as well as family members of combat veterans (U.S. Department of Veterans Affairs [DVA], undated b). In 1989, the VA created the National Center for PTSD with the mission of advancing the clinical care and social welfare of American veterans through research, education, and training in the science, diagnosis, and treatment of PTSD and stress-related disorders.

In 1987, GAO, at the behest of the chairman of the Senate Veterans Affairs Committee, undertook a detailed review of the vet center program. GAO found that

> [m]any veterans who served in Vietnam experienced readjustment problems resulting in family difficulties, unemployment, alcohol or drug dependency, and other forms of social or economic impairments. These veterans were often reluctant to seek evaluation or treatment from established VA facilities. The Readjustment Counseling Program was designed to overcome this reluctance by making VA's mental health services available to these veterans on an outpatient, storefront basis, avoiding the implication of mental illness. As of April 1987, 188 vet centers had been opened. (Fogel, 1987, p. 10)

The report also noted that "[n]one of the vet centers [were] located in existing VA health-care facilities" (Fogel, 1987, p. 17).

One reason at the time for the GAO study was the need to assess a number of proposals to relocate the storefront facilities to existing VA medical centers. GAO found that

> (1) the relocation would probably not have a significant effect on program costs; (2) veterans' access to readjustment counseling would probably not be significantly affected, but their willingness to seek that care might be lessened if the vet centers were absorbed into existing VA facilities; and (3) . . . the quality of readjustment counseling would be adversely affected if the vet centers were relocated to existing VA facilities and the medical center staff provided the counseling instead of the vet center staff. (Fogel, 1987, p. 19)[100]

A critical question was, who were the vet centers serving?

After 1984, with the passage of the Veterans' Health Care Act of 1984 (Pub. L. 98-528, October 19, 1984), the VA established special inpatient units at 13 of its medical centers for the diagnosis and treatment of PTSD. These services were to be coordinated with services provided by the vet centers. GAO found, however, that hospital beds were not available at many VA facilities, and the average waiting period was six months. Moreover, one requirement made integration of the two programs problematic: that the veteran be "free from substance abuse and acute psychiatric illnesses . . . to be considered for admission." Moreover, veterans were sometimes reluctant, not wanting "to be away from their families or jobs for an extended period of time. . . . most PTSD units plan for their patients to stay for from 3 to 5 months" (Fogel, 1987, p. 69).[101]

In 1989, Congress directed the VA to establish the National Center for PTSD as a center of excellence in research and education on PTSD. The center receives support from the VA but also from other sources. As a sign of how things have changed, the center recognizes that PTSD affects more than just the military and combat veterans and sees its mission "to advance the clinical care and social welfare of America's Veterans and others who have experienced trauma, or who suffer from PTSD"[102] (National Center for PTSD, undated).

---

[100]To determine willingness to seek care, GAO surveyed 328 vet center clients. While 53 percent said that they would go to a vet center if it were "located at the nearest VA facility and run by vet center staff," 43 percent said they would not. Thirty-two percent said they would go to a VA facility "even if the program was run by VA facility staff rather than the vet center staff," but the majority, 63 percent, said they would not. See Fogel, 1987, p. 20.

[101] For a discussion of inpatient treatment, see Arnold, 1985, pp. 241–261.

[102] According to the VA, the center was

> organized to facilitate rapid translation of science into practice, ensuring that the latest research findings inform clinical care; and translation of practice into science, and ensuring that questions raised by clinical challenges are addressed using rigorous experimental protocols. (National Center for PTSD, undated)

How Extensive Was PTSD Among Vietnam Veterans?

When the vet centers were first established, it was hoped that they would be a temporary measure that could address the problem and then be closed. Rather than seeing an initial surge and then a falloff of new clients, veterans kept coming, so Congress reauthorized the program in 1981 for an additional two years. In 1983, ten years after American troops left Vietnam (and 15 years after the first large numbers of troops were deployed), Congress again reauthorized the program, but this time wanted to know, once and for all, whether PTSD was a transitory problem that would eventually come to an end or whether it would require a continuing, long-term commitment. Accordingly, to determine the "prevalence, incidence, and effects of PTSD,"[103] the VA hired a research team lead by the Research Triangle Institute (RTI) in September 1984 to undertake the NVVRS.

The timing of the study was judicious because the publication of DSM-III in 1980 offered a definitive diagnosis of a specific psychiatric disorder that allowed the team to apply very specific criteria to determine whether a veteran was suffering from PTSD.[104] Also, Washington University in St. Louis had recently developed a new survey technique, the Diagnostic Interview Schedule, "to detect specific mental disorders gleaned from interviews conducted by survey research interviewers, rather than by mental health professionals" (Kulka et al., 1990, p. xxv).

In 1988, the RTI team reported its results. Like the Egendorf study (Egendorf et al., 1981) almost a decade before, RTI found that "the majority of Vietnam theater veterans had made a successful reentry into civilian life and currently experience few symptoms of PTSD or other readjustment problems" (Kulka et al., 1988, p. 1). However, this study was the first to be able to give definitive estimates of the extent of PTSD in the Vietnam population:

- NVVRS findings indicate that 15.2 percent of all male Vietnam theater veterans are current cases of PTSD. This represents about 479,000 of the estimated 3.14 million men who served in the Vietnam theater. Among Vietnam veteran women, current PTSD prevalence is estimated to be 8.5 percent of the approximately 7,200 women who served, or about 610 current cases. . . .

---

[103] The study also needed to "be of sufficient size, scope complexity and design to provide national estimates of the extent of Vietnam veterans' mental health and other health needs. The study also needed to permit sophisticated analysis of the nature scope, covariation, and etiology of Vietnam veterans' readjustment difficulties" (Kulka et al., 1990, p. 6).

[104] The study actually used the definition of PTSD that was eventually incorporated into DSM-III-R and published by the American Psychiatric Association in 1987. DSM-III-R described PTSD as a syndrome characterized by

> four major criteria: (1) the occurrence of an event that is "outside the range of usual human experience and that would be markedly distressing to almost everyone"; (2) persistent, intrusive and distressing re-experiencing of that event; (3) persistent avoidance of stimuli associated with the event; and (4) persistent symptoms of increased arousal, . . . [e.g.,] difficulty falling or staying asleep, irritability or outbursts of anger. (Kulka et al., 1990, pp. 32–33)

- An additional 11.1 percent of male theater veterans and 7.8 percent of female theater veterans—350,000 additional men and women—currently suffer from "partial PTSD." That is, they have clinically-significant stress reaction symptoms of insufficient intensity or breadth to qualify as full PTSD, but may still warrant professional attention.
- NVVRS analyses of the *lifetime* prevalence of PTSD indicates over one-third (30.6 percent) of male Vietnam theater veterans (over 960,000 men) and over one-fourth (26.9 percent) of women serving in the Vietnam theater (over 1,900 women) had the full-blown disorder at some time during their lives. Thus, about one-half of the men and one-third of the women who have ever had PTSD *still* have it today. . . .
- The prevalence of PTSD and other postwar psychological problems is significantly, and often dramatically, higher among those with high levels of exposure to combat and other war-zone stressors in Vietnam . . . .
- . . . PTSD has a substantial negative impact not only on veterans' own lives, but also on the lives of spouses, children, and others living with such veterans.
- . . . Such veterans have also made greater use of mental health services in general, both from the VA and from other sources . . . . Nevertheless, very substantial proportions of Vietnam veterans with adjustment problems have *never* used the VA or any other source for their mental problems. (Kulka et al., 1988, pp. 1–4, emphasis in the original)[105]

The RTI study team answered the question Congress had posed: PTSD was "a chronic, rather than an acute disorder" (Kulka et al., 1990, p. xxviii). In 2014, 25 years after the initial NVVRS results were published, that answer was reiterated by a follow-up assessment covering approximately 80 percent of those who had participated in the original NVVRS: "PTSD is not going away. It is chronic and prolonged, and for Veterans with PTSD, the war is not over" (Abt Associates, 2014).

The reassessment, now called the National Vietnam Veterans Longitudinal Study (NVVLS), was conducted by Langone Medical Center Department of Psychiatry at New York University and Abt Associates. Their initial results seemed to echo those reported after World War II,[106] that for most with PTSD, the impact on their lives

---

[105] Kulka's report that "substantial proportions of Vietnam veterans with adjustment problems" had never used the VA (Kulka et al., 1990, p. xxvii) was consistent with what was reported after World War II. While there was no recognition of PTSD per se at that time, the National Research Council did study soldiers who had been diagnosed with psychoneurotic disorders during their service in 1944 and were followed after the war. The study found that "treatment had been obtained through the VA by [only] 11 percent of the men . . . [although] about 40 percent . . . were drawing VA compensation for psychiatric disability" (Brill and Beebe, 1955, pp. 135–136). This suggests that the VA never saw the vast majority of veterans with some degree of neuropsychiatric impairment; even then, the VA at the time had all that it could handle treating those who did seek its help.

[106] The National Research Council 1955 follow-up study also found "there is no evidence that treatment played an important role in the general improvement which occurred between separation and follow-up" (Brill and Beebe, 1955, p. 135).

did not get better or worse as time progressed, regardless of whether they received treatment. The Langone-Abt team reported that only 4.6 percent of the PTSD cases reported a decrease in symptoms, while 13 percent reported substantial increases. Furthermore, it had been reported in 1988 that PTSD was connected to other negative health outcomes—e.g., "Vietnam theater veterans with service connected disabilities were almost 50 percent more likely than those without [service-connected disabilities] to have PTSD" (Kulka et al., 1988, p. 15)—but it was now reported that those with PTSD had "greater risk of heart disease and other chronic diseases and . . . a nearly two times higher risk of death than Veterans not suffering with PTSD" (Abt Associates, 2014), even after accounting for demographic factors, such as sex and ethnicity. The VA also reported that "PTSD was associated with increased mortality due to cancer and external causes of death" (DVA, Office of Research and Development, undated).

Another View on the Prevalence of PTSD

Another view on the prevalence of PTSD comes from Israel and the work of Zahava Solomon. Her important contribution comes from a unique study that carefully matched soldiers who had participated in the war in Lebanon in 1982; her subjects all came from the same units and, to the extent possible, had been exposed to the same wartime conditions. They included soldiers who had broken down in combat—had shown signs of combat stress at the time of the campaign—and those who had not. Armed with the American Psychiatric Association's new definition of PTSD, as published in DSM-III,[107] she and her colleagues at the Israel Defense Force Medical Corps and Tel Aviv University constructed a 13-item inventory of PTSD symptoms. The responses to the inventory were grouped into three categories, corresponding to the criteria of DSM-III diagnosis of PTSD: " (a) re-experiencing of the trauma, (b) numbing of responsiveness, and (c) a combination of miscellaneous symptoms" (Solomon, 1993, pp. 55–56). Figure 5.25 presents the results.

Solomon found that, while the differences between the combat stress group and the non–combat stress group were significant, both groups showed substantial rates of PTSD but that these rates declined over time. Not reflected in the summary presentation depicted in Figure 5.25 was the fact that there was some fluctuation in the composition of the group with PTSD; not everyone with PTSD had it for all three years of the study. Among the combat stress group, 28 percent had PTSD for all three years, while only 3 percent of non-CSR had PTSD all three years.[108] Moreover, 75 percent of the group with combat stress had some PTSD during the three years of the study, compared with only 28 percent for the group without combat stress.

---

[107] She found that, "since the publication of DSM-III, clear criteria have been available for the diagnosis of PTSD. Its uniform definition permits, for the first time, meaningful comparison of data gathered by different researchers and clinicians" (Solomon, 1993, p. 55).

[108] For a more complete discussion of the results, see Solomon, 1993, Ch. 5, and Solomon, Benbenishty, and Mikulincer, 1988.

Figure 5.25
Percentage of Israeli Soldiers Diagnosed with PTSD with Combat Stress Reaction During the Lebanon War of 1982 and by Time Since the War

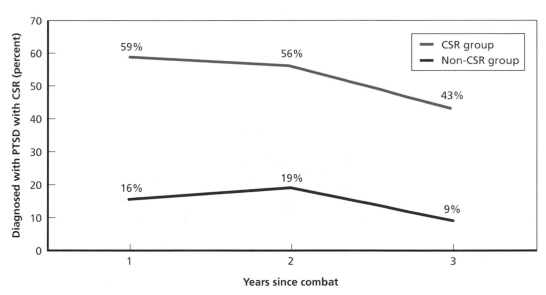

SOURCE: Solomon, 1993, p. 57.

In 1987, Solomon and her colleagues asked whether delayed PTSD was real.[109] Looking at a sample of 150 cases of veterans who had sought help between six months and five years after their active service in summer 1982, she found that true delayed onset PTSD was "quite rare," amounting to about 10 percent of those who asked for help. However, 33 percent of her sample consisted of veterans whose subclinical symptoms had become progressively worse who had now sought help and been diagnosed with full PTSD. A somewhat larger group, 40 percent of her sample, had had full-blown clinical PTSD all along but had lived with it and now sought help. She found that another 13 percent of those who had asked for help after the war could trace their PTSD to combat stress in previous engagements and 4 percent to other causes.

With the psychiatric community's acceptance of PTSD in the late 1970s, Solomon's work provides a perspective on the future, and a critique of the past, for the nature of combat and PTSD as an enduring consequence of war:

> Combat stress reaction, often followed by a lifetime of posttrauma, is the psychological price that some soldiers pay for the proclivity of the human race for war. The price is high, and it is also inevitable. There is no way that men can kill and maim, see their friends killed and maimed, and fear being killed or maimed themselves without at least some of them breaking down. The best way to prevent combat-induced psycho-pathology is to stop making war. (Solomon, 1993, p. 256)

---

[109]The question is posed as the title of Solomon, 1993, Ch. 13.

Agent Orange

In 1977, it may have seemed that the emerging consensus about PTSD might calm the troubled waters between Vietnam veterans and the VA. But a new tempest was brewing as the first lawsuit alleging damages stemming from the use of and exposure to an herbicide known as *Agent Orange* was filed in federal court (see Hansen, 1981, p. 29). The VA was receiving the first of what would eventually be thousands of claims that illness and disabilities had been caused by exposure to Agent Orange. By the end of June 1985, the VA had examined some 200,000 Vietnam veterans to determine whether they were being adversely affected by exposure to the herbicide (Bowsher, 1986, p. 2). The controversy continues to this day.[110]

The Use of Agent Orange in Vietnam

Between 1962 and 1971, and especially after 1967, U.S. military forces sprayed nearly 19 million gallons of herbicides in Vietnam to strip the jungle canopy, destroy the enemy's crops, and clear tall grass and bushes from around U.S. positions.[111] Agent Orange accounted for approximately 60 percent of herbicide sprayed (see Table 5.9). It was mainly applied from airplanes and helicopters but also from boats and ground vehicles, and some was even applied by soldiers wearing back-mounted sprayers. Figure 5.26 shows an aerial application in progress.

Agent Orange is a 50-50 mixture of two biodegradable phenoxy acids (2,4,5-T and 2,4-D) that, individually, were used as agricultural herbicides. These components were initially thought to be relatively benign,[112] but by 1969, they had been "reported

---

[110] In late 2014, the Congressional Research Service reported that,

> [n]early 40 years after the American military presence in Vietnam ended, the controversy surrounding Agent Orange and its possible association with various illnesses of Vietnam veterans and their offspring continues unabated. In general, no other presumption of service connection has had so many congressional hearings, or has been so extensively studied and debated as has establishment of presumption of service connection for diseases associated with exposure to Agent Orange. (Panangala, Shedd, and Moulta-Ali, 2014, p. 9)

[111] In a 1994 report, the Institute of Medicine (IOM) summed up the use of Agent Orange:

> The military use of herbicides in Vietnam began in 1962, was expanded during 1965 and 1966, and reached a peak from 1967 to 1969. Herbicides were used extensively in Vietnam by the U.S. Air Force's Operation Ranch Hand to defoliate inland hardwood forests, coastal mangrove forests, and, to a lesser extent, cultivated land, by aerial spraying from C-123 aircraft and helicopters. Soldiers also sprayed herbicides on the ground to defoliate the perimeters of base camps and fire bases; this spraying was executed from the rear of trucks and from spray units mounted on the backs of soldiers on foot. Navy riverboats also sprayed herbicides along riverbanks. The purpose of spraying herbicides was to improve the ability to detect enemy base camps and enemy forces along lines of communication and infiltration routes, and around U.S. base camps and fire bases. Spraying was also used to destroy the crops of the Vietcong and North Vietnamese. (Committee to Review the Health Effects in Vietnam Veterans of Exposure to Herbicides, 1994, p. 24)

[112] The development of herbicides dates back to the 1890s, but field tests date to the early 1940s. In 1948, the Department of Agriculture approved one component of Agent Orange, 2,4,5-T. It was inexpensive to produce and easy to apply. By the early 1970s, it was "the most widely used herbicide in the United States" (Committee to Review the Health Effects in Vietnam Veterans of Exposure to Herbicides, 1994, p. 35). The results of numerous tests on animals and on men who had been exposed, either while producing the 2,4,5-T and 2,4-D or as

Table 5.9
Application of Herbicides in the Vietnam War, by Year

Agent	Millions of Gallons Applied per Year								
	1962–July 1965	Aug–Dec 1965	1966	1967	1968	1969	1970	1971	Total
Orange	—[a]	0.37	1.64	3.17	2.22	3.25	0.57	0.00	11.22
White	—[a]	0.00	0.53	1.33	2.13	1.02	0.22	0.01	5.24
Blue	—[a]	0.00	0.02	0.38	0.28	0.26	0.18	0.00	1.12
Total	1.27[a]	0.37	2.19	4.88	4.63	4.53	0.97	0.01	18.85[b]

SOURCE: Committee on the Effects of Herbicides in Vietnam, 1974, p. S-3.

NOTE: A number of herbicides were used in Vietnam. These were identified by color-coded names—Orange, White, Blue, Purple, Pink, and Green—taken from the color the band around the 55-gallon drums that contained the chemicals. The defoliation program used Agents Orange, White, and Blue from early 1966 to 1970 but only Agents White and Blue in 1970 and 1971. Agent Orange was the most extensively used herbicide (Committee to Review the Health Effects in Vietnam Veterans of Exposure to Herbicides, 1994, p. 27). For a more complete discussion of herbicides used in Vietnam, see Committee on the Effects of Herbicides in Vietnam, 1974, pp. II-3 to II-10.

[a] Amounts making up the total unavailable.

[b] Overall total includes the 1.27 from the first column.

to produce birth defects in laboratory animals" (Committee on the Effects of Herbicides in Vietnam, 1974, p. S-4).[113] The use of Agent Orange was suspended the following year (see Table 5.9). What was of great concern to the scientific community was the realization that, as an unavoidable by-product of its manufacture, Agent Orange was inherently contaminated with a highly toxic chemical, dioxin (also known as 2,3,7,8-Tetrachlorodibenzodioxin [TCDD]).

Dioxin

The amount of dioxin found in Agent Orange depended on the manufacturing process, with different manufacturers producing different concentrations. After the war, the levels of dioxin found in samples of Agent Orange were up to 1,000 times higher than

---

farmworkers using the herbicides, are summarized in Committee on the Effects of Herbicides in Vietnam, 1974, pp. II-22 to II-33. The committee compared these herbicides with

> a number of other chemicals. The two herbicides [the main components of Agent Orange] . . . are compounds which are distinctly toxic but which must be consumed in quite substantial quantities to have any overt effect. They are clearly much less toxic than well-known poisons such as strychnine and arsenic. (Committee on the Effects of Herbicides in Vietnam, 1974, II-31)

[113] In 1965, the National Cancer Institute contracted with Bionetics Research Laboratory in Maryland to investigate the possible effects of a number of pesticides and herbicides. The study released in 1969 found that a component of Agent Orange caused malformations and stillbirths in mice when administered in high doses. Bionetics later reanalyzed data used for its initial study and revealed that the cause of toxicity was the contaminant dioxin (Committee to Review the Health Effects in Vietnam Veterans of Exposure to Herbicides, 1994, p. 30).

Figure 5.26
Operation Ranch Hand: UC-123 Special Aerial Spray Missions

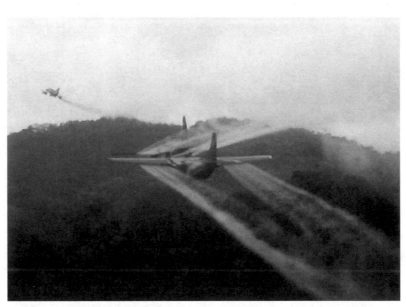

SOURCE: U.S. Air Force photo.

those found in herbicides for domestic use in the United States.[114] However, awareness of the extreme toxicity of dioxin dates only to the early 1970s,[115] with extensive epidemiological, environmental, and case-controlled studies starting in the mid-1970s.[116] At that point, when the claims about Agent Orange started to draw national attention in the late 1970s, the VA recognized only disability claims related to chloracne, a skin disease resembling severe acne. All other claims were rejected. A comprehensive list of health outcomes became available only when the IOM, part of the National Academy of Sciences (NAS), published *Veterans and Agent Orange: Health Effects of Herbicides Used in Vietnam* (Committee to Review the Health Effects in Vietnam Veterans

---

[114] Analysis of samples of Agent Orange available after the war tested dioxin levels as high as almost 50 ppm and averaging 1.98 and 2.99 ppm. Domestic manufacturing standards at the time required dioxin levels to be less than 0.05 ppm (Committee to Review the Health Effects in Vietnam Veterans of Exposure to Herbicides, 1994, p. 91).

[115] As the committee reported,

> [t]he public became aware of the potential health effects of exposure to TCDD in tandem with the increased concern over possible health effects of exposure to herbicides sprayed in Vietnam. As studies were completed that demonstrated the toxicity of TCDD in animals, scientists began to realize that numerous individuals may have been exposed to TCDD. (Committee to Review the Health Effects in Vietnam Veterans of Exposure to Herbicides, 1994, p. 36)

[116] See Chs. 8 and 9 of Committee to Review the Health Effects in Vietnam Veterans of Exposure to Herbicides, 1994, pp. 300–590.

of Exposure to Herbicides, 1994). The list has been reassessed biannually since then (National Academies of Sciences, Engineering, and Medicine, 2016). Drawing on evidence from occupational, environmental, and case-controlled studies of exposure to a variety of herbicides and herbicide components, the review committee allocated particular health outcomes to categories of relative certainty of association (see Box 5.1).

Veterans and the Institute of Medicine Connect Agent Orange with Cancer

Groups of scientists, including the Federation of American Scientists and the American Association for the Advancement of Science, had expressed concerns when herbicides were first employed in Vietnam in the 1960s. But it took seven years after Agent Orange's last use in 1970 for veterans to first suspect that the herbicide might be the cause of the cancers they were having. In 1977, Maude deVictor, a benefits counselor in the Chicago VA regional office, started to research the possible link between cancer and Agent Orange after the VA denied a claim by the widow of a Vietnam veteran who had died of cancer. To the great consternation of the VA, her research found its way into a local television documentary, *Agent Orange, the Deadly Fog*, which aired on March 23, 1978, with follow-on national media coverage (see Schuck, 1986, p. 23). For Paul Reutershan, another Vietnam veteran dying of cancer, the account rang true. Eventually, before his death, he founded Agent Orange Victims International and initiated a lawsuit against the manufacturers of Agent Orange. A month after his death, his lawsuit was taken over by a class-action lawsuit filed in U.S. federal court.[117]

In May 1984, the suit against the manufacturers of Agent Orange was settled for $180 million. However, because the case never went to trial, "no causal relationship was ever established between the alleged health effects in Vietnam veterans and their exposure to Agent Orange" (Committee to Review the Health Effects in Vietnam Veterans of Exposure to Herbicides, 1994, p. 35).

The Federal Government's Response to the Concerns of the Public

In April 1970, the Senate Committee on Commerce, with oversight on the environment, was the first congressional committee to hold what would be scores of hearings related to the use and health effects of herbicides employed in Vietnam.[118] The following November, Congress passed Pub. L. 91-441, which led to a NAS study, *The Effects of Herbicides in South Vietnam*. NAS mainly focused on the environmental effects of herbicide use but did report that it was "unable to gather any definitive indication of direct damage by herbicides to human health" (Committee on the Effects of Herbicides in Vietnam, 1974, p. x).

---

[117] In September 1978, attorney Edward Gorman filed a $10 million damage suit against Dow Chemical and two other manufacturers of Agent Orange on behalf of Paul Reutershan, a Vietnam veteran stricken with cancer. Reutershan died of abdominal cancer on December 14, 1978 (Nicosia, 2001, p. 434). Veterans of the Vietnam War and the Veterans Coalition, undated, provides a timeline of these legal actions.

[118] Committee on the Effects of Herbicides in Vietnam, 1974, pp. 48–49, Table 2-1, provides a list of hearings on Agent Orange and dioxin.

Box 5.1
Summary of Findings of Associations Between Exposure to Herbicides and Specific Health Outcomes

Sufficient Evidence of an Association

- Soft-tissue sarcoma (including heart)
- Non-Hodgkin's lymphoma
- Chronic lymphocytic leukemia (including hairy cell leukemia and other chronic B-cell leukemias)
- Hodgkin's lymphoma
- Chloracne

Limited or Suggestive Evidence of an Association

- Laryngeal cancer
- Cancer of the lung, bronchus, or trachea
- Prostate cancer
- Multiple myeloma
- Amyloid light-chain amyloidosis
- Early-onset peripheral neuropathy
- Parkinson's disease
- Porphyria cutanea tarda
- Hypertension
- Ischemic heart disease
- Stroke (category change from update 2010)
- Type 2 diabetes (mellitus)
- Spina bifida in offspring of exposed people

Inadequate or Insufficient Evidence to Determine an Association

- Esophageal cancer
- Stomach cancer
- Colorectal cancer (including small intestine and anus)
- Hepatobiliary cancers (liver, gallbladder, and bile ducts)
- Pancreatic cancer
- Bone and joint cancer
- Melanoma
- Nonmelanoma skin cancer (basal cell and squamous cell)
- Breast cancer
- Cancers of reproductive organs (cervix, uterus, ovary, testes, and penis; excluding prostate)
- Urinary bladder cancer
- Renal cancer (kidney and renal pelvis)
- Cancers of brain and nervous system (including eye)
- Endocrine cancers (thyroid, thymus, and other endocrine organs)
- Leukemia (other than chronic B-cell leukemias, including chronic lymphocytic leukemia and hairy cell leukemia)
- Cancers at other and unspecified sites
- Infertility
- Spontaneous abortion (other than after paternal exposure to TCDD, which appears not to be associated)
- Neonatal or infant death and stillbirth in offspring of exposed people
- Childhood cancer (including acute myeloid leukemia) in offspring of exposed people
- Neurobehavioral disorders (cognitive and neuropsychiatric)
- Neurodegenerative diseases, excluding Parkinson's disease
- Chronic peripheral nervous system disorders
- Hearing loss
- Respiratory disorders (wheeze or asthma, chronic obstructive pulmonary disease, and farmer's lung)
- Gastrointestinal, metabolic, and digestive disorders (changes in hepatic enzymes, lipid abnormalities, and ulcers)
- Immune system disorders (immune suppression, allergy, and autoimmunity)
- Circulatory disorders (other than hypertension, ischemic heart disease, and stroke)
- Endometriosis
- Disruption of thyroid homeostasis
- Eye problems
- Bone conditions

SOURCE: Committee to Review the Health Effects in Vietnam Veterans of Exposure to Herbicides, 2014, p. 8-10.

The VA initially met the claims of a variety of negative health outcomes associated with the use of Agent Orange with skepticism. The 1974 NAS report had not made a case for an association between exposure and negative health outcomes. Moreover, claims were hard to verify because there was no way to definitively determine which veterans had actually been exposed.[119] Even for the relatively few who had actually handled Agent Orange, there was no way to determine the extent of the exposure, especially exposure to dioxin, because it was not consistently found in samples of Agent Orange.[120] Nevertheless, in 1978, to calm fears that many veterans had that their health may have been compromised by exposure to Agent Orange, the VA initiated a program to provide any veteran who wanted it a comprehensive physical examination and an opportunity to record self-reported possible exposures while serving in Vietnam. The objectives of the program, however, were very limited, and its execution was uneven.[121] This added to, rather than ameliorated, the frustration Vietnam veterans felt in dealing with the VA.[122]

---

[119] The Comptroller General found that a

> large number of U.S. Army and Marine Corps ground troops were in and close to sprayed areas during and shortly after spraying. The names and last known addresses of marines assigned to these units can be identified. However, Army personnel cannot be identified because Army records are incomplete. At that time, the Department of Defense (DOD) did not consider herbicide orange toxic or dangerous to humans and took few precautions to prevent exposure to it. (Comptroller General of the United States, 1979, p. 1)

[120] In 1982, the Air Force initiated a longitudinal study of the almost 1,200 Air Force personnel who were part of the Ranch Hand program and sprayed herbicides from the air in Vietnam. They were compared with about 1,800 Air Force personnel who were not involved in the spraying and who were matched to the Ranch Hands in terms of age, race, and military occupation. The study itself became controversial as veterans' groups "alleged that government officials delayed and withheld information on the study's findings, improperly influenced the study's design and implementation, and failed to provide adequate veterans' representation on the Advisory Committee" (GAO, 1999, p. 4). In 1996, birth defects among the offspring of veterans who served in Operation Ranch Hand were a factor in the IOM placing spina bifida on the list of health outcomes for which there was "limited or suggestive evidence" of an association (Rivera, 2014, p. 22; GAO, 1999, p. 21).

[121] According to GAO, managers of the VA Agent Orange Registry said that, because the program was voluntary, the registry could not be

> viewed as being representative of Vietnam veterans as a whole and cannot be used as an epidemiological tool or to make statistically valid comparisons with other groups. According to VA, the registry's purposes are to
> - identify veterans concerned about the possible health effects of exposure to agent orange in Vietnam,
> - permit VA to contact veterans to provide further information or for further testing,
> - provide a means of detecting veterans' specific health problems in the event unusual health trends show up in the veterans, and
> - describe the characteristics of veterans in the registry. (Baine, 1986, p. 28)

For further discussion of the many problems, see Baine, 1986.

[122] Four years after the registry program was started and after almost 90,000 Vietnam veterans had been examined, the Comptroller General reported that about 55 percent of the veterans responding to a questionnaire

> were dissatisfied with their agent orange examination. Generally, veterans complained that
> - their examinations were not thorough,
> - VA provided them little or no information on the potential health effects of exposure to agent orange,
> - VA personnel did not show enough interest in their health, and
> - they did not get an examination as soon as they wanted. (Comptroller General of the United States, 1982, p. i)

Although the examinations were more thorough than veterans perceived, GAO's evaluation of the examination programs at 14 of the VA's 178 medical facilities generally confirmed veterans' complaints.

Fearful of opening the government up a wide range of health claims, the VA took a conservative stand. In May 1978, the administrator instructed that, when veterans thought they might have a problem because of exposure to Agent Orange, his staff should take detailed medical histories of any "symptoms and signs which are not explicable in terms of definable diseases in terms well-known medical entities, . . . [including] such details the veteran man may remember concerning his exposure to defoliant agents" (Cleland, 1978). The staff, however, was also admonished that,

> [i]n view of the remaining uncertainties on the long-term effects of the defoliants, all VA personnel should avoid premature commitment to any diagnosis of defoliant poisoning. Similarly, entries in medical records should not contain statements about the relationship between a veteran's illnesses and defoliant exposure unless unequivocal confirmation of such connection has been established. (Cleland, 1978)

In 1980, the VA administrator went even further, telling Congress that,

> [u]nless or until some such latent effects of Agent Orange or its derivative components are scientifically documented, there are intrinsic limitations to VA's authority to allow these [Agent Orange] claims under current law. Though I cannot emphasize enough our policy to resolve reasonable doubt as to service incurrence of disabilities in favor of claimants, there is currently no medical basis upon which adverse health effects of late-post-exposure onset can be reasonably tied to Agent Orange. (Cleland, 1980, p. 11)

The VA's position notwithstanding, and despite repeated requests from Congress for the VA and, later, the Center for Centers for Disease Control and Prevention to conduct an epidemiological study of the health effects of exposure to Agent Orange,[123] Congress eventually took matters into its own hands. On November 3, 1981, the Veterans' Health Care, Training, and Small Business Loan Act (Pub. L. 97-72) became law. Congress clearly intended to give veterans the benefit of the doubt. Even though the government did not acknowledge a link between Agent Orange and diseases, with the exception of chloracne, the act instructed the VA to recognize a veteran's own report of exposure as sufficient proof to receive medical care, absent specific evidence to the

---

[123]In fact, numerous government agencies have studied Agent Orange, including the White House, Office of Technology Assessment, GAO, Department of the Air Force, Centers for Disease Control, Environmental Protection Agency, National Research Council, IOM, and the VA (Committee to Review the Health Effects in Vietnam Veterans of Exposure to Herbicides, 1994, pp. 45–63). However, the many methodological problems have frustrated attempts to undertake a full epidemiological study of Vietnam veterans and Agent Orange, as reported to Congress as early as 1981 (Peterson, 1981) and summarized by GAO in 1990 (GAO, 1990).

contrary.[124] In 1996, Congress clarified this access by passing the Veterans' Health Care Eligibility Reform Act (Pub. L. 104-262); thereafter, "a veteran does not have to demonstrate a link between a certain health condition and exposure to Agent Orange; instead, medical care is provided unless the VA determines that the condition did not result from exposure to Agent Orange" (Panangala and Shedd, 2014, summary).

Access to health care was one thing, but monetary payments to compensate for disabilities caused by exposure to Agent Orange were another. One of the VA administrator's objections to the Veterans' Dioxin and Radiation Exposure Compensation Standards Act of 1984 (Pub. L. 98-542) was that it ordered the VA to establish guidelines, standards, and criteria for the resolution of benefit claims and disability compensation but did not provide a presumption of service connection for any specific disease based on exposure to dioxin.[125] Veterans, however, still had to "provide proof of a service connection that established the link between herbicide exposure and disease onset" (Panangala and Shedd, 2014, p. 5). It was expected that the regulations would reflect the intent of Congress that the VA grant "claimants the benefit of the doubt when there is an approximate balance of positive and negative evidence regarding any issue material to resolution of a claim" (DVA, 1993, p. 68). However, this was not what happened, and the regulations were soon being litigated.

In *Nehmer v. U.S. Veterans' Administration* (1989), the U.S. District Court for the Northern District of California found that the VA's "cause and effect" standard for determining which diseases would qualify was too stringent. The court said that the VA should use a more lenient "significant statistical association" standard and ordered the VA to reconsider thousands of claims it had rejected. With the court ruling in hand and to clarify the issue, Congress passed the Agent Orange Act (Pub. L. 102-4) in 1991, which established in law a presumption of service connection when a positive statistical association exists between Agent Orange exposure and the occurrence of a disease.[126] At the time, Pub. L. 102-4 was described as a "historic compromise" between two competing factions in Congress. The view from the Senate side of Capital

---

[124]Before the passage of Pub. L. 97-72, veterans who complained of Agent Orange–related illnesses had the lowest priority for VA treatment because their illnesses were not considered to be service connected. The new law instructed the VA to give priority status based on a veteran's own report of exposure unless there was evidence to the contrary.

[125]The VA Administrator told Congress,

> The compensation program must be attuned to justifiable conclusions about the connection between Agent Orange exposure and disorders possibly arising from that exposure. At the same time we must do our best to avoid taking steps that have the potential for undermining the program's credibility and legitimacy because of inconclusive scientific evidence. . . . In view of the current state of scientific findings, enactment [of H.R. 1961] would compromise the integrity of the compensation program. (as quoted in Panangala, Shedd, and Moulta-Ali, 2014, p. 12)

[126]It should be noted that medical conditions associated with Agent Orange were not the only ones for which such a presumption of service connection was made. For example, Pub. L. 98-223, 1984, clarified a presumption concerning depressive neurosis for former POWs (DVA, 1993, p. 55).

Hill was that there was a "sizable and growing body of scientific evidence suggest[ing] that exposure to agent orange is associated with the development of various diseases in Vietnam veterans," while the view from the House side was that "exposure to herbicides in Vietnam is not responsible for the health effects now experienced by Vietnam veterans" (as quoted in DVA, 1993, p. 74). The law gave responsibility for reviewing the scientific literature on the association between herbicide exposure during Vietnam and health outcomes exclusively to the IOM. Congress intended that an "independent scientific organization will make independent scientific judgments and recommendations, while the policymaker—the Secretary—will make the policy decision that determines whether VA must establish a presumption of service connection" (as quoted in DVA, 1993, p. 74).

Given the acrimonious history of relations between the VA and veterans over the issue of Agent Orange, one might suspect that it would not be so simple for an ill veteran who had served in the Republic of Vietnam between January 9, 1962, and May 7, 1975, and had a disease determined to be associated with exposure to Agent Orange to receive disability compensation. Soon, veterans and the VA were back in court, litigating the meaning of "served in the Republic of Vietnam." For the VA, the term referred only to veterans who had actually set foot on the landmass or served in the inland waterways of Vietnam; for example, the presumption of exposure would not extend to those who had served aboard ships off the coast of Vietnam. Eventually, the federal courts sided with the VA, requiring those who served offshore to prove they had actually been exposed to Agent Orange.[127] Table 5.10 lays out the extensive use of the presumptions of exposure to Agent Orange to qualify for VA's disability compensation for a number of conditions, the diseases covered, and the severity of disability ratings. The actual cash payments a veteran receives, however, vary by the percentage of disability.[128]

The Presumption of Service Connection

Providing medical services and disability compensation based on a presumption of service connection was key to achieving a semblance of peace between Vietnam veterans and the VA, as it would again be when it came to veterans' claims concerning unexplained illnesses associated with service in Kuwait and Iraq during the Gulf War of 1991–1992.[129] The presumption of a service connection, first used in 1921, relieves

---

[127] See the discussion of blue-water veteran litigation in Panangala and Shedd, 2014, pp. 9–11.

[128] In 2016, disability payments ranged from $130 per month for a 10-percent disability, $822 per month for a 50-percent disability, and $1,714 for a 90-percent disability. The payment for a 100-percent disability was $2,585 per month (DVA, 2016b).

[129] According to an IOM report,

> The Gulf War presumption process was heavily influenced by the Agent Orange presumption history. . . . The history of the government's sluggish response to radiation and herbicide exposure concerns played a role in the establishment of Congress' Gulf War presumptions for undiagnosed illnesses and chronic multisymptom ill-

Table 5.10
Presumptions in VA's Disability Program for Herbicide Agents

Condition	Number of Veterans	Disability Severity Rating
Type II diabetes	197,000	Most are 10% and 20%
Prostate cancer	30,000	One-third at 100%, average 40%
Respiratory cancer	5,000	One-half at 100%
Non-Hodgkin's and Hodgkin's lymphoma	5,000	One-half at 100%, balance at 50%

SOURCE: Samet and Bodurow, 2008, p. 62.

veterans of the burden to prove that a disability or illness was caused by a specific exposure and often contains a specified period for which the presumption would be in force and a threshold level of disability.[130] Presumptions have resulted from both regulatory and legislative action. According to the VA,

> [p]resumptions were enacted into law in response to difficulties veterans experienced with their claims for service connection. The suggestion that VA base determinations regarding service connection on "sound medical principles," while appearing reasonable, fails to recognize that medical science does not always know the exact cause, the time of onset or the aggravating circumstances of a condition.

> There is no incontrovertible evidence that any of the presumptive conditions could not be aggravated or have the onset precipitated by military service. Likewise, there is no scientific basis for questioning the manifestation periods set by law. (DVA, 1993, p. ii)

> Presumptions play an important role in both the philosophical basis for service connection and in the actual administration of the compensation program. They serve to fill in the holes in scientific and medical knowledge, as well as resolve complex policy questions and simplify determinations of service connection for VA. (DVA, 1993, p. iii)

Congress set the pattern for using the presumption of service connection on August 9, 1921, when it passed the Veterans' Bureau Act (Pub. L. 67-47), which included presumptions of service connection for active pulmonary tuberculosis and

---

ness. Following Congress' experiences with establishing radiation and Agent Orange legislation in the 1980s and early 1990s, Congress did not want to wait to lend aid to the first Gulf War veterans. (Samet and Bodurow, 2008, pp. I-77 to I-78)

[130] For example, VA Technical Bulletin 8-43, dated August 19, 1947, stated that for "malaria and chronic diseases characteristically tropical in origin" the presumption of service connection is authorized "when the disease is shown by satisfactory evidence to have been present to 10 percent disabling degree within one year from date of termination of active wartime service" (DVA, 1993, p. 22).

neuropsychiatric disease. The purpose of the change, according to the senator who proposed it, was to rectify "the sharp and altogether unjustifiable annoyance [in law] requiring the disabled soldier to prove that the disease from which he is suffering was contracted in line of service" (as quoted in DVA, 1993, pp. 6–7).[131] Within a year, the administrator of the Veterans' Bureau extended the presumption of service connection to other "chronic constitutional diseases" manifesting within one year of separation from active service "unless there [is] affirmative evidence to the contrary or evidence establishing that some intercurrent disease or injury which is a recognized cause of the disorder was suffered between the date of separation from service and the onset of the chronic disease" (DVA, 1993, p. 10). Since 1921, nearly 150 health outcomes have been presumed to be service connected.[132]

There are a number of arguments for and against the use of presumptions. Some find that presumptions "simplify and streamline the adjudication process . . . promote accuracy and consistency in adjudications" (Samet and Bodurow, 2008, p. 39). The use of the presumption of service, however, has its critics. As early as 1956, the Bradley Commission, established by President Eisenhower and chaired by the former administrator of the VA, General Bradley, recommended,

> the presumption of service connection for chronic diseases, tropical diseases, psychoses, tuberculosis, and multiple sclerosis as now listed should be withdrawn [because] there is otherwise in the law sufficient protection for the veteran to establish service connection of any and all diseases. (Bradley Commission, 1956a, p. 178)

The veterans' service organizations strongly opposed the elimination of presumptions. The National Commander of Disabled American Veterans called the commission's recommendation "downright ridiculous in the present state of medical knowledge" (as quoted in DVA, 1993, p. 42), and Olin E. Teague, chairman of the House Committee on Veterans' Affairs, explained that "the reason we passed [the presumption statute] was because Congress did not agree with many of the medical findings [of VA doctors]" (as quoted in DVA, 1993, pp. 41–42). Even the VA challenged the very premise of the recommendation of the Bradley Commission, noting that

> [i]t has been suggested in the past that presumptions are not necessary and that they can be eliminated, basing service connection strictly on "sound medical principles." . . . The problem is, however, that the impressive term, "sound medical principles," becomes less impressive upon examination. . . . Studies do not necessarily exist which definitively pinpoint the inception or even the cause of the

---

[131] Senator David Walsh (D-Massachusetts) also said, "In my opinion, that provision of the law which places the burden upon the disabled veteran of connecting his disease with his service has been responsible for more complaints, dissatisfaction, and disappointment . . . than any other single provision" (as quoted in DVA, 1993, p. 7).

[132] For a review of the history of presumptions of service connection, see DVA, 1993.

chronic conditions for which presumptive service connection is established. (DVA, 1993, pp. 95–96)

Over time, however, the use of presumptions has remained controversial, particularly as it has been extended to distinct groups of veterans—veterans exposed to radiation from aboveground nuclear tests and the atomic bombs detonated in Japan; POWs from World War II, the Korean War, or the Vietnam War who suffered from dietary deficiencies, forced labor, or inhumane treatment; Vietnam veterans serving on the Vietnam mainland, for Agent Orange exposure; environmental presumptions for Gulf War veterans with medical signs and symptoms that cannot be explained or diagnosed; and veterans of the wars in Afghanistan. In 2006, the Veterans' Disability Benefits Commission asked the IOM whether there was a better way to make these determinations. The commission expressed its concern about the current system this way:

> Leaving aside questions of the possible effect of psychic injuries inflicted by war . . . , it seems that science cannot easily or quickly resolve . . . issues particularly where (1) chemical/radiation exposure levels are often unknowable or difficult to ascertain and (2) the effect of exposure on diseases experienced is scientifically unsettled.
>
> Notwithstanding this uncertainty, the intense emotions surrounding those genuinely suffering and the perceived unfairness of forcing veterans to "prove" the environments or places where they served related to their possible exposure has led Congress and the Executive Branch to create presumptions. Certain studies (not even necessarily involving veterans), for example, showing that those exposed to dioxin have slightly higher rates of diabetes or prostate cancer, have resulted in an inexorable push to compensate all veterans with diabetes/prostate cancer even if it is likely that dioxin exposure is a determinative factor in only a small percentage of cases. Since it is impossible to know what role dioxin played in any particular case, all Vietnam veterans with diabetes and prostate cancer have been and are being granted presumptive service connection. Is this presumption fully supported by medical evidence? What amount of increase in occurrence rate is enough to warrant compensation? What approaches could be considered to alleviate this costly result? (Samet and Bodurow, 2008, pp. 341–342)

Harkening back to the same issue that was adjudicated in *Nehmer v. United States Veterans' Administration*, the IOM recommended a four-level classification scheme incorporating a *causal effect standard* rather than, as the commission called it, *the less-precise statistical standard* (Veterans' Disability Benefits Commission, 2007, p. 11).[133] The commission generally endorsed the IOM's recommendation "with a few caveats," saying it was "concerned over the use of causal effect rather than [a statistical] associa-

---

[133] See recommendation 5 in Samet and Bodurow, 2008, p. 333.

tion as the criteria for decision and encourages further exploration" (Veterans' Disability Benefits Commission, 2007, p. 113).

The use of a causal standard or a statistical standard notwithstanding, the process of establishing a presumption of service connection is ultimately political, as the IOM's case study of Gulf War presumptions shows (Samet and Bodurow, 2008, pp. 177–187), which Chapter Six will discuss more fully. Suffice it to say, the IOM argued that,

> [w]hen a presumption of service connection for a disease or health condition is legislated by Congress . . . rather than through the accrual and evaluation of scientific evidence, there is the potential to diminish the credibility of a presumptive decision-making process that is evidence based. A misperception then may arise that the decision was evidence based, even though it was actually driven by other considerations. (Samet and Bodurow, 2008, p. I-83)

Reconsidering the Role of the VA in the Care of Veterans—Again

As noted previously, President Eisenhower established a commission in 1955, under the chairmanship of General Bradley, the former administrator of the VA, to seek principles on which a modern veterans' system could be built. A letter of instruction from President Eisenhower highlighted "the broad social security programs to provide economic assistance to the aged and the needy" that did not exist when the Veteran's Bureau was created after World War I and the fact that "many of our veterans will be able to qualify both for non–service-connected pensions and social security benefits when they reach age 65" (Eisenhower, 1955). A year later, the Bradley Commission reported that the justification for non–service-connected benefits was "weak and their basic philosophy is backward looking rather than constructive. Our society has developed more equitable means of meeting most of the same needs and big strides are being made in closing remaining gaps" (Bradley Commission, 1956a, p. 138).[134] Two decades later, in 1977, the National Research Council attempted to answer the same question President Eisenhower had asked.

The National Research Council reported that, historically,

> VA facilities were justified on the grounds that they were needed to provide care to veterans with service-connected disabilities. Veterans without service-connected disabilities who are eligible for care may receive it only if excess capacity exists after meeting the needs of veterans with service-connected disabilities. The Congress did not provide the capacity to take care of *all* eligible veterans—only those with service-connected disabilities. At present, less than 30% of the patients treated by the VA have service-connected disabilities, and many of them are being treated

---

[134]The Bradley Commission recommended that "non–service-connected benefits should be limited to a minimum level and retained only as a reserve line of honorable protection for veterans whose means are shown to be inadequate and who fail to qualify for basic protection under the general Old-Age and Survivors Insurance system" (Bradley Commission, 1956a, p. 138).

for health problems that are unrelated to their service-connected disabilities. More than 80% of all the medical care provided is for non–service-connected disabilities. . . .

[After World War I,] Congress continued to amend the VA health care eligibility laws to make it easier for veterans without service-connected disabilities to obtain health care from the VA. It also authorized expansion of the range and comprehensiveness of specialized services offered by VA hospitals. . . . (National Research Council, 1977, p. 4, emphasis in the original)

Moreover, with the expansion of third-party hospital insurance coverage and the advent of Medicare and Medicaid, "decisions on resources for the VA health-care system can hardly be discussed responsibly without explicit recognition of these major changes in social conditions and public policy" (National Research Council, 1977, p. 5).

Legacy

If the Korean War was, as historian Clay Blair has suggested (Blair, 1987), the war that Americans forgot, the war in Vietnam may well be the war that Americans wish they could forget. Looking back on the war, historian Robert Timberg said that the "Vietnam War bruised American Society like nothing else in this century. The nation split over the war" (Timberg, 1995). The outward signs of the split were the "draft card burning, campus riots, and violent protest demonstrations of the late 1960s and early 1970s" (U.S. Senate, 1978, p. 50). Besides the legacy of medical advances, the Vietnam War changed our notion of the long-term consequences of combat service with a focus on PTSD, readjustment assistance, and Agent Orange. In addition, the collective guilt of the American people concerning the war and how the soldiers who fought in Vietnam were treated when they returned home resulted in a new appreciation for those who serve and heightened commitment to their long-term care. Finally, the advent of the all-volunteer force, which was fostered as a response to the antidraft, antiwar movement, had a somewhat unexpected result: the professionalization and expansion of the career medical force.

Lessons Learned by the Army Medical Department

The Army Medical Department highlighted eight notable advances in combat care as a result of the Vietnam War, as shown in Box 5.2.

Trauma Care

The publication of (Committee on Trauma and Committee on Shock, 1966) is considered to be the inaugural event in the establishment of trauma care, "a sustained effort sponsored by government to control 'accidental injury'" (Mullins, 1999). The authors

> **Box 5.2**
> **Army Medical Department Advances in Combat Care from the Vietnam War**
>
> General use of helicopters for patient transport
> Monitoring of organ function in theater of operations
> Blood gas measurements
> Serum chemistries
> Portable radiology equipment
> Use of mechanical ventilators in theater of operations
> Effective topical antimicrobial chemotherapy for burns
> Staged intercontinental aeromedical transport of burn patients
> Identification of Acute Respiratory Distress Syndrome
> Established Vietnam Vascular Registry
>
> SOURCES: Murray, Hitter, and Jones, 2016, p. 2; Pruitt, 2008, p. S7.

saw the impact of advances made during the Korean and Vietnam wars as a catalyst for change:

> Expert consultants returning from both Korea and Vietnam have publicly asserted that, if seriously wounded, their chances of survival would be better in the zone of combat than on the average city street. . . . Probably no American community can lay claim to maintenance of a model of first aid, sorting, communication, and transportation comparable to that of the Armed Services. (Committee on Trauma and Committee on Shock, 1966, p. 12)[135]

While such references often lump Korea and Vietnam together, the legacy of each conflict is, in fact, distinct and very different.

As noted earlier in this chapter, in Vietnam, the deployment of forces, the changing technology, and the fluidity of combat operations modified the traditional five-level medical support model even more than the advent of MASH units had during Korean conflict. In Vietnam, while divisions with extensive air ambulance assets, such as the 1st Cavalry Division, continued to adhere to the traditional evacuation model, the divisions that did not have their own organic air ambulances units, such as the 25th Division, followed a different model and evacuated their wounded directly to surgical hospitals using helicopters assigned to and operating from the hospital—what were called Dust Off helicopters. As a result, to a large extent, the MASH units of Korean War, which had brought the skills of the surgeon up to the front line, were no longer needed. Helicopters in Vietnam transported the wounded to physicians working in modern facilities, where teams of medical specialists could deliver outstanding care. Civilian trauma care centers adopted this new model, which was also incorpo-

---

[135] The authors also reported that the

> [e]xcellence of initial first aid, efficiency of transportation, and energetic treatment of military casualties have proved to be major factors in the progressive decrease in death rates of battle casualties reaching medical facilities, from 8 percent in World War I, to 4.5 percent in World War II, to 2.5 percent in Korea, and to less than 2 percent in Vietnam. (Committee on Trauma and Committee on Shock, 1966, p. 12)

rated into the "development of the JTS [Joint Trauma System] over the course of the wars in Afghanistan and Iraq, demonstrating a continual ebb and flow between the two sectors" (Berwick, Downey, and Cornett, 2016, p. 15).

The Long-Term Consequences of War

Unlike previous generations of veterans, Vietnam veterans were in open conflict with the VA, the very agency created to support them, over the long-term health consequences of their service.

PTSD

From the vantage point of the 50th anniversary of Tet offensive in Vietnam, one could argue that the recognition of the long-term psychological consequences of war—PTSD—is Vietnam's most enduring legacy. As highlighted in this chapter, the very acceptance of PTSD as a consequence of war was the result of a bitter intergenerational battle that pitted veterans of World War II against those of the Vietnam conflict and shook the very foundations of the psychiatric profession. In 1970, Vietnam appeared to validate the Army's approach to dealing with soldiers that had problems adjusting to combat.[136] Soon, that assessment would change with the recognition that the Army and the VA needed to "gear themselves to the need for treatment of the large number of emotional problems, ignored or postponed in active duty, but often thrust into prominence upon return" (Bourne, 1972, p. 23, abstract). Accommodating this new reality was particularly difficult for the VA.

Given the creeping escalation of American involvement in Vietnam, the VA was very slow to recognize and accommodate the new generation of veterans. The new veterans were markedly different from the World War II generation that dominated the VA, both as patients and as providers. As a result, the VA resisted the development of programs to meet their needs. Nowhere was this more evident than in the struggle within the VA, and within the psychiatric community, to recognize what was initially called *Vietnam Syndrome*, later *PTSD*. The discussion in this chapter recounts the decade-long battle that finally saw the American Psychiatric Association include a diagnosis of PTSD in DSM-III. With the validation of PTSD, progress was possible and led to the creation of vet centers and the National Center for PTSD.

---

[136] As previously noted, Dr. Peter Bourne, the chief of the neuropsychiatric section, U.S. Army Medical Research Team–Viet Nam, Walter Reed Army Institute of Research wrote,

> Viet Nam experience has shown that we now successfully identified most of the major correlates of psychiatric attrition in the combat zone. . . . As a result, there is reason to be optimistic that psychiatric casualties need never again become a major cause of attrition in the United States military in a combat zone. (Bourne, 1970, p. 487)

Readjustment Assistance

One manifestation of PTSD was problems readjusting to civilian life, such as difficulties in obtaining employment and homelessness. As noted, the role of vet centers has expanded, and the centers today serve more than just Vietnam veterans:

> Vet Centers across the country provide a broad range of counseling, outreach, and referral services to combat Veterans and their families. Vet Centers guide Veterans and their families through many of the major adjustments in lifestyle that often occur after a Veteran returns from combat. Services for a Veteran may include individual and group counseling in areas such as Post-Traumatic Stress Disorder (PTSD), alcohol and drug assessment, and suicide prevention referrals. All services are free of cost and are strictly confidential. (DVA, 2018)

Agent Orange

It was not only the issue of recognizing the validity of a psychiatric reaction—PTSD— that pitted Vietnam veterans against the VA. Claims that some Vietnam veterans were ill and disabled as a result of being exposed to the herbicide known as Agent Orange were also bitterly contested. Unlike with PTSD, however, Congress became heavily involved. With the passage of the Veterans' Health Care, Training and Small Business Loan Act (Pub. L. 97-72) of 1981, Congress gave veterans the benefit of the doubt, while not acknowledging a link between Agent Orange and disease, and instructed the VA to recognize a veteran's own report of exposure to Agent Orange as sufficient proof to receive medical care at a VA facility. A decade later, Congress passed the Agent Orange Act (Pub. L. 102-4), which took responsibility for reviewing the scientific literature on the association between herbicide exposure during Vietnam and health outcomes out of the hands of the VA and gave it to an independent scientific organization, the IOM. Moreover, the acrimony over Agent Orange affected decisions on concerns about unexplained illnesses that veterans of the 1991 Persian Gulf War later raised (see Chapter Six).

In 1995, President Clinton, at the annual meeting of the Veterans of Foreign Wars, acknowledged that many veterans were apparently suffering from disabling illnesses, saying that "neither they nor their doctors know how they got it." He further stated that "treatment for these veterans couldn't be delayed as it was for Vietnam veterans who were exposed to Agent Orange. That's why we moved to provide medical care and to compensate fully and fairly these Gulf veterans while making every effort to find the answers" (Clinton, 1995).

Professionalization of Military Medicine

In 1973, shortly after becoming a U.S. Senator, Sam Nunn (D-Georgia) told the Georgia General Assembly that "the concept [of the all-volunteer force] is a clear result of the Vietnam war because it caused the President and Congress to yield to the tremendous pressure to end the draft at almost any price" (Nunn, 1973). With the end of the draft, DoD established new programs to ensure that new physicians and other health professionals would join both to support the peacetime military establishment and to meet wartime requirements. Accordingly, Congress passed the Uniformed Services Health Professions Revitalization Act of 1972 (Pub. L. 92-426, 1972), authorizing the Armed Forces Health Professions Scholarship Program and establishing USUHS. In May 1974, Congress also approved a program of incentives—the Uniformed Services Variable Incentive Pay Act for Physicians (Pub. L. 93-274, 1974), and a new incentive pay package was initiated the following September. By the end of FY 1976, the number of new physicians was almost three and one-half times that of the previous year. Moreover, physician losses were down by 27 percent, thanks to medical scholarships and bonuses for physicians and other critical health professionals.

In 1995, GAO reported to Congress on USUHS and the Health Profession Scholarship Program, saying that, while USUHS is the most expensive source of military physicians by most measures, the university costs nearly the same as the regular scholarship program, when all federal costs are considered, and is less costly than the deferred scholarship program. GAO reported that the quality of USUHS medical education compares well with that of all medical schools and that its graduates' abilities are as good as or better than those of other military physicians. Graduates appear to be better trained in military medicine than their civilian peers; the university

> provides training in the special needs of military medicine as an integral part of its medical school curriculum. By the time University students graduate and begin active duty, they have received at least 784 hours of medical readiness training. Other new military physicians take specific medical readiness training courses once they are on active duty; however, the initial training they receive is less extensive than that provided to University graduates. (Baine, 1995)

Importantly, GAO told Congress that

> the University engages in several activities in addition to operating its School of Medicine. These activities include providing overseas medical personnel required continuing medical education, serving as the academic affiliate for several military graduate medical education programs, and offering graduate education programs for allied health professionals. The University has established research and archival programs in such areas as casualty care, preventive medicine, and psychiatric responses to trauma and disaster. (Baine, 1995)

GAO also reported that USUHS "graduates are likely to meet DOD's needs for an experienced cadre of military physicians" (Baine, 1995).

CHAPTER SIX

The Unraveling of the Middle East: Operation Desert Shield and Operation Desert Storm, August 1990–February 1991

From the vantage point of the second decade of the 21st century, it seems clear that the years since the end of World War II can be divided into two periods: the Cold War with the Soviet Union and the oil wars in the Middle East in the late 20th and early 21st centuries. The next four chapters recount the second period. This chapter covers the initial conflict in the Persian Gulf, which was the shortest and least costly in terms of American military casualties in our history. The conflict in Afghanistan and Iraq following the events of 9/11 is presented in the next three chapters: Chapter Seven covers the military and the medical care for casualties in theater during the longest period of conflict in our history; Chapter Eight examines medical and care issues related to amputations, the provision of mental health services to the force, and the issues related to TBI; and Chapter Nine deals with the interface between the departments of Defense and Veterans Affairs and the VA's changing role in providing long-term care for those who served our country in the military.

For the United States, the conflicts in Korea and Vietnam were the hot battles of the Cold War. While the fall of the Soviet Union in 1989 and the triumph of democratic capitalism held the promise of a new *pax Americana* (see Fukuyama, 1992), the transition into the period of wars in the Middle East was swift. The first Gulf War in 1990, our conflict with al-Qaeda, the events of September 11, 2001, and the wars in Afghanistan and Iraq are the events that mark this second period.

The root cause of the wars during this second period was the world's thirst for petroleum.[1] A geographic accident placed a significant portion of the world's oil supply in an unstable region of "artificial states" created from the remnants of the Ottoman

---

[1] Toby Craig Jones makes the point that, "the Iraq War was the outgrowth of several decades of strategic thinking and policy making about oil" (Jones, 2012, p. 209). Specifically, the connection between oil and al-Qaeda can be found in bin Laden's 1996 fatwa:

> the latest and the greatest . . . aggression, incurred by the Muslims since the death of the Prophet . . . is the occupation of the land of the two Holy Places . . . by the armies of the American Crusaders and their allies. . . . The presence of the USA Crusader military forces on land, sea and air of the states of the Islamic Gulf is the greatest danger threatening the largest oil reserve in the world. (bin Laden, 1996)

Empire after World War I.[2] A case in point is the creation of Iraq and Kuwait as independent countries, with Kuwait blocking Iraq's access to the Persian Gulf.[3]

During the Cold War, the United States committed troops to enforce its strategy of containment,[4] with open conflict in Korea and Vietnam. In retrospect, these conflicts had much in common, including the fact that neither was officially classified as a war because Congress never passed a declaration of war, which the Constitution requires.[5] Similarly, the first oil war in the Middle East, often referred to as the *Gulf War*,[6] was not a war but two designated military operations: operations Desert Shield and Desert Storm. Unlike the two world wars of the first half of the 20th century, the post–World War II conflicts were fought for limited ends by limited means. These were "business as usual" conflicts without full mobilization of either the economic or human resources of the country.[7]

---

[2]   Scott Anderson provides a description of the creation of these artificial states in the Middle East:

> The process began at the end of World War I, when two of the victorious allies, Britain and France, carved up the lands of the defeated Ottoman Empire between themselves as spoils of war. In Mesopotamia, the British joined together three largely autonomous Ottoman provinces and named it Iraq. . . . To the west of Iraq, the European powers took the opposite approach, carving the vast lands of "greater Syria" into smaller, more manageable parcels. Falling under French rule was the smaller rump state of Syria—essentially the nation that exists today—and the coastal enclave of Lebanon, while the British took Palestine and Transjordan, a swath of southern Syria that would eventually become Israel and Jordan. Coming a bit later to the game, in 1934, Italy joined the three ancient North African regions that it had wrested from the Ottomans in 1912 to form the colony of Libya. . . .
>
> [j]ust beneath the sectarian and regional divisions in these "nations" there lay extraordinarily complex tapestries of tribes and subtribes and clans, ancient social orders that remained the populations' principal source of identification and allegiance. . . . The Europeans eventually left, but the sectarian and tribal schisms they fueled remained. (Anderson, 2016, pp. 8–9)

[3]   Joe Stork and Ann M. Lesch maintain, however, that

> Iraq's claim to all of Kuwait was not the reason Baghdad invaded in August 1990. Rather, it served as a justification after the fact. What gives the Iraqi argument currency in the Arab world is less the merits of this territorial claim than the powerful sense that the political and economic order prevailing in the region as a whole has been constructed and maintained primarily for the benefit of the Western powers. Behind this perception is oil. Many of the political arrangements that characterize the region—borders, ruling families, economic structures and more—exist and persist because of the stake that oil has represented for Western industrialized countries. (Stork and Lesch, 1990, p. 13)

[4]   George F. Kennan, a career Foreign Service officer, formulated the policy of containment, the basic U.S. strategy for fighting the Cold War (1947–1989) with the Soviet Union (adapted from U.S. Department of State, Office of the Historian, c. 2010).

[5]   The conflict in Korea was officially classified as a "police action." The war in Vietnam is often referred to as a "conflict," whose legal basis rested on a number of congressional resolutions (U.S. Department of State, Office of the Historian, undated).

[6]   At various times, it has also been referred to as *Persian Gulf War*, *First Gulf War*, *Gulf War I*, *Kuwait War*, *First Iraq War*, and *Iraq War*.

[7]   At the height of World War II in 1945, the Army's strength was 8.26 million. At the height of the Korean war in 1952, the Army's strength was 1.6 million—less than one-fifth the size of the World War II force.

On the Eve of Operations Desert Shield and Desert Storm

The Army

During the early morning hours of August 2, 1990, the lead elements of two Iraqi divisions entered Kuwait, precipitating the Persian Gulf War of 1990–1991. In response, at 10 a.m. on August 8, the first element of the American 82nd Airborne Division from Fort Bragg, North Carolina, departed neighboring Pope AFB to take up defensive positions to protect the Kingdom of Saudi Arabia. By the end of the next week, a full brigade of 4,600 paratroopers and their equipment was on the ground, and the remainder of the division had deployed by August 24 (Scales, 1993).

The American army that deployed in August 1990 was a far cry from the army that had fought in Vietnam, which MG Robert Scales, Jr., who was later commandant of the Army War College, described as being an army "cloaked in anguish."[8] The Army of 1990 had "fundamentally changed its character from the mass conscripted army of World War II, Korea, and Vietnam to a small body of high-quality, long-service professionals" (Scales, 1993). Moreover, it was an army that changed almost everything—how it recruited soldiers, how it thought about and trained for combat, how it educated its commissioned and noncommissioned officers, and how it operated with its sister services, especially after the Goldwater-Nichols Defense Reorganization Act reforms of 1986 (Pub. L. 99-433, 1986). With a focus on the Soviet threat in Europe, and to complement the newly developed concepts of AirLand Battle, the Army fielded a new generation of combat equipment, dubbed the Big Five, which included the UH-60 Blackhawk transport helicopter, the M1 Abrams Main Battle Tank, the AH-64 Apache Attack Helicopter, the Patriot Air Defense Missile, and the M2/3 Bradley Fighting Vehicle troop carrier.[9] This was the Army that faced the Soviet-trained and -equipped army of Saddam Hussein in fall and winter 1990–1991.

The Gulf War occurred at a unique moment in post–World War II history. Despite the planned reductions in Army strength following the collapse of the Berlin Wall in November 1989 (see Grissmer and Rostker, 1992), the United States still retained most of the forces it had built up during the Cold War and moved the Army's VII Corps from Germany to Saudi Arabia with little concern for the Soviet threat to Western Europe. Nevertheless, when offensive ground operations were initiated on February 24, 1991, the United States and its coalition partners faced a formidable foe, which

---

[8]   General Scales described the U.S. Army of the early 1970s as

   an institution fighting merely to maintain its existence in the midst of growing apathy, decay, and intolerance. Forty percent of the Army in Europe confessed to drug use. . . . Between 1969 and 1971, Army investigators recorded 800 instances of attacks involving hand grenades in which 45 officers and noncommissioned officers were killed. (Scales, 1993)

[9]   Scales, 1993, and Kirkpatrick, 1991, discuss these changes.

the Defense Intelligence Agency estimated to consist of 545,000 troops; 4,280 tanks; 3,100 artillery pieces; and 2,800 armored personnel carriers (DoD, 1992a, p. 254).[10]

The American Soldier

In the final report to Congress on the conduct of Gulf War, Secretary of Defense Dick Cheney said,

> Warriors win wars, and smart weapons require smart people and sound doctrine to maximize their effectiveness. The highly trained, highly motivated all-volunteer force we fielded in Operations Desert Shield and Desert Storm is the *highest quality fighting force the United States has ever fielded*. (DoD, 1992a, p. xviii; emphasis added)[11]

The decision to end conscription in 1970 and the program to transition to an all-volunteer force by 1973 fundamentally changed the way America selected the people who would staff the armed services. With the end of conscription, the armed forces no longer could rely on the Selective Service to deliver to each the manpower it needed to maintain the strength Congress had authorized. The services had to offer prospective recruits a package of pay and benefits, including vocational training, that would entice qualified people to join voluntarily. The new system, however, enabled the services to establish new and higher standards than had existed under conscription. This was particularly true for the Army, which, after an initial rocky start, learned how to recruit a high-quality force of young men and women.[12] The evolution of the all-volunteer force is reflected in Figures 6.1–6.3 and in Table 6.1, which document the changing personnel profile of the armed forces from 1973 to 1991.

---

[10] The U.S. Army Central Command (ARCENT), which "consisted of the XVIII Airborne Corps and VII Corps, was on the western flank of the theater. Positioned on ARCENT's left flank was the XVIII Airborne Corps; VII Corps was to the right. These two corps covered about two-thirds of the line occupied by the multinational force" (DoD, 1992a, p. 257). A total of 697,000 U.S. forces deployed, and peak personnel strength was 541,400. Other coalition forces totaled 259,700 at peak personnel strength (Hernandez et al., 1999). ARCENT's strength was reported to be 280,000 (Englehardt, 1991).

[11] This was reflected in an op-ed piece by Congressman G. V. (Sonny) Montgomery (D-Mississippi), at one time one of the foremost critics of the all-volunteer force:

> We have the best and brightest young men and women in the armed forces today that we have had at any time in the 35 years I have been associated with the military. . . . The bottom line is that we have a more representative sample of middle America in the volunteer force of 1990 than can be associated in any draft, and we don't have the morale and discipline problems that accompany conscription through their two-year hitches. (Montgomery, 1990, p. A17)

[12] The turnaround in the Army's fortunes in terms of the success of the all-volunteer forces is generally attributed to the efforts of Army GEN Maxwell Thurman (Rostker, 2007). Thurman noted 13 major actions that he believed had turned the Army's 1979 recruiting failure into a success story in the 1980s. As he saw it, there were nine internal management changes, including establishing quality goals, and four that required congressional action, including better pay, the postservice college fund, and a new G.I. bill.

Figure 6.1
Non–Prior-Service Active Component Accessions with at Least a High School Diploma,
FYs 1973–1991

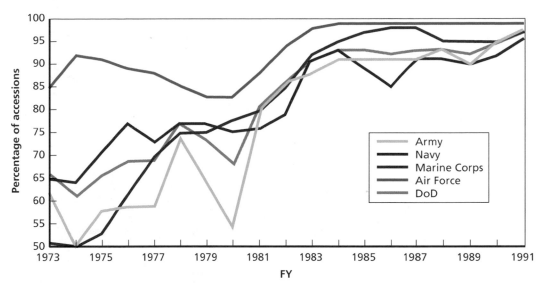

SOURCE: Office of the Assistant Secretary of Defense for Force Management and Personnel, 1992, p. 19.

Figure 6.2
Non–Prior-Service Active Component Accessions in Armed Forces Qualification Test
Categories I–III, FYs 1973–1991

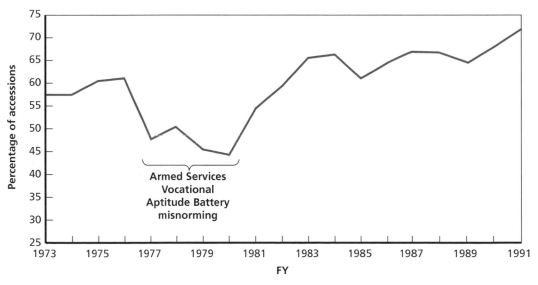

SOURCE: Office of the Assistant Secretary of Defense for Force Management and Personnel, 1992, p. 22.
NOTE: For four years in the late 70s, the Armed Services Vocational Aptitude Battery tests were being
scored in a way that allowed low-aptitude men to enlist in the military. This is referred to as *misnorming*.

Figure 6.3
Average Age and Months in Service for the Active Component Enlisted Force, FYs 1973–1991

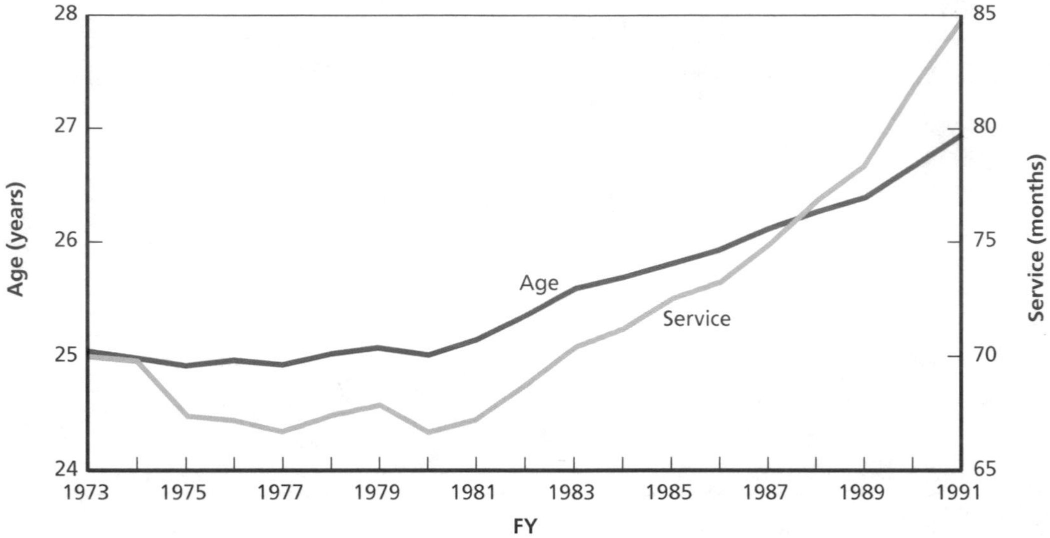

SOURCE: Office of the Assistant Secretary of Defense for Force Management and Personnel, 1992, p. 50.

Demographics of Deployed Troops

The demographic composition of the military force deployed to the Persian Gulf reflected the many changes that had been initiated after Vietnam with the advent of the all-volunteer force. As shown in Table 6.2, women made up almost 7 percent of the deployed force, and about 17 percent of the force came from National Guard and reserve units. The mean age was 28; 70 percent were non-Hispanic or white, 23 percent black, and 5 percent Hispanic.

Medical Support During Operations Desert Shield and Desert Storm

While subsequent events would bring this assessment into question, the general consensus at the time of the invasion of Kuwait was that the Iraqi armed forces were a formidable and battle-tested fighting force. Iraq began the crisis with one of the world's larger armies, equipped with great numbers of tanks, armored personnel carriers, and artillery, some of which were reported to be state of the art. The Iraqi armed forces were structured similarly to the British forces, but their operations were modeled more closely on Soviet armed forces. Military units were reported to be well equipped, with ample supplies of ammunition, water, food, and fuel, and were backed by extensive supply and transportation infrastructures. The regular army comprised more than 50 divisions, with additional special-forces brigades, and specialized maneuver and artillery units. The elite Republican Guard Forces Command—eight divisions and almost

Table 6.1
Army Active Component Enlisted Accessions and Force,s FY 1991

	Army (%)	DoD Total (%)	Civilian Population (%)
Active component enlisted accessions			
Males	85.5	87.5	49.3[a]
White	73.9	77.4	81.5[a]
Black	20.1	16.7	14.3[a]
Hispanic	6.1	7.3	11.4[a]
Education of active component enlisted accessions			
Diploma high school graduate	97.6	97.3	81.1[a]
GED certificate	1.9	2.5	
Some college	8.2	6.1	38.9[a]
AFQT category of male accessions			
I	5.0	4.8	10.0[b]
II	39.2	38.6	29.4[b]
IIIA	29.9	27.4	14.4[b]
IIIB	24.2	27.7	16.0[b]
IV	1.0	0.6	20.4[b]
V	0	0	9.9[b]
Mean reading grade level of active component accessions	11.4	11.3	10.3[b]
Education of active component enlisted force			
Diploma high school graduate	90.7	93.2	88.0[c]
GED certificate	6.8	4.8	
Some college	7.1	6.8	47.9[c]
Active component enlisted force			
Males	88.8	89.2	54.5[c]
African American	60.5	70.5	84.9[c]
Black	31.9	23.1	11.6[c]
Hispanic	4.5	5.2	8.9[c]

SOURCE: Office of the Assistant Secretary of Defense for Force Management and Personnel, 1992.

NOTE: Percentages may not sum to 100 due to rounding.

[a] 18–24-year-old civilians.

[b] 1980 civilian youth population.

[c] 18–44-year-old civilians.

Table 6.2
Demographic Characteristics of Persian Gulf War Veterans

Characteristics	Percentage with Characteristics (n = 697,000)
Gender	
Male	93
Female	7
Age in years	
17–25	55
26–30	20
31–35	12
35–65	13
Race/ethnicity	
White	70
African American	23
Hispanic	5
Other	2
Rank	
Officer	10
Enlisted	90
Military branch	
Army	50
Navy	23
Marine	15
Air Force	12
Military status	
Active duty	83
Reserve or National Guard	17

SOURCE: Joseph et al., 1997, p. 151.

20 percent of the ground force—was Iraq's most capable and loyal force, receiving the best training and equipment. The Iraqi Air Force was the largest in the Middle East, with more than 700 combat aircraft. Iraq annually produced thousands of chemical weapons, including those containing mustard and the nerve agent, Sarin, and was the first nation in history to use nerve agents on the battlefield (DoD, 1992a, pp. 9–16; Scales, 1993).

Planners at U.S. Central Command (USCENTCOM) initially expected a "sizable" number of combat casualties (DoD, 1992a, p. 230). GEN Norman Schwarzkopf, USCENTCOM's commander, told the Senate after the war that he had expected 10,000 to 20,000 wounded and dead, but to be on the safe side, he had ordered over 16,000 body bags. (The actual casualties were 146 battle deaths, 145 nonbattle deaths, and 470 WIA.) To care for the expected casualties, USCENTCOM followed the prescribed joint Health Service Support Concept of five levels of care from Level I—"medical support . . . provided by individual soldiers; by specifically trained individuals; or by elements organic to combat, combat support . . . , and designated medical units"— through Level V hospitals in Europe or the United States (DoD, 1992a, p. 452). Overall, 65 major hospital units from the Army, Navy, and Air Force were deployed to the Kuwait theater of operations (KTO) to provide Level III and IV support, with a capacity of over 18,000 beds,[13] staffed by over 41,000 medical support personnel. This in-theater capacity was backed up by a theater evacuation policy that anticipated that the Air Force would move the most critically wounded to Germany, where the Air Force and Army had readied an additional 5,500 beds, and "up to 22,000 beds in CONUS" (DoD, 1992a, p. 456).

Army Medical Deployments

The Army deployed to the KTO some 23,000 medical personnel, 198 separate medical units, including 44 Army hospitals,[14] in addition to the medical personnel in the individual combat units, e.g., medical aides and battalion aid station staff (see GAO, 1992, p. 2). Included were station hospitals, evacuation hospitals, combat support hospitals (CSHs), and the traditional MASHs. The most immediate need was for air ambulances, and this was provided by the first Army medical unit to deploy to the KTO, the 45th Medical Company. The first element of six UH-60 Black Hawk helicopters arrived in Dhahran, Saudi Arabia, on August 27, 1990. By the end of the August, the 44th Medical Brigade, the 47th Field Hospital, the 28th CSH, and the 5th MASH were on their way. In addition, the Army accelerated the conversion of deployed field hospitals to the Deployable Medical System design, incorporating the most up-to-date medical equipment available, which was completed by December 1990 (Ledford, 1992).[15] Eventually, the Army deployed 44 hospitals: eight MASHs with 60 beds;

---

[13] DoD also noted that, when "the land campaign began on 24 February, all assets to support the 18,530-bed requirement were in theater and 15,430 beds were operational" (DoD, 1992a, p. 456).

[14] The Army hospitals included "17 Reserve hospitals, 11 National Guard hospitals, and 16 Active Component hospitals. Nine hospitals were in host nation fixed facilities" (Ledford, 1992, p. 3).

[15] After the war, the commander of the 7th Medical Support Command noted,

One of the problems that we did experience was that very few of our active units had worked or trained in DEPMEDS [Deployable Medical System] and did not know what facilities and equipment they would actually have to work with in a wartime scenario. This was partly due to the fact that during peacetime there were only a very limited number of fully-equipped DEPMEDS fielded, and partly because of the competing requirement

nine CSHs with 200 beds; 22 evacuation hospitals, three field hospitals, and one station hospital—each with 400 to 500 beds—and one general hospital with 1,000 beds (GAO, 1992, p. 13).

The Impact of Medical Deployments

To facilitate the deployment of Army medical personnel and to ensure continued medical support for nondeployed troops and military families, the first callup of reserve personnel augmented military hospitals in the United States, freeing active military medical personnel for deployment. To fill the resulting vacancies, the Professional Officer Filler System matched vacancies in deploying medical units with available reserve medical personnel (see Schubert and Kraus, 1995, pp. 84–89; Blanck and Bell, 1991, p. 858). By February 1991, when the ground offensive began, 87,487 medical personnel were on active duty, the largest force since World War II (Ledford, 1992, p. 3). These actions notwithstanding, the growing deployment stretched the medical establishment *nearly* to the breaking point, especially in Europe.

In Europe, with the decision to deploy the VII Corps to the KTO—the 1st and 3rd Armored Divisions, the 2nd Armored Cavalry Regiment, and a robust corps support command—it became clear that the total number of medical personnel was inadequate to carry out the U.S. Army Europe's three medical missions: providing wartime medical support to the deploying corps; providing rear-area medevac, treatment, and logistical base for USCENTCOM; and maintaining adequate medical services for the approximately 200,000 military personnel and family members who remained in Europe. According to the 7th Medical Command's planners,

> the units that should deploy with VII Corps were short 184 doctors, 56 dentists, 237 nurses, 94 medical service personnel, and 1,417 other personnel for a total personnel shortage of 1,988. . . .
>
> [Therefore,] it was necessary to reduce some peacetime services at least temporarily, while filling vacancies as quickly and fully as possible [with mobilized personnel]. . . . (Gehring, 2002, p. 180)
>
> By the end of the first week of January 1991, USAREUR [U.S. Army Europe] had received 3,447 newly assigned medical personnel. (Gehring, 2002, p. 182)

These were primarily Army Reserve and National Guard medical personnel. Looking back, the Army Surgeon General, LTG Frank F. Ledford, Jr., noted that this was "the fastest mobilization of medical assets in history—we did in three months what took us three years in Korea" (as quoted in DoD, 1992a, p. 451).

---

to provide peacetime care to our beneficiaries, which reduces the amount of time available for field training for our clinical personnel. However, since we had several months to prepare before the ground war started, . . . we managed to have our medical personnel trained and familiar with the equipment and materiel available. (Sosa, 1992)

Operation Desert Storm

The Ground Offensive: The 100-Hour Ground War

On January 17, 1991, the defensive Operation Desert Shield ended, and the offensive Operation Desert Storm began, with an air campaign designed to destroy Iraq's air force and air defenses and to inflict as much damage as possible on Iraqi ground forces. On January 18, the Iraqis retaliated with Scud missile attacks on Saudi Arabia and Israel. Concurrently, General Schwarzkopf deployed his troops, positioning the VII Corps and XVIII Airborne Corps on the Iraqi border, with the U.S. Marine Central Command and two coalition forces commands to their right, facing Kuwait (see Figure 6.4).[16] The ground attack began at 0100 hours on February 24 by elements of the XVIII Airborne Corps securing the coalition's left flank (Schubert and Kraus,

Figure 6.4
Operation Desert Storm, February 24–27, 1991

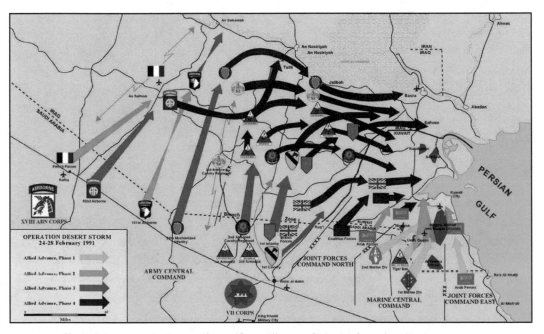

SOURCE: Office of the Special Assistant for Gulf War Illnesses (OSAGWI), undated.

---

[16] The VII Corps consisted of "one British and four American heavy divisions, four self-propelled artillery brigades, an armored cavalry regiment, a combat aviation brigade, and expanded numbers of combat service and combat service support units under an enlarged support command" (Gehring, 2002, p. 189). The XVIII Airborne Corps consisted of the 82nd Airborne Division, the 101st Airborne Division (Air Assault), the 24th Infantry Division (Mechanized), the French 6th Light Armored Division, the 3rd Armored Cavalry, and the 12th and 18th Aviation Brigades (Schubert and Kraus, 1995, p. 173).

1995, p. 174). Some 100 hours later, a "cease-fire" was ordered with coalition forces well inside Iraq, their achievement staggering, as noted:

> In ninety hours of continuous movement and combat, VII Corps had . . . destroyed more than a dozen Iraqi divisions, an estimated 1,300 tanks, 1,200 infantry fighting vehicles and armored personnel carriers, 285 artillery pieces, and 100 air defense systems, and captured nearly 22,000 men. At the same time, the best Iraqi divisions destroyed only 7 M1A1 Abrams tanks, 15 Bradleys, 2 armored personnel carriers, and 1 Apache helicopter. And while killing unknown thousands of enemy troops, VII Corps lost 22 soldiers killed in action. (Schubert and Kraus, 1995, p. 197)

> The U.S. Army had contributed the bulk of the ground combat power that defeated and very nearly destroyed the Iraqi ground forces. The Iraqis lost 3,847 of their 4,280 tanks, over half of their 2,880 armored personnel carriers, and nearly all of their 3,100 artillery pieces. . . . [The American Army took] an estimated 60,000 prisoners. And these surprising results came at the cost of 148 Americans killed in action. In the theater of operations Army Central Command had won the fastest and most complete victory in American military history. (Schubert and Kraus, 1995, p. 201)

Casualties

In total, nearly 700,000 U.S. troops deployed to the Persian Gulf region in support of operations Desert Shield and Desert Storm. In 1992, DoD reported to Congress that there had been a "total of 613 US military battle casualties in Operation Desert Storm, 146 service personnel were killed in action, including 35 killed by fire from friendly forces, and 467 were wounded, including 72 by fire from friendly forces" (DoD, 1992a, p. 589).[17] DoD further noted that, "[b]efore the ground offensive began, 15 servicemen were killed and 18 were wounded" in nine incidents involving friendly fire; the remaining friendly fire casualties "occurred during the ground offensive, in which 20 servicemen were killed and 54 were wounded in 11 separate incidents" (DoD, 1992a, p. 591).[18] A Scud missile attack on a barracks in February 24, 1991, inflicted more U.S. casualties—38 Army Reservists from Pennsylvania—than any other single engagement. In addition, "[d]uring Operation Desert Storm, 173 C-130 missions were flown which transported 2,375 patients, including Coalition and Iraqi casualties" (DoD, 1992a, pp. 463–464).

---

[17] Various but similar numbers have been reported for total KIA. Note that the total KIA in this quote differs from that in the previous quote.

[18] Note that there were also 225 deaths due to disease or accidents (Presidential Advisory Committee [PAC] on Gulf War Veterans' Illnesses, 1996, Ch. 1).

Assessment of Medical Support

The impressive overall performance notwithstanding, given the very short duration of the war, a number of support systems were not stressed or even adequately tested, none more so than the medical system.[19] In the latter part of 1991, the DoD Inspector General (IG) visited 131 medical installations to assess "medical mobilization planning and execution [capabilities] in support of military contingency operations" (DoD IG, 1993, p. 3). Noting that operations Desert Shield and Desert Storm provided the only example since Vietnam involving the large-scale activation of medical units and the logistical support system, the IG concluded that

> DOD could not ensure the deployability of medical personnel during contingencies for several reasons, including outdated methods for determining personnel requirements, assignment of personnel to incorrect skill areas, and inadequate training of medical personnel. The report also stated that DOD's deployable hospitals lacked sufficient mobility and had incompatible communication capability that limited their ability to prepare for incoming casualties. (Gebicke, 1996, p. 4)

Similarly, GAO was concerned that these units lacked mobility, and surgical capabilities could not move forward to provide timely support.[20] And DoD, in its report to

---

[19] One example was combat psychiatry, as the Commander of the U.S. Army Medical Research Unit, Europe noted:

> Corps and division mental health teams (and the evacuation hospitals) did not have to cope with large numbers of battle fatigue casualties in SWA [Southwest Asia]. If significant casualties had occurred, these teams would have found it very difficult to carry out their mission. They were not adequately staffed, equipped or trained in peacetime to perform their wartime role. (Martin, 1992, p. 44)

[20] GAO argued that a MASH should have enough internal transportation assets to be 100-percent mobile and should have enough transportation assets to move about 20 percent of the unit. During Operation Desert Storm, MASH and CSH units moved only portions of their hospitals because of the weight of the hospital sets, the speed of the battle, and the shortage of trucks and materiel-handling equipment. GAO stated that, "[a]ccording to Army reports, over 40 percent of the bed capacity of these units was left behind the line of departure, and only half the surgical capability moved forward" (GAO, 1992, p. 40). One MASH commander

> said that his unit could set up 4 operating tables and 36 beds in 12 hours and be ready to receive patients. However, when the ground war started, it became apparent that the unit would have to be made lighter and more mobile so that it could keep up with the advancing forces. His MASH downsized to 12 beds and 4 operating tables. (GAO, 1992, p. 43)

According to Army after-action reports,

> hospitals had been inadequately designed to perform their doctrinal missions. Personnel . . . [who] moved forward with combat troops reported that they had simply been unable to carry out their missions due to problems with mobility. They stated that during their move to Iraq, under no enemy fire, with no air threat, with roads and essentially flat terrain, they had been unable to move, set up, or prepare to take patients before the ground war was over. They said that, in fact, their unit had been so far behind that they had not even unloaded their equipment. (GAO, 1992, p. 44)

Army doctrine required a 60-bed MASH to be 100-percent mobile and a 200-bed CHS to be 50-percent mobile (Ross, 1990, p. 38). Ross, 1990, p. 36, notes that "European/NATO scenarios for battle expect the MASH to

Congress, also said, "mobility of MASH and CSH assets in a rapidly changing environment may require further analysis" (DoD, 1992a, p. 469). In fact, the Army was well aware of these issues and had started to address them with the design for a new, smaller forward surgical team (FST). However, while a number of the new FSTs were deployed to the KTO, they were still thought of as "a small sub-unit of a MASH that can break away and move, with minimal organic equipment, as far forward as needed" (Ledford, 1992, p. 4), rather than as a replacement for the MASH units.[21]

The Development of Forward Surgical Team Storm

Between the end of Vietnam War and 1990, several minor combat deployments pointed to the need for a small, easy-to-insert surgical capability. During the U.S.-led invasion of Grenada in 1983, known as Operation Urgent Fury, the first MASH unit did not arrive until four days after the invasion began.[22] The Army then began developing the concept of an FST,[23] as a small, easily deployable surgical facility that could perform

---

require 3–7 days to complete a displacement (teardown, move, reopen) and the CSH to require 17 days to complete a displacement." Ross, 1990, p. 9, reports that comparison of the "total cargo and personnel requirements with the total cargo and personnel capacity shows the MASH is not 100 percent mobile" and has an effective mobility of only 43 percent.

[21] For example, COL Kenneth K. Steinweg, the commander of the 5th MASH during operations Desert Shield and Desert Storm, saw the FST as providing "forward peacetime trauma support," not "combat casualty support," and considered it to be an

> organic part of the 5th MASH. The FST was envisioned as an advance element of the MASH. Highly mobile, and with a 2-hour set-up time, the FST was designed to move quickly to an area of conflict, allowing time for the remainder of the MASH to travel and set up. The FST uses a general purpose large tent and has special lightweight operating room tables and the capacity to carry sixty units of blood. It is powered by lightweight 15-kW portable generators. (Steinweg, 1993, p. 734)

The FST had a staff of only 22, including four physicians in three vehicles. Steinweg argued that "it could not operate much longer than 24 hours before personnel became exhausted, limiting capabilities" (Steinweg, 1993, p. 734).

[22] The Grenada operation was characterized as having a "[s]hortage of medical personnel and confusion over Medevac procedures," which "sometimes held up treatment of the injured. Army helicopter pilots carrying wounded men had to learn the techniques for landing on naval vessels" (Cole, 1997, pp. 67–68); see also Stinger and Rush, 2006, p. 269. The delay in deploying the MASH can be attributed to the substantial amount of airlift it requires, i.e., "eight C-141s are required to deploy an airborne infantry battalion, while 20 C-141s are required to deploy a MASH" (Nolan, 1990, p. 109).

[23] The Army took lessons from many nations. The French had parachutist surgical units, and the British had parachute clearing troop and army field surgical teams (Broyles, 1987, pp. 56–58, 66). During the Lebanon War, 1982, the Medical Corps of the Israel Defense Forces provided its mobile surgical units with sophisticated equipment, enabling them to perform advanced resuscitation and lifesaving surgical procedures, followed by prompt evacuation to rear hospitals (Gasko, 1984). Stinger and Rush also noted that the

> late Dr. Charles Rob, a world-renowned vascular surgeon then serving in the Royal Army Medical Corps in World War II, pioneered the first airborne [FSTs] with the British 1st Airborne Division in the North Africa campaign. Dr. Rob made two combat jumps with his FST in World War II. He set up his FSTs under very austere conditions, and they were very successful in saving wounded British paratroopers. After a long and distinguished surgical career, Dr. Rob passed away in 2001. (Stinger and Rush, 2006, p. 269)

trauma surgical procedures from the moment the fighting began. By 1986, two surgical airborne squads had been trained: the 274th Medical Detachment (Airborne) from Fort Bragg and the 250th Medical Detachment Surgical (Airborne) at Fort Lewis. In 1989, personnel from these units parachuted into Panama as part of Operation Just Cause. Unfortunately, the surgical teams could not set up their operating rooms until their operating tables, anesthesia machines, and other heavy equipment arrived by air transport (Stinger and Rush, 2006, p. 269). Nevertheless, the Army's assessment of FSTs was "exceptionally positive," with an after-action recommendation that the Army reexamine "conventional military medical doctrine to evaluate the costs and benefits of the decreased logistical requirements of far-forward surgical resuscitation and immediate far-back evacuation" (Marble, 2014, p. 33). That reexamination was ongoing in August 1990 when Saddam Hussein's Iraqi Republican Guard invaded Kuwait.

In response to the IG and GAO assessments of operations Desert Shield and Desert Storm, the Army's Surgeon General initiated a medical reengineering program in early 1993. Then, in March 1995, DoD published *Medical Readiness Strategic Plan 1995–2001* (Joseph, 1995) to serve as an overall road map for attaining and sustaining military medical readiness promising that things would be different the next time the Army deployed (see Chapter Seven).

Gulf War Illness

In early 1992, members of an Indiana Army National Guard unit that had deployed to the Persian Gulf reported suffering from fatigue, muscle and joint pain, memory loss, and severe headaches,[24] blaming their symptoms on exposure to a toxic environment during their deployment.[25] In response, the VA established a health registry where veterans could report their symptoms. The DoD then conducted an epidemiologic study, and a number of government panels were formed to examine the claims

---

[24] The IOM provided a more complete list:

> An undiagnosed illness, which may be associated with the following chronic symptoms: fatigue; symptoms involving skin, headache, muscle pain, joint pain, neurological symptoms, neuropsychological symptoms; symptoms involving the respiratory system, sleep disturbances, gastrointestinal symptoms, cardiovascular symptoms, abnormal weight loss, or menstrual symptoms. Also included are the following medically unexplained chronic multi-symptom illnesses that are defined by a cluster of signs or symptoms: Chronic Fatigue Syndrome, Fibromyalgia, and Irritable Bowel Syndrome. (Samet and Bodurow, 2008, p. 44)

[25] The VA's Research Advisory Committee on Gulf War Veterans' Illnesses notes:

> In addition to the many physical and psychological challenges common to other wartime deployments, military personnel who served in the 1990–1991 Gulf War were exposed to a long list of potentially hazardous substances. Many possible "causes" of Gulf War illness have been suggested and even promoted in different quarters since the war. Understanding the causes of Gulf War illness has been particularly challenging because of the lack of hard data on individual exposures in theater. (Research Advisory Committee on Gulf War Veterans' Illnesses, 2008, p. 6)

(see Figure 6.5). While none found evidence linking the reported illnesses to service in the gulf, reports of negative postdeployment symptoms spread and continued to be received from soldiers from additional units. On March 6, 1995, at the annual conference of the Veterans of Foreign Wars in Washington, D.C., President Bill Clinton acknowledged that many veterans were now apparently suffering from disabling illnesses, which "neither they nor their doctors know how they got" (Clinton, 1995, p. 4). He said that, to "avoid the kinds of problems that delayed care and compensation for those exposed to Agent Orange" (Clinton, 1995, p. 4), he had committed to increasing medical evaluations, research, and compensation and to appointing a Presidential advisory committee to review and make recommendations regarding the government's efforts to find the causes of undiagnosed illnesses and chronic multisymptom illness and improve the care Gulf war veterans were receiving.

Medical Evaluation of Gulf War Veterans and Research

In an effort to better understand what might be affecting the troops that returned from the Persian Gulf, the departments of Defense and Veterans Affairs undertook clinical and comparison studies and sponsored a wide range of research. DoD examined the immediate health of deployed soldiers who were still on active duty, and the VA monitored long-term effects.

DoD's Comprehensive Clinical Evaluation Program

On June 7, 1994, DoD instituted the Comprehensive Clinical Evaluation Program to provide clinical and research information related to Gulf War health questions. The evaluation program's protocol consisted of clinical evaluation supervised by a board-certified physician in either family practice or internal medicine. All participants were asked about (1) medical and family histories, (2) symptoms, (3) number of days of work lost due to illness during the 90 days prior to examination, and (4) any self-perceived exposure in the Persian Gulf to a full panoply of environmental hazards and potentially harmful substances, including petroleum products, pyridostigmine bromide pills, oil-well fire smoke, insect repellents, and anthrax and botulinum vaccinations. As of April 1996, 20,000 veterans had completed the evaluation program examinations.[26] From this group, the most common primary diagnosis reported was "diseases of the musculoskeletal system and connective tissue" (18.6 percent), with "pain in joint" (31 percent) being the most common specific diagnosis. Among the 3,558 participants with a primary diagnosis of "symptoms, signs, and ill-defined conditions," no single disease was predominant. Participants reported a wide variety of symptoms, with fatigue,

---

Research Advisory Committee on Gulf War Veterans' Illnesses, 2008, pp. 7–9, highlights exposures to psychological stressors, Kuwaiti oil-well fires, depleted uranium, vaccines, pyridostigmine bromide, pesticide, nerve agents, infectious disease, and combinations of exposures.

[26] The following results were reported in Joseph, 1997.

Figure 6.5
Key Responses to Reports of Ill Veterans of the Gulf War, 1992–1995

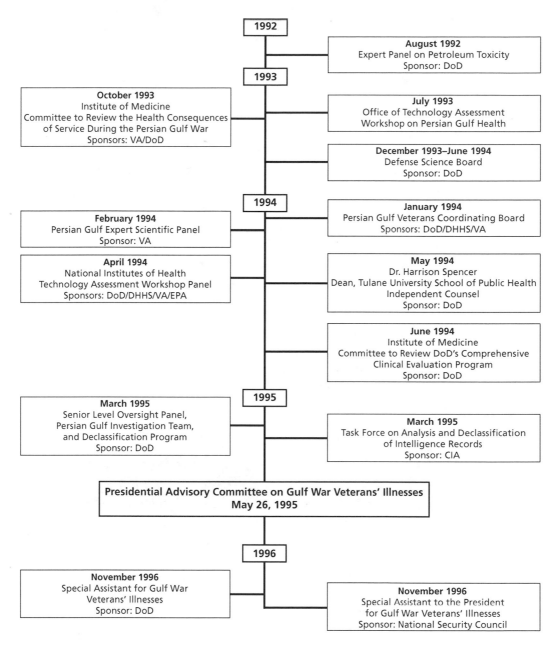

SOURCE: Presidential Advisory Committee on Gulf War Veterans' Illnesses, 1996, p. 3.
NOTE: EPA = Environmental Protection Agency.

headache, memory problems, and sleep disturbances being the most frequent complaints. However, there was no clinical indication of a new or unique syndrome.[27]

The VA's National Health Survey of Gulf War Era Veterans and Their Families

In 1995, at the direction of Congress, the VA funded the National Health Survey of Gulf War Era Veterans and Their Families research project, which compared the health of 15,000 deployed veterans with that of 15,000 nondeployed veterans. Unlike the DoD clinical study of the deployed, the VA's study compared mail and telephone survey responses and found that, "in comparison with their peers, Gulf veterans had a higher prevalence of functional impairment, health care utilization, symptoms, and medical conditions and a higher rate of low general health perceptions" (Kang et al., 2000). A subsequent follow-up, undertaken in 2001, reported that, "[t]en years after the Gulf War, the physical health of deployed and nondeployed veterans is similar. However, Gulf War deployment is associated with an increased risk for fibromyalgia, chronic fatigue syndrome, skin conditions, [and] dyspepsia" (Eisen et al., 2005, p. 881).[28] In 2001, the VA Secretary "determined that there [was] no basis to establish a presumption of service connection for any disease based on service in the Persian Gulf during the Persian Gulf War" (Principi, 2001, p. 325702).

Gulf War Health Research

Since the end of the Gulf War, the federal government, through DoD, VA, and the Department of Health and Human Services (DHHS), has funded more than 480 distinct projects, ranging from small pilot studies to large-scale epidemiological studies involving large populations, and major center–based research programs. Funding for the FY 2006 through FY 2015 period was $245.8 million (Kalasinsky and Jaeger, 2016, p. 2).

The Presumption of Illnesses Associated with Service in the Persian Gulf War

With the recent experience with Agent Orange fresh on their minds, and in the face of Gulf War veterans' complaints rising on October 8, 1992, Congress passed the Veterans Health Care Act of 1992 (Pub. L. 102-585, 1992), establishing the Persian Gulf War Veterans Health Registry (Environmental Agents Service, 1992, p. 1). The

---

[27] The IOM drew the same conclusion in reviewing the health effects of serving in the Gulf War. They reported that

> Gulf War veterans do not all experience the same array of symptoms has complicated efforts to determine whether there is a "Gulf War syndrome" or overlap with other symptom-based disorders. The nature of the symptoms suffered by many Gulf War veterans does not point to an obvious diagnosis, etiology, or standard treatment. (Committee on Gulf War and Health, 2005, p. 17)

[28] In 2014, the VA reported:

> While 12 percent of all pre-9/11 Veterans had at least one service-connected disability and received health care from VA, 17 percent of Veterans who deployed to the Persian Gulf have at least one service-connected disability and received health care from VA. (Gulf War Veterans' Illnesses Task Force, 2014, p. 8)

following March (1993), the VA established "a 'blue ribbon' panel of experts to examine these concerns, including multiple chemical sensitivity, chronic fatigue syndrome, and post-traumatic stress disorder."[29] This was followed on December 20, 1993, with enactment of the Priority VA Health Care for Persian Gulf Veterans Act (Pub. L. 103-210), which authorized VA to provide health-care services on a priority basis.[30] In late 1994, Congress passed the Veterans' Benefits Improvements Act of 1994 (Pub. L. 103-446), which authorized the VA to compensate veterans

> suffering from a chronic disability resulting from an undiagnosed illness or combination of undiagnosed illnesses that became manifest either during active duty in the Southwest Asia theater of operations during the Persian Gulf War or to a degree of ten percent or more within a presumptive period following such service. ("Secretary Brown Praises Congress for Passage of Persian Gulf Legislation," 1995, p. 1)

Originally, these adverse health effects had to manifest within two years of service in the Persian Gulf, but the presumptive period was extended a number of times. Compensation is now authorized for Gulf War veterans who show

> signs or symptoms that may be a manifestation of an undiagnosed illness or a chronic multisymptom illness [including] the following:
>
> (1) Fatigue.
> (2) Unexplained rashes or other dermatological signs or symptoms.
> (3) Headache.
> (4) Muscle pain.
> (5) Joint pain.
> (6) Neurological signs or symptoms.
> (7) Neuropsychological signs or symptoms.

---

[29] At the time the VA secretary said,

> While most of the Persian Gulf veterans we are treating have health problems no different from those of other veterans, a number of them have conditions that may be related to Gulf service which, so far, have eluded diagnosis. I am determined that VA discover exactly just what is causing these problems and develop treatment approaches to help these veterans. ("Secretary Brown Establishes 'Blue Ribbon' Panel . . . ," 1993, p. 1)

[30] According to the VA,

> Prior to enactment of this legislation, . . . Persian Gulf War veterans who claimed exposure to toxic substances and/or environmental hazards did not have the priority for VA medical services accorded to veterans who receive services for conditions possibly related to exposure to Agent Orange or ionizing radiation. . . . Public Law 103-210 equalized the entitlement.
>
> [The law] . . . gave VA authority to waive the copayment requirement for . . . a Persian Gulf veteran for any condition that the treating physician medically determines is possibly related to that veteran's Persian Gulf service.
>
> The legislation also authorizes VA to, upon request, reimburse any veteran who paid a copayment, excluding prescription copayments, for hospital care, nursing home care, or outpatient services, furnished by VA before enactment of this law. ("President Signs Legislation Authorizing Priority Treatment," 1994, p. 4)

(8) Signs or symptoms involving the upper or lower respiratory system.
(9) Sleep disturbances.
(10) Gastrointestinal signs or symptoms.
(11) Cardiovascular signs or symptoms.
(12) Abnormal weight loss.
(13) Menstrual disorders. (38 U.S.C. § 1117)

The FY 2008 National Defense Authorization Act (NDAA) established a presumption of service connection for Gulf War veterans who develop an active mental illness. The domain of symptoms presumptively linked to Gulf War service was extended by Congress with the passage of the Veterans Education and Benefits Expansion Act of 2001, which expanded the definition of "qualifying chronic disability" to include a "medically unexplained chronic multisymptom illness (such as chronic fatigue syndrome, fibromyalgia, and irritable bowel syndrome) that is defined by a cluster of signs or symptoms" (Pub. L. 107-103, 2001, Subsec. 202 (a)).

Importantly, the basis for presumption was extended in 1994, from outcome (i.e., unexplained illnesses) to exposure to toxic agents, such as fumes and smoke from military operations, oil well fires, diesel exhaust, paints, pesticides, depleted uranium, infectious/biological agents, chemical, or other toxic agents, environmental or wartime hazard, and vaccines. (Samet and Bodurow, 2008, p. I-81). And, in 2010, nine specific infectious diseases were added.[31]

Even as Congress was authorizing compensation for undiagnosed illnesses, it ordered VA to commission a scientific review of what have been contributing to the health effects veterans were experiencing. The reviews were done by the IOM, and summary findings were reported in 2005, 2010, and 2016.[32] Box 6.1 shows the IOM's final conclusions regarding the association between deployment to the Gulf War and specific health concerns. On the association between illness and specific environmental exposures, IM found that

> efforts to model or otherwise reconstruct the exposures that Gulf War veterans experienced during deployment are also unlikely to yield useful results. . . .

> Without definitive and verifiable individual veteran exposure information, further studies to determine cause-and-effect relationships between Gulf War exposures and health conditions in Gulf War veterans should not be undertaken. (Committee on Gulf War and Health, 2016, p. 10)

---

[31] The infectious diseases are brucellosis, campylobacter jejuni, coxiella burnetti (Q fever), malaria, mycobacterium tuberculosis, nontyphoid salmonella, shigella, visceral leishmaniasis, and West Nile virus (Emrey-Arras, 2017, p. 6).

[32] The summary findings were reported in Committee on Gulf War and Health, 2005; Committee on Gulf War and Health, 2010; and Committee on Gulf War and Health, 2016.

Box 6.1

Summary of Conclusions Regarding Associations Between Deployment to the Gulf War and Specific Health Conditions

Sufficient Evidence of a Causal Relationship
- Posttraumatic stress disorder (PTSD)

Sufficient Evidence of an Association
- Generalized anxiety disorder, depression, and substance abuse (particularly alcohol abuse)
- Gastrointestinal symptoms consistent with functional gastrointestinal disorders such as irritable bowel syndrome and functional dyspepsia
- Chronic fatigue syndrome
- Gulf War illness

Limited/Suggestive Evidence of an Association
- Amyotrophic lateral sclerosis (ALS)
- Fibromyalgia and chronic widespread pain
- Self-reported sexual difficulties

Inadequate/Insufficient Evidence to Determine Whether an Association Exists
- Any cancer
- Cardiovascular conditions or conditions of the blood and blood-forming organs
- Endocrine and metabolic conditions
- Neurodegenerative diseases other than ALS
- Neurocognitive and neurobehavioral performance
- Migraines and other headache disorders
- Other neurologic outcomes
- Respiratory diseases
- Structural gastrointestinal diseases
- Chronic skin conditions
- Musculoskeletal system diseases
- Genitourinary conditions
- Specific birth defects
- Adverse pregnancy outcomes such as miscarriage, stillbirth, preterm birth, and low birth weight
- Fertility problems
- Increased mortality from any cancer, any neurologic disease (including multiple sclerosis, Alzheimer's disease, Parkinson's disease, and ALS), respiratory disease, or gastrointestinal disease

Limited/Suggestive Evidence of No Association
- Objective measures of peripheral neurologic conditions
- Multiple sclerosis
- Mortality from cardiovascular disease or parasitic diseases
- Decreased lung function
- Mortality due to mechanical trauma or other external causes

SOURCE: Quoted from Committee on Gulf War and Health, 2016, p. 263.

The Presidential Advisory Committee on Gulf War Veterans' Illnesses

On May 26, 1995, President Clinton issued EO 12961, which established the PAC on Gulf War Veterans' Illnesses, to "conduct an independent, open, and comprehensive review of all facets—risks, diagnosis, treatment, and research—related to health issues and Gulf War service [and] . . . to make sure the government was doing all it could as quickly as it could" (PAC, 1996, pp. 2–4). On December 31, 1996, the committee submitted its final report to the secretaries of DoD, VA, and DHHS, concluding that, in "all areas save one, the government has responded with a comprehensive series of measures to address Gulf War veterans' illnesses" (PAC, 1996, p. iii). Speaking for the committee, the chair, Dr. Joyce Lashof, said the following:

> Many veterans clearly are experiencing medical difficulties connected to their service in the Gulf War. First and foremost, continuing to provide clinical care to evaluate and treat veterans' illnesses is vital. At the same time, however, a causal link between a single factor and the symptoms Gulf War veterans currently report remains elusive. And while the Committee finds that stress is likely to be an important contributing factor to Gulf War veterans' illnesses, the story is by no means complete: Veterans, their physicians, and policymakers clearly stand to benefit from the broad array of ongoing research. . . .

> The Committee is pained by the current atmosphere of government mistrust that now surrounds every aspect of Gulf War veterans' illnesses. It is regrettable—but also understandable. Our investigation of the Department of Defense's efforts related to chemical weapons led us to conclude these early efforts have strained public trust in our government. Hence, evidence of possible chemical warfare agent exposures during the Gulf War must be thoroughly evaluated by a group independent of DOD. This process must be conducted in an open manner and include veterans. The Committee recognizes that in November 1996 DOD announced it was expanding its efforts related to low-level CW [chemical weapon] agent exposure. These initiatives—combined with independent, vigorous oversight—could begin to restore public confidence in the government's investigations of possible incidents of CW agent exposure. (PAC, 1996, p. iii)

Office of the Special Assistant for Gulf War Illnesses

The "atmosphere of mistrust" Lashof referred to was the result of changing assessments by the CIA and DoD on the possible exposure of troops to chemical weapons. The initial assessment was that American troops had not been exposed to chemical weapons during their deployment to the Persian Gulf. In September 1995, the certainty of that conclusion began to change when a reassessment of intelligence information from the CIA and the Defense Intelligence Agency suggested that chemical agents may have been released at the Iraqi weapon depot at Khamisiyah during the U.S. occupation of the area. In May 1996, UN inspectors confirmed that 122 mm chemical rockets had been stored at Khamisiyah. In June 1996, DoD changed its long-held position and announced that, in March 1991, American troops had unknowingly destroyed sarin-filled rockets.

To say the least, the senior leadership of the Pentagon was not pleased with the quality of the staff analysis they had previously relied on, which was now so clearly wrong. In September 1996, the Deputy Secretary of Defense, Dr. John White, asked the Assistant Secretary of the Navy (Manpower and Reserve Affairs), Dr. Bernard D. Rostker—the author of this volume—to field a team to look at everything the department was doing concerning Gulf War illnesses. On November 12, 1996, White announced the establishment of OSAGWI, to be headed by Rostker, to "do everything possible to understand and explain Gulf War illnesses, to inform the Gulf War veterans and the American public of our progress, and then to ensure that DoD makes whatever changes are required in equipment, policy and procedures" (OSAGWI, 1998, p. 4). White gave Rostker broad authority to coordinate all aspects of DoD's Gulf War investigations but wanted him to focus on the war's operational aspects and future force protection issues. He emphasized the need for a communications program that would reach out to the veterans and learn from them what went on during the Gulf War. He stipulated that health-related programs—specifically, the clinical and health research programs—would remain the responsibility of the Office of the Assistant Secretary of Defense for Health Affairs. In OSAGWI's first annual report, Rostker highlighted the changes that were immediately introduced to meet President Clinton's charge to "leave no stone unturned":

- We are listening to our veterans and incorporating what they tell us into our investigations. We received almost twelve hundred postal letters and twenty-seven hundred e-mail letters through the Internet. Our "veteran contact managers" spoke with almost twenty-nine hundred veterans by phone.
- We have developed an outreach program including GulfLINK, GulfNEWS and met with veterans at thirteen "Town Hall" meetings and four national veterans conventions throughout the United States. We also frequently meet with Veterans Service Organizations and Military Service Organizations to discuss topics of interest to them.
- We are systematically investigating and reporting on possible chemical and biological agent exposures. This included substantial field testing to determine the likely level of exposure resulting from the detonations of sarin filled rockets at Khamisiyah [an Iranian weapon depot]. We have published four information papers and nine case narratives.
- We have extended our inquiries to "other causes" for Gulf War illnesses, such as the fumes from oil well fires, depleted uranium and pesticides. (OSAGWI, 1998, pp. 1–2)

In addition to spearheading the new focus on Gulf War illnesses, White provided the resources to carry out the expanded mission. The Persian Gulf Illnesses Investigation Team, which OSAGWI replaced, had had a staff of four government employees and eight contractors. Plans for the new office originally called for a staff of 110, a ninefold increase. By FY 1999, however, OSAGWI had grown to 196 personnel, 26 of whom were government employees, and the remainder were contractors. These added resources allowed an expanded program in support of concerned veterans. In its first four years, OSAGWI released 17 reports, called case narratives, on possible exposures to chemical weapons, four environmental exposure reports, and nine information papers. In addition, OSAGWI commissioned the RAND Corporation to conduct eight reviews of scientific literature pertaining to Gulf War illnesses.[33] By 1999, the GulfLINK website was being viewed by more than 200,000 visitors per month, and in May 1998, *Government Executive Magazine* selected GulfLINK as one of the "Best Feds on the Web." *GulfNEWS* circulation expanded from its original 2,000 in 1997 to nearly 20,000 in 1999. To discuss the results of its investigations and to learn about and respond to veterans' concerns, OSAGWI staff conducted town hall meetings at 17 military installations and in 13 cities throughout the country and overseas. OSAGWI answered approximately 11,500 hotline calls; fielded 6,991 emails; and sent notification letters to some 162,500 veterans who served in the Gulf. It also worked with individual Gulf War veterans to help them obtain their outpatient records from the National Personnel Records Center in St. Louis, Missouri (OSAGWI, 2000).

Noting these, a PAC special report from October 1997 acknowledged that "DOD has expanded significantly the resources it is devoting to Gulf War veterans' illnesses, . . . [and] the considerable improvement DOD has made in outreach to Gulf War veterans, particularly VSOs [veterans' service organizations]" (PAC, 1997, p. 17). However, the PAC reiterated its "recommendation that an entity other than DOD (e.g., the President's Foreign Intelligence Advisory Board or, again, NSF [National Science Foundation]) perform oversight" (PAC, 1997, p. 21). The PAC report said that

> the government's credibility in addressing the health concerns of Gulf War veterans continues to be challenged. To be sure, room for improvement exists. The government's efforts have yielded significant improvements in services and essential, new knowledge—but, still, progress is gradual. Unfortunately, however, such progress now often is viewed skeptically, at best. There remains a widespread and deeply held view that the government is failing to adequately address the health concerns of Gulf War veterans. In fact, the Committee perceives public mistrust about the government's handling of Gulf War veterans' illnesses not only has endured, but has expanded since the *Final Report*. This persistent atmosphere of distrust ill serves the Nation. . . .

> [T]he primary focus of the government's efforts needs to shift from investigations to the nth degree of individual incidents, to a process that will ensure that research data and clinical improvements with a direct impact on veterans' lives can be regularly accounted for and integrated into VA's disability compensation and medical benefits programs. (PAC, 1997, p. 23).

Special Oversight Board for DoD Investigation of Gulf War Chemical and Biological Incidents

In accordance with the PAC's recommendation—"to ensure full public accountability and reinforce the commitment to an independent review, an entity other than DoD

---

[33] The reports that emerged from this review can be found via the RAND's webpage on Gulf War illnesses (RAND Corporation, undated).

should perform any oversight" (Rudman, 2000)—President Clinton signed EO 13075 on February 19, 1998, establishing the Special Oversight Board for Defense Department Investigation of Gulf War Chemical and Biological Incidents, with former U.S. Senator Warren Rudman (R-New Hampshire) as its chairman. This board focused on OSAGWI, and in its final report found the following (quoted from Rudman, 2000, Ch. 9, "Findings" section):

- The Department of Defense and OSAGWI have worked diligently to fulfill the President's directive to "leave no stone unturned" in investigating the possible causes of Gulf War illnesses.
- DoD has made no effort to deliberately withhold information from the general public or from veterans concerning its investigations or findings related to Gulf War illnesses. On the contrary, DoD has made an extraordinary effort to publicize its findings through the publication of reports and newsletters, public outreach meetings, briefings to veterans and active duty servicemembers, the creation of a toll-free hotline, and the creation of an actively updated website.
- The Board finds that the revised case narrative methodology fully reflects OSAGWI procedures and, more important, provides the most accurate method for assessing the likelihood that chemical warfare agent exposures may have occurred in the Persian Gulf.
- The Board finds that in each of its case narratives, OSAGWI makes assessments regarding the presence of chemical and biological warfare agents that are consistent with available evidence.
- The Board finds that in each of its environmental exposure reports, OSAGWI makes assessments regarding environmental exposures that are consistent with available evidence.
- The Board finds that the Department of Defense appropriately implemented ten of the twelve recommendations contained in the PAC Special Report. (DoD was not required to act on two of the recommendations.)

In a summary, the board said that "DoD and VA have met the spirit of the PAC recommendations to search for the cause(s) of Gulf War illnesses" (Rudman, 2000, Ch. 2, "New Directions" section).

The Institutional Legacy of Gulf War Illness: Looking Toward the Future

In September 1999, the special oversight board asked DoD to expand OSAGWI's "focus from strictly Gulf War issues to the development of a 'future oriented' organization that would also address the multiple aspects of military operations before, during, and after a deployment" (Rudman, 2000, Ch. 2, "New Directions" section). As a result, the Secretary of Defense established the Office of Special Assistant to the Secretary of Defense for Gulf War Illnesses, Medical Readiness, and Military Deployments.

In 2001, the new administration of President George W. Bush took steps to consolidate and institutionalize the focus on deployment health. The new special assistant, Dr. William Winkenwerder, Jr., was also the Assistant Secretary of Defense for Health Affairs, and he soon incorporated the staff of the former special assistant's office into the established Deployment Health Support Directorate, reporting to the Deputy Assistant Secretary of Defense for Force Health Protection and Readiness.[34]

After American troops had been deployed to Afghanistan, DoD leadership told Congress that the "experiences of the Gulf War focused our attention on traditional and nontraditional challenges to deployment health" (Embrey, 2002) and that the department was committed to implementing many of the strategies the IOM had recommended in its comprehensive three-year study, *Strategies to Protect the Health of Deployed U.S. Forces* (Joellenbeck, Russell, and Guze, 1999). That report highlighted (1) Joint Staff actions to create and establish a vision for force health protection to support Joint Vision 2020; (2) the designation of the U.S. Army Center for Health Promotion and Preventive Medicine as the department's lead agency to provide a comprehensive environmental surveillance program; (3) continued efforts to coordinate and collaborate on medical research among DoD, VA, and DHHS through the Research Working Group of the Military Veterans' Health Coordinating Board; (4) sponsorship of the Millennium Cohort Study, a longitudinal study to assess the health impact of major elements of military service, especially deployments and their associated risks;[35] and (5) the establishment of three deployment health centers—one each for health surveillance, health care, and health research—focusing on the prevention, treatment, and understanding of deployment-related health concerns. Two centers are at Walter Reed, and the third is at the Naval Health Research Center in San Diego.

Gulf War Illness Circa 2016

In 2016, the IOM published its tenth report on the Gulf War and health, noting that reported health outcomes for Gulf War veterans

> have been hampered by the relatively amorphous nature of the disorder and its multiple definitions over the past two decades, including chronic multisymptom illness, Gulf War syndrome, and multiple unexplained physical symptoms. Even though the evidence base for Gulf War illness has increased over the past few years, it has provided little new information that has increased our understanding of the disease or how to effectively treat or manage it. . . .
>
> The time that has elapsed since the war—25 years—brings with it the potential to impact veterans' recall of events, . . . [and] advancing age can provoke new health

---

[34] As reported to Congress in Winkenwerder, 2002.

[35] This study involves a cross-sectional sample of over 140,000 military personnel who will be followed prospectively every three years over a 21-year period, through 2022.

concerns and the development of new diseases long after the war. In any population, it can be difficult to distinguish aging-related effects from those caused by a war many years ago. (Committee on Gulf War and Health, 2016, p. ix)

About the same time that the IOM was looking at the medical evidence, the VA reported the results of the 2012 survey of Gulf War and nondeployed Gulf War–era veterans, that "Veterans of . . . [the Gulf] war continue to report poorer health than those who served at the same time but did not see service in the Gulf" (DVA, 2016a). More specifically,

Diseases that have been associated with Gulf War service—such as Gulf War Illness presenting as chronic multisymptom illness, chronic fatigue syndrome, and fibromyalgia and dermatitis—were also significantly more likely to be reported by the Gulf War deployed. Gulf War veterans also reported more health care utilization than Gulf Era veterans. (Dursa et al., 2016, p. 43)

Accordingly, the VA renewed its call for Gulf War veterans with these symptoms to apply for disability compensation, as the following notice in the *Gulf War Newsletter* made clear:

For Gulf War Veterans, VA presumes that unexplained symptoms are related to Gulf War service if a Veteran has experienced them for six months or more. The "presumptive" illness(es) must have first appeared during active duty in the Southwest Asia theater of military operations or by December 31, 2016, and be at least 10 percent disabling.

If you are a Gulf War Veteran who may experience a cluster of medically unexplained chronic symptoms that can include fatigue, headaches, joint pain, indigestion, insomnia, dizziness, respiratory disorders, and memory problems, VA presumes that some health conditions were caused by military service. In practical terms, Gulf War Veterans who meet certain criteria don't have to prove an association between their illness and military service. By assuming a link between symptoms and military service, it can simplify and speed up the application process for benefits. (VHA, 2016c, p. 7)

What the VA did not tell veterans was that the likelihood of their claim receiving a positive response was very low. Very few of the 700,000 veterans of the Gulf War appear to have been successful in pressing disability claims based on the medical issues the VA highlighted. Generally, the VA does not track the number of presumptive service-connected disability claims filed, granted, or denied. However, in 2006, the VA did report to the IOM that, of the roughly 700,000 who served in the Gulf, 3,259 Gulf War veterans with undiagnosed illness were receiving disability payments as a result of a presumption of a service connection and that the "typical" disability severity rating was 10 percent (Samet and Bodurow, 2008, p. 62).

More recently, the GAO examined the VA's processing of Gulf War veterans' disability claims for three medical issues: undiagnosed illnesses, medically unexplained chronic multisymptom illnesses, and nine specific infectious diseases. The GAO reported that, during FYs 2010–2015, the overall approval rate for Gulf War veterans with these medical issues was 17 percent,[36] compared with 57 percent for non–Gulf War veterans. The average approval rates were approximately 13 percent for undiagnosed illness medical issues, 29 percent for medically unexplained chronic multisymptom illness medical issues, and 14 percent for medical issues related to certain infectious diseases (Emrey-Arras, 2017, p. 18). In 2015, the approval rate for medically unexplained chronic multisymptom illness was 22.6 percent, and that for undiagnosed illness was 10.2 percent.[37]

VA officials told the GAO, "These Gulf War Illness medical issues may be denied at a higher rate, in part, because . . . Gulf War illness is not always well understood by the VA staff,[38] and veterans sometimes do not have the medical records to adequately support their claims" (Emrey-Arras, 2017, p. 19). It may also be that the level of disability-associated medically unexplained chronic multisymptom illnesses and undiagnosed illnesses among the Gulf War veterans filing claims is less than what is required to warrant compensation.[39] However, VA did tell the GAO that "many of the veterans with denied Gulf War medical issues had other related medical issues approved, and, as a result, many veterans still received some disability compensation from VA" (Emrey-Arras, 2017, p. 18).

---

[36] A single veteran claim can contain many medical issues, and each issue is adjudicated separately. The 2010–2015 Gulf War illness approval rate of 17 percent reflected 18,000 positive judgments on 102,000 medical issues rated. Overall, the VA considered 24.7 million medical issues from all veterans and determined that compensation should be awarded for 14 of them (Emrey-Arras, 2017, p. 18).

[37] Computed from Table 1, "Approval Rates by VBA Regional Office for Medically Unexplained Chronic Multisymptom Illness and Undiagnosed Illness Medical Issues Completed in Fiscal Year 2015," in Emrey-Arras, 2017, pp. 39–40.

[38] For example, GAO reported that,

> [a]ccording to several VBA [Veterans Benefits Administration] claim rating staff we interviewed, VHA [Veterans Health Administration] medical examiners sometimes provide a medical opinion related to service connection when one is not necessary because the veteran has a presumptive condition . . . If VBA claim raters do not recognize that the medical examiner has provided an unnecessary medical opinion about service connection for a presumptive condition, they may inadvertently deny a claim. (Emrey-Arras, 2017, p. 22)

[39] To qualify for disability compensation under a presumptive service connection based on symptoms of undiagnosed illness or medically unexplained chronic multisymptom illness, Gulf War veterans need to present evidence of a disabling condition with a 10 percent or greater disability rating, and their illness(es) or symptom(s) must be "chronic," i.e., exhibited intermittently or constantly for 6 months (Emrey-Arras, 2017, p. 8).

The Continued Unraveling of the Middle East: Operation Enduring Freedom, Operation Iraqi Freedom, and Beyond

On June 21, 2001, Secretary of Defense Donald H. Rumsfeld told the Senate Armed Service Committee:

> Today America is strong; we face no immediate threat to our existence as a nation or our way of life; we live in an increasingly democratic world, where our military power working in concert with friends and allies helps contribute to peace, stability, and growing prosperity. (Rumsfeld, 2001)

He warned, however, that

> recent history should make us humble. It tells me that the world of 2015 will almost certainly be little like today and, without doubt, notably different from what today's experts are confidently forecasting. (Rumsfeld, 2001)

Less than three months later, Rumsfeld's doubt about the durability of his forecast came to pass.[1] On September 11, 2001, the United States was attacked by al-Qaeda, a militant Sunni Islamist global organization founded in 1988 by Osama bin Laden that, at the time of the attack, was based in Afghanistan. For the American people, the hijacking of four airplanes and the subsequent attacks on the World Trade Center in New York and the Pentagon in Washington, D.C., and the loss of Flight 93 in Shanksville, Pennsylvania, were as traumatic as the attack on Pearl Harbor, which had brought the United States into World War II. For the military, however, it proved to be a pivotal shift that rivaled the dropping of the atomic bomb on Hiroshima that ushered in the atomic age.[2] The American military had long maintained the basic structure and doctrine that had been honed during World War II and employed and

---

[1] Rumsfeld would later write, "surprise was inevitable" (Rumsfeld, 2011, p. 297).

[2] Harry Laver drove home this point:

> In September 2001, government officials, members of the military, and citizens across the United States drew parallels between the terrorist attacks on the American homeland and the December 1941 bombing of Pearl Harbor. . . .

improved during the conflicts in Korea, Vietnam, and the lighting 100-hour campaign of Desert Storm. Over the next decade and a half, during OEF in Afghanistan and OIF in Iraq, the U.S. military learned to fight a new kind of war against new kinds of enemies.[3] But in September 1991, all this lay ahead.

On the Eve of 9/11

The Army

The end of the Cold War precipitated a rethinking of America's role in the world and reconsideration of the military force structure, a "rethink" that predated even the first Gulf War of 1991 (see Bush, 1990). By the time of 9/11, the resulting drawdown and restructuring (see Rostker, 2007, pp. 653–711) had produced an Army whose end strength was 40 percent lower than it had been after Vietnam and one-third smaller than during Operation Desert Storm (see Figure 7.1). With these reductions came cuts in the Army's medical programs.[4] Nevertheless, this smaller Army was designed to fight a conventional enemy, with some defense planners pressing for an even smaller Army transformed by emphasizing informational warfare and standoff technologies, one that did not stress the physical presence of soldiers, "boots-on-the ground," at

---

A more appropriate and useful point of comparison, especially from a strategic planning perspective, is 6 August 1945, when the detonation of an atomic bomb signaled a sea change in warfare. . . .

On 11 September 2001, another paradigm shift occurred. Terrorism was added to the post-1945 conventional and nuclear strategic equation as an equally significant third factor. The Bush Administration faced a challenge similar to that which strategic planners had encountered at the opening of the nuclear age, to create an effective and rational defense policy in a world that had been radically altered, one by atomic weapons, the other by terrorism. (Laver, 2005, pp. 107–108)

[3]   OEF began on October 7, 2001, when the United States launched military operations in Afghanistan, including airstrikes against Kabul and Kandahar. In sustaining military operations for more than a decade, American troops continued to fight a widespread insurgency and establish a viable government. U.S. combat operations in Afghanistan ended on December 31, 2014. As part of Operation Freedom's Sentinel, U.S. forces remain in the country to participate in a coalition mission to train, advise, and assist Afghan National Defense and Security Forces and to conduct counterterrorism operations against the remnants of al-Qaeda, the Taliban, and the Islamic State. At the end of the first quarter of FY 2018, "there were roughly 14,000 U.S. troops in Afghanistan" (Lead Inspector General for Overseas Contingency Operations, 2017, p. 2).

On March 20, 2003, the U.S. and coalition forces launched OIF. U.S. troops seized Baghdad after just 21 days. A broad insurgency followed over the next seven years. U.S. combat operations ended on September 1, 2010. American troops remained in the country to advise Iraqi security forces as part of Operation New Dawn (OND) until the final withdrawal on December 15, 2011. Operation Inherent Resolve (OIR) is the U.S. and coalition effort to support Iraqi Security Force operations with limited military operations against the Islamic State, starting on August 8, 2014.

[4]   For a discussion of the reductions in the Army's medical program during the 1970s, 1980s, and the post–Cold War 1990s, see Marble, 2015.

Figure 7.1
Army End Strength from the End of Vietnam to 9/11

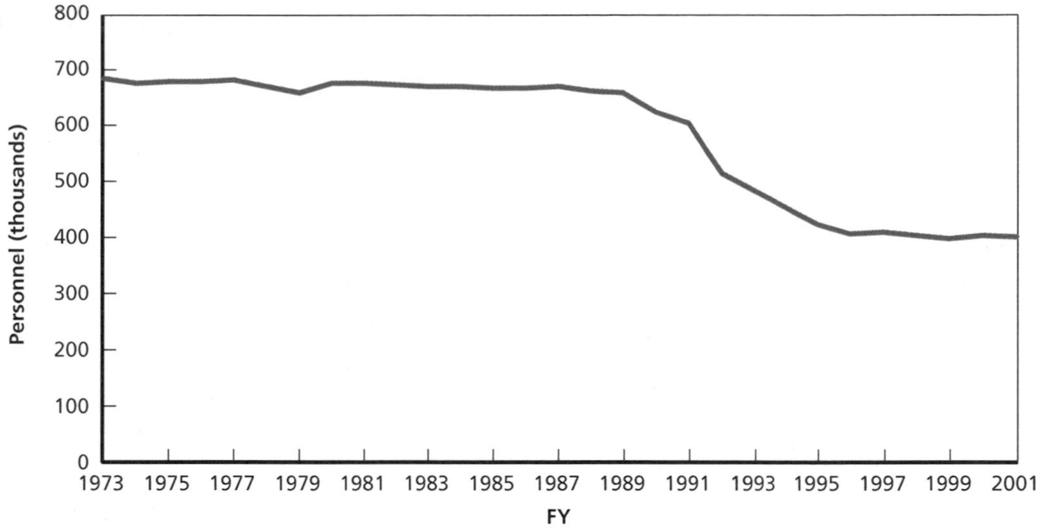

SOURCE: Office of the Under Secretary of Defense for Personnel and Readiness, 2003, Table D-15.

which the traditional Army excelled.[5] Here is how the 1990s, the decade after the Gulf War, unfolded for the Army and the situation the Army faced on the eve of 9/11.

President George H. W. Bush's Base Force

In January 1990, President George H. W. Bush proposed that the nation "transition to a restructured military" that would incorporate "a new strategy that is more flexible, more geared to contingencies outside of Europe while continuing to meet our inescapable responsibilities to NATO [the North Atlantic Treaty Organization] and while maintaining the global balance."[6] The Joint Chiefs of Staff, led by its chairman, General Colin Powell, developed a concept of a minimum, or *base*, force (see DoD, 1992b, p. 19). With the end of the Cold War, Powell thought it possible for the United States to cut defense spending by 25 percent and maintain an ability to fight two major theater wars simultaneously, without help from any of our allies, against an enemy whose forces were qualitatively equal to ours. This vision of future warfare was largely modeled after Operation Desert Storm, which to some, including Marine Corps Gen. Anthony

---

[5] Michael E. O'Hanlon reports:

> Early in Rumsfeld's tenure, the secretary's study groups were talking about slashing the active duty Army from 10 to eight divisions or even less. . . . Predictably, the Army fought very hard against this idea . . . [and] won the debate, and the September 2001 QDR [Quadrennial Defense Review] preserved Clinton's Army virtually intact. (O'Hanlon, 2003)

[6] As quoted by Senator Sam Nunn in his March 22 floor speech (Nunn, 1990).

Zinni, Commanding General of USCENTCOM, was a mistake.[7] "Desert Storm . . . was an aberration," he wrote:

> In the high- and top-level war colleges, we still fight the Saddam Hussein type of adversary, an adversary stupid enough to confront us symmetrically with less of everything, so we always win. But we are confronted with the likes of a wiser Saddam Hussein and a still-elusive Osama bin Laden—just a couple of the charmers out there who no longer will take us on with a symmetric force matchup.
>
> In still trying to fight our kind of war, be it Desert Storm or World War II, we ignore the real warfighting requirements of today. (Zinni, 2000)

Zinni's concerns notwithstanding,[8] the Army embarked on its own transformational program through the rest of the decade.[9] Small-scale contingencies and operations, such as counterdrug operations and humanitarian support, were the "lesser included cases" of a force still primarily designed to fight and win a conventional war.

President Bill Clinton's Bottom-Up Review Force

The legacy the Bush administration left for the new Clinton administration that took office in January 1993 was the Base Force. Even with American troops struggling in Somalia; the recognition of the importance of peacekeeping and peace enforcement; and humanitarian operations reflected in the new tagline, the *Full Spectrum Force* (see DoD, 1997, p. 21), the focus was still on conventional forces winning "two major regional contingencies" (DoD, 1995, p. 15). That focus did not change even after a terrorist attack on the World Trade Center in New York in 1993, the bombing of our embassies in East Africa in 1998, and the attack on the USS *Cole* in the Yemeni port of Aden in 2000. What did undermine the complacency of the Army was its disappointing performance in orchestrating the deployment of troops to Albania to prepare for a

---

[7]   A 2000 National Defense University report commented on the divergent views of future warfare, noting

> the relative rarity of American military involvement in major theater warfare against cross-border aggression. From this perspective, *Desert Storm* is an exception rather than a rule. Given the apparent increase in the number and frequency of nonstate threats and the potential for asymmetric operations, it has been suggested that the primacy of the DoD focus on preparing for classic MTWs [major theater wars] is a mistake. The threats of the future, according to this view, will be significantly different and will require a different emphasis in preparations. (Tangredi, 2000, pp. 100–101; emphasis in the original)

[8]   Zinni's admonition rang true in Afghanistan, as the Army's account notes:

> The Army's COIN [counterinsurgency] doctrine had languished over the previous two decades. With the exception of the Army's Special Forces (SF), no units had trained to conduct COIN. While commanders in late 2003 and 2004 made the transition to COIN with enthusiasm and flexibility, there was still a gap in knowledge and experience that had to be overcome. (Wright et al., 2010, p. 324)

[9]   For a comprehensive discussion of the Army's transformation during the 1990s, see Brown, 2011.

possible military action in Kosovo in 1999.[10] It brought into question the Army's plans for transformation, leading Secretary of Defense William Cohen to direct the new Chief of Staff of the Army, GEN Eric Shinseki,[11] to develop plans for a lighter, more deployable force.[12] For most of the Clinton years, however, under the rubric of Force XXI,[13] transformation meant the Army moving forward along traditional lines based on digital information technologies, e.g., sensors and digital command and control systems. Some in the Office of the Secretary of Defense (OSD) wanted to reduce the Army's force structure even further than planned by jettisoning two divisions to free funds for modernization and to shift funds from ground to air and naval forces,[14] even as some cautioned that the information age would not necessarily mean fewer boots on the ground,[15] and others argued "that no foreseeable technology offered 'silver bullets' reliable enough to justify doing away with balanced combinations of arms" (Brown, 2011, p. 226).

President George W. Bush's Transformational Force

The path that George W. Bush's administration followed was laid out in his policy speech at The Citadel, the military college in South Carolina, on September 23, 1999, almost two years to the day *before* the attack on America. The then–Republican candidate for President promised to transform the American military. He promised "a revolution in the technology of war" in which size would be replaced by "mobility and swiftness." As he saw it, "[t]his revolution perfectly matches the strengths of our country—the skill of our people and the superiority of our technology. The best way to

---

[10] The history of the Army's operations in support of 1999's Operation Joint Guardian recounts the following:

> The awkward deployment of Task Force Hawk and problems with the initial U.S. insertion into Kosovo troubled military commanders. Both tasks were completed, but because contingency plans for rapid deployment were inflexible, yet not always defined in full, nothing went as smoothly as expected. (Phillips, 2007, p. 53)

[11] Shinseki became Chief of Staff immediately after Kosovo, and one of his first tasks was to "parlay criticisms of Task Force Hawk into a mandate for accelerated transformation" (Brown, 2011, p. 191).

[12] At the time, I was Under Secretary of the Army and was privy to the letter of instruction General Shinseki received from Secretary Cohen when he assumed the position of Chief of Staff.

[13] In 1994, Force XXI developed along two lines. Army's Training and Doctrine Command redesigned operational forces, and the newly established Army Digitization Office developed and field-tested digital information technologies. This was later extended and called the Army After Next. See Donnelly, 2007, pp. 5–9.

[14] Brown notes that the debate was contentious "in the Quadrennial Defense Review that reported out in 1997 (QDR1997), [and] remained robust and lively during the Quadrennial Defense Review that reported out in 2001 (QDR2001)" (Brown, 2011, pp. 224–225).

[15] For example, in 1995, a group of information-age enthusiasts gathered at the Army's Arroyo Center at RAND to discuss the implications of the information revolution for the future of the Army. They saw a future in which "sensors, not communications or computing, will be the bottleneck on information" and argued that "[t]he best broad-bandwidth sensor on the battlefield may be the soldier, not a coupled electronic device" (Nichiporuk and Builder, 1995, p. 65), particularly "in forested, hilly terrain, . . . in canopied jungle, or in urban areas . . . finding the enemy, especially when he operates in small units, is difficult at a distance" (Nichiporuk and Builder, 1995, p. 67).

keep the peace," he told his audience, "is to redefine war on our terms" (Bush, 1999). In the Presidential debates of that year, he railed against "nation building" and policies that extended our troops to carry out what he saw as nonmilitary missions. He carried forward this vision after becoming President, telling the graduating class at the Naval Academy that

> [w]e must build forces that draw upon the revolutionary advances in the technology of war that will allow us to keep the peace by redefining war on our terms. I'm committed to building a future force that is defined less by size and more by mobility and swiftness, one that is easier to deploy and sustain, one that relies more heavily on stealth, precision weaponry, and information technologies. (Bush, 2001)

On June 21, 2001, the new Secretary of Defense, Donald Rumsfeld, expanded on Bush's ideas, telling the Senate Armed Services Committee that it was his goal to build a defense strategy that would prepare us "for the emerging threats we will all face in this new and still dangerous century" (Rumsfeld, 2001). By one account, this included discarding the "two major war" strategy in favor of a strategy for "handling murkier situations," a change that one observer thought had the "gravest implications for the Army, the most manpower-intensive service in wartime" (Ricks and Pincus, 2001).[16]

The Army had very different views on how transformation should be carried out from those of Bush and Rumsfeld. For the Army, transformation was evolutionary, and it intended to be ready to fight, "at any given time . . . at any level of intensity." Its leaders thought that technologies needed to be "proven before they were relied upon" and that "many functions might never be particularly amenable to technological solutions, requiring the steadiness and collective individual efforts of 'boots on the ground'" (Brown, 2011, p. 236).

By contrast, for Bush and Rumsfeld, transformation was revolutionary. Rumsfeld, a former naval officer with a strong background in airpower and missile defense, saw the revolution in military affairs in terms of "networked systems, information dominance, remote sensors, and precision-guided munitions" and a diminished role for "manpower-intensive ground combat power, particularly that of the Army's heavy forces" (Brown, 2011, p. 226). He was "willing to 'skip a generation' in development to free up funding for 'leap ahead' technologies" (Brown, 2011, p. 236). Indeed, as one observer notes, Bush and Rumsfeld

> were willing to take risks and force their vision on contemporary battlefields, believing technology was already far enough along to do away with much of the mass the Army considered prudent. Ground forces seemed destined to be bit play-

---

[16] The 2001 QDR noted the shift in the "focus of U.S. force planning from optimizing for conflicts in two particular regions—Northeast and Southwest Asia—to building a portfolio of capabilities that is robust across the spectrum of possible force requirements, both functional and geographical" (DoD, 2001, p. 17).

ers in their futuristic vision. Some of the missions most consumptive of boots on the ground were dismissed as "washing windows," best contracted out to lesser allies. This overlooked the historical phenomenon that allies are seldom willing to risk the blood of their soldiers if the United States is not willing to do so as well. (Brown, 2011, p. 236)

The differences in approach and philosophy led to debates not only over military strategy but also over future defense plans, as envisioned in the 2001 QDR (DoD, 2001); after 9/11, on what forces were to be deployed in Afghanistan; and later, on how the wars in Afghanistan and Iraq would be prosecuted. The dispute eventually cost Secretary of the Army Thomas White his job and alienated Army Chief of Staff Eric Shinseki from the Bush administration.[17] However, on 9/11, the Bush-Rumsfeld vision of a transformed military relying more on technology than manpower had not yet taken hold. The Army that was available to go into battle was not the high-tech force Bush and Rumsfeld envisioned but the conventional one honed during the Clinton years and geared to fight a conventional enemy. As a result, it was largely unprepared for the COIN and nation-building missions that would so consume it in the decade to come. The one exception was the special operations forces (SOF), which had been strengthened with the creation of U.S. Special Operations Command (USSOCOM). But, even then, at the time of the 9/11 attack, there was no "Unconventional Warfare . . . plan for Afghanistan" (USSOCOM, 2007, p. 87).

The American Soldier on the Eve of 9/11

In 2001, the American military had operated without conscription for 28 years. Over that time, the personnel structure of the Regular Army had changed dramatically. The enlisted force of 2001 was more senior, with more experienced soldiers in its ranks and many more females (see Figure 7.2), than the force of 1973, when the draft ended. Although women constitute a smaller proportion of the Total Force than men, their representation has grown greatly since the inception of the all-volunteer force, increasing by an average of four-tenths of a percentage point each year (see Office of the Under Secretary of Defense for Personnel and Readiness, 2003). While women were not given positions in the ground combat arms, they were assigned combat support jobs that would put them in harm's way (Williams and Staub, 2005).

---

[17] The Army's history of its transformation efforts notes that the

> differences in approach and philosophy led to recurrent debates [that] . . . inevitably spilled out of the Pentagon and into public forums. . . . When Baghdad fell, Rumsfeld and his colleagues considered themselves vindicated. Despite a few misgivings about residual messiness, most commentators saw the campaign as a brilliant victory and perhaps, like Afghanistan, yet another harbinger of the new way of war. Within a few weeks, President Bush would pilot a fighter onto an aircraft carrier grandly bearing the banner "Mission Accomplished." Rumsfeld chose not to continue his contention with the Army leadership. He fired White, a political appointee, on 1 May. Shinseki was to retire a little over a month later; Rumsfeld did not attend his 12 June departure ceremony. (Brown, 2011, p. 236)

Figure 7.2
U.S. Army: Years of Service Groups and Gender, FYs 1973–2001

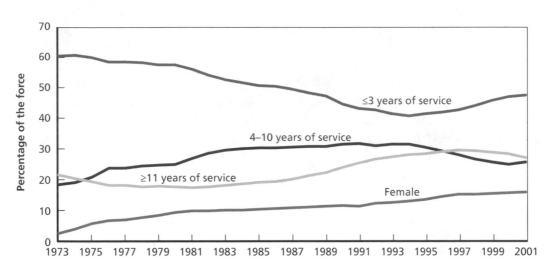

SOURCE: Office of the Under Secretary of Defense for Personnel and Readiness, 2016, Tables D-12 and D-13.

In 2001, the all-volunteer force was ethnically *diverse* but "not an exact replica of society as a whole" (Office of the Under Secretary of Defense for Personnel and Readiness, 2003, summary). The yearly report on *Population Representation* noted,

> [a]mong the enlisted ranks, the proportion of African Americans continues to exceed population counts of the civilian labor force. Hispanics are underrepresented in the military, but their percentages have increased over the years. Minorities comprise proportionally less of the officer corps; however, their representation levels are in keeping with minority statistics among the pool of college graduates from which second lieutenants and ensigns are drawn. Women continue to be underrepresented in the military, compared to their proportion in civilian society. However, accession statistics show that women continue to gain in both numerical and proportional strength. (Office of the Under Secretary of Defense for Personnel and Readiness, 2003)

This enlisted force came from all socioeconomic levels, even as members "from the lowest-income and highest-income families are less likely to be represented" (Golding and Adedeji, 2007, p. 30), as shown in Table 7.1.

It was an enlisted force with above-average aptitudes (see Table 7.2), but slightly fewer recruits were in the top group, Category I, which comprised only 7 percent of

Table 7.1
Distribution of Active-Duty Enlisted Personnel, by Family Income Category Prior to Military Service

Family Income Category	Families of Enlisted Personnel (%)	Families with Recruit-Age Youth (%)
Lowest 10 percent	6	10
10–25 percent	18	15
25–50 percent	28	25
50–75 percent	24	25
75–90 percent	17	15
Highest 10 percent	7	10

SOURCE: Adapted from CBO, 2007, p. 30.
NOTE: Percentages may not sum to 100 due to rounding.

Table 7.2
Distribution of Army Non–Prior-Service Accessions and Corresponding Civilian Population, by Armed Forces Qualification Test (AFQT) Category, FY 2001

	I (%)	II (%)	IIIA (%)	IIIB (%)	IV (%)	High Quality I+II+IIIA and High School Diploma (%)
Army non–prior-service accessions	3.84	32.44	29.23	33.65	1.86	52.47
18–23 years old	7.94	28.16	15.30	18.28	21.03	51.40

SOURCE: Office of the Under Secretary of Defense for Personnel and Readiness, 2003, Tables B-5, B-9.

those taking the Armed Forces Qualification Test (AFQT).[18] Particularly noteworthy was the fact that the Army took in almost no one classified as Category IV. In total, the percentage of the Army's non–prior-service accessions considered to be "high quality" was slightly higher than in the general population.

Medical Support on the Eve of 9/11

The post–Cold War transformation of the American military establishment was not restricted to combat forces; it also included medical support. In 1997, the Chairman of the Joint Chiefs of Staff published his vision of the future, calling for a transition to deploy "small, mobile, and capable [medical] units to provide essential care in theater,"

---

[18] AFQT scores are percentiles that are normalized to the 1997 American youth population. For example, a score of 92 represents the 92nd percentile and means that 92 percent of the youth population scored at or below that score. It is standard to report these AFQT score percentiles in these categories: Cat I: 100–93, Cat II: 92–65, Cat IIIA: 64–50, IIIB: 49–31, Cat IV: 30–10, and Cat V: 9–1.

with a focus on "first response, forward resuscitative surgery, theater hospital, and en route care" (Joint Staff, 1997, p. 31). This vision was a radical departure from the way medical care had been provided in Vietnam and even during Operation Desert Storm, just six years earlier. By the time troops were deployed to Afghanistan in 2001, significant changes had been taken in the way forward resuscitative surgery was performed on the battlefield, in the way trauma medical personnel were trained, and the care that wounded soldiers would receive during their evacuation back to the United States.

Forward Surgical Teams

As a direct result of operations Desert Shield and Desert Storm, the Army's Surgeon General initiated a medical reengineering program in early 1993 that called for the phaseout of the MASH in favor of smaller hospital modules that could provide a full range of services, be self-sufficient, and be ready for rapid response. In September 1993, the commanding general of the U.S. Army Medical Department Center and School told the Surgeon General, "I do not believe that the 30-bed MASH is a viable organization for the force structure and should be replaced with the Forward Surgical Team [FST]" (as reported in Marble, 2014, p. 24). The envisioned FSTs had

> twenty personnel, two OR tables, and no beds—truly a team, not a hospital. It would be attached to combat brigades, would deploy with the brigade, work in the battle zone, do short surgeries, and only hold postoperative patients for short periods. It . . . would rely on the brigade's medical company for key equipment such as X-ray machines and would also use the company's minimal care ward for postoperative holding. (Marble, 2014, p. 34)

In September 1996, with the concurrence of the Army Surgeon and the Chief of Staff of the Army, the new concept was officially adopted. A year later, FM 8-10-25, *Employment of Forward Surgical Teams Tactics, Techniques, and Procedure*, was published, providing the rationale for the change:

> Historically, 10 to 15 percent of wounded in action require surgical intervention to control hemorrhage and to provide stabilization sufficient for evacuation. A surgical capability as far forward as the brigade support area . . . is required to reduce mortality of those soldiers. . . . The evolving, increasingly nonlinear battlefield requires proximate medical care (to include surgical capability) to ensure that stabilization of casualties is sufficient for evacuation to a corps-level hospital. Hospitals are complex organizations that do not have the mobility of the units supported. (FM 8-10-25, 1997, p. 1-3)

The new concept was fully in accord with Joint Vision 2010.[19] As envisioned, the mission of the FST was to

> provide a rapidly deployable immediate surgery capability, enabling patients to withstand further evacuation. It provides surgical support forward in division, separate brigade, and ACR [armored calvary regiment] operational areas. The requirement to project surgery forward increases as a result of the extended battlefield. This small, lightweight surgical team is designed to complement and augment emergency treatment capabilities for the brigade-sized task force. (FM 8-10-25, 1997, p. 2-3)

The first 20-man FST under the new concept, the 274th Medical Detachment, Forward Surgical (Airborne), was established in March 1997. It was capable of continuous operations for 72 hours and only "limited by personnel fatigue/exhaustion and available supplies" (FM 8-10-25, 1997, p. 2-1). While FSTs would ideally have a lightweight shelter system with an environmental control unit for heating and cooling, they were initially deployed using general-purpose tentage configured as in Figure 7.3.

The new FST was designed to implement the concept of *phased combat casualty care*, performing only procedures necessary to stabilize patients for evacuation. Care was to be provided only to casualties with one or more of 57 specific conditions.[20] Typical of these conditions were "major chest and/or abdominal wounds; continuing hemorrhage; severe shock; wounds causing airway compromise or respiratory distress; and acutely deteriorating level of conscious with closed head wounds" (FM 8-10-25, 1997, p. 1-5). By one account, this would be the "10% to 15% of wounded who would otherwise not survive transport to the CSH in the rear, while at the same time recognizing who cannot be saved. Lesser injured and expectant patients are treated by

---

[19] The future laid out in Joint Staff, 1997, was further expanded on in Medical Readiness Division, J-4, 1997. The 2003 revision to FM 8-10-25 (rebranded as FM 4-02.25) describes the FST as

> a 20-man team, which provides far forward surgical intervention to render non-transportable patients sufficiently stable to allow for medical evacuation to a Level III hospital combat support hospital . . . . There are 57 patient condition codes . . . that identify patients with the type of injuries that would benefit most from FST intervention. Surgery performed by the FST is resuscitative surgery; additional surgery may be required at a supporting Level III hospital in the [area of operations]. Patients remain at the FST until they recover from anesthesia, once stabilized they are evacuated as soon as possible. The postoperative intensive care capacity of the FST is extremely limited, there is no holding capability. The FST is not a self-sustaining unit and must be deployed with or attached to a medical company or hospital for support. Further, the FST is neither staffed nor equipped to provide routine sick call functions. (FM 4-02.25 [FM 8-10-25], 2003, p. iv)

[20] In practice, it was not possible to strictly adhere to this prohibition. During its deployments to Afghanistan and Iraq, the 250th FST reported that,

> [i]n OEF 22 (47%) casualties sustained injuries meeting at least one of the 57 specific injury categories in Field Manual 8-10-25(4), in OIF 37 (63%) met the criteria. Entry criteria were less stringent in OEF due to stand-alone employment of the FST, whereas in OIF the unit was consistently integrated with a forward support medical platoon that would care for minor injuries. (Rush et al., 2005, p. 566)

Figure 7.3
Sample Layout for a Forward Surgical Team Using Two Large General-Purpose Tents

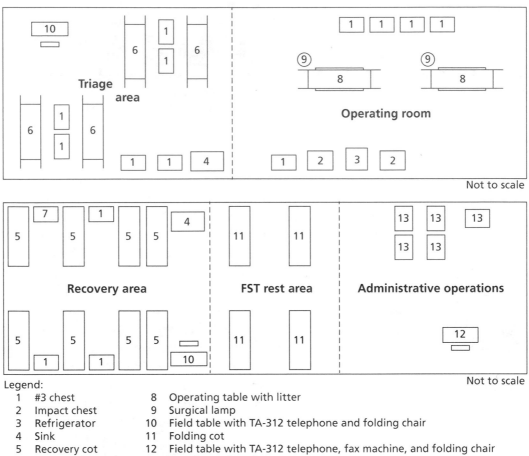

Not to scale

Not to scale

Legend:
1	#3 chest	8	Operating table with litter
2	Impact chest	9	Surgical lamp
3	Refrigerator	10	Field table with TA-312 telephone and folding chair
4	Sink	11	Folding cot
5	Recovery cot	12	Field table with TA-312 telephone, fax machine, and folding chair
6	Litter with stand	13	Supplies and equipment
7	Medical chest		

SOURCE: Adapted from FM 4-02.25 [FM 8-10-25], 2003, p. 4-3.
NOTE: The two large general-purpose tents may be placed end to end, connecting the operating room and recovery area. This can be done either by using a fabricated connective vestibule or by tying the end poles of the two tents together and rolling up the end flaps.

the co-located brigade medical company or battalion aid station" (Rush et al., 2005, p. 565). As envisioned,

> surgery performed at the FST . . . [was] generally not complete surgery rather it . . . [was] an initial effort to save life and limb, prevent infection, and render the patient transportable. Surgical procedures, not essential to resuscitation and stabilization, . . . [were to] be avoided. (FM 4-02.25 [FM 8-10-25], 2003, p. B-1)

Trauma Training

The second major change after Operation Desert Storm, going hand-in-hand with the establishing of FSTs, was improving trauma training. After Operation Desert Storm, the Army reported that

> surgical teams identified to complement the rapid movement of troops during the war and provide emergency surgical services consisted of physicians who were not surgeons, such as obstetrician/gynecologists. . . [who] could not have provided life-saving definitive surgery. (Gebicke, 1998, p. 12)

In March 1995, DoD published *Medical Readiness Strategic Plan 1995–2001*, which, among other things, was to deal with the "persistent medical support problems" (Joseph, 1995, p. iii) highlighted in operations Desert Shield and Desert Storm. However, the Congressional Budget Office found that this document did not adequately address the issue of medical training for the demands of combat. At the time, only two military hospitals, Brooke Army Medical Center and the Air Force's Wilford Hall Medical Center, had staffs that were qualified to provide Level I trauma care. As part of an informal agreement with civilian hospitals in San Antonio, Texas, the emergency rooms in both hospitals routinely saw civilian patients with "blunt and penetrating injuries caused by vehicle accidents, fires, falls, and gunshot and knife wounds" (Davidson, 1995, p. 9).

In 1996, Congress held hearings on the need for DoD to address trauma training, and Section 744 of the FY 1996 NDAA (Pub. L. 104-106, 1996) required the Secretary of Defense to implement a demonstration program to evaluate the feasibility of providing shock trauma training for military medical personnel in civilian hospitals. As a result, in August 1996, DoD established the Combat Trauma Surgical Committee and, in February 1997, promulgated training standards for hands-on experience and continuing education for trauma care. In May 1997, the surgeons general of the three medical departments endorsed these recommendations. However, establishing demonstration programs under Section 744 proved slow going (see Gebicke, 1998, p. 17). It was not until July 1999 that the Joint Trauma Training Center was established at the Texas Medical Center, Ben Taub General Hospital, with the mission to "train doctors, nurses and medics to care for trauma patients and soldiers in forward military medical operations" (Begnoche, 2001, p. 3). The program lasted only two years because of a disagreement between the Texas State Medical Board and the federal government over malpractice coverage (see Thorson et al., 2012, p. S484). In 2001, the U.S. Army Trauma Training Center (ATTC) was established at the University of Miami Miller School of Medicine Ryder Trauma Center, the only Level I trauma center in Miami-Dade County (serving a population of 2.5 million). The ATTC was staffed by ten active-duty physicians who trained upwards of 11 FSTs in two-week courses per year. The first team completed training in January 2002; between then and

2015, more than 112 FSTs—2,000 soldiers—were trained (Valdiri, Andrews-Arce, and Seery, 2015, p. e17).

Initially, the program centered on hands-on clinical training, but this changed over time:

> While the overall mission of the program to provide predeployment trauma training and validation at the end of a unit's normal training readiness cycle has remained fairly consistent over the past 14 years, the vision and philosophy has evolved. The three main goals are to provide basic and advanced trauma refresher training, combat trauma unique concepts and skills, and develop the group into a strongly functioning team to improve patient outcomes on the battlefield. There are new team-building exercises, mobile learning modules, major changes in the mass casualty exercise, new lectures and skills stations that better match current theory, and lessons learned from recent patient injuries. (Allen et al., 2016, p. 554)

Initially, rotations lasted anywhere from seven to 28 days, ending with a simulated mass-casualty exercise. Over time, the program morphed into three phases over a 14-day period. During the five days of Phase I, FST members review principles of trauma resuscitation and shock, with an emphasis on teamwork (see Figure 7.4). Phase II was the seven-day clinical phase, with the five-person teams caring for incoming traumatic patients. The capstone of the program was Phase III, in which the entire

Figure 7.4
Five-Person Trauma Team Approach Taught at U.S. Army Trauma Training Center

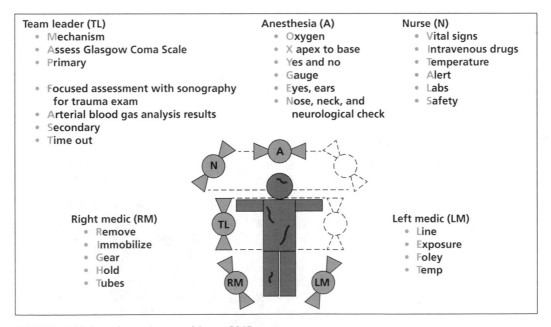

SOURCE: Valdiri, Andrews-Arce, and Seery, 2015.

20-person FST took control of all patients arriving at the trauma center during a 48-hour period. Oversight was provided by ATTC and Ryder Trauma Center hospital staffs. Following the "train as you fight" paradigm, the team tested its work-rest cycles and patient flow management skills when situations exceeded the team's capability.

The "professional excellence and personal dedication [of medical and health services support personnel] . . . [and] transformational advances in trauma care" (Berwick, Downey, and Cornett, 2016, p. 255) notwithstanding, the IOM reported that,

> [a]t the start of Operation Enduring Freedom and Operation Iraqi Freedom, the military medical force was overstaffed with specialists in pediatrics and obstetrics/gynecology but understaffed in specialties critical for combat casualty care. . . . During the latter years of the wars, additional general surgeons completed trauma and surgical critical care fellowships and deployed to forward areas . . . , but it was still common for nontrauma specialists . . . to fill in to meet the trauma care needs of forward surgical teams and combat support hospitals. . . . (Berwick, Downey, and Cornett, 2016, p. 258)

> From the first year of the war to the last . . . , the military's ability to deliver trauma care showed great variability, due in part to deployed military providers learning on the job rather than entering the combat zone prepared. A survey of military-affiliated physicians, many of whom had experienced multiple deployments, found that more than 50 percent felt that their deployed trauma team was inadequately prepared to operate in the combat environment. (Berwick, Downey, and Cornett, 2016, p. 259)[21]

The Management of Intertheater Medical Evacuation

The third major change after Operation Desert Storm was the emphasis on management of intertheater medevac. The rapidity with which the operation came to an end and the fact that the massive casualties anticipated never materialized meant that the medical system as a whole, including the AE system, was never stressed, as the GAO reported:

> The medical and evacuation units requested by the U.S. Central Command and provided by the Air Force would not have been sufficient to handle the large number of predicted casualties. Further, even though the units had to treat fewer casualties than were predicted, the units still experienced difficulty accomplishing their mission. Deployed units did not have enough or the right mix of personnel; supplies were often incompatible with the equipment, missing, or outdated; many personnel were not appropriately trained; and the system used to regulate the movement of patients did not function adequately. (Gebicke, 1993, p. 2)

---

[21] Berwick, Downey, and Cornett, 2016, Ch. 5, provides a more complex discussion of the military trauma care workforce.

Initial steps were taken in 1993 to improve the management of the AE system when the Assistant Secretary of Defense for Health Affairs established a task force of more than 130 military and civilian experts from throughout DoD.[22] Their findings, recommendations, and action items were contained in the *Medical Readiness Strategic Plan 1995–2001* (Joseph, 1995).[23] Their work was particularly timely because war games conducted in December 1994 and in March 1995 showed that the Air Force would not be able to provide adequate lift capability to move medical supplies and deployable hospitals to support the planning scenarios of fighting two nearly simultaneous major regional conflicts. As a result, the Joint Staff pressed the services to "approach medical operations from a joint perspective and redesign their medical systems assuming smaller and lighter deployable hospitals and quicker evacuation of patients to the United States for treatment" (Gebicke, 1996, p. 3). The clear emphasis was on the need for "jointness," something GAO argued was conspicuously lacking:

> current medical planning is [still] based on Cold War assumptions in which the services planned to fight the former Soviet Union individually rather than jointly. This lack of a joint approach made the DOD medical system unresponsive to the full continuum of anticipated contingencies, including major regional conflicts, peacemaking, and disaster relief. (Gebicke, 1996, p. 5)[24]

Even though the U.S. Transportation Command was established in 1992 as the single manager for DoD transportation, it was another four years before the requirements for joint planning of patient movement were established, with the publication of *Joint Tactics, Techniques and Procedures for Patient Movement in Joint Operations* (Joint

---

[22] The task force focused on nine functional areas: planning; requirements, capabilities, and assessment; command, control, communications, computers, and information management; logistics; medical evacuation; personnel; training; blood supply; and readiness oversight (Joseph, 1995; Gebicke, 1996, p. 1). A follow-on report was issued in 1998 (Bailey, 1998).

[23] DoD highlighted the need for a new strategic plan (Joseph, 1995, p. iii):

- Radical changes in the international security environment beginning in 1989 signaled the end of the Cold War and the beginning of a New World Order. The implications of this shift in focus are apparent in many actions underway for some time: development of new military strategies; major armed forces reductions; and the revision of Service missions, roles and responsibilities.

- Operations Desert Shield and Desert Storm, 1990–1991, although successful, highlighted persistent medical support problems. Several reports by the DoD Inspector General . . . , General Accounting Office . . . , and other agencies called for dramatic changes and improvements.

- Congress and a new administration initiated sweeping changes and management initiatives to realign and streamline the military. The Bottom-Up Review, Defense Planning Guidance, Section 733 Study and aggressive health care reform initiatives mandated changes to accommodate declining defense budgets and structure.

[24] See also Gebicke, 1995.

Publication [JP] 4-02.2, 1996).[25] In 1998, a series of DoD instructions, directives, and regulations further refined the requirements and responsibilities.[26]

En Route Care

The fourth major change after Operation Desert Storm was the emphasis on en route care. After Vietnam, the intertheater AE mission "remained relatively stable in its routes, airframes, and missions" (Vanderburg, 2003, p. 12). While some thought the lack of en route advanced trauma life support capabilities was a potential problem, others saw it as a problem too hard to solve.[27] During Operation Just Cause in Panama in 1989, the potential problem became a reality when casualties had to be airlifted before they were stable, and in-flight care was a "challenge for the usual crew of two flight nurses and three aeromedical evacuation technicians" (Mabry, Munson, and Richardson, 1993, p. 943).[28] Although no major doctrinal, manning, training, or equipment changes came about after Operation Just Cause, it was clear that a system designed to transport stable casualties was unprepared to meet the rigors and uncertainty of combat when unstable patients might need to be transported over long distances.[29]

---

[25] JP 4-02.2 states that

> [i]ntertheater patient evacuation is usually supported by. . . [U.S. Transportation Command] airlift resources. . . . Air Mobility Command dedicated, preplanned, opportune, or retrograde aircraft missions . . . pick up patients from staging facilities at designated theater AE interface airfields. . . . (JP 4-02.2, 1996, p. vii)

> JFCs [Joint Force Commanders] will establish a system that integrates the available capabilities of the patient movement system, synchronizes their application, and prepares to employ air, land, and sea forces to achieve patient movement objectives. (JP 4-02.2, 1996, p. viii)

[26] In January, *Health Services Operations and Readiness* (DoD Directive 6000.12, 1998) established patient movement policy and gave the Commander, Transportation Command the responsibility for establishing and maintaining a system for medical regulating and movement of patients (other than intratheater). Several months later, *Air Transportation Eligibility* (DoD Regulation 4515.13-R, 1998) set guidelines to determine eligibility for patient movement. Finally, on September 9, 1998, *Patient Movement* (DoD Instruction 6000.11) established "procedures for the movement of patients, medical attendants, and related patient movement items on DoD-provided transportation, [and] . . . aeromedical evacuation patient priorities."

[27] In 1984, the Military Airlift Command's surgeon questioned the capability to care for "marginally stable patients" at a time when "even starting an I.V. in flight can at times be as much of a challenge as catheterizing a running horse" (as quoted in Mabry, Munson, and Richardson, 1993, p. 942).

[28] Mabry, Munson, and Richardson, 1993, p. 943, goes on to say that, "[u]ltimately, one physician was released to act as a medical attendant on every flight, even though it meant the loss of physicians from an overwhelmed facility. Some of these were not trained in critical care or the flight environment."

[29] Lt Gen Paul K. Carlton, Jr., father of the Air Force's Critical Care Air Transport Team (CCATT), also highlighted the experience in Operation Just Cause:

> Beginning with Operation Just Cause in Panama (1989), it became apparent that our troops would, at times, suffer injury in a location where only minimal stabilizing medical care is available. In such situations, AE is absolutely critical to assure we can quickly move patients to state-of-the-art trauma centers, even though such centers are hundreds or thousands of miles away. (Carlton, 2003, p. v)

During the initial phase of Operation Desert Shield, in late August 1990, the 1611th AE Squadron was deployed to Saudi Arabia. By all accounts, it was unprepared to perform its mission to provide advanced trauma life support because its personnel lacked critical care training and the unit did not have the right equipment.[30] Extraordinary steps were needed. By February 1991, when offensive action commenced, the 1611th had expanded from an original complement of 75 members to more than 1,300, and AE crews had been given "an abbreviated advanced trauma life support course" (Mabry, Munson, and Richardson, 1993, pp. 943–944).

Soon after the end of Operation Desert Storm, on May 16, 1991, the Air Force addressed the issue of en route quality of care at a flight surgeons' conference at Brook AFB. The consensus recommendation from the conference was that, in the future, the Air Force should have "designated flight surgeons . . . capable of providing critical care support within the [AE] system and . . . [that they be] qualified in Advanced Trauma Life Support (ATLS) and Advanced Cardiac Life Support" (as quoted in Mabry, Munson, and Richardson, 1993, p. 946). This recommendation notwithstanding, there was again a lack of dedicated resources during military operations in Somalia in 1993, and "the most critical could not be immediately evacuated" because the sending hospital could not spare personnel for a long evacuation flight without seriously degrading its capability (Beninati, Meyer, and Carter, 2008, p. S370).[31]

After Somalia, in 1994, the Air Force Surgeon General called for a new concept of transporting casualties that moved the paradigm from "stable" to "stabilized" and put new emphasis on "replace" versus the traditional "return to duty."[32] There was also a new focus on achieving a smaller theater footprint.[33] These were radically new concepts for how to care for casualties with

---

[30] Mabry, Munson, and Richardson, 1993, p. 943, noted:

> The 1611th was faced with the prospect of moving large numbers of fresh casualties, as had been the experience in Operation Just Cause, with an AE system designed for stable casualties. Its personnel were trained but largely inexperienced, and few had critical care or ATLS [advanced trauma life support] training. . . . Ten flight surgeons were initially deployed to Saudi Arabia in August 1990 to support the USAF AE system. None had specific training; they had been arbitrarily selected without special requirement for ATLS or AE experience, and they lacked a well-defined role or mission beyond contingency medical support.

[31] Even after Operation Desert Storm, a significant limitation in the AE system was that it lacked the intrinsic capability to manage critically ill casualties. It relied on medical attendants, supplies, and equipment provided by the sending medical facility, which was not practical in many cases because sending these personnel on a long evacuation flight would seriously degrade their capability to provide care at their field locations.

[32] This is often referred to as a philosophy of "evacuate and replace" (Berry, 2002, p. 10; Critical Care Air Transport Team, 2016).

[33] Carlton, 2003, p. v, ties the need for a smaller footprint to Operation Desert Storm:

> During Operation Desert Shield/Desert Storm (1990 to 1991), the amount of sealift required to move "mobile hospitals," together with the time required to set them up, mandated that the medical services of all military branches find a new way to deliver medical care to combat troops.

a truly light, lean, mobile, and capable array of medical forces that can arrive quickly on-scene for medical support of virtually any deployment anywhere in the world, . . . equipped only for stabilization-type procedures and . . . far less capable than the old fixed facilities . . . deployed in Europe during the Cold War. (Carlton, 2003, p. v)

By 1997, this concept found its way into the Chairman of the Joint Chiefs of Staff's vision of the future (Joint Staff, 1997; Medical Readiness Division, J-4, 1997), which called for "deploying small, mobile, and capable units to provide essential care in theater" and a strategy that focused on "first response, forward resuscitative surgery, theater hospital, and en route care" (Joint Staff, 1997, p. 31).

Calling for enhanced en route care is one thing, but having the ability to provide it was another. In the early 1990s, Col P. K. Carlton and Col Chris Farmer created the first written concept of operations for expanding the Air Force's aeromedical critical care transport system, with the design of a new unit and plan of action. In May 1994, the CCATT pilot program—the 59th Medical Wing—was established at Wilford Hall Medical Center. Its goal was the

air transportation of **stabilized** (rather than stable) patients as soon as possible after treatment adequate to assure the movement to definitive care without adverse sequelae. At a minimum, a stabilized patient has an assured airway and stabilized fractures, all hemorrhage is controlled, and fluid resuscitation has begun. (Hurd and Jernigan, 2003, p. 3; emphasis in the original)

With the successful deployment of the CCATT in 1995 and 1996, the Air Force formally made the three-person CCATT a part of the AE system.[34] Complementing the establishment of the CCATT was the development and deployment of a new long-range aircraft particularly well suited for the AE mission, the C-17 (see Klesius, 2012). First operational in January 1995, the C-17 was initially used in support of operations in Bosnia in late 1995. It is most noteworthy for its ability to land on almost any semi-improved airfield and is "ideal for moving patients from almost any location directly back to the United States without en route stops. Its litter stanchions will accommo-

---

. . . [T]he Surgeons General of the Army and Navy . . . worked throughout the 1990s to streamline our medical forces.

[34] According to Critical Care Air Transport Team, 2016,

The CCAT team is a three-person medical team consisting of a physician specializing in an area such as critical care, pulmonology, surgery, etc., along with a critical care nurse and a respiratory technician. The team is experienced in the care of critically ill or injured patients with multi-system trauma, shock, burns, respiratory failure, multiple organ failure and other life-threatening complications. The complex, critical nature of the patient's condition requires continuous stabilization, advanced care, life-saving invasive interventions during transport, and life or death decisions.

date 36 litter patients and a variable number of ambulatory patients depending upon the types of seats used" (Jernigan, 2003, p. 103). See Figure 7.5.

The New Five Echelons of Medical Care

In the decade between Operation Desert Storm and OEF—1991 to 2001—medical care for the combat wounded changed from a system widely seen as ineffective to one that could rapidly move patients off the battlefield to a far forward advanced surgical treatment facility, then provide rapid air evacuation to facilities outside the war zone. The AE portion of that system has been described as "a 6,000-mile-long intensive care unit [ICU] in the sky, stretching from staging areas in the Middle East to the continental United States" (Buckenmaier and Bleckner, 2008, p. 113). As a result, the familiar five echelons of care schematic that took 45 days to traverse during the Vietnam War has been reduced to three days or less (see Figure 7.6).

The new system allowed battle casualties to be treated almost immediately after being wounded, moving to an Echelon II FST within minutes, then onward to an Echelon III CSH within hours. When medevac flights are short, casualties can be taken directly to a CSH, skipping over the FST echelon. For the most crucial casualties, the transfer out of the combat zone to an Echelon IV facility could now occur in as little as 12 hours. For those returning to the United States, the stay at the Echelon IV facility at Landstuhl, Germany, routinely lasted no longer than two or three days, less if needed.[35]

Afghanistan—Operation Enduring Freedom

Three days after the attack on the World Trade Center, President Bush flew to New York. At the site of the World Trade Center, now known as Ground Zero, he addressed the recovery workers: "I can hear you! The rest of the world hears you! And the people—and the people who knocked these buildings down will hear all of us soon." Thirty-five days later, America's all-volunteer Army, backed by a new medical support system, initiated military operations against al-Qaeda in Afghanistan.

Operations

The official U.S. Army history of the initial military response to 9/11 is titled, *A Different Kind of War* (Wright et al., 2010), which it was and would remain. While the military services had been preparing to fight two major theater wars and while the Bush

---

[35] The critical condition of most evacuees is reflected in the fact that about one-half of casualties returning to CONUS require additional surgery after they return (Stephenson, 2008, pp. 10–12).

Figure 7.5
Aeromedical Evacuation on a C-17

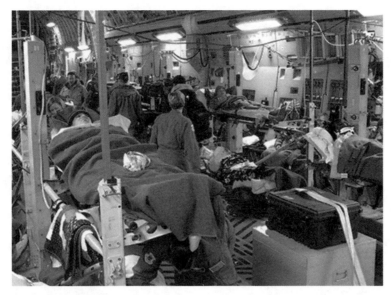

SOURCE: U.S. Air Force Photo.
NOTE: 36th Aeromedical Evacuation Squadron personnel attend to wounded soldiers on a trip from Ramstein Air Base, Germany, to Andrews AFB, Maryland.

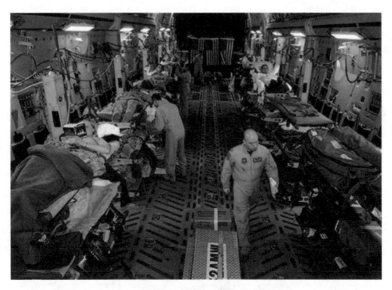

SOURCE: U.S. Air Force Photo/Master Sgt. Scott Reed.
NOTE: Monitoring patients during a C-17 aeromedical evacuation mission from Balad Air Base, Iraq, to Ramstein Air Base, Germany.

Figure 7.6
Evacuation Chain for Combat Casualties

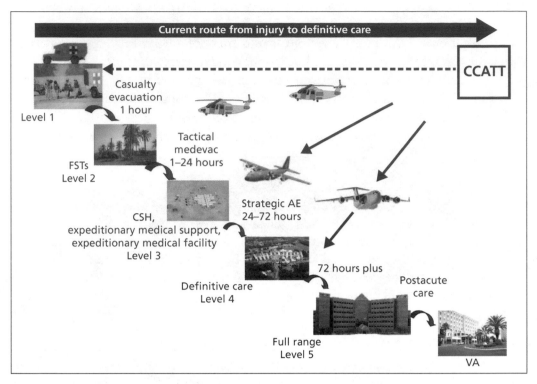

SOURCE: Adapted from Bailey et al., 2012, p. 26.

administration wanted to pivot to a more technologically advanced force, the enemy that presented itself on 9/11 required a completely different response.[36]

On September 15, 2001, four days after the attacks, President Bush assembled his senior national security advisors at Camp David to consider his options. By that time, it was known that the attack had been planned and executed by Osama bin Laden, the head of al-Qaeda, operating from his sanctuary in Afghanistan, under the protection of the Taliban. The options presented to the president that day included (1) cruise missile strike; (2) a cruise missile strike backed up by manned aircraft raids— or what Rumsfeld would later call "pounding sand a little harder" (Rumsfeld, 2011, p. 359); (3) a cruise missile strike backed by stealth bombers and some boots on the ground. It was only the last that appealed to Bush, who, as Rumsfeld later reported, wanted "American military forces on the ground in some fashion as soon as an effective

---

[36] At the time of the attack on 9/11, even after having dealt with al-Qaeda after previous attacks on the World Trade Center in New York, embassies in East Africa, and the USS *Cole*, the United States did not have either a plan to mount an offensive against terrorist targets in Afghanistan or "diplomatic arrangements for basing, staging, over flight and access . . . with Afghanistan neighbors" (Franks, 2004, p. 251).

response would be prepared" (Rumsfeld, 2011, p. 359). The problem was that conventional forces would take months to prepare, leaving America at risk of another attack. Something more immediate was called for, and it came in a plan to deploy SOF to work with local anti-Taliban forces inside Afghanistan. While the complete response to the attack would be an international effort involving not only the UN and NATO but also non-NATO countries, such as the Republic of Georgia,[37] the job of developing the detailed military plans fell to GEN Tommy Franks, commander of USCENTCOM.[38]

USCENTCOM planners developed more-detailed plans for the three options presented to President Bush at Camp David. Preferring the third plan, which used SOF, the USCENTCOM staff expected that small SOF teams

> would provide intelligence support and air support to . . . [the anti-Taliban Northern Alliance, which controlled territory in northeast Afghanistan]. US Army SF possessed the requisite training and experience in a myriad of tasks, including advising foreign armies, and SF teams were prepared to act quickly and covertly while operating in the austere environment of Afghanistan. The Air Force combat air controllers could identify enemy targets and guide ordnance onto these targets using laser target designators and other devices, making these teams a lethal joint combination. (Wright et al., 2010, pp. 44–45)

A fourth option was also developed, "a broader intervention with larger conventional units," or what General Franks called a *sequel* that would follow the initial phases of option three and "exploit the gains made by the NA [Northern Alliance] and ensure remaining enemy concentrations were defeated" (Wright et al., 2010, p. 45).[39] This would eventually include an effort to "Prevent the Re-Emergence of Terrorism and Provide Support for Humanitarian Assistance Efforts" (Wright et al., 2010, p. 46)—the last of the four phases in USCENTCOM's campaign plan. In Franks' view, this would take three to five years. He was "certain that surviving Taliban and al-Qaeda units would resort to guerrilla combat once their large formations had been destroyed . . . [and that] stabilizing and rebuilding Afghanistan . . . would require both counterinsurgency and civil affairs military forces" (Franks, 2004, pp. 271–272). This was

---

[37] Wright et al., 2010, pp. 31–36, describes the development of the Coalition, including NATO and the UN.

[38] As Wright et al., 2010, p. 42, noted,

> CENTCOM did not have a developed plan on the shelf for conventional ground operations in Afghanistan, nor did its planners have the type of detailed information required to immediately construct a detailed plan. . . . The leadership of CENTCOM and the planning teams thus began scrambling to learn as much as they could about Afghanistan's history, culture, and terrain.

[39] The Afghan Northern Alliance was an anti-Taliban coalition that controlled territory in northeast Afghanistan and that had been established in late 1996, after the Taliban took over Kabul, the capital. The Northern Alliance fought a defensive war against the Taliban government. The alliance received support from Iran, Russia, Turkey, India, and Tajikistan, while the Taliban were backed by al-Qaeda and Pakistan.

just the kind of mission President Bush had railed against when he was a candidate for president (Miller, 2010; "Bush a Convert . . . ," 2008).[40]

Given Afghanistan's landlocked geographic location, there was an immediate need to make sure American forces had ready access to the country from Uzbekistan, Tajikistan, and Pakistan for forward operating bases for combat search and rescue (CSAR) units, communication relay stations, and medevac units. As plans developed, medical support was to be provided not only to American and Coalition forces but also to the Afghan population.[41] The initial U.S. military response, OEF,[42] began on October 7, 2001, with air strikes against targets in Afghanistan. The first insertion of Special Force's Operational Detachment–Alpha teams occurred on October 19. The Army's history recounts:

> [J]ust over 5 weeks had passed since the World Trade Center buildings had fallen. Within those 5 weeks, the Coalition had planned a complex response to the 9/11 attacks and then launched the initial deployment of forces . . . . Unlike preceding American wars, SOF would be the main effort for this fight. Instead of selecting the US military's powerful conventional units as the American vanguard on the ground, leaders at the Pentagon and at CENTCOM had chosen these small teams to deal the fatal blows to the Taliban and al-Qaeda. It would indeed be a different kind of war. (Wright et al., 2010, pp. 67–68)

It took a little more than six weeks for approximately 100 SF soldiers, some of whom are shown in Figure 7.7, to empower the Northern Alliance and decisively defeat the Taliban in northern Afghanistan. This was followed by victories at Mazar-e-Sharif and Kabul in November 2001 and Kandahar on December 7, 2001. This led to the formation of a new interim government as coalition forces engaged al-Qaeda in the

---

[40] At The Citadel in South Carolina on September 23, 1999, presidential candidate Bush said:

> As president, I will order an immediate review of our overseas deployments—in dozens of countries. . . . The problem comes with open-ended deployments and unclear military missions. In these cases, we will ask, "What is our goal, can it be met, and when do we leave?" As I've said before, I will work hard to find political solutions that allow an orderly and timely withdrawal from places like Kosovo and Bosnia. We will encourage our allies to take a broader role. We will not be hasty. But we will not be permanent peacekeepers, dividing warring parties. This is not our strength or our calling. (Bush, 1999)

[41] The Army's history recounts:

> Because the Coalition campaign was focused on al-Qaeda and the Taliban rather than against the Afghan people, the United States wanted to ensure the war did not deprive the innocent people of Afghanistan of food and other necessities. President Bush stipulated that humanitarian assistance be a vital component of the campaign. (Wright et al., 2010, p. 50)

> In addition to the bombing, on the first night of the air campaign C-17 Globemasters, flying from Ramstein Air Base in Germany, began dropping food and medical supplies to the Afghan population. (Wright et al., 2010, p. 64)

[42] After 2014, U.S. military operations in Afghanistan, both noncombat and combat, continued under the name Operation Freedom's Sentinel.

Figure 7.7
Hamid Karzai with U.S. Special Forces During Operation
Enduring Freedom in 2001

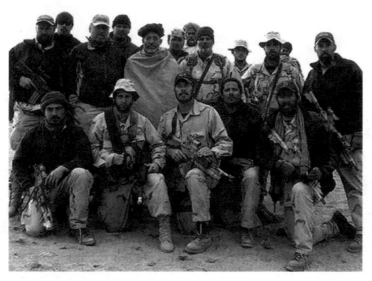

SOURCE: U.S. Army photo.

mountains of Tora Bora. The action at Tora Bora not only failed to kill or capture Osama bin Laden, it also showed the limits of unconventional warfare. Three months later, in an action known as Operation Anaconda, conventional U.S. Army forces engaged the Taliban and al-Qaeda for the first time.[43]

After Operation Anaconda, the nature of OEF fundamentally changed. The Taliban and al-Qaeda "scattered and sought refuge in remote corners of Afghanistan or across the border in Pakistan" (Wright et al., 2010, p. 181), altering their tactics from conventional to unconventional warfare. For the Coalition, accomplishing its mission became challenging because, as the Army would later note, the Taliban and al-Qaeda "were actually better suited to unconventional tactics rather than the conventional operations they [had previously] tried to conduct."[44] While fighting a war of insur-

---

[43] As to the use of conventional forces, see Wright et al., 2010, pp. 136–137.

[44] In retrospect, the Army came to understand that,

> Once driven out of or otherwise freed from fixed positions, they [the Taliban and al-Qaeda] would become a more potent fighting force. No longer would they have to wait for attacks against them; they could seize the initiative, at least locally, deciding where and when to attack. This transformation of the Taliban and al-Qaeda from conventional fighters to the unconventional began at Tora Bora. Bin Laden, Mullah Omar, and their military commanders realized that they could not stand up to US military might and melted into the mountains of southern and eastern Afghanistan and the tribal regions of Pakistan to escape. In these sanctuaries, they would begin to reconstitute and eventually sally forth to strike US and Coalition forces then disappear back into the mountains to blend in with the local population. (Wright et al., 2010, pp. 120–121)

gency was new for the Americans, it was familiar for the Taliban, as summed up by an Afghan leader hundreds of years before: "When you encounter a stronger enemy force, avoid decisive engagement and swiftly withdraw only to hit back where the enemy is vulnerable. By this you gain sustainability and the ability to fight a long war of attrition" (Wright et al., 2010, p. 181).

After Operation Anaconda, it was also clear that the new government in Kabul would need both military and economic support, and the United States took on the very mission of nation-building that President Bush had so denounced just a few months before.[45] In the future, military support would be very different; the Americans came to understand that the war in Afghanistan would take a "different mindset and different capabilities than . . . that focused on defeating an adversary militarily" (JP 3-24, 2013, p. xi). Eventually, the Coalition, while still employing conventional units, shifted its focus from just defeating the enemy on the battlefield to COIN operations.

There was another change in the works, one that would put OEF on the back burner in favor of toppling the regime of Saddam Hussein in Iraq. Even before Kandahar fell on December 8, 2001, Secretary of Defense Rumsfeld was pressing Franks to prepare a "commander's concept" for war against Iraq.

A complete accounting of military operations in Afghanistan is well beyond the scope of this book, but suffice it to say the United States "enjoyed less success in achieving the Coalition's ultimate objective—the creation of a stable Afghanistan" (Wright et al., 2010, p. 317) than it had in the initial campaign against al-Qaeda and the Taliban. After the initial defeat of the Taliban in December 2001, the number of U.S. troops doubled, from 10,000 in 2002 to 20,000 in 2005 (see Figure 7.8).[46] Even as

---

[45] In his autobiography, President Bush explains:

> Over time, the thrill of liberation gave way to the daunting task of helping the Afghan people rebuild—or, more accurately, build from scratch. . . . When I ran for president, . . . I worried about overextending our military by undertaking peacekeeping missions. . . . But after 9/11, *I changed my mind*. Afghanistan was the ultimate nation-building mission. We had liberated the country from a primitive dictatorship, and we had a moral obligation to leave behind something better. We also had a strategic interest in helping the Afghan people build a free society. The terrorists took refuge in places of chaos, despair and repression. A democratic Afghanistan would be a hopeful alternative to the vision of the extremists. (Bush, 2010, pp. 204–205; emphasis added)

See also Bush, 2002, and Dao, 2002. While President Bush clearly had changed his mind,

> senior officials in the Pentagon told him [LTG Dan K. McNeill, the Combined Joint Task Force–180 commander] to plan for US forces to be in Afghanistan for a very limited period and to ensure that American Soldiers did not become involved in nation building. . . . The strong antipathy toward large-scale reconstruction and governance efforts at high levels in the US Government persisted through 2002 and into 2003, shaping the development of OEF as well as the nascent plans to overthrow the Saddam regime in Iraq. (Wright et al., 2010, p. 319)

[46] There are many ways to measure the number of troops deployed to fight the Afghan and Iraq wars. The counts of boots on the ground in Figure 7.8 are based on a once-a-month headcount limited to U.S. troops in country that is compiled by the Joint Staff using inputs from the services. Other measures are based on "operational reports, combat pay records, average strength reports, and location reports," with DMDC preparing the last two.

Figure 7.8
Boots on the Ground in Afghanistan, 2001–2018

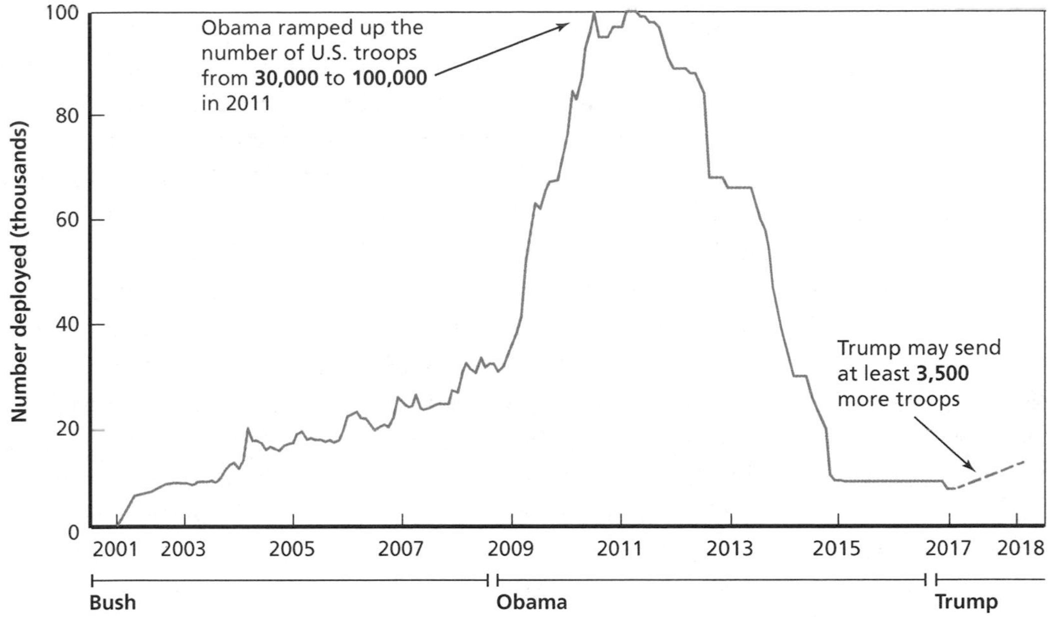

SOURCE: Frostenson and Lin, 2017. Used with permission.

U.S. troop levels surpassed 35,000 in 2008, the security situation on the ground was judged to be unsatisfactory; before leaving office in 2009, President Bush initiated the so-called "Afghanistan surge," authorizing a further increase up to 45,000 troops.

Soon after taking office in 2009, President Barack Obama approved the deployment of an additional 21,000 service members to Afghanistan.[47] In November 2009, with the goal to "cripple the Taliban, train the Afghan military, stabilize government then withdraw the U.S. forces by the . . . [end of his] second term" (Kurtzleben, 2016), he added another 20,000 troops to the surge (see Baker, 2009). In December 2009, he agreed to an additional 30,000 troops—boots on the ground—with deployed troop levels peaking at 100,000 in May 2011. At the end of July 2011, President Obama announced that the surge would be reversed and that the U.S. troops would move to limit their combat role and focus on training and assisting the Afghan Army. In February 2013, he announced that the number of U.S. troops in Afghanistan would be reduced to 33,000 by the end of 2013. On May 27, 2014, President Obama announced that the last day of OEF would be December 31, 2014, even as he planned for some

---

Following the lead of the Congressional Research Service, the numbers reported here are boots on the ground or in-country troop levels. The differences between the various measures can be significant (Belasco, 2009, pp. 21–23).

[47] Belasco, 2009, pp. 1–3, offers a detailed discussion of President Obama's actions.

9,800 troops to remain in Afghanistan for another year as part of Operation Freedom's Sentinel. In June 2016, the House of Representatives passed the FY 2017 Defense Authorization Act, which contained a "sense of Congress" resolution that the United States should keep 9,800 troops in Afghanistan after 2016 (see Katzman, 2016, p. 30). In July 2016, President Obama announced that 8,400 American troops would remain in Afghanistan through the end of his term in office, a significantly larger number than he had originally hoped (see Landler, 2016). However, as late as the end of 2017, there were 14,000 American troops in Afghanistan, with U.S. forces exercising "expanded combat authorities . . . to conduct offensive operations against the Taliban, rather than only engage with the militants in self-defense" (Lead Inspector General for Overseas Contingency Operations, 2017, p. 2).

Initial Battlefield Medical Support for the Combat Troops in Afghanistan: The First Test of the New System

The first test of the new medical system put in place after Operation Desert Storm came during the initial phases of OEF with the initial deployment of the 274th and 250th FSTs and the later deployment of the 102nd FST. Given the small number of U.S. soldiers deployed and the low-intensity nature of the initial conflict, medical support was largely provided by the organic capabilities of the deployed units (see Holt and Jones, 2015, p. 36). Overall American casualties were modest (see Figure 7.9), and the tempo of casualties did not provide a robust test of the new medical support system.

The 274th FST was the first to deploy. It covered the northern part of Afghanistan from Uzbekistan, then moved to Bagram Airfield in Afghanistan after the fall of Kabul. The 250th FST initially covered the southern part of Afghanistan from Oman, then moved to Kandahar after the fall of that city. The first Echelon III facility in the combat zone was the 86th CSH, originally posted to Uzbekistan. The 339th CSH, a reserve unit, was the "first U.S. hospital in Afghanistan" (Beitler et al., 2006, p. 189). After six months, the reserve unit was replaced by the multicomponent 48th CSH.

274th Forward Surgical Team

The 274th FST from Fort Bragg, North Carolina, was deployed to Uzbekistan on October 14, 2001 (see Peoples et al., 2005a; Peoples et al., 2005b). Figure 7.10 shows an FST in operation. The 274th FST saw its first combat casualties on November 26, 2001, and dispatched a five-man surgical team to Kandahar, Afghanistan, on December 5, 2001, to care for soldiers injured from a friendly fire incident. On December 7, 2001, the FST sent a five-man team and an operating room to Bagram, Afghanistan, with the rest of the team following shortly. The 274th Forward Surgical Hospital was redeployed to CONUS on May 8, 2002.

During its seven months in support of OEF, the 274th cared not only for U.S. soldiers but also for soldiers from the other coalition countries, Afghan militia, and even enemy soldiers. Of the 153 American soldiers the FST classified as combat casual-

Figure 7.9
Army Casualties During the Initial Phase of Operation Enduring Freedom, October 2001–March 2003

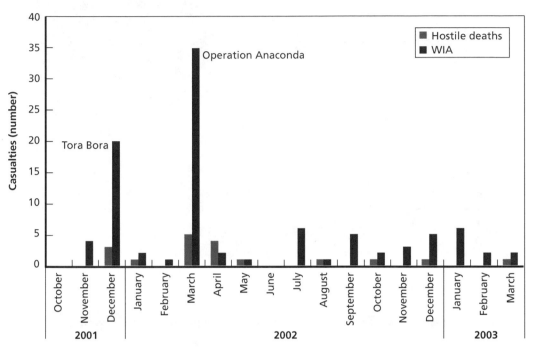

SOURCE: DMDC, 2016.

ties, 14 were classified as KIA; 108 were WIA; 14 had diseases; and 17 had nonbattle injuries. Fragments, mainly from mines, caused about one-half of the casualties, and wounds were predominantly of the extremities, with few significant head, chest, and abdominal wounds. Gunshot wounds were the most common cause of death, accounting for 57 percent of all deaths. The surgical team performed 54 major combat-related trauma surgeries. It performed total of 33 vascular procedures, with 13 amputations; six of these were traumatic amputations, and seven were nontraumatic amputations.[48] The unit attributed the relatively few penetrating head, chest, and abdominal wounds and the resulting low mortality rate to the low-intensity nature of the conflict and the use of personal protective equipment—body armor.

As one might expect, the tempo of activities at the 274th FST was very much geared to the tempo of battle, with Operation Anaconda being the most challenging (see Table 7.3). By one account, the 274th was at times overwhelmed by waves of casualties, suggesting the need not only for predeployment training but also for further training of deployed FSTs received (Pereira et al., 2010, p. 985).

---

[48] *Traumatic amputation* refers to the loss of a body part, usually a finger, toe, arm, or leg, that occurs as the result of an accident or injury. In combat, the majority of these are due to explosions (Clasper and Ramasamy, 2013).

Figure 7.10
Forward Surgical Team in Afghanistan

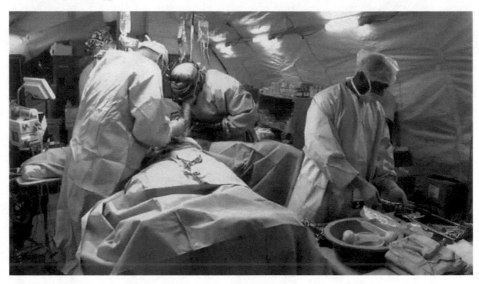

SOURCE: Still image from Usher, 2011.

Table 7.3
U.S. Combat Related Casualties Cared for by the 274th FST in Support of Operation Enduring Freedom

	274th FST		Army	
Period	KIA	WIA	KIA	WIA
Before Operation Anaconda, October 2001–February 2002	6	56	4	27
During Operation Anaconda, March 2002	8	88	5	35
During Operation Anaconda, April 2002–May 2002	0	3	5	3
Total	14	147	14	65

SOURCES: Numbers for 274th FST from DMDC, 2016; those for the Army from Peoples et al., 2005a, pp. 452, 454, 456.

NOTE: Note that the distribution of KIAs, and the absolute number of WIA numbers reported by the 274th FST and those recorded by the Defense Casualty Analysis System are different.

Even with the few U.S. casualties sustained during the initial phase of OEF, there were lessons to be learned. In a published report recounting the deployment to Afghanistan, the surgical staff of the 274th FST suggested that, in the future, FSTs needed to be more "flexible, well trained, and well equipped," with a "compact, portable, ultrasound system for focused abdominal sonography for trauma examinations and the new portable, digital, X-ray system" (Peoples et al., 2005b, p. 468). The team had lacked sufficient sterilization equipment; generator capacity; heaters; tentage; and, most important, radiographic capability (Fischer, 2003, p. 3). The 274th FST reported that it was able to overcome the shortage of radiographic equipment by using a British portable digital X-ray system.[49]2

250th Forward Surgical Team

Initially, the 250th FST from Fort Lewis, Washington (see Place, Rush, and Arrington, 2003),[50] was deployed to Seeb Air Base near Muscat Oman (SABO), with the Air Force's 320th Expeditionary Medical Group, then moved forward to Kandahar International Airport in Afghanistan after the city was taken. At Kandahar, it "provided stand-alone surgical support for the CJSOTF-S [Combined Joint Special Operations Task Force–South] (Task Force K-Bar), the 26th Marine Expeditionary Unit, 3rd Brigade/101st Airborne Division (Air Assault), Coalition Forces, and local Afghan militia" (Rush et al., 2005, p. 565). The unit stayed at Kandahar until April 2, 2002, when it returned to CONUS.[51] During its six-month deployment, the 250th FST performed 68 surgical procedures on 50 patients (see Rush et al., 2005, p. 564).

The workload at both sites was low, even for a low-intensity special operations conflict. While there were sporadic peaks, the surgical team saw no more than eight casualties per day at SABO and five casualties per day at Kandahar. On the busiest day, the team performed 12 operations at SABO and seven operations at Kandahar. In total, only 57 specific injuries required emergent resuscitative surgery.[52]

The deployment to SABO was "significantly different from the Army doctrine that states the FST should be one terrain feature away from the battle" (Place, Rush, and Arrington, 2003, p. 421). As a result, the time from wounding to treatment ranged between 6 and 12 hours. After the unit redeployed forward to Kandahar, the mean time from wounding to treatment fell to less than three hours. However, the redeployment put the unit in harm's way, performing surgical procedures while under fire. (see Figure 7.11).

---

[49] Specifically, at peak times, the British 34th Field Hospital assisted with many of the combat wounded, and the 274th made use of the British X-ray equipment before receiving its own new field digital X-ray system (Peoples et al., 2005b, p. 467).

[50] As part of a feasibility study for the Joint Trauma Training Center program in 1999, some members of the 250th FST received training at the Level 1 trauma center at Ben Taub Hospital (Houston, Texas). However, they were not allowed to function as a team or to use their equipment. The conclusion was that "[b]ecause the real and opportunity costs are significant, this program does not justify trauma sustainment for FST surgeons from military trauma centers" (Place et al., 2001, p. 93).

[51] Rush et al., 2005, p. 565, describes the initial deployment of the 250th in more detail.

[52] The 250th FST reported that, similar to the experience of the 274th FST, the majority of injuries (55 percent) resulted from blasts, with gunshots making up only 17 percent of all injuries (Place, Rush, and Arrington, 2003, p. 421).

Figure 7.11
Surgery Under Live Fire in Afghanistan

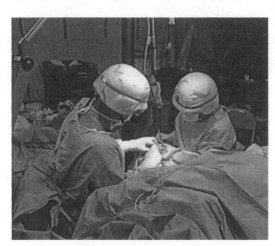

SOURCE: Pratt and Rush, 2003.
NOTE: The 250th Forward Surgical Team performs
surgery on a wounded special operations soldier
while under live fire at Kandahar, Afghanistan.

102nd Forward Surgical Team

In August 2002, the 102nd FST, which had been created soon after 9/11 in fall 2001, deployed to Kandahar (see Beekley and Watts, 2004). The unit's primary mission was to provide trauma surgical support to units of the 101st and 82nd Airborne Divisions, to coalition special operations units, and to allied Afghan militia forces. The FST's mission was expanded to include humanitarian assistance. This was the first unit to be trained at the Army's new Advanced Trauma Training Center at the Ryder Trauma Center of the University of Miami. The team consisted of three general surgeons, one orthopedic surgeon, two nurse anesthetists, one critical care nurse, one emergency room nurse, one operating room nurse, one executive officer, and five emergency medical technicians or scrub technicians. The team was supported by a five-person Air Force Critical Care Aeromedical Transport Team also stationed at Kandahar. It was supported by 48th CSH at Bagram Airfield, near Kabul. Over its seven months in theater, the 102nd FST performed 112 operations on 90 patients, of whom 79 percent were trauma patients. Most of the patients it saw, however, were Afghan militia or civilians; less than 30 percent were American soldiers. Wounds were commonly caused by high-velocity gunshots or blast fragmentation.

48th Combat Support Hospital

A contingent of the 48th CSH established the first integrated multicomponent hospital ever deployed to a combat zone. The blended unit of active duty and reserve soldiers was mobilized on October 21, 2002, arrived at Bagram Airfield near Kabul at the beginning of December and saw its first patient on December 6, 2002. It saw its last patient on June 7, 2003. The unit initially consisted of 124 personnel, about 23 percent of its parent unit,[53] to staff "a 28-bed hospital with 12 intensive care unit (ICU) and 16 intermediate care ward beds. . . . There were two operating rooms, equipped and staffed to perform a total of three simultaneous procedures" (Beitler et al., 2006, pp. 189–190). Figure 7.12 shows the deployed 48th CSH.

In the six months the 48th CSH was deployed, it saw 10,679 U.S. and coalition forces, civilian contractors, Afghan military, and Afghan civilian patients, the vast majority for routine problems in sick call. There were 477 hospital admissions, of which 208—44 percent—were American or coalition soldiers. A total of 358 surgical procedures were performed on 168 trauma patients, including 62 amputations on 48

Figure 7.12
Aerial View of the 48th Combat Support Hospital Deployed at Bagram Airfield, Near Kabul, Afghanistan, December 2002–June 2003

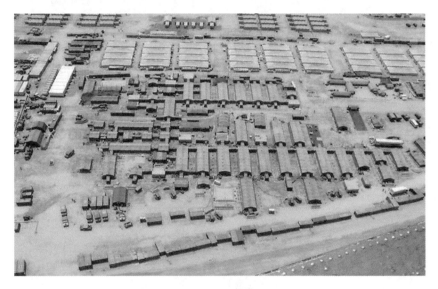

SOURCE: Strite, 2010.

---

[53] The initial deployment included:

There were 92 (74%) men, 32 women, 77 (62%) enlisted soldiers, and 47 officers. Seventy-three (59%) individuals were assigned to the unit and the remaining 51 were active duty professional fillers assigned from hospitals belonging to the Army's North Atlantic and Southeast Regional Medical Commands. The professional staff included six surgeons (general, one; general/vascular, one; general/surgical oncology, one; orthopedic, two; oral maxillofacial, one), four anesthesia providers (a combination of anesthesiologists and certified registered nurse anesthetists), one emergency medicine physician, two family physicians, one internist (initially a gastroenterologist and later an infectious disease specialist), one pediatrician, one radiologist, and one physician's assistant. The nursing staff consisted of 16 registered nurses. Radiology capabilities included computed tomography, ultrasound, and plain films while the laboratory contained a blood bank, microbiology section, and hematology and chemistry elements. An active three-man pharmacy was also an integral part of the unit. (Beitler et al., 2006, p. 189)

individuals. The most common causes of injury were land mines and unexploded ordnance. The most common injuries were to the extremities. The value of body armor
was apparent.[54]

Within the Army's five-level echelons-of-care organization (see Figure 7.6), the
Echelon III 48th CSH supported the two Echelon II FSTs. Over the six months, 91
patients were evacuated from the FSTs to the 48th CSH, and 25 trauma patients were
evacuated from the 48th CSH to the Echelon IV facility at Landstuhl Regional Medical Center in Germany, typically within three to five days of arriving at the CSH.

Over the six months, the limitations of the CSH became clear, especially given
that it performed many of the functions of a community hospital, for which it was not
designed. As the unit later noted,

> [t]he CSH was designed, equipped, and supplied to provide care to U.S. and coali-
> tion forces. The inclusion of Afghan patients and U.S. contractors added pediatric
> and more elderly individuals. In addition, an institution designed for short patient
> stays was compelled to provide care over protracted periods of time. These patients
> frequently required advanced ICU care followed by rehabilitation. Medical supply
> was problematic throughout the deployment, and this necessitated ingenuity and
> resourcefulness to optimize patient care. Finally, patients were evacuated to the
> CSH from a variety of rural locations throughout the nation. Faced with lim-
> ited local medical infrastructure, a steady influx of Afghan patients and paucity
> of resources for medical outreach, discharge planning, transport, and placement
> proved very challenging. (Beitler et al., 2006, p. 192)

Iraq—Operation Iraqi Freedom

Although responding to Osama bin Laden, al-Qaeda, and the Taliban in Afghanistan
was the first order of business after 9/11, it was hardly the only military action on President Bush's mind. On September 26, 2001, just 15 days after 9/11 and a week *before*
American forces went into battle in Afghanistan, President Bush asked Secretary of
Defense Rumsfeld to "take a look at our war plans on Iraq" (Rumsfeld, 2011, p. 425).
On November 27, 2001, Secretary Rumsfeld asked General Franks to prepare a "commander's concept" for war against Iraq. On December 4, 2001, even as Coalition forces
were pressing the final attack on Kandahar, the first version of the campaign against

---

[54] The unit later reported:

> The benefits of body armor were clearly apparent when comparing coalition and Afghan patients. The protec-
> tive equipment frequently prevented potentially lethal torso wounds. Land mine injuries provide a valuable
> case in point. Although Afghan patients often sustained multiple injuries, the wounds of soldiers wearing body
> armor were generally confined to the extremities. (Beitler et al., 2006, pp. 192–193)

Iraq was presented to Rumsfeld. President Bush was briefed on December 12, 2001, and again on December 28, 2001.[55]

General Franks knew from the start that "Iraq would differ in complexity from Afghanistan by several orders of magnitude" (Franks, 2004, pp. 335–336) He would later say that, while the challenge in Afghanistan "had been to remove the Taliban and destroy al Qaeda's base of operations, . . . Iraq represented a vastly more difficult challenge" (Franks, 2004, p. 336). The goal would be to "to remove the regime of Saddam Hussein" (Franks, 2004, p. 330).

Operations

The military campaign Secretary Rumsfeld and General Franks envisioned, the first major combat of the 21st century, would challenge the old maxim that "the attacking force should have a 3-to-1 numerical advantage over the entrenched defender" (Franks, 2004, p. 415). As Franks saw it, "strength would derive from the mass of effective firepower, not simply the number of boots or tanks on the ground" (Franks, 2004, p. 415).[56]

Military actions against Iraq—OIF—commenced on March 19, 2003, with the main ground attack kicking off on March 21. Less than three weeks later, on April 9, Baghdad fell. Prophetically, Franks later noted that "[t]he media would report the war was won. And the major battles *were* over. But not the war" (Franks, 2004, p. 523). OIF would last for another seven years.

Officially, U.S. combat operations ended on September 1, 2010. American troops, however, remained to support Iraqi security forces as part of OND until the final withdrawal on December 15, 2011. On August 8, 2014, OIR saw the return of American and Coalition forces to support the Iraqi Security Forces against the Islamic State.

Military engagement in Iraq was, to a great extent, a replay of Afghanistan. Military planners effectively produced a quick and decisive defeat of Iraqi military forces, yet were "ineffective in preparing for postwar operations" (Perry et al. 2015, p. 53).[57]

---

[55] Franks, 2004, pp. 346–356, and Rumsfeld, 2011, p. 431, provide details of the briefing.

[56] As Franks saw it,

> Our ground forces, supported by overwhelming air power, would move so fast and deep into the Iraqi rear that time-and-distance factors would preclude the enemy's defensive maneuver. And this slow-reacting enemy would be fixed in place by the combined effect of artillery, air support, and attack helicopters. (Franks, 2004, p. 415)

[57] RAND's comprehensive report on OIF for the Army concluded that it

> was not a lack of planning for either combat (also called Phase III) or postwar (also called Phase IV) operations that led to the coalition's military forces—triumphant in all major combat operations—being unprepared for the immediate postwar challenges. Instead, problems arose from the failure of the planning process to identify resource requirements for the transition from combat to post-combat operations, as well as from the failure to challenge assumptions about what postwar Iraq would look like. (Perry et al., 2015, pp. xx–xxi)

As Figure 7.13 shows, the U.S. troop level was still at 149,000 six months after the invasion of Iraq; by year's end, the level fell to about 124,000 and remained there for the next three years. As in Afghanistan, the security situation on the ground deteriorated. By October 2006, weekly security incidents in Iraq reached 1,400.[58] In January 2007, President Bush announced that five additional brigade combat teams (BCTs), an increase of 30,000 troops, would be deployed; the surge would peak at 165,000 troops in November 2007.[59] By July 2008, troop levels were back to 147,000. In January 2009, with U.S. forces emphasizing advising and assisting, rather than engaging in combat, President Obama reduced the troop level to 141,000 as of March 2009; by September 2010, the troop level was at 49,000. With the failure to a sign a new bilateral security agreement, only a handful of U.S. troops would be in Iraq at the start of 2012.[60]

Deployments

The number of boots on the ground in country shown in Figure 7.13 does not reflect the total number of American military personnel deployed, particularly Air Force and Navy personnel operating offshore or outside Afghanistan and Iraq. Starting in May 2008, DoD reported not only the number of troops in country but also the number of U.S. troops deployed in the surrounding area to provide in-theater support, as well as those conducting other counterterror operations. In addition, a large number of American civilian contractors supported the troops in both Afghanistan and Iraq. Table 7.4 shows the total number of Americans, troops and contractors, deployed in support of operations in Iraq and Afghanistan at critical points during the conflict. By 2016, in Afghanistan, American contractors outnumbered deployed troops.

Given the nature of the conflict, the majority of the 260,000 troops deployed were Army. Figure 7.14 shows the contribution each military component made to OEF and OIF/OND in FY 2008. The total deployed amounted to about 12 percent of the 2.2-million active-duty and reserve U.S. military personnel serving. Overall, some 17 percent of active-duty forces were deployed, compared to 7 percent of reserve forces. The highest deployment rate was for Army active-duty forces, with more than one-

---

Most notable was the absence of any serious discussion of the size of the force required to secure the peace following major combat operations. . . . Optimistic assumptions about how coalition forces would be greeted, the postwar viability of Iraqi institutions, and the continuing existence of the Iraqi army led planners to underestimate the number of coalition troops and the different kinds of effort (e.g., nation-building, counterinsurgency) needed to achieve peace. (Perry et al., 2015, p. xxi)

[58] The number reported weekly peaked at close to 1,600 in June 2007 (DoD, 2009, p. 19).

[59] The Army had limited options to increase troop levels quickly in reaction to a deteriorating situation. As unpopular as it was, the Secretary of Defense extended the tours of troops already deployed from 12 to 15 months. In April 2008, Army tours in Iraq returned to 12 months. See Belasco, 2009, pp. 38–39.

[60] Belasco, 2014, p. 10, notes that, as of 2014, 230 U.S. military remained in Iraq as part of the Office of Security Cooperation.

Figure 7.13
Boots on the Ground in Iraq, FYs 2001–2017

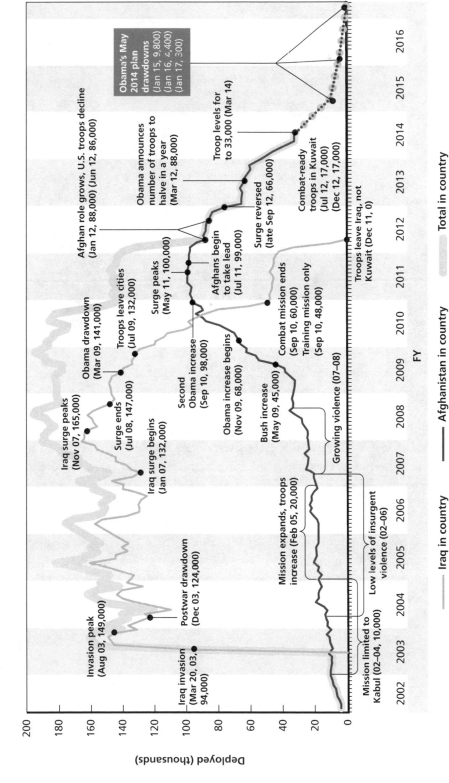

SOURCE: Adapted from Belasco, 2014, p. 9.
NOTE: Dotted lines are projections.

Table 7.4
Americans Deployed in Support of OEF and OIF/OND at Critical Times in the Conflict

Personnel	September 2007	June 2008	March 2009	March 2011	December 2011	June 2016
	Peak of OIF Surge	End of OIF	OIF Drawdown; Beginning of OEF Surge	Peak of OEF Surge	End of OIF/OND	Sense-of-Congress Resolution
OEF						
In country	24,056	33,902	38,350	99,800	94,100	8,730
In theater	NR	14,348	13,950	29,800	2,700	NR
U.S. contractors	3,387	4,724	10,036	20,413	25,287	8,837
OIF/OND						
In country	165,607	158,900	141,300	45,660	11,455	4,087
In theater	NR	28,760	27,450	42,150	42,855	NR
U.S. contractors	26,869	29,611	29,611	20,413	11,237	1,605

SOURCES: Belasco, 2014, Table A-1; Peters, Schwartz and Kapp, 2016, Tables 1 and 3.
NOTE: NR = not reported.

quarter being deployed (26 percent).[61] The deployment of some 7 percent of the Army National Guard and Army Reserve strengths "allowed the Army to reduce deployments of active-duty soldiers" and thereby increase the time at home between deployments (Bonds, Baiocchi, and McDonald, 2010, p. 25).[62]

OEF and OIF/OND were not only the longest wars in our history but the first fought with an all-volunteer force employing significant numbers of career soldiers. As a result, many soldiers were deployed multiple times. Over a period of 14 years, from September 2001 through September 2015, 2.7 million *individual* service men and women were deployed (see Table 7.5). The largest number of individuals deployed was from the Army (47.8 percent), and most of those (64.5 percent) were Regular Army soldiers. Of the 855,000 Regular Army troops deployed, almost one-half (49.4 percent) were deployed two or more times; the average length of a deployment was 9.3 months (see Wenger, O'Connell, and Cottrell, 2018, p. 4).

---

[61] Deployment rates were 16 percent for the Marine Corps, 12 percent for the Navy, and 8 percent for the Air Force (Belasco, 2009, p. 43).

[62] Rotation-planning goals are reflected in ratios. For deploying active-duty units, the ratio is the amount of time deployed to the amount of time not deployed. For deploying National Guard and Army Reserve units, the ratio is measured as time mobilized to time not mobilized (Geren and Casey, 2009).

Figure 7.14
Service and Component Shares of OEF and OIF Troops in FY 2008

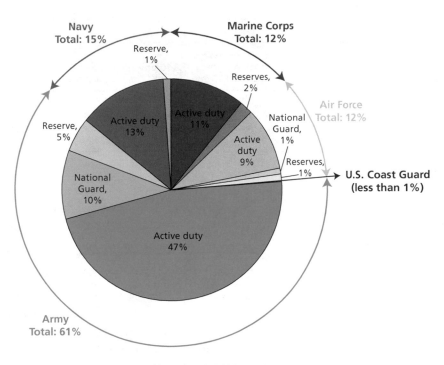

SOURCE: DMDC, as reported in Belasco, 2009, p. 41.
NOTE: Percentage of total average strength.

Battle and Nonbattle Casualties

Battle casualties refers to both those who died from injuries inflicted in combat—either immediately (KIA) or later (DOW)—and those who are wounded in combat.[63] *Nonbattle casualties* refers to those who are killed or incapacitated while deployed but not while engaged in combat.

Hostile and Nonhostile Deaths

Disease has been the scourge of armies throughout history. Up to and including World War I, more soldiers died of disease than from combat.[64] While it is rare today for soldiers to actually die from an illness, the large number of deployed soldiers and the

---

[63] As of February 2017, hostile deaths were 1,920 KIA and 610 DOW for OIF; 999 KIA and 329 DOW for OEF; and 22 KIA and 16 DOW for OND (Defense Casualty Analysis System, 2017). *DOW* refers to individuals who died as a result of their wounds even after having been successfully evacuated to the attention of a surgeon at an Echelon II/III medical facility (Army Dismounted Complex Blast Injury Task Force, 2011, p. 7).

[64] Despite the great advances in medicine after the Civil War, disease once again claimed more American lives during World War I than the enemy did. The Army's immunization programs could not control influenza or its respiratory complications, especially pneumonia; the flu and respiratory disease accounted for 80 percent of the 55,868 nonhostile deaths during the war (Rostker, 2013, pp. 129–132).

Table 7.5
Individual Service Members Deployed, by Component and Service,
September 2001–September 2015

Component	Army	Air Force	Marine Corps	Navy	All Services
Regular	855,000	397,000	333,000	515,000	2,100,000
Reserve	156,000	47,000	38,000	55,000	295,000
National Guard	344,000	84,000	N/A	N/A	428,000
Total[a]	1,326,000	518,000	367,000	563,000	2,774,000

SOURCE: Wenger, O'Connell, and Cottrell, 2018, p. 3. The authors used data from RAND Arroyo Center Analysis of DMDC's Contingency Tracking System Deployment File (September 2001 through September 2015; 2001 and 2015 represent partial calendar years).

[a] Total figures are lower than the sum across rows because some service members deployed with multiple components or ranks.

relatively small number of combat deaths mean that a significant number of deaths still occur from nonhostile causes. Figures 7.15 and 7.16 show hostile (KIA and DOW) and nonhostile deaths during recent operations in Afghanistan and Iraq.

Today, accidents among deployed troops are by far the leading cause of non–combat-related deaths (see Table 7.6). Illnesses and personal injuries account for only 2.4 percent of all deaths among troops deployed to Afghanistan and Iraq since 2002.

Battle and Nonbattle Hospitalizations and Medical Evacuations

Even as deaths from disease have largely been eliminated as a significant problem for today's Army, disease and nonbattle injuries remain "leading causes of morbidity during wars and military operations" (Hauret et al., 2016, p. 15). As measured by hospitalization rates and medevacs from theater, disease and nonbattle injuries were the second most prevalent causes for hospitalizations and the most prevalent causes of medevacs (see Table 7.7). Among the 75,000 medevacs, 12,000 were soldiers WIA; 11 percent were "urgent" evacuations; and the remainder were classified as "priority"—40 percent—or "routine"—49 percent (Carino, 2017a, p. 13).

Hostile Deaths and Wounded-in-Action

During OEF, those WIA accounted for 91.45 percent of all battle casualties (both WIA and KIA). Figure 7.17 shows how the wounds occurred over time. Figure 7.18 presents a similar picture for operations in Iraq, with WIA accounting for 89.7 percent of all battle casualties (WIA and KIA).

Causative Agent

With the exception of the first three weeks of OIF, combat in both Afghanistan and Iraq was highly unconventional, which was fully reflected in the agents that caused the wounds and in the wounds themselves. Moreover, the prevalence of gunshot wounds

Figure 7.15
Army Hostile and Nonhostile Deaths Operation Enduring Freedom, by Month

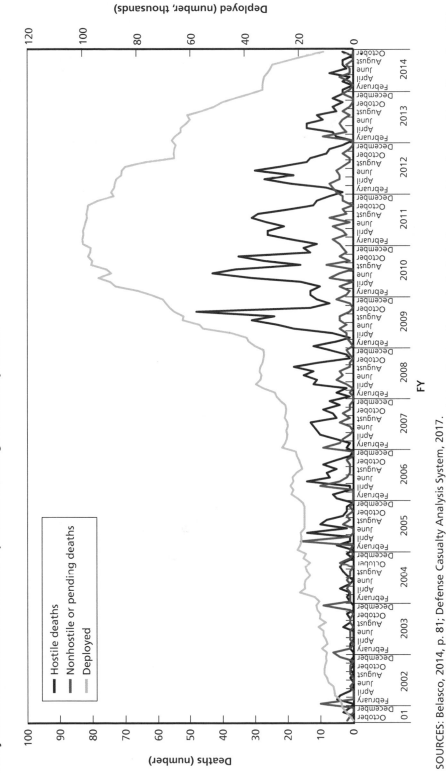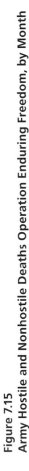

SOURCES: Belasco, 2014, p. 81; Defense Casualty Analysis System, 2017.
NOTES: *Hostile* deaths include KIAs, DOWs, and deaths from terrorist activities. *Nonhostile* deaths include those resulting from accident, illness, homicide, a self-inflicted wound, or undetermined causes and those still under investigation (pending). *Deployed* refers to the number of individuals deployed to the region and counted as part of the operation.

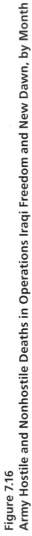

Figure 7.16
Army Hostile and Nonhostile Deaths in Operations Iraqi Freedom and New Dawn, by Month

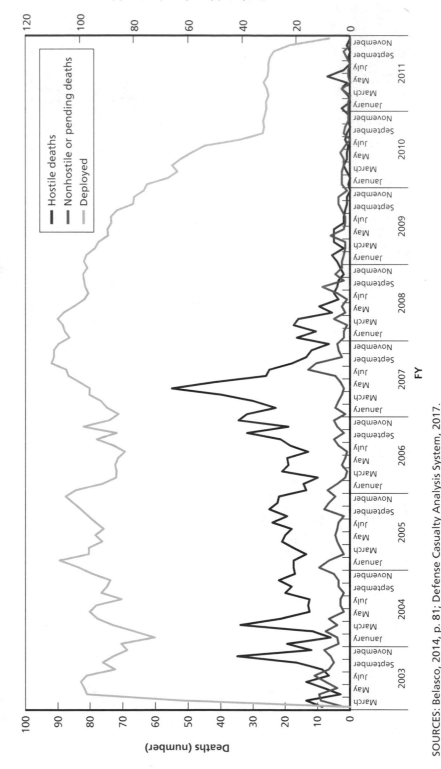

SOURCES: Belasco, 2014, p. 81; Defense Casualty Analysis System, 2017.
NOTES: *Hostile* deaths include KIAs, DOWs, and deaths from terrorist activities. *Nonhostile* deaths include those resulting from accident, illness, homicide, a self-inflicted wound, or undetermined causes and those still under investigation (pending). *Deployed* refers to the number of individuals deployed to the region and counted as part of the operation.

Table 7.6
Army Nonhostile and Hostile Deaths, by Conflict, 2001–2017

	OEF	OIF	OND
Accident	194	413	3
Illness or injury	39	72	8
Homicide	10	23	3
Self-inflicted	83	180	10
Undetermined	7	9	1
Total nonhostile deaths	333	697	25
Total hostile deaths	1,328	2,536	38

SOURCE: Defense Casualty Analysis System, 2017.

Table 7.7
Distribution of In-Theater Hospitalizations and Medical Evacuation from Afghanistan and Iraq, CYs 2001–2016

	Hospitalizations		Evacuations	
	OEF	OIF/OND	OEF	OIF/OND
Battle Injuries (%)	36	21	17	16
Nonbattle injuries (%)	18	19	31	34
Digestive disorders (%)	11	15	6	6
Ill-defined conditions (%)	10	10	8	9
Behavioral health (%)	3	6	12	10
Total (number)	12,251	23,299	27,207	47,647

SOURCE: Hauret et al., 2016, pp. 17–19.

decreased over time; blast wounds increased sharply, as did severe limb injuries. One analysis compared the severity of injuries and the causes of death from March 2003 to April 2004 against those from June 2006 to December 2006 and found that casualties resulting from gunshot wounds fell from 30 percent to 24 percent, while casualties from explosions—IEDs, rocket-propelled grenades, mortars, mines, bombs, and grenades—rose from 56 percent to 76 percent (Kelly et al., 2008, p. S23). The authors attributed these changes to

> the change in the enemy forces and tactics during the time course studied. The early conflict was more of a traditional war with most injuries resulting from small arms wounds, to the present insurgency characterized by ambushes, IEDs, and other explosive devices. IEDs now contain more explosive power, produce more

Figure 7.17
Army Battle Casualties—Killed in Action, Died of Wounds, and Wounded in Action—During Operation Enduring Freedom in Afghanistan, CYs 2001–2014

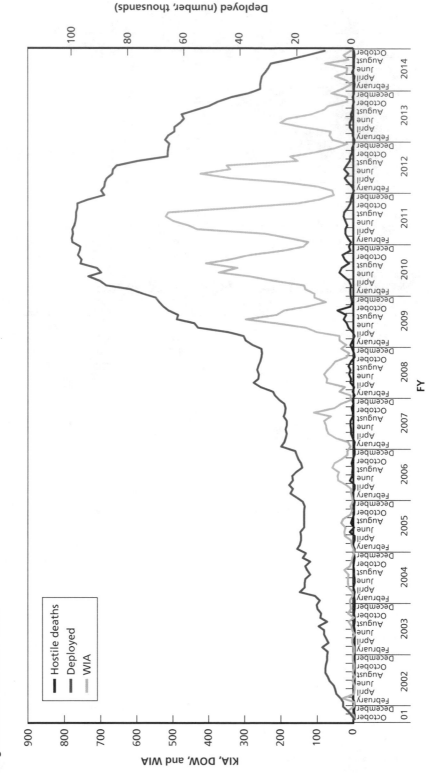

SOURCES: Belasco, 2014, p. 81; DMDC, 2016.
NOTES: *Hostile* deaths include KIAs, DOWs, and deaths from terrorist activities. *Nonhostile* deaths include those resulting from accident, illness, homicide, a self-inflicted wound, or undetermined causes and those still under investigation (pending). *Deployed* refers to the number of individuals deployed to the region and counted as part of the operation.

Figure 7.18
Army Battle Casualties—Killed in Action, Died of Wounds, and Wounded in Action—During Operation Iraqi Freedom and Operation New Dawn in Iraq, CYs 2003–2011

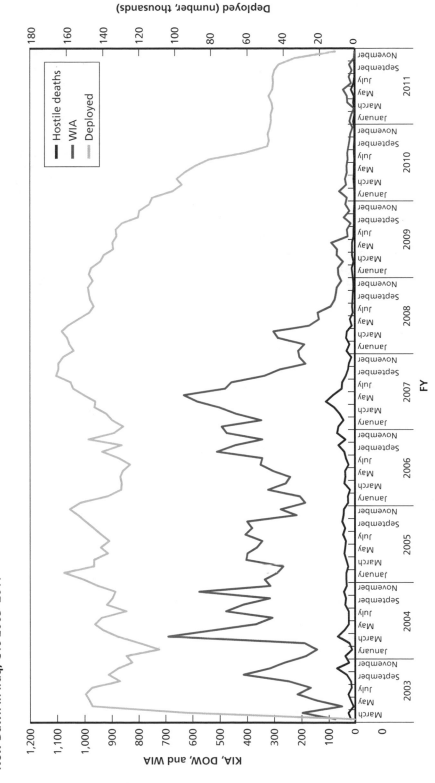

SOURCES: Belasco, 2014, p. 81; DMDC, 2016.
NOTES: *Hostile* deaths include KIAs, DOWs, and deaths from terrorist activities. *Nonhostile* deaths include those resulting from accident, illness, homicide, a self-inflicted wound, or undetermined causes and those still under investigation (pending). *Deployed* refers to the number of individuals deployed to the region and counted as part of the operation.

and deadlier fragmentation, and use more fuel to increase the size of the fireball produced. (Kelly et al., 2008, p. S24)

A 2012 review of combat casualties showed the predominance of wounds caused by explosions, particularly from IEDs (see Table 7.8). These results are significantly different from those for previous conflicts (see Figure 7.19). A complementary analysis of KIAs based on autopsy records from the Mortality Trauma Registry of the Armed Forces Medical Examiner System shows a similar pattern:

> [B]etween October 2001 and June 2011, 4,596 battlefield fatalities were reviewed and analyzed. The causes for the lethal injuries were 73.7% explosive, 22.1% gun-shot wounds, and 4.2% other (vehicle crash, industrial, crush, etc.). The stratification of mortality was notable that 87.3% of all injury mortality occurred in the pre-MTF [military treatment facility] environment . . . . Of the composite of all battlefield deaths, 35.2% ($n = 1,619$) were instantaneous, 52.1% ($n = 2,397$) were acute (minutes to hours) pre-MTF, and 12.7% (n = 580) of casualties died of wounds after reaching an MTF. Of the pre-MTF deaths, 75.7% ($n = 3,040$) were classified as NS [nonsurvivable], and 24.3% ($n = 976$) were deemed potentially survivable [PS]. (Eastridge et al., 2012, pp. S432–S433)

Improvised Explosive Devices

Although land mines, booby traps, and other devices had been used in previous wars, the IED has become the particular weapon of choice of insurgents in Afghanistan and Iraq (see Cordesman, Loi, and Kocharlakota, 2010). By 2007, "IEDs, roadside bombs, and suicide car bombs, [had] caused over 60% of all American combat casualties in Iraq and 50% of combat casualties in Afghanistan, both killed and wounded" (Wilson, 2007, p. 1). Table 7.9 shows the relative prevalence of IED compared to other weapons used against American troops in Afghanistan and Iraq as of 2017.

Table 7.8
Casualties in Afghanistan and Iraq, October 7, 2001–May 7, 2012

Mechanism of Injury	Afghanistan		Iraq		Total	
	Deaths (%)	WIA (%)	Deaths (%)	WIA (%)	Deaths (%)	WIA (%)
Artillery, mortar, or rocket	2.0	5.9	17.7	10.3	10	9
Explosive device	64.7	69.3	24.4	80.4	45	77
Grenade	0.1	0.0	0.0	0.3	0	0
Gunshot	29.4	16.7	53.4	9.1	41	12
Rocket-propelled grenade	3.9	8.2	4.5	2.9	4	5

SOURCE: Hayes, 2015, p. 88.

Figure 7.19
Mechanisms of Injury from Previous U.S. Wars

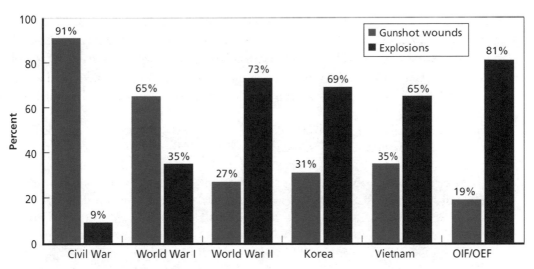

SOURCE: Data from Owens et al., 2008, p. 297.

Table 7.9
Causes of Injuries

Cause of Injury	Total	Afghanistan	Iraq
Number			
IED	14,751	7,744	7,007
Landmine, grenade, mortar, artillery, rocket-propelled grenade	13,507	3,423	10,084
Gunshot wounds	3,643	1,887	1,756
Other combat injury	4,978	1,290	3,688
Total	36,879	14,344	22,535
Percent			
IED	40.0	54.0	31.1
Landmine, grenade, mortar, artillery, rocket-propelled grenade	36.6	23.9	44.7
Gunshot wounds	9.9	13.2	7.8
Other combat injury	13.5	9.0	7.8

SOURCE: Carino, 2017c.

NOTE: Percentages may not sum to 100 because of rounding.

In Afghanistan, Russian land mines and other munitions left over from the 1980 Russo-Afghan War provided a ready supply. In Iraq, the ammunition depots left unguarded after the initial invasion were looted, and the munitions were converted into IEDs (see Figure 7.20).

Figure 7.20
Improvised Explosive Device in Eastern Baghdad, November 7, 2005

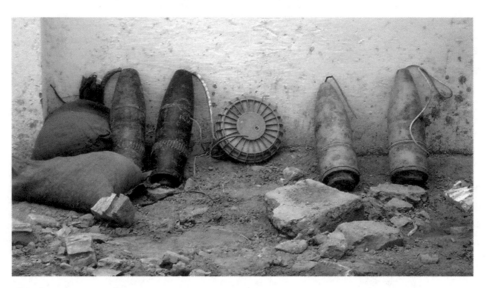

SOURCE: U.S. Army photo.

A typical IED might consist of several 155-mm Howitzer shells tied together and altered with a detonator and cell telephone, so it could be detonated remotely, or it might have a pressure switch, so that it would explode when a soldier stepped on it or vehicle drove over it. Such a device could tip over an Abrams tank or destroy a Humvee or even a Mine-Resistant, Ambush-Protected (MRAP) vehicle (Figure 7.21). Obviously, it could seriously maim or kill infantry soldiers (Trunkey, 2012, pp. 883–884).

The lethality and devastating effects of the high-explosive blast injuries from IEDs demonstrate "wounding patterns consisting of a preponderance of extremity injuries and a high mortality rate for penetrating head injuries . . . consistent with historical data from previous conflicts" (Nelson et al., 2008, p. 215). Close-proximity IED blasts often resulted in complex injuries and mortality rates as high as 50 percent, even among soldiers wearing Kevlar helmets, ballistic eye protection, and full body armor. Injuries were not limited to those on foot patrol; those traveling in armored vehicles were suddenly propelled upward, injuring the ears, lungs, bowels, brain, and other organs. Debris fragments would cause secondary injuries. Figure 7.22 illustrates the results of an IED exploding beneath an armed vehicle.

Blast injuries to dismounted soldiers became such a problem that, in 2006, DoD established the Joint IED Defeat Organization to investigate countermeasures. In January 2011 the Surgeon General of the Army established the Complex Battle Injury Task Force to examine

IED- or land mine–related blast injury to a dismounted Warrior that includes at least one lower extremity amputation and also includes severe injuries to other

Figure 7.21
A Mine-Resistant, Ambush-Protected Vehicle Hit by a 300–500 lb. IED in Iraq, September 7, 2007

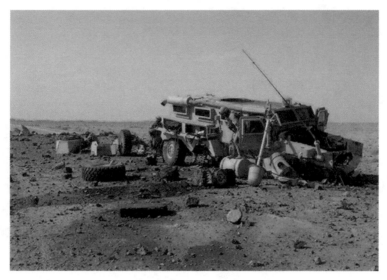

SOURCE: U.S. Marine Corps photo.

limbs, GU [genitourinary] system, pelvis, and/or abdomen. This description is based more on the inclusion of several severe injuries compounding complexity, and not intended to be exclusive of injuries of similar severity, sustained from other mechanisms. (Army Dismounted Complex Blast Injury Task Force, 2011, p. i)

In June 2011, the Task Force reported that "extremities . . . are at greatest risk for complex blast injuries, especially among dismounted Warriors" (Army Dismounted Complex Blast Injury Task Force, 2011, p. ii).[65] Figure 7.23 illustrates the destructive power of a land mine–induced traumatic limb amputation.

Locations of Wounds

The locations of wounds reported for October 2001 through January 2005, for both OEF and OIF, shows a very high incidence of head and neck wounds (see Table 7.10). For this group of 3,102 wounded soldiers, about one-half of the head and neck wounds were caused by IEDs.

---

[65] The Task Force noted that, in 2010, battlefield injuries in the Afghanistan theater of operation exceeded those in the Iraqi theater of operation and that

[t]he primary injury in the ATO [Afghanistan Theater of Operation] often resulted from enemy contact with ground-emplaced IEDs and land mines. The injury of interest, DCBI [Dismounted Complex Blast Injury], has increased significantly. A significant number of these injuries, but not all, were sustained by Warriors on dismounted patrols. (Army Dismounted Complex Blast Injury Task Force, 2011, p. 4)

Figure 7.22
Impact of an IED Blast Underneath an Armed Vehicle

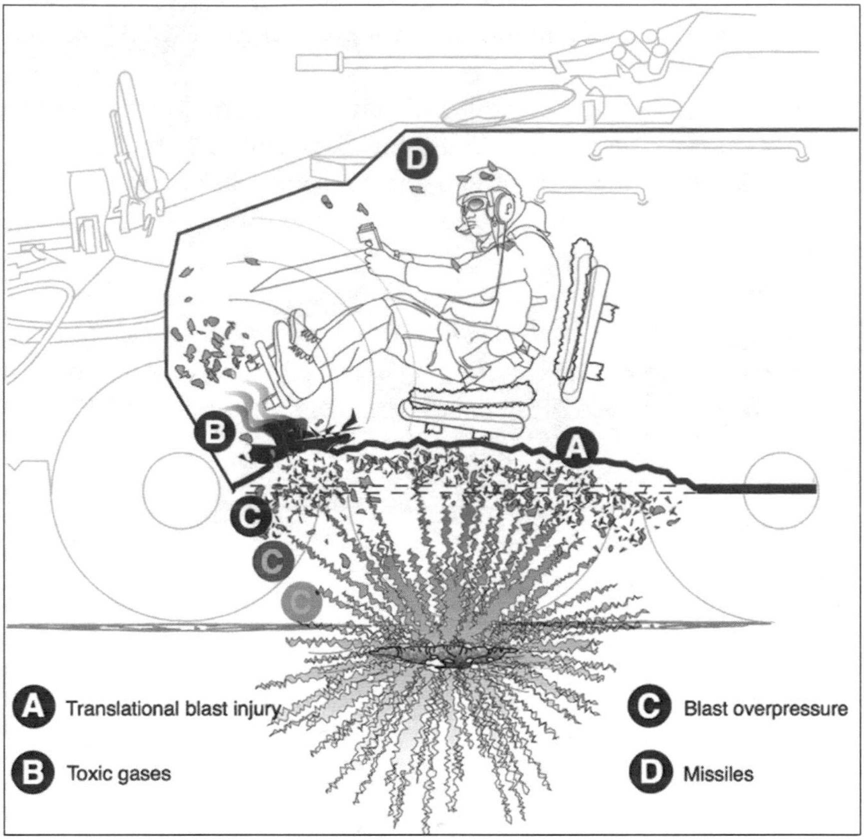

A Translational blast injury		**C** Blast overpressure	
B Toxic gases		**D** Missiles	

SOURCE: Brevard, Champion, and Katz, 2012, p. 55.

Facial wounds accounted for 61 percent of the wounds in the head and neck region; the face is one of the few remaining exposed regions not protected by improvements in body armor. Such wounds are often associated with TBI,[66] although "closed brain injuries outnumber penetrating ones" (Okie, 2005, p. 2045).

---

[66] A case in point is the experience of Army Sergeant David Enne:

> [A]n improvised explosive device (IED) went off right next to Emme's truck, knocking him out.

> Emme's version of what happened next is patched together, from his own memories and what others told him later. "I remember waking up and wondering who the hell I was, where the hell I was, and why can't I see or hear? My soldier was screaming for me to get out of the truck and I told him no, because it hurt too much. So he literally threw me out of the truck and guided me to a Stryker," a lightweight armored vehicle.

> The blast wave and fragments from the explosion had blown out Emme's left eardrum, fractured his skull, injured his left eye, and caused a severe contusion in the left frontotemporal area of his brain. His fellow soldiers rushed him to the nearby military base, where he partially regained his vision and tried to walk before again losing consciousness. He was medically evacuated, first to a combat support hospital in Balad and then to one

Figure 7.23
Impact of a Blast from a Land Mine

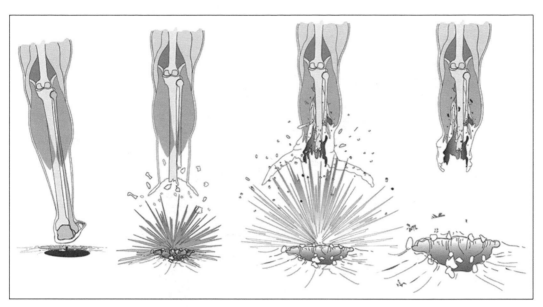

SOURCE: Brevard, Champion, and Katz, 2012, p. 48.

Table 7.10
Distribution of Wounds, by Body Region

Region	World War II (%)	Korea (%)	Vietnam (%)	OEF/OIF[a] (%)
Head and neck	21.0	21.4	16.0	29.4
Thorax	13.9	9.9	13.4	5.6
Abdomen	8.0	8.4	9.4	10.7
Extremities	58.0	60.2	61.1	54.1

SOURCE: Owens et al., 2008, pp. 295–296.

[a] From 3,102 casualties, resulting in 6,609 wounds, as recorded in the Joint Theater Trauma Registry (JTTR) for October 2001 through January 2005.

in Baghdad. There, neurosurgeons performed a craniectomy, removing a large piece of skull from the left temporal region to give Emme's brain room to swell. They implanted the bone under the subcutaneous tissue of his abdomen, hoping that it could be replaced later—if Emme survived. He remained unconscious and remembers nothing about his stops in these hospitals. (Okie, 2005, p. 2043)

Overall Measures of Survival

Overall, a larger proportion of wounded personnel survived in Iraq and Afghanistan than during the Vietnam War.[67] The survival rates of 89.8 percent in Iraq and 91.4 percent in Afghanistan were higher than in any previous American conflict (see Figure 7.24).

It is important to note that, as medical support has evolved over the most recent conflicts, the KIA rate has decreased, and the DOW rate has increased. These changes are attributed to improved protection for mounted and dismounted soldiers and to advances: "improved hemorrhage control and increased focus on prehospital Tactical Combat Casualty Care training coupled with rapid evacuation" (Holcomb et al., 2006, p. 400). However, these changes may be exaggerated because many of the more severely injured casualties who in the past would have died on the battlefield before reaching a medical treatment facility (and would then have been classified as KIAs) now die at the MTF or shortly thereafter and are thus classified as DOWs.

Figure 7.24
Survivability Rates

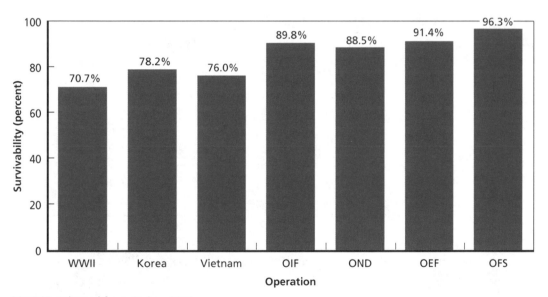

SOURCE: Adapted from Carino, 2016.
NOTES: OFS = Operation Freedom's Sentinel. The survivability percentage is equal to 100 percent minus the total KIA and DOW, divided by total WIA, KIA, and DOW for the theater of interest, i.e.,

$$Survivability = 1 - \frac{KIA + DOW}{KIA + DOW + WIA}.$$

---

[67] Goldberg argues that the survival rate of 75.8 percent for Vietnam reported by the Army Surgeon General's office understates the actual survival rate because it does not count the WIAs who did not require hospitalization; that is, the actual survival rate for Vietnam was about 86 percent (Goldberg, 2016, p. 11). See also Holcomb et al., 2006.

Initial Battlefield Medical Support for the Combat Troops in Iraq

If the initial use of FST and CSH in Afghanistan did not follow doctrinal lines, the same could not be said of battlefield medical support during the initial days of OIF. In March 2003, the experience the 274th and 250th FSTs gained in Afghanistan was employed in Iraq in support of OIF. Between March and May 2003, as the battle progressed in a traditional linear fashion, the FSTs and their supporting CSHs were used, for the *first and only time*, as prescribed by doctrine.

The 274th FST traveled 1,100 miles "setting up in Nasiriyah, Najaf, Karbala, and points along the way in the southern desert, then in Mosul in the north, and finally in Baghdad" (Gawande, 2004, p. 2472). This FST cared for 132 U.S. and 74 Iraqi military and civilian casualties, with 80 percent of casualties having gunshot wounds, shrapnel injuries, or blast injuries.

The 250th FST parachuted into northern Iraq with the 173rd Airborne Brigade on the night of March 26, 2003.[68] After treating minor injuries at the drop zone,[69] the 250th FST supported the 173rd, the 10th SF, and the Kurdish militia in taking the northern oil city of Kirkuk on April 11, 2003. After that, the 250th FST

> initiated a massive civil affairs campaign to rebuild the city's infrastructure and win the hearts and the minds of the people. The 250th integrated with the local surgical community and initiated an array of reconstruction projects, while still providing far forward surgical capability to the maneuver units of the 173rd task force fighting the insurgency until redeployment in March 2004. (Rush et al., 2005, p. 565)

During the 11 months of its deployment, the 250th FST performed 59 surgical procedures on 48 patients (Rush et al., 2005, p. 564).

In the south, the 555th FST supported the 2nd BCT of the 3rd Infantry Division. The 555th FST employed the Chemical Biological Protective Shelter System (CBPSS; see Figure 7.25).[70] Over the 24 days of the main assault, the 555th FST treated 79

---

[68] As Rush et al., 2005, p. 565, reported,

> [a]fter redeployment the 250th re-equipped, further modernized, and updated techniques and procedures based on lessons learned from the OEF experience. In late January 2003 the unit was called upon again, this time in support of OIF and the 173rd Airborne Brigade out of Vicenza, Italy. The unit moved to Vicenza just as the invasion of Iraq started in the south where the 2-day, pre-war link up with the 173rd's forward support medical platoon occurred. On the night of March 26, 2003, while the 555th FST out of Fort Hood, TX was supporting the 3rd Infantry Division's drive toward Baghdad in the south . . . , echelon one of the 250th FST jumped into northern Iraq with 1000 men of the 173rd ABN BDE [Airborne Brigade] to provide drop zone surgical support for the assault on the airfield at Bashur, thus officially opening the Northern Front in OIF.

[69] There were "only 9 injuries among 1000 paratroopers during the airborne assault on the Bashur airfield. The worst of these were a tibia-fibula fracture and a paratrooper with bilateral dislocated shoulders" (Rush et al., 2005, p. 568).

[70] The CBPSS consists of a modified high-mobility multipurpose-wheeled vehicle (properly abbreviated as "HMMWV" but commonly referred to as a "Humvee") with a lightweight multipurpose shelter mounted on the

Figure 7.25
The 555th FST During Operation Iraqi Freedom: A Chemical Biological
Protected Shelter System in the Desert of Southern Iraq and Operational
in a Suburb of Baghdad

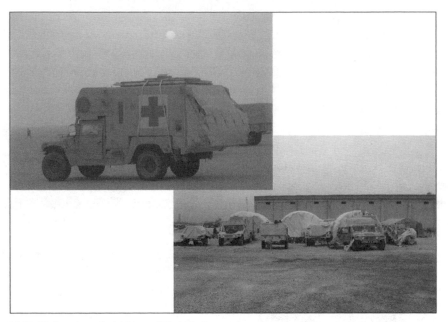

SOURCE: Patel et al., 2004, p. 203. U.S. Army photos.

Americans, 52 Iraqi combat casualties, and 23 Iraqi civilians and performed 24 major
surgical operations. "The most frequent cause of injuries encountered in all groups was
high energy bullet and fragmentation injuries. The most commonly injured regions in
U.S. soldiers were the upper (32%) and lower (30%) extremities, followed by head and
neck" (Patel et al., 2004, p. 203).

With the end of conventional hospitalities at the beginning of May 2003, "a
period of unconventional warfare and unstable peace commenced. As in Afghanistan,
combat surgical units were once again used in a non-doctrinal manner, occupying
fixed facilities in remote outposts, as well as Baghdad" (Schoenfeld, 2012, p. 381).
Nevertheless, experiences during the initial assault provided valuable lessons, confirming and challenging expectations and doctrine. The establishment of highly mobile
surgical teams far forward on the battlefield clearly saved lives. As the 555th FST
reported, "the overall mortality rate of patients presenting to the FST was 1.9% (3/154)

---

back, a 300-ft. semicylindrical airbeam supported soft shelter, and a towed high-mobility trailer with a 10-kW
tactical quiet generator. The Humvee's engine or the 10-kW generator provides the necessary power to support
surgical operations. An environmental support system mounted on the front of the lightweight multipurpose
shelter provides heating, cooling, airbeam inflation, chemical and biological filtration, and air ventilation. These
vehicles were arranged so that the tents could be connected to create three adjoining rooms (Patel et al., 2004).

and the mortality rate for those patients who underwent operations was 12% (3/25). Of the twenty-five major operations performed, only one patient died on the operating room table" (Patel et al., 2004, p. 204).

Confirming the *forward* medical support the FSTs provided, the 555th FST reported several engagements with the enemy, including one in which they captured seven POWs. This led to an important point:

> The days when medical personnel were located in the rear are over. Medical personnel attached to FSTs need to be trained not only in their respective fields but also in combat skills such as weapons training and management of prisoners of war. (Patel et al., 2004, p. 207)

The mobility of the FST was confirmed; the 55th FST reported that,

> [d]uring the movement to Baghdad, the FST's CBPSSs were set up and taken down multiple times. There were periods when the FST would be set up for less than 12 hours. One of the strengths of the FST is its ability to become operational quickly. The CBPSS can be inflated in 4 minutes and the FST can be made fully operational in less than 30 minutes. The CBPSS is an example of technology making a tremendous impact on the ability of the FST to deliver rapid far forward surgical care. (Patel et al., 2004, pp. 205–206)

While noting that the FST operational concept is based on selectivity, transportability, and limited resuscitative surgery and given the doctrinal limitations on what should be done at an FST, Patel et al. found that "there are times when difficult decisions to amputate must be made at the FST level due to the type of injury, risks of subsequent infection and availability of evacuation based on enemy activity" (Patel et al., 2004, p. 205). They particularly noted that, while there was often a need to address vascular injuries, teams lacked appropriate equipment to provide such critical care.[71]

After May 2003, Echelon II and III surgical support was provided at combat surgical units occupying fixed facilities in remote outposts, as well as in major cities.[72] From 2008 to 2009, the 772nd FST undertook the first mobile surgical support mis-

---

[71] The 555th FST noted:

> If there is a concern for the possibility of a vascular injury and evacuation is not possible secondary to enemy activity, these patients may need to undergo operative exploration to ensure no vascular injury is present. The risks associated with surgery are less than the poor outcomes associated with delayed treatment or missed vascular injuries. Future deployments will need the doppler ultrasound to be added to the MTOE [Modified Table of Organization and Equipment] which will help in the management of extremity injuries. (Patel et al., 2004, p. 205)

[72] For example, in

> August of 2003, the 28th CSH, which mobilized in support of the Iraqi invasion, established permanent residence at Ibn Sina Hospital in Baghdad and was designated the burn care center for OIF.

sions since the 2003 invasion of Iraq in support of SOF and U.S. Marines in Afghanistan. The FST divided itself into a highly mobile light team supporting Marines in western Afghanistan and a more robust heavy surgical resuscitation team supporting an infantry BCT in the eastern Afghanistan (Remick, 2009).

New Emphasis on Tactical Combat Casualty Care

Research during and after Vietnam concluded that as many as 8 percent of KIAs were preventable, with the leading cause of these deaths being severe loss of blood from extremity wounds (Maughon, 1970; Bellamy, 1984).[73] However, little action was taken to address these findings until 1994, when USSOCOM funded a study that, after two years, recommended "a basic casualty-management protocol that is appropriate for the battlefield" (Butler, Haymann, and Butler, 1996, p. 3). It soon became clear that the medical practices being taught to military medics, corpsman, and pararescuemen, which were based on civilian trauma practices, were not completely transferable to a battlefield environment. As a result, a new set of guidelines that was to be "woven into a comprehensive set of battlefield trauma care strategies" (Blackbourne et al., 2012, p. S389) was promulgated in 1996 and called Tactical Combat Casualty Care (TCCC).[74] The guidelines were adopted by the Navy SEALs and the Army's 75th Ranger Regiment.[75] However, when the United States next went to war, in 2001, "most US military units had not made the transition to TCCC-based concepts for managing trauma in the prehospital tactical environment" (Butler and Blackbourne, 2012,

---

The 31st CSH relieved the 28th at Ibn Sina and between 2003 and 2004 treated 3,426 combat-wounded patients. . . . (Schoenfeld, 2012, p. 381)

More recently, members of the 86th CSH reported on their experience at Ibn Sina hospital from 2007 to 2009. With the OIF conflict winding down, the most common procedures reported by this CSH were appendectomy, hernia repair, and incision and drainage of abscesses. In contrast, the 541st FST, deployed to Afghanistan and used in a nondoctrinal split capacity (two 10-man teams perform surgery in remote locations), reported treating 761 patients with combat-related injuries. In this experience, nearly half of the treated population was Afghani, and only a quarter of the combat-injured were American. (Schoenfeld, 2012, p. 382)

[73] Bellamy reported that, among "277 casualties who were killed in action by hemorrhage from arterial wounds, no less than 38 per cent had a site at which hemorrhage could have been controlled at least temporarily by simple first aid measures" (Bellamy, 1984, p. 60).

[74] TCCC is divided onto three distinct phases: (1) care under fire, (2) tactical field care, and (3) tactical evacuation care (Gerhardt et al., 2012, p. 93).

[75] Today, "the TCCC guidelines include tourniquets, hemostatic dressings, new prehospital fluid resuscitation and analgesic strategies, and many other advances over prehospital care as it was practiced in 2001" (Butler, Smith, and Carmona, 2015, p. 322). In 2011, the 75th Ranger Regiment reported that,

[d]espite the lethality of modern-day warfare, the 75th Ranger Regiment's implementation of a comprehensive casualty response system sustained by focused training directed by tactical leaders using data from a unit-based PHTR [prehospital trauma registry] has resulted in historically low casualty rates for a frontline unit of its type, to include virtual elimination of preventable combat death. (Kotwal, Montgomery, et al., 2011, p. 1356)

p. S396). Several studies later found "a significant incidence of potentially preventable death was still present in US combat fatalities" (Blackbourne et al., 2012, p. S389).[76]

In 2001, USSOCOM established the triservice Committee on TCCC "to ensure that emerging technology and information is incorporated into the TCCC guidelines on an ongoing basis" (Butler and Blackbourne, 2012, p. S396). In 2004, USCENT-COM incorporated TCCC into its new Joint Theater Trauma System (JTTS), with LTC Brian Eastridge as the first JTTS deployed theater trauma medical director (Defense Health Board, 2015, p. ES-1; Bailey et al., 2012, p. 6).[77]

In November 2007, TCCC received official recognition when the Assistant Secretary of Defense for Health Affairs directed that the Committee on TCCC become a subgroup of the Trauma and Injury Subcommittee of the Defense Health Board. This board is the senior external medical advisory group to the Secretary of Defense. The JTS became an official DoD program under the U.S. Army Institute of Surgical Research in 2010.[78]

TCCC has, over time, gone from being used primarily by USSOCOM and 18th Airborne Corps units to being used throughout Afghanistan and Iraq, but "the evolution has . . . occurred unevenly and sporadically" (Kotwal, Butler, et al., 2013a, p. 12). An assessment by the U.S. Army Institute of Surgical Research in 2013 found that TCCC concepts, medications, and equipment had been incompletely applied as a result of "divided and overlapping responsibilities" (Butler, Smith, and Carmona, 2015, p. 323). "Combat commanders typically act on the advice of their unit surgeons, but most military physicians have limited training in administering a prehospital trauma care system, and many have little or no knowledge of TCCC concepts" (Butler, Smith, and Carmona, 2015, p. 324). It has been recommended that, in the future, "line commanders should have casualty response training provided as part of their initial and refresher training in combat leadership" (Eastridge et al., 2012, p. S435). In 2015, the Defense Health Board published a report on lessons learned that included recommen-

---

[76] See also Kelly et al., 2008, and Holcomb et al., 2007.

[77] JTTS originally focused on care of the injured within the theater and at the primary out-of-theater receiving MTF, located at Landstuhl Regional Medical Center, Germany. The system was ultimately expanded to include CONUS and VA facilities. A number of military physicians have played critical and continuing roles in the development of TCCC, JTTS, JTS and the Joint Theater Trauma Registry (JTTR), the most notable being Drs. Frank Butler, John Holcomb, and Brian Eastridge.

[78] While JTTS is limited to the USCENTCOM theater of operations, JTS focuses on the entire U.S. military. JTS coordinates with the civilian American College of Surgeons Committee of Trauma and is the "enduring organization in the DoD that promotes improved trauma care to U.S. wounded warriors and other DoD eligible trauma victims . . . [and] the chief organization for consultation on the care of the injured for the Services, COCOMS [combatant commanders] and entire DoD, to include its senior leadership" (Bailey et al., 2012, p. 2). See also Defense Health Board, 2015, pp. 12–14, for a discussion of the respective roles of JTS and JTTS.

dations for improvement as the system continues to evolve. Box 7.1 highlights the 15 "evidence-based practice guidelines."[79]

The Joint Theater Trauma Registry

The JTTR has been the backbone of the entire JTS program (Costanzo and Spott, 2010, p. 21). It is the data repository about the prehospital management of combat casualties and has "led to the development of more than 30 evidence-based battlefield relevant clinical practice guidelines, and decreased morbidity and mortality from combat injury" (Eastridge, 2012, p. xiii). It was developed by the Army's Institute of Surgical Research, in partnership with the U.S. Air Force and U.S. Navy, in response to a December 2003 DoD directive to capture and report battlefield injury. It was renamed the DoD Trauma Registry (DoDTR) in 2012. The registry provides the data for "performance improvement studies and gap analyses for medical capabilities to direct ongoing and future combat casualty care research, trauma skills training, and direct combat casualty care" (U.S. Army Institute of Surgical Research, 2016a). For example, analysis of data from the DoDTR was used to benchmark casualty care,

---

Box 7.1
Current State of Battlefield Trauma and Injury Care: Tactical Combat Casualty Care Guidelines

- Phased care in the tactical environment, including care under fire, tactical field care and tactical evacuation care.
- Use of blood or blood components for resuscitation from hemorrhagic shock when feasible.
- Needle decompression to treat tension pneumothoraces, with a 14-gauge, 3.25 needle/catheter.
- Use of vented chest seals to treat open pneumothoraces.
- Use of fluoroquinolones and ertapenem or cefotetan for battlefield antibiotics.
- Use of fluid resuscitation and supplemental oxygen to maintain high oxygen saturation when treating moderate/severe TBI.
- Use of tourniquets, including junctional tourniquets, to control life-threatening external hemorrhage from sites amenable to tourniquet placement.
- Use of Combat Gauze to control external hemorrhage from sites not amenable to tourniquet placement.
- Use of tranexamic acid if there is an anticipated need for significant blood transfusion.
- Use of intraosseous techniques when vascular access is difficult to obtain.
- Use of the Ready-Heat Blanket/Heat-Reflective Shell and warm fluids if intravenous fluids are required.
- Use of nasopharyngeal airways, protective airway positioning (including sitting up and leaning forward), and surgical cricothyroidotomies for airway management.
- Use of oral analgesics, ketamine, morphine, and fentanyl citrate lozenges as described in the TCCC "triple-option analgesia" plan.
- Documentation of care by using TCCC Casualty Cards and TCCC electronic After-Action Reports.
- Tactical, scenario based combat training

SOURCE: Quoted from Defense Health Board, 2015, p. 6.

---

[79] Butler and Blackbourne, 2012, compares battlefield trauma care in 2001, at the start of the current conflicts, with what was provided a decade later and provides a time line showing the progress of TCCC over the decade.

beginning at Level III medical facilities, and to establish metrics for 24-hour mortality in casualties with polytrauma and a moderate or severe blunt TBI (O'Connell et al., 2012). Between 2007 and 2014, more than 1,500-peer review studies were published using data from the JTTR/DoDTR (U.S. Army Institute of Surgical Research, 2016b).

With regard to the early findings of Maughon and, later, those of Bellamy concerning preventable deaths on the battlefield, it was clear by 2007 that there was a lack of data on prehospital care. At that time, fewer than 10 percent of the records documenting the care 30,000 casualties had received were reaching an MTF because the Field Medical Card, DD Form 1380, "was not . . . optimally configured for documenting first responder care on the battlefield" (Kotwal, Butler, et al., 2013b, p. 2). It was decided that JTTS would adapt the casualty card that the 75th Ranger Regiment had developed (U.S. Army Institute of Surgical Research, 2016a). The 2014 version of this card is shown in Figure 7.26.

The Defense Health Board has endorsed use of the card, and the Army has adopted it servicewide, although the Army Surgeon General's Dismounted Complex Blast Injury Task Force found that, as of by 2011, "only 14% of casualties have prehospital care documented upon arrival at a Role II/III facility" (Army Dismounted

Figure 7.26
Tactical Combat Casualty Care Card, 2014 Version

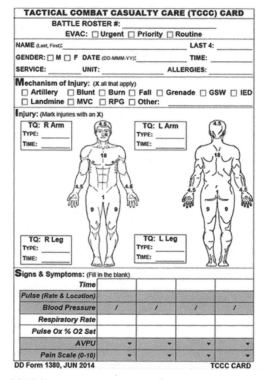
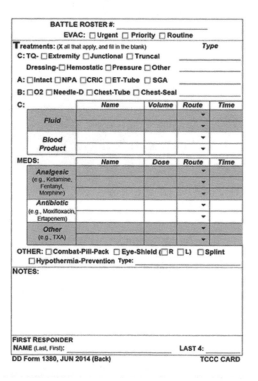

SOURCE: U.S. Army Institute of Surgical Research, 2016a.

Complex Blast Injury Task Force, 2011, p. 21). Nevertheless, analysis using JTTR data has been instrumental in "proving the Golden Hour evacuation policy saves lives, [and] provided the supporting evidence to prompt a doctrinal change of Army flight medics from Emergency Medical Technician (EMT)–Basic to an EMT-Paramedic to improve the survivability of combat casualties" (U.S. Army Institute of Surgical Research, 2016a). The analysis of the reduction in preventable deaths that the 75th Ranger Regiment had achieved was partially documented from data recorded in JTTR (Kotwal, Montgomery, et al., 2011).

Combat Life Saving Care: Hemorrhage Control Using Tourniquets and Hemostatic Agents and Combat Lifesaver Training

Today, "hemorrhagic death is the leading preventable cause of mortality in combat casualties" (Perkins and Beekley, 2012, p. 124). Despite the pioneering work of Maughon (1970) and Bellamy (1984), which pointed out that the leading cause of preventable deaths was the severe loss of blood from extremity wounds, most military trauma care in 2001 was based on civilian practices that prioritized airway, breathing, and circulation, with "avoidance of tourniquet use for fear of causing ischemic damage to extremities" (Blackbourne et al., 2012, p. S389). Two important evidence-based changes to medical protocols incorporated in Afghanistan and Iraq concerned the use of tourniquets and hemostatic, clot-promoting agents to control bleeding and reduce preventable death. Advanced lifesaving skills are also promulgated as a "bridge between the self-aid/buddy-aid [first aid] training given all soldiers during basic training and the medical training given to the combat medic" (Army Institute of Professional Development, 2012).

Tourniquets

The analysis of SOF operations during 1993's Operation Restore Hope in Somalia suggested that the use of tourniquets—one of the most ancient of medical devices[80]— could save lives. In 1997, U.S. Navy SEALs and the 75th Ranger Regiment adopted new trauma guidelines, including the use of tourniquets, under the TCCC program. These efforts notwithstanding, when U.S. forces were deployed to Afghanistan, "most went without tactical tourniquets, and most users had been trained not to use any tourniquet at all" (Kragh et al., 2013, p. 8).

Even for those who understood the need to control hemorrhaging, the tourniquets that were available were ineffective, slow, clumsy, and inaccessible in an emergency. Given this lack of an effective tourniquet, preventable fatalities continued. A study of the SOF fatalities conducted between 2001 and 2004 concluded that as many as 15 percent of all fatalities were "potentially survivable," with 50 percent dying from

---

[80] The use of tourniquets throughout history is well documented; see Kragh et al., 2012, and Mabry, 2006.

truncal hemorrhaging, 19 percent from compressible hemorrhaging, and 13 percent from a "hemorrhage amenable to tourniquet" (Holcomb et al., 2007, p. 986).[81]

By early 2003, before the invasion of Iraq, the Committee on TCCC took up the issue of tourniquet use, formally recommending that soldiers carry and be trained in the proper use of a modern tourniquet. In early 2004, the new combat application tourniquet (CAT) became available, but disagreements remained on how the CATs should be used. The popular press soon highlighted the muddle over tourniquets,[82] with the *Baltimore Sun* noting in March 2005 that the Army had "ordered an additional 172,000 modern tourniquets for soldiers in Iraq and Afghanistan, . . . [so] each soldier will be equipped with the life-saving device" (Bowman, 2005). Subsequent research showed the reintroduction of the tourniquets improved survival rates,[83] as noted in a 2012 summary report:

> Modern tourniquets were initially fielded to conventional US forces in late 2005. Implementation was ubiquitous after 2007. Before the introduction of tourniquets,

---

[81] These results were consistent with a later study of 4,596 battlefield fatalities between October 2001 and June 2011, which found that

> 87.3% of all injury mortality occurred in the pre-MTF environment. Of the pre-MTF deaths, 75.7% (n = 3,040) were classified as nonsurvivable, and 24.3% (n = 976) were deemed potentially survivable (PS). The injury/physiologic focus of PS acute mortality was largely associated with hemorrhage (90.9%). The site of lethal hemorrhage was truncal (67.3%), followed by junctional (19.2%) and peripheral-extremity (13.5%) hemorrhage. (Eastridge et al., 2012, p. S431)

Similar results were reported by Kelly et al., 2008.

[82] The *Baltimore Sun* laid out the story:

> Since at least a month before the war in Iraq began, medical experts in the Army and other services have called on the Pentagon to equip every American soldier in the war zone with a modern tourniquet. . . . The cost would not likely exceed $2 million, or about two thousandths of a percent of the $82 billion proposed for the war this year. . . .

> Army and Pentagon officials contacted by The Sun were at a loss to explain why every American soldier is not carrying a tourniquet, referring questions to other departments or declining to comment. . . . [t]he Army's deputy surgeon general, said that the service has embraced the concept of issuing tourniquets to everyone in Iraq and that he was surprised to learn that some don't have them. He also said he is not familiar with the purchasing and logistical procedures necessary to make it happen.

> Even though the Army has approved a new soldier first-aid kit that would include a tourniquet and manufacturers say they are ready to produce as many as 100,000 tourniquets a month, the Pentagon has not placed an order. One obstacle seems to be the slow-churning military bureaucracy, which has forced soldiers to wait on the development of new training manuals and a pouch for carrying the tourniquet. (Little, 2005a)

[83] Research has also found that, with the use of tourniquets,

> prehospital death rates from isolated limb exsanguination have dropped to 2%, compared to 9% in the Vietnam War. Tourniquets can control limb hemorrhage, a leading cause of death on the battlefield, with more frequent tourniquet use attributed to fewer deaths from this cause. In the Vietnam War, when tourniquet use was uneven, about 9% of casualties died from isolated limb exsanguination. (Kragh et al., 2009, p. 5)

For a comprehensive overview, see Holcomb, Butler and Rhee, 2015.

the death rate from peripheral-extremity hemorrhage was 23.3 deaths per year, which was reduced to 17.5 deaths per year during the training and dissemination period from 2006 to 2007. After full implementation, this number was reduced to 3.5 deaths per year, an 85% decrease in mortality. If not for the innovative and improvised tourniquets used by Special Operations Forces and unit-based initiatives of some conventional forces before modern tourniquet fielding, this reduction in mortality would have probably been even greater. (Eastridge et al., 2012, p. S433)

Today, newly designed tourniquets, such as the one shown in Figure 7.27, are part of every soldier's personal equipment.

Hemostatic, Clot-Promoting Agents

Hemostatic agents are designed to stem blood loss by promoting clotting. These agents include Celox blood-clotting granules and gauze impregnated with either chitosan or kaolin. But which agents work the best in a combat environment? Are they cost effective?

Figure 7.27
Modern Combat Tourniquet

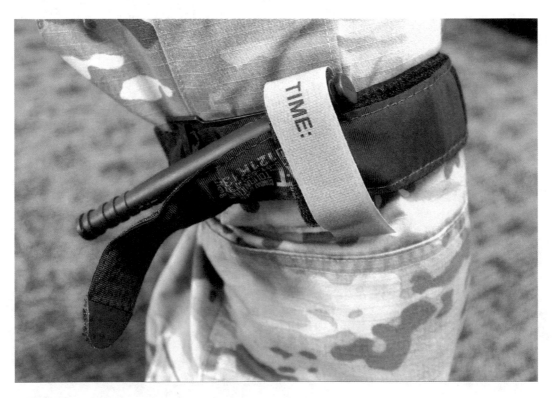

SOURCE: U.S. Army photo.

In reaction to the story in the *Baltimore Sun*, senior members of the U.S. Senate Committee on Appropriations wrote Defense Secretary Rumsfeld:

> We are deeply concerned by reports that the Pentagon has failed to identify and fulfil urgent requests for equipment essential to saving lives of our troops in the field. This type of delay is disturbing during times of peace, but in the midst of the armed conflicts in Iraq and Afghanistan, it is nothing short of appalling. (As quoted in Little, 2005b)

The Army was on notice that delays in fielding lifesaving material would not be tolerated. However, just eight months later, the *Sun* was questioning whether the Army, in its zeal to see potentially life-saving innovation fielded as soon as possible, was not rushing things too fast:

> [T]he U.S. Army is launching a multimillion-dollar campaign to equip all its combat troops with a futuristic bandage designed to stop massive bleeding from battlefield injuries, despite doubts about its effectiveness and the development of a cheaper product that many scientists believe works better. (Little, 2005c)

Then, in 2009, the *Sun* reported that "the U.S. Army in recent years has rushed a number of medical innovations onto the battlefields in Iraq and Afghanistan with little testing or data to support them, and then altered or abandoned them when they didn't live up to expectations" (Little, 2009). Pointing to the disagreements among the military services on which hemostatic agents work best, the *Sun* told its readers that "the aggressive push is a point of pride to some Army doctors and officials, but others deride it as reckless and say they felt pressured to defy their own judgments in favor of the military's favored, but unproven, treatments" (Little, 2009).

While an evaluation of various hemostatic agents is far beyond the scope of this discussion, it should be noted that the 2014 version of the TCCC guidelines did recommend the use of combat gauze "for compressible hemorrhage not amenable to tourniquet use or as an adjunct to tourniquet" (U.S. Army Institute of Surgical Research, 2014, p. 3).

Advanced Combat Lifesaver Training

In today's mobile environment across a widely dispersed battlefield, the Army has realized that it is not always possible for trained medical personnel, including combat medics, to be available at all times. As a result, the Army has developed a five-day course, consisting of 40 hours of blended classroom and hands-on training (see Flynn, 2014), to provide a limited number of combat soldiers with additional combat lifesaving skills. The objective is to provide "a bridge between the self-aid/buddy-aid [first aid] training given all soldiers during basic training and the medical training given to the combat medic. . . . Normally, one member of each squad, crew, or equivalent-sized unit will be trained as a combat lifesaver" (Army Institute of Professional Development, 2012, p. 1-2).[84]

Evacuation from the Battlefield

The evacuation of casualties from the battlefield has been a critical early step in providing effective care for casualties. As noted previously, the use of helicopters in Korea and Vietnam reduced the time between wounding to reception of the wounded at a medical facility. During World War II, the average time from wounding to definitive treatment was 10.5 hours; during the Korean War, it dropped to 6.3 hours; and in Vietnam, it was 2.8 hours (Arnold, 2015, p. 222). By 2001, there was a general expectation that care should be provided within the *golden hour*, so called because, it was claimed, morbidity and mortality increase significantly after an hour. The concept, generally attributed to Dr. R. Adams Cowley, founder of the Baltimore Shock Trauma Institute, had achieved the status of dogma by 2001, "despite a lack of clear supporting evidence" (Clarke and Davis, 2012, p. 1261).[85]

The tactical geometry in Afghanistan made achieving the goal of evacuation within an hour particularly challenging, and the conclusion drawn at a NATO conference in 2008 was that the one-hour standard was "just not feasible . . . even if we could enhance the number of helicopters and medical treatment facilities significantly" (Hartenstein, 2008, p. 5-6). That conclusion notwithstanding, Defense Secretary Robert Gates set the American goal at one hour—the golden hour—in 2009 (Shanker, 2009).[86] To accomplish this, he directed an increase in the number of helicopters assigned to medevac in Afghanistan by 25 percent, with some of the helicopters previously dedicated to the search-and-rescue missions for downed pilots reconfigured and reassigned to medevac. The availability of additional aircraft and the prior-

---

[84] Combat lifesavers are trained to treat the casualty for shock, control bleeding, initiate intravenous infusions, apply splints to fractured limbs, insert an oropharyngeal airway in an unconscious casualty, manage battle fatigue, transport a casualty using various litter carries, and load casualties onto military vehicles (Miller, 2018).

[85] At least two research teams had tried and failed to validate the claim attributed to Dr. Cowley that "the first hour after injury will largely determine a critically-injured person's chances for survival" (Cowley, 1975). See Rogers and Rittenhouse, 2014, and Lerner and Moscati, 2001. The lack of direct evidence notwithstanding, an analysis of Vietnam casualties suggested that, because of

> [t]he deleterious effects of delayed evacuation to treatment facilities capable of providing definitive surgical care; . . . [a] six-hour delay would increase the number of casualties who died before reaching medical treatment facilities to 26 per cent, and a 24- hour delay would mean that at least 32 per cent of the total number of casualties will have died. (Bellamy, 1984, p. 60)

[86] It should be noted that the golden hour program was not without its detractors. It has been argued that a

> strict and arbitrary adherence to this "golden hour" may be at odds with optimal patient care in the current conflict in Helmand Province and may have the potential to result in additional morbidity and mortality. This may occur by suboptimal tasking of MEDEVAC assets, triage to a less resourced medical facility and/or aviation mishaps. (Clarke and Davis, 2012, p. 1261)

ity given the medevac missions improved mission performance substantially, as seen in Table 7.11, and had a positive impact on casualty statistics, as shown in Table 7.12.

Results of Changes in Tactical Combat Casualty Care

Overall, with the emphasis on TCCC—hemorrhage control and rapid evacuation—76 percent of all combat-related deaths that occurred before casualties were admitted to a combat hospital in 2012, which was substantially less than the "prehospital mortality in Korea (91% of combat deaths) and Vietnam (88% of combat deaths)," as well the 87 percent reported for 2011 (Rasmussen et al., 2015, p. S61).

Table 7.11
Mean Time Intervals for Prehospital Helicopter Transport of U.S. Military Casualties in Afghanistan Before and After the Golden Hour Mandate

Timing	Before Golden Hour Mandate	After Golden Hour Mandate
Injury to call (minutes)	15.9	13.4
Call to launch (minutes)	26.1	22.7
Launch to scene arrival (minutes)	30.9	16.3
Scene to treatment facility arrival (minutes)	50.4	25.1
Overall mission time (minutes)	110.0	66.0
Missions achieving transport in 60 minutes or less (%)	24.8	75.2

SOURCE: Kotwal, Howard, et al., 2016, Table 2.

Table 7.12
U.S. Casualty Statistics in Afghanistan Before and After the Golden Hour Mandate

Combat Casualty Statistics	Before Golden Hour Mandate[a]	After Golden Hour Mandate[a]	Overall October 2001– December 2015[b] (%)
Returned to duty (%)	33.5[c]	47.3[c]	—
Killed in action (%)	16.0[c]	9.9[c]	7.1
Died of wounds (%)	4.1	4.3	2.4
Case fatality rate	13.7[c]	7.6[c]	9.3

[a] Kotwal, Howard, et al., 2016, Table 1.

[b] Rasmussen et al., 2015, p. S61.

[c] Comparison is significant before versus after the mandate (p < 0.05) X2 with Yates correlations.

Intertheater en Route Care

The U.S. Air Force is responsible for transporting combat casualties from the theater of operations back to the United States. As previously noted, as the Army was revising the way it provided trauma care, with the creation of FSTs, the Air Force was simultaneously revising its evacuation capabilities, using new aircraft and creating three-person CCATTs consisting of an ICU physician, ICU nurse, and respiratory therapist. Initially, the Air Force plan was to stabilize patients after initial surgery for 72 to 96 hours before transporting them out of country, but "by the time of the heavy casualty surge during OIF (2004–2006), movement of patients by CCATTs within hours of their field stabilization surgery became increasingly common" (Ingalls et al., 2014, p. 808). Subsequent analysis of data from the JTTR has validated that decision and the benefits of early AE. A review of the medical records of almost 1,000 casualties showed that 93 percent of the most grievously injured combat casualties transported by the Air Force arrived at Landstuhl Regional Medical Center within 72 hours and 98.5 percent by 96 hours after wounding. The mean time was 38 hours after wounding. The overall 30-day mortality for this group of patients was 2.1 percent, with mortality en route being less than 0.02 percent. The analysis showed no statistically significant difference between survivors at 30 days and decedents with respect to time from injury to arrival at Landstuhl. The following account vividly tells the story:

> By early 2005, combat and medical operations had reached a significant level of maturity. Rapid evacuation from the point of injury by rotary wing medical evacuation promptly delivered casualties within minutes to awaiting operating rooms at surgically capable facilities (level II or level III). . . . Combat casualties underwent 1 or more surgical stabilization procedures within the first 12 hours of wounding as a matter of routine. The first procedure might occur at a forward operating base with a smaller level II facility followed by rapid evacuation to the larger, central level III combat support/theater hospital. Further surgery was undertaken as necessary at the level III facility and/or the patient was rapidly prepared by awaiting CCATTs for subsequent transcontinental transport to Germany. The CCATT mission of accompanying patients who were within hours of wounding and surgery provided the challenge and the opportunity to continue postoperative critical care and resuscitation, literally on the fly. The progressively shorter intervals from wounding to arrival in Germany offered the advantage of delivering the casualty an increasing level of medical sophistication in a much cleaner, resource-intensive, and controlled environment of care. (Ingalls et al., 2014, p. 812)

Protection for the Soldiers

The desire to protect soldiers from penetrating projectiles is as old as recorded history. Paintings on Egyptian tombs, carvings on Babylonian walls, medieval tapestries showing knights in armor, and temple facades at Angkor Wat depict soldiers with shields, armor, and helmets. Often, it is not just the soldier that is protected but also his means of transportation, whether that be a horse, a carriage, or a motor vehicle. Equally old are the complaints that the armor does not provide sufficient protection and that what protection it does provide is costly and the adds weight, further burdening the soldier. All these complaints reappeared during the latest campaigns in Afghanistan and Iraq.

Body Armor

By 2001, the Army had developed a new body armor, known as the Interceptor Body Armor system, that was a significant improvement over its 1990s predecessors in terms of both weight and protection. It weighed "16 pounds, a third lighter than the previous 20-year-old bulky design that protected only against shrapnel but couldn't stop bullets" (Stern, 2003). It consisted of an outer tactical vest containing two ceramic plates known as small-arms protective inserts. However, over time, as the threat changed and as the desire for additional protection increased, additional components were added. While this increased the body area covered, it doubled the weight of the body armor, which was then twice as heavy as what soldiers carried in 2003.[87] The outer tactical vest now consists of a base vest assembly, front yoke and collar assembly, back yoke and collar assembly, lower back protector assembly, groin protector assembly, and deltoid protector component (see Figure 7.28).

Given that today's average combat load far exceeds the 50-lb maximum goal set in 2001, with the Interceptor Body Armor making up a significant part of the weight,[88] is the additional weight and the apparent decrease in combat performance worth it?[89] Does body armor save lives? More specifically, given the threat environment, particularly in Afghanistan with the heavy use of IEDs, is body armor—which was initially designed to protect against penetrating projectiles, such as shrapnel and bullets—effective? The data shown earlier, in Table 7.10, indicates a substantial reduction in thoracic injuries, which has been attributed to "improvements in body armor" (Beekley, Bohman, and Schindler, 2012, p. 11).[90] However, as both conflicts pro-

---

[87] Originally, the Interceptor Body Armor System weighed 17.86 pounds, with the vest weighing 9.86 pounds, and two plate inserts weighing four pounds each. This was lighter than the previous body armor, which weighed 25.1 pounds. Due to the increased danger from IEDs, a newer version was developed. With all the components, the improved system weighs 33.1 lbs. (See U.S. Army, 2013, pp. 160–161.)

[88] In 2003, the average combat load for an Army soldier in Afghanistan was 63 lbs.; by 2007, it was reported to be 97 lbs. (Horn et al., 2012, p. 5; Bachkosky, 2007, p. 11).

[89] By one account, "[f]or a rifleman, increasing his load from 50 pounds (goal) to 95 pounds (actual today) reduces the marching distance that a soldier/marine can traverse in eight hours by 35 percent (from approximately 17 to 11 miles)" (Horn et al., 2012, p. 8).

[90] Peoples noted "the small number of wounds to the abdomen and chest, areas that were protected by the new body armor currently being worn by our soldiers in battle. There were only 12 chest/abdominal penetrating wounds documented in this series. Some of these occurred among soldiers who were not wearing body armor at the time" (Peoples et al., 2005b, p. 464). It was also reported that "analysis of casualties from January to July 2004, [showed] the rate of thoracic injury was 18% in patients without body armor and <5% in soldiers wearing armor" (Eastridge et al., 2006, p. 1367).

Figure 7.28
Interceptor Body Armor System and Outer Tactical Vest with Components

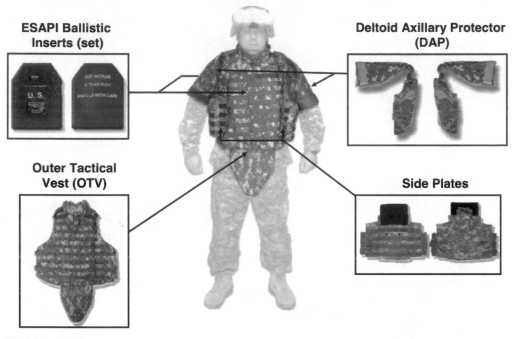

SOURCE: DoD IG, 2009, p. 2.

gressed from conventional warfare, with a predominance of gunshot wounds, to an insurgency characterized by IEDs, wounding patterns changed and so did the relative effectiveness of body armor. Now, injuries to the unprotected parts of the body—head; extremities; and the junctions between the torso, arms, neck, and legs—were more common. In a perverse way, improvements in body armor may have helped more wounded survive, but with serious wounds to less-protected regions, such as the head and extremities. However, a systematic review of the major journals, reference texts, and published abstracts found "no evidence to suggest that by virtue of wearing body armor the likelihood of sustaining a head, neck or face . . . injury increases as such, but a higher incidence of fragment injuries to the HFN [head, face, and neck] region may be due to the more common use of IEDs and other explosive devices" (Tong and Beirne, 2013, p. 425).

Up-Armored Humvees and Mine-Resistant, Ambush-Protected Vehicles

A September 30, 2007, headline in the *Washington Post* proclaimed: "The IED Problem Is Getting Out of Control. We've Got to Stop the Bleeding" (Atkinson, 2007). The accompanying story, with supporting graphs and charts, told the story of a rising tide of deaths and wounded soldiers caused by IEDs and the resulting heightened congressional concern. The year before, DoD had created the Joint IED Defeat Organization to investigate countermeasures and had sent electronic warfare officers to Iraq and Afghanistan to work on such countermeasures as electronic jammers and predetonators, radars, X-ray equipment, and robotic explosive ordnance disposal equipment. Many thought more could be done to protect soldiers themselves. Initially, the Army added armor to its Humvees, the modern replacement for the venerable jeep. These "up-armored" Humvees (see Figure 7.29) were built on a heavier chassis, with an improved engine to handle the added weight of the armor. It proved essential for cross-country, off-road movement. They reportedly cost three times what the original had (see Keyes, 2011).

By 2005, however, commanders in the field were clamoring for a more robust mine-protected vehicle. In November 2006, the Marine Corps awarded a contract for the first 144 of a new class of MRAPs, which incorporated a "V"-shaped hull (see Figure 7.30). In February 2007, the Navy approved initial production using the expedited procedures of the Warfighting Rapid Acquisition Program. The following September, DoD made the MRAP a major defense acquisition program (see Sullivan, 2009). Production grew from an initial Marine Corps order for 1,169 vehicles to an authorized level of 25,700 split among the Army, Marine Corps, Navy, Air Force, and Special Operations Command. By January 2011, 13,624 MRAPs had been delivered to Afghanistan, including more than 6,500 of the newer version, designed to meet the challenges of Afghanistan's rugged terrain. While the MRAPs could not move off road, they provided much better protection against IEDs underneath road paving or on the close sides of the roads than the up-armored Humvees. The total cost of the program had grown to almost $44 billion (Feickert, 2011).

In 2010, *USA Today* reported that

> [n]early 80% of roadside bomb attacks on Humvees from January 2009 through the end of July 2010 killed occupants . . . . That figure dropped to 15% for attacks on [MRAPs] . . . .
>
> The military estimates that MRAPs have reduced deaths and injuries by 30%. (Brook, 2010)

The following year, the Congressional Research Service told Congress that the MRAP had "significantly reduced troop deaths from roadside bombings in Afghanistan even as insurgents have stepped up their use of IEDs" (Feickert, 2011, p. 2).

Figure 7.29
Up-Armored Humvee

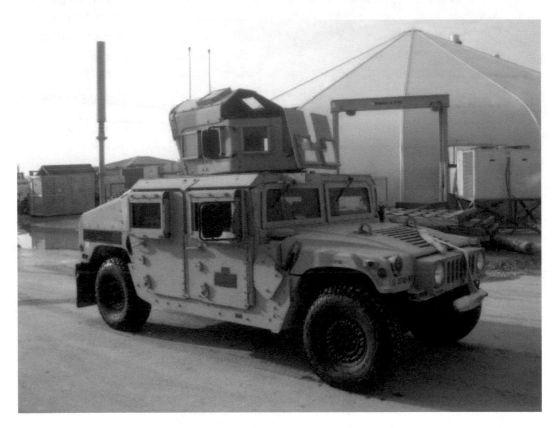

SOURCE: U.S. Air Force photo/Todd Spencer.

Legacy

In 2016, the U.S. Army Medical Department held a three-day conference to explore the advances that have occurred in military medicine since 9/11. The 47 lectures were eventually published in a comprehensive issue of the *United States Army Medical Department Journal* highlighting the medical legacy of advances in medical care during operations in Afghanistan and Iraq (West, 2016). Box 7.2 lists the 15 advances in combat casualty care highlighted by the Army.

Figure 7.30
Mine-Resistant, Ambush-Protected Vehicle

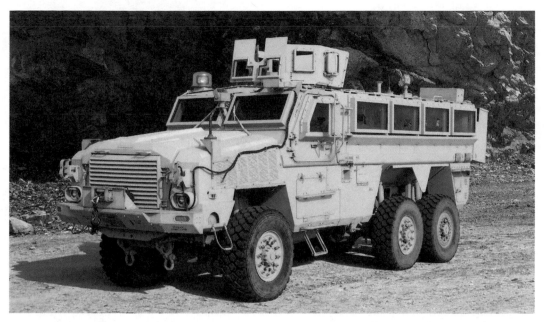

SOURCE: Promotional image from BAE Systems.

Of particular note were advances made in trauma care on the battlefield. While the combat settings often differ radically from what is found in the civil sector,[91] the IOM found that the "organized civilian trauma system . . . is well positioned to assimilate and distribute the recent wartime trauma lessons learned and to serve as a repository and incubator for innovation in trauma care" (Berwick, Downey, and Cornett, 2016, p. 9), and that the

> [p]artnership across the military and civilian systems can facilitate the transfer of lessons learned and encourage the continued advancement of trauma care in both

---

[91] Gerhardt and colleagues offered an example:

> [I]n civilian sector emergency medical services . . . , a typical motor vehicle collision scene might include an ambulance crew routinely consisting of two or even three emergency medical technicians (EMTs), with at least one being an EMT-Paramedic. . . . In the majority of cases, significant resources will be brought to bear upon one or two patients. In addition, civilian sector out-of-hospital careproviders do not typically face hostile gunfire and are able to fully focus on patient care.
>
> In contrast . . . a combat medic or other careprovider responding to casualties after a roadside bomb . . . [may carry the] medical equipment . . . in a rucksack. . . . There is likely to be only one medic assisting casualties that were injured by a combination of high-explosive ordnance, vehicle fires, or small-arms fire. The medic is appropriately focused on patient care but must also be cognizant that the overarching priorities are the combat unit's integrity and mission. While working, the medic may become the target of hostile fire and may have to return fire. (Gerhardt et al., 2012, p. 91)

Box 7.2
Army Medical Department Advances in Combat Care from Operations in Afghanistan and Iraq

Development of a military trauma registry
"Low volume" resuscitation fluids—colloids and red blood cells
Hemostatic agents
- Systemic
- Topical

Use of "damage control" initial surgery
Use of endovascular stents
Common use of external fixators
Improved tourniquets
CAD/CAM limb prostheses
Pain control
Concussion care
Established clinical practice guidelines for combat casualty care
Identification of coagulopathy in injury
Challenges of treating infections with fungus and multidrug-resistant bacteria
Deployed Electronic Health Record
Reach back capability with telehealth and programmatic email communication

SOURCES: Murray, Hitter, and Jones, 2016, p. 2; Pruitt, 2008, p. S7.
NOTE: CAD/CAM = computer-aided design and computer-aided manufacturing

sectors. While interface between the military and civilian sectors is hardly a new phenomenon, a number of collaborative platforms have recently been developed to encourage the bidirectional translation of best practices. (Berwick, Downey and Cornett, 2016, p. 106)

CHAPTER EIGHT

The Changing Nature of War Casualties: Amputations, Traumatic Brain Injury, Psychological Casualties, and PTSD

Chapter Seven covered the military and the medical care for casualties in Afghanistan and Iraq during the longest period of conflict in our history; this chapter examines medical and care issues related to amputations, the provision of mental health services of the force, and the issues related to TBI. Chapter Nine will cover the care war casualties receive after leaving the military.

Throughout the two volumes of *Providing for the Casualties of War,* particular attention has been paid to two conditions that have epitomized the changing nature of warfare, medical science, and the long-term support provided disabled veterans: loss of a limb (amputation) and the psychological consequences of war. The amputee has been a focus of attention for centuries. As recently as the American Civil War, the so-called signature wound was amputation of a major limb, and a veteran with an artificial arm or leg was the living reminder of the traumatic consequences of battle. Today, things have changed. TBI and PTSD arguably have the distinction of being the signature wounds of the most recent conflicts. Psychological impairments have been recognized as a significant consequence of war, the manifestations of which can be "lifelong and pervade all aspects of a service member's or veteran's life, including mental and physical health, family and social relationships, and employment" (Committee on the Assessment of Ongoing Efforts in the Treatment of Posttraumatic Stress Disorder et al., 2014, p. 1).

This chapter examines how, since 9/11, the Army has dealt with amputees, soldiers with TBIs, psychological casualties, and PTSD. In terms of absolute numbers of soldiers affected, the number of amputees is very small relative to the number of soldiers reported to have TBI or PTSD. Nevertheless, concern for amputees remains high, and the issue is still one veterans' service organizations cover most frequently on their websites, ranking third, just behind PTSD and above TBI in a recent analysis of the webpages of these organizations.[1] Moreover, until recently, the Army's definition of

---

[1] A qualitative content analysis of 15 veteran-relevant health content areas on the websites of 34 veteran service organizations showed that, between July 2011 and January 2012, of 277 health topics, "the top five . . . [were] insurance/Tricare/Veterans Administration issues (28.2%), posttraumatic stress disorder (PTSD; 15.5%),

a wounded warrior—admission to its wounded warrior program—was almost exclusively reserved for amputees. The story of how the Army's amputee program changed is highlighted here, as is the Army's TBI program and how psychological impairments, including PTSD, are managed today. Unlike amputations, which are, in general, an immediate consequence of a battle injury, TBIs and PTSD may not be immediately obvious, resulting in a whole new set of issues that affect both the Army and the Department of Veterans Affairs, which are covered in Chapter Nine.

Amputations

The loss of a limb—a major amputation—is now relatively rare, but still in line with recent experience (see Table 8.1). Since the beginning of combat in 2001 through February 2017, more than 1.3 million Army soldiers have been deployed to Afghanistan and Iraq. Among Army casualties are more than 3,900 "hostile deaths" and more than 36,000 WIA (Defense Casualty Analysis System, 2017), compared with 1,098 major limb amputations and 179 minor limb amputations.[2] (Army soldiers accounted for 66.1 percent and marines for 29.8 percent of major amputations.) Figure 8.1 shows the distribution of major limb amputations for the Army in Afghanistan and Iraq over time.

One thing that sets the current conflicts off from former wars and the amputations of civilians is the high rate of multilimb amputations, as Figure 8.2 shows.[3] The percentage of amputees with multiple amputations, i.e., the multilimb amputation rate, was 39 percent for OEF, and 24 percent for OIF and OND, which was much higher than the 2 to 20 percent multiple-amputee rates reported from World War I, World War II, the Korean War, and the Vietnam War (Krueger, Wenke, and Ficke, 2012, p. S443). For all the services, from the beginning of hostilities through 2016,

---

disability/amputation/wounds (13.4%), Agent Orange (10.5%), and traumatic brain injury (9.0%)" (Poston et al., 2013, p. 88).

[2]   As of February 1, 2017 (Carino, 2017a). Major limbs include legs, arms, and full hands and feet. Minor limbs include fingers and toes. Note that the numbers reported do not include "limb salvage," which is performed to give patients an alternative to amputation.

[3]   Scoville, 2003h, makes the distinction:

> The wounding patterns resulting from military conflict are very different from civilian injuries and have a great impact on the management of the associated amputations. The high kinetic energy delivered by modern munitions results in extensive soft tissue zones of injury, causing wounds that are subject to more complications, and may take longer to heal. . . .

> Wounds related to war surgery are initially left open because of the high risk of infection. . . . Because of the severe nature of war wounds, reconstructive procedures are often done later, even months after injury . . . .

> Blast injuries also may have associated mild-moderate traumatic brain injuries (TBI) that are concomitant with amputations.

Table 8.1
Army Amputation Survivors, Civil War, World Wars I and II, Korean War, Vietnam Conflict, and Recent Operations in Afghanistan and Iraq

Conflict	Extremities Wounded	Individuals Wounded	Surviving Amputees	
			Number	Percentage of Surviving Wounded
Civil War	Upper	83,536	12,860	15.4
	Lower	89,528	8,002	10.2
	Total	173,064	20,862	12.1
World War I	Upper	55,000	2,359	4.3
	Lower	69,000	2,044	3.0
	Total	124,000	4,403	3.6
World War II	Upper	167,000	3,152	1.9
	Lower	248,000	11,760	4.7
	Total	415,000	14,912	2.5
Korea	Upper	21,002	454	2.2
	Lower	26,270	1,023	3.9
	Total	47,272	1,477	3.1
Vietnam	Total	96,802	5,283	5.4
Afghanistan and Iraq	Major limb	—	1,098	3.0
	Minor limb	—	179	—
	Total	36,810	1,277	3.5

SOURCES: Beebe and DeBakey, 1952, p. 194; Reister, 1975, p. 400; Otis and Huntington, 1883, p. 877; Reister, 1973, pp. 48, 160; "Vietnam War Statistics," 2015; and Carino, 2017a.

NOTE: The World War II and Korea numbers include nonbattle amputations; the World War I numbers do not. In Korea, there were also 1,120 traumatic amputations (Reznick, Gambel, and Hawk, 2009, p. 33).

there were 1,134 single-limb amputations, 463 two-limb amputations, 56 three-limb amputations, and six four-limb amputations. It was reported that the most common cause of injuries leading to an amputation was an explosive device (93 percent). The vast majority of the amputations, more than 80 percent, were done the same day as the wounding, with 10 percent occurring more than 90 days after the date of injury. This suggested "that the medical personnel who are initially caring for the injured Service Members have been consistent in determining which limbs should undergo an acute amputation and those that should undergo an attempted salvage" (Krueger, Wenke, and Ficke, 2012, p. S442).

Figure 8.1
Army Major Limb Amputations, 2001–2016

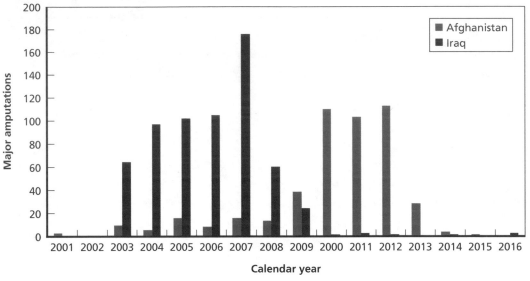

SOURCE: Carino, 2017a.

Figure 8.2
Multilimb Amputations, 2001–2016

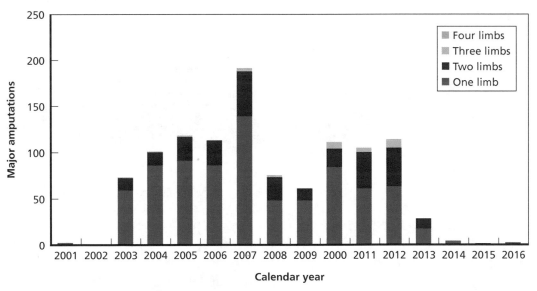

SOURCE: Carino, 2017a.

Rehabilitation Reconsidered

As noted in Chapter Five, the respective roles of the Army and the VA/DVA were clear in theory once the amputee was returned to the United States. The Army was responsible for initial treatment of the seriously wounded. But for casualties whose continuing service was unlikely, such as amputees, the stated policy was to transfer them to a VA hospital. As noted, during the Vietnam War, the actual handoff from the Army to the VA depended on "administrative policy, whim, physical considerations, staffing patterns, and bed availability" (Brown, 1994, p. 193). The stories of the two senators discussed in Chapter Five illustrated how far, during Vietnam, the Army had moved away from the model of extended care provided to officers after World War II. After 9/11, with a career-oriented all-volunteer force in place and with the prospect of further conflict in the Middle East, the Army Surgeon General, LTG James Peake, asked "for an estimate on the number of amputee patients that could be expected from a war in Afghanistan" (Scoville, 2007a, p. 4) and a plan for how amputees should be handled in the future.

When the United States was attacked on 9/11, the Army and the entire DoD were unprepared to provide rehabilitation services to combat amputees because their focus had been on circulatory, rather than on combat-related, orthopedic issues.[4] Unfortunately, this was not a new situation; the Army Medical Department has seldom been prepared for a major conflict, whether the Civil War, the Spanish American War, World War I, or World War II.[5] Nevertheless, the staff of the Office of the Surgeon General understood the challenges as it prepared recommendations for the Surgeon General:

> In past armed conflicts, the combat amputee has been a significant clinical problem for the military medical care system due to the severity of the injuries, the associated morbidity, and prolonged hospitalization. The likelihood of military operations using ground forces in landmine filled Afghanistan require [sic] proactive planning for multiple amputee casualties. The Russian's [sic] reported on their experience in Afghanistan that in 1978 land mines accounted for 4% of all injuries—the rates in 80, 82, 84, and 86 were 8%, 18%, 21% and 24% respectively as the use of land mines proliferated. The time to medical treatment because of the mountainous terrain and transport difficulties was: under 6 hrs 4% of patients received medical treatment (other than initial first aid) 6–12 hrs 21% 12–24 hrs 25% 2 days or greater 50% of patients. (Scoville, 2001b, p. 1)

---

[4] In CY 2001, DoD cared for 99 patients from the Circulatory Services and 57 patients from Orthopaedic Services. In CY 2002 the numbers were 76 and 46, respectively, within DoD (Scoville, 2006a, p. 1).

[5] Rostker, 2013, discusses the unpreparedness of the Army Medical Department at the outbreak of a major conflict at length.

Within a matter of days, a team from the Office of the Surgeon General and the Walter Reed Medical Center was working to reestablish an Army amputee center like those that had been established during World War I, World War II, and Vietnam.[6] As the team saw it, the Army needed a designated amputee center to provide the "special care needed by amputees in the transition from a wounding to final prosthetic fitting, . . . before a patient is treated by the VA System" (McHale, 2001a, p. 2). In a marked departure from Army policy during Vietnam, McHale and her team argued that, before transitioning to the VA, the military should provide this care because

> [f]irst, no civilian institution has experience in treating open wounds of the upper and lower extremity while simultaneously fitting for a pylon/practice prosthesis. . . . [L]eaving the wounds open is the safest means to care for a patient on the battlefield. This is not common practice at civilian hospitals. Second, establishment of a separate amputee service and ward at a military hospital has several benefits for the patient. He is able to see how others of similar age progress with rehabilitation including walking (lower extremity) and performing activities of daily living (upper extremity). Amputees from previous conflicts cite the informal group therapy that occurs in such a setting. This is a tremendous reassurance to the patient. By parceling out patients to civilian facilities or several military hospitals on a general orthopedic service such an environment would be lost. Finally, all patients will need a medical board towards the completion of their treatment. Simply retiring these patients, without the benefit of seeing how well they will rehabilitate, does no service for the amputee. (McHale, 2001a, p. 3)[7]

They thought that amputee care required "a team approach of surgeons, nurses, therapists, psychiatrists, prosthetists, and social workers to help not only in the physical transformation of the patient but be able to provide vocational or other opportunities to make the amputee a productive member of society" (McHale, 2001a, p. 2). McHale and her colleagues recommended that "the most likely site for establishing a center for amputee care would be Walter Reed Army Medical Center. . . . [It was] the most likely place for evacuation for an upcoming conflict. . . . Walter Reed Army Medical Center already has a modern brace and limb service that could easily be expanded" (McHale, 2001b).

---

[6]   Amputee centers were initiated by the U.S. Army in World War I and II. During the Vietnam War, Valley Forge Army General Hospital maintained a separate amputee service. During World War II,

> the United States military established five "amputation centers" at ports of debarkation. . . . Since these centers were responsible for the amputee's full rehabilitation, as well as early care, longer military hospital stays were required. By 1944, two additional centers were established to handle the workload. (Flood and Saliman, 2002, p. 18)

[7]   Doukas, 2003a, and Polly, 2003, also forcefully make the case for an Army amputee care center.

On October 31, 2001, the Surgeon General approved plans to develop a "virtual" amputee system to keep the level of care consistent across the Army,[8] with a center of care at Walter Reed and the new Extremity War Trauma Surgery Course to train surgeons prior to deployment (Scoville, 2003f). By the beginning of December 2001, a panel of outside experts was

> [developing] a consensus doctrine for the care of military amputee care [sic] from injury in theater to rehabilitation to return to duty/discharge, . . .
>
> [reviewing] space and patient flow at WRAMC [Walter Reed Army Medical Center] for amputee care, . . .
>
> [and reviewing] available equipment . . . to verify ability to provide state of the art amputee care and identify additional requirements. (Scoville, 2001a)[9]

Unfortunately, however, the new system was not in place when the first amputees arrived. The first group of ten amputees stayed an average of 51 days before being transferred to the VA or home base; the

> majority of patients were discharged from out-patient care with a temporary prosthesis, physical therapy routines in pamphlet form, limited to no occupational therapy and the basic ability to ambulate independently in a wheelchair, crutches or initial prosthesis. Some patients returned to their home of record after their definitive surgery. Servicemembers were totally dependent on Tricare Benefits for all of their orthotic and prosthetic care and depended on VA or Military clinics for any physical therapy or occupational therapy. Servicemembers were not assigned to a medical hold company and remained assigned to the deployed unit. (Scoville, 2006a)

This was totally unsatisfactory, especially compared with later practices, in which

> patients [were] assigned to local medical hold commands at the Medical Centers, with an average stay time of a year or more. Most patients have several definitive prostheses for a variety of activities, the proper therapy for use and care of them-

---

[8]   In this virtual system, Walter Reed was to be

at the center of a multi-site, coordinated complex of facilities that include regional medical centers in Europe, Brooke Army Medical Center in San Antonio, the Department of Veterans Affairs, and other military and civilian treatment facilities. Wherever in the virtual system that amputee patients receive care, the goal of the USAAPCP [U.S. Army Amputee Patient Care Program] . . . is to ensure that they receive the kind of care that will allow them to lead lives unconstrained by their amputation. (Office of the Surgeon General, Department of the Army, 2004, p. i)

[9]   Initial meetings took place at Walter Reed on December 2–3, 2001, to identify requirements for amputee care and develop plans for managing light, medium, and heavy casualty loads. A second symposium for amputee care providers was held at USUHS on August 19, 2002, sponsored by Walter Reed's Department of Orthopaedics, again involving leaders in amputee care from both the civilian health-care sector and the VA. See Scoville, 2003d.

selves and their prosthetics and most are commonly returned to the highest levels of sports and function. (Scoville, 2006a)

A Building a New System of Care for the Combat Amputee

Planning went forward during spring and summer 2002; on August 22, 2002, the Surgeon General gave final approval for Walter Reed to be the Army's primary site, with a capacity for ten acute inpatients and 50 long-term advanced-function outpatients, and for Brooke Army Medical Center at Fort Sam Houston, Texas, to be the secondary site (Scoville, 2003d).[10] Funding for the program was to come immediately from the Chief of Staff of the Army—$2.5 million—for renovations to Walter Reed in 2002, with the following appropriated funds from Congress: FY 2003, $2.4 million; FY 2004, $10 million; FY 2005, $7.8 million; and FY 2006, $3.9 million (Scoville, 2006a, p. 2). In addition, an outside Amputee Care Program Board of Directors was established to "serve in an advisory capacity to broaden the scope of vision for the amputee care program, [and to] make such suggestions for the improvement of the program as it deems necessary" (Commander, Walter Reed Army Medical Center, 2003; see also Doukas, 2003b).

Administratively, things were also changing. It was usual for amputees to receive primary care from a variety of different medical specialties, as needed to meet immediate medical or surgical needs. However, "their holistic and amputee-specific care was less than consistent" (Pasquina et al., 2009, p. 8). A new Department of Orthopedics and Rehabilitation soon brought all critical subspecialties needed for the care of amputees (orthopedics, physical medicine and rehabilitation, occupational therapy, physical therapy, and prosthetics and orthotics) together into a single united department that followed a new patient flow protocol (see Figure 8.3), and new team guidelines were being developed for the rehabilitation (Scoville, 2002a; Scoville, 2002b).

A New Paradigm for the Army

By November 2003, prior to OIF, 53 soldiers had sustained major amputations, with 11 involving multiple extremities, in Afghanistan. Walter Reed had treated 47 of these patients (Scoville, 2003b), and "approximately 25% . . . of all amputee patients treated at WRAMC . . . also received care in VA health care system" (Scoville, 2003d). If the respective roles of the Army and VA had been clear before 9/11, with the ultimate responsibility for amputees being with the VA, the Army now saw it quite differently, as the Chief of the Amputee Patient Care Center at Walter Reed explained:

> After previous military conflicts, soldiers who underwent an amputation typically received immediate life-saving medical treatment and limb stabilization in a military medical facility. Once a patient was stable, the trend was to medically dis-

---

[10] The Brooke Army Medical Center amputee patient care site held a formal opening ceremony on January 14, 2005 (Scoville, 2005a).

Figure 8.3
Walter Reed Army Medical Center Amputee Service Patient Flow

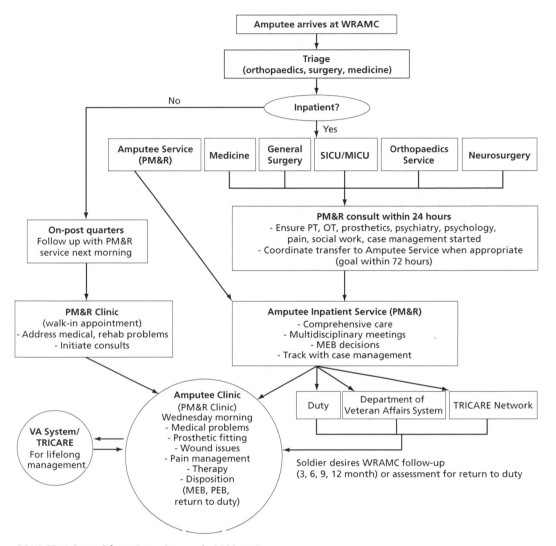

SOURCE: Adapted from Pasquina et al., 2009, p. 9.
NOTES: MICU = medical ICU; OT = occupational therapy; PM&R = physical medicine and rehabilitation;
PT = physical therapy; SICU = surgical ICU.

charge soldiers w/amputations and transition them over to the Veteran's Administration healthcare system for rehabilitation and prosthetic care. After Operation Desert Storm, we realized that an amputation was not necessarily a career-ending injury, especially with the evolution of new prosthetics that allow soldiers to run, jump, etc. Now, after Operations Enduring Freedom and Iraqi Freedom, the military's attitude toward rehabilitation of the soldier/amputee has evolved into a proactive team-effort approach. The Walter Reed Army Medical Center has established the Amputee Center of Excellence. This center provides a full spectrum of state-of-the-art care for soldiers who sustain traumatic amputations on the battle-field. This team is dedicated to the rehabilitation and restoration of soldiers; the end goal is to provide soldiers the option to remain on/return to active duty and complete their military careers. (Scoville, 2003e)

But it was more than just giving amputees the opportunity to return to active duty. The Army saw that it had a role in the continued care of amputees even after they had left service: Amputees were generally medically retired and therefore would have access to the military health care system, if they chose to use it, for the rest of their lives:

Patients . . . may elect to continue their care at Walter Reed, or may seek additional care at facilities closer to their home. The amputee care program provides the opportunity for patients to return to WRAMC periodically for re-evaluation, revisions or refinements to their prosthetic devices, and an intensive rehabilitation program. (Polly et al., 2003)

Moreover, the Army saw that soldiers were different from most civilians in key ways:

a. All of the individuals sustaining combat amputations are high-level athletes and the goal is to return them to the highest level of activity that they wish to achieve. These physiologically young individuals differ from the average amputees in the civilian sector who often are lower level activity patients that function well with basic prosthetic appliances.

b. The standard of care on the civilian sector, and in the Veteran's Health Administration, is to return the amputee patient to a community ambulation level with capabilities to perform all activities of daily living. The standard of the US Army Amputee Patient Care Program is to return all individuals to the highest level of activity achievable. This includes running and ambulation on uneven terrain for the lower extremity amputee patient, and strenuous upper body activity, including overhead skills for the upper extremity amputee.

c. It is projected that these patients will return to WRAMC on numerous occasions for advanced skills training and prosthetic enhancements. (Scoville, 2003c)

To some extent, this was a replay of what the Army had wanted to do at the end of World War I. In 1917, the Surgeon General of the Army unsuccessfully tried to keep recovering soldiers on active duty until they had obtained the "maximum cure" (see Rostker, 2013, pp. 150–152). This time, the goal was to "return each patient to the highest level of function possible" (Scoville, 2003g), or as the Army explained it in a report to Congress, the "goal of the USAAPCP [US Army Amputee Patient Care Program] . . . is to return patients to their pre-injury level of activity, called 'tactical athleticism'" (Office of the Surgeon General, Department of the Army, 2004, p. 4-1).

This time, the Army was not trying to keep draftees in service but members of the all-volunteer force, who, if they were medically retired, could select care from the VA, the Army, *or both*. This time, the Army also had the President of the United States on its side. On December 18, 2003, President Bush spoke at the Amputee Patient Center at Walter Reed:

> Americans would be surprised to learn that a grievous injury, such as the loss of a limb, no longer means forced discharge. In other words, the medical care is so good and the recovery process is so technologically advanced, that people are no longer forced out of the military. When we're talking about forced discharge, we're talking about another age and another army. This is a new age, and this is a new army. Today if wounded service members want to remain in uniform and can do the job, the military tries to help them stay. (Bush, 2003)

Now, with the implied support of President Bush, there was a new emphasis on retaining these *wounded warriors,* and a new Army program to do just that.

U.S. Army Wounded Warrior Program

To facilitate amputees remaining on active duty in April 2004, the Army initiated the Disabled Soldier Support System program—renamed the U.S. Army Wounded Warrior Program in November 2005—to help "disabled soldiers cut through red tape to seek out the help or information they need until they can return to active duty or receive a medical retirement from the military" (Miles, 2004). The program provided "disabled soldiers a single starting point for help with their financial, administrative, medical, vocational and other needs. It also helps them sort out the medical and vocational entitlements and other benefits for which they quality" (Miles, 2004). As envisioned the program incorporated and integrated

> several existing programs to provide holistic support services for our severely disabled Soldiers and their families throughout their phased progression from initial casualty notification to their return to home station and final career position. DS3 [The Disabled Soldier Support System] will also use a system to track and monitor severely disabled Soldiers for up to five years beyond their medical retirements to provide appropriate assistance through an array of existing service providers. ("Disabled Soldier Support System," 2005)

To be eligible for the program, a wounded soldier needed to have a 30-percent or greater disability from a *single* cause. The single-cause provision was critical in limiting the number of wounded soldiers that were eligible for the program to those who unambiguously needed special care from the time of initial casualty notification. Technically, eligibility extended to soldiers who had become blind or deaf or had vision or severe hearing loss; suffered amputations, spinal cord injuries and paralysis, severe burns, or TBI; had been permanently disfigured; had PTSD; and/or had contracted a fatal, incurable disease with limited life expectancy (Hudak et al., 2009, p. 567). In practice, however, as the director of the Disabled Soldier Support System emphasized, the program was limited to casualties that involved paralysis or the loss of limbs or eyes. During 2004, the first year of the program, 340 soldiers were eligible, with 179 being eligible because of major limb amputations (see Hudak et al., 2009; Carino, 2017a).

Given the kind of services provided, eligibility had to be clear. While eligibility was clear for those who had suffered a major limb amputation, it was not so clear for others, who were then excluded. The example of one soldier with a TBI illustrates the point. His 30-percent disability rating was the result of 10 percent for cognitive disorder secondary to the TBI, 10 percent for posttraumatic headaches caused by the TBI, and 10 percent for the loss of part of the skull. While the evaluation reached the critical 30-percent disability level, the Physical Evaluation Board (PEB) placed this soldier on the TDRL, subjecting him and his family to "periodic reexaminations and reevaluations," which as his wife explained, filled the family "with dread that at some point in the future, they might suddenly decide to drop him below the crucial 30 percent total rating" (Williams, 2014, pp. 119–120).

In 2008, eligibility for the program was changed to include "Soldiers who have received, or are expected to receive, a 50% or higher combined disability rating from the Army because of combat or combat-related injuries" (Hudak et al., 2009, p. 567). The number of soldiers in the program grew from 2,432 in 2007 to 4,329 by April 1, 2009, with most of the growth coming from soldiers suffering from PTSD and TBI.[11] Nevertheless, given the relative prevalence of PTSD, TBI, and major limb amputations, the Army Wounded Warrior Program was covering all amputees, about 4 percent of those with PTSD, and about 28 percent of those with severe or penetrating TBI.[12]

Returning Amputee Patients to Active Duty

Historically, few soldiers who have had limbs amputated have remained on active duty. While there is a long history of invalid soldiers continuing to serve—with noted examples being the 150 French *companies detaches d'invalides* in the 1760s (Snyder, Gawdiak, and Worden, 1991, p. 6), the American Invalid Corps during the Revolution (Forman, 1965, p. 19), and the Civil War's Veteran Reserve Corps—amputees do not often remain in active service (Kishbaugh et al., 1995). After Vietnam, however, several who did remain made significant contributions, including now-retired GEN Frederick Franks, a lower leg amputee, who commanded the VII Corps during

---

[11] The Army reported that, of the 4,329 soldiers who were enrolled in the Army Wounded Warrior Program on April 1, 2009, approximately 1,300 had PTSD; 700 had TBI; and just under 700 had amputations (Army Wounded Warrior Program, 2009).

[12] Between October 2001 and December 2008, the Army reported 33,198 cases of PTSD among soldiers who had been deployed to Afghanistan and Iraq; 2,489 cases of severe or penetrating TBI; 6,954 cases of moderate TBI; and 671 soldiers who had a major limb amputation (Carino, 2017a, p. 2).

Operation Desert Storm (Scales, 1993, p. 133), and former Chief of Staff of the Army, GEN Eric Shinseki, a partial-foot amputee. It was General Shinseki who provided the initial funds to support the U.S. Army Amputee Patient Care Program at Walter Reed.

Generally, amputees are considered unfit for military service, but the discharge process is rather convoluted and involves determinations by the Medical Evaluation Board (MEB) and the PEB.[13] At the time the Army Amputee Patient Care Program was established, Army Regulation 40-501 directed that an amputee of the upper or lower extremities be referred to an MEB for evaluation of his or her condition and that the evaluation be forwarded to a PEB, which determines "fitness or unfitness . . . [considering] the results of the MEB, as well as the requirements of the soldier's MOS [military occupational specialty], in determining fitness" (Army Regulation 40-501, 2011, p. 21). Given the new emphasis on retaining as many amputees as was practical, the regulation was changed,[14] and amputees were given "temporary profiles," allowing them to remain in rehabilitation longer so they might achieve a higher level of function. At the end of rehabilitation, the temporary profile was updated. In a few cases, amputees were able to demonstrate that they could fully meet all the physical requirements of their military occupations and were found fit for duty. In such cases, they were assigned to a job appropriate for their rank and skills. In most cases, PEBs found amputees not fit for duty, and a permanent medical retirement was appropriate. However, amputees were allowed to request a Continuance on Active Duty waiver, which was normally granted if the amputation was the result of combat, and if the soldier could "demonstrate a higher level of function with a prosthesis and have the recommendation of two medical officers" (Stinner et al., 2010, p. 1476). An analysis of 395 combat-related major limb amputations between October 1, 2001, and June 1, 2006, showed that 65 amputees—16.5 percent—remained on active duty: PEBs had determined that 11 were fit for duty, and 54 received Continuance on Active Duty waivers. These results are consistent with more-recent data (see Figure 8.4), which shows longer-term retention of 14 percent for all amputees, 17 percent for amputees who had lost one limb, and 5 percent for amputees who had lost more than one limb. The retention of 17 percent for all amputees, however, is somewhat lower than what Army Amputee Patient Care Program considered possible, which was that "nearly 40% of patients could reach a level of function necessary to return to active duty military service if they so choose" (Scoville, 2004a). This meant that a little less than one-half the amputees who were considered physically retainable chose to continue serving.

---

[13] Gambel, 2014, provides a useful guide.

[14] Chapter 3 in Army Regulation 40-501, describes how a soldier with significant limb loss is to be evaluated; this was changed to provide that:

> Soldiers with amputations will (assuming no other disqualifying medical conditions) be provided a temporary profile not less than 4 months (but not to exceed 1 year) to enable the Soldier to attain maximum medical benefit. (Army Regulation 40-501, 2011, p. 24)

Figure 8.4
Retention on Active Duty of Army Major Limb Amputees, October 2001–April 2016

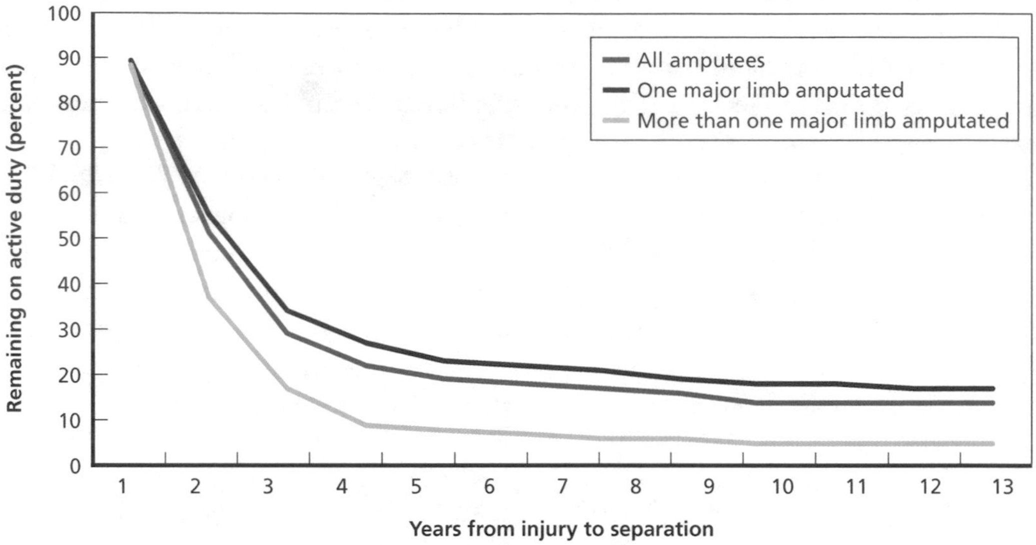

SOURCE: Carino, 2016.

Vietnam and OIF/OEF Compared

In 2010, the VA reported the results of the first national survey of amputees from the Vietnam War and the conflicts in Afghanistan (OEF) and Iraq (OIF). The Survey for Prosthetic Use, conducted in 2007 and 2008, identified "level(s) of limb loss . . . , concurrent injuries and illnesses, health status, quality of life, and physical function" and documented the "use, replacement, rejection, and abandonment of prosthetic devices and . . . satisfaction with prosthetic and assistive devices" (Smith and Reiber, 2010, p. vii). The survey provided detailed data on an extensive sample of amputees from Vietnam and OEF/OIF.

The results of the survey clearly showed how much the rehabilitation of amputees had changed in the quarter century that separated Vietnam from OIF/OEF and highlighted the paradigm shift for DoD and the VA (see Table 8.2).[15] After 9/11, DoD initiated "holistic rehabilitation care . . . [at] specialized centers . . . designed to achieve the highest level of physical, psychological, and emotional function in servicemembers with limb loss" (Smith and Reiber, 2010, p. viii). Care from the VA for Vietnam amputees was clearly less ambitious. Traditionally, at the VA, all veterans with limb loss "receive[d] prosthetic devices according to their functional level if deemed medically appropriate by their managing physician" (Blough et al., 2010, p. 388). And the VA took "a narrow view of amputation care, focusing only on managing prosthetic devices" (Smith and Reiber, 2010, p. vii); "the rehabilitation approach was to offer a

---

[15] Pasquina, 2010, and Sigford, 2010, use the term *paradigm shift* to describe the change.

Table 8.2
Provision of Prosthetic Devices Among Participants in the 2007–2008
Survey for Prosthetic Use

Conflict	Respondents Currently Using Prosthetics (%)	Of Those Currently Using Prosthetics, Percentage Who Received a Prosthetic from			
		Private Sources[a]	VA	DoD	Multiple Sources
Vietnam	78.2	78	16	1	5
OIF/OEF	90.5	42	9	39	10

SOURCE: Berke et al., 2010, p. 361.

[a] Under contract with VA.

veteran with a lower-limb loss either a prosthetic device or a wheelchair" (Smith and Reiber, 2010, p. ix). Moreover, combat amputees notwithstanding, the "majority of veterans with amputations receiving care in VA medical facilities have sustained their amputations because of medical conditions such as diabetes and peripheral vascular disease" and were very different from the new "young, highly trained group of individuals committed to an active lifestyle who are early in their developmental life cycle" (Sigford, 2010, p. xv). Following DoD's lead, VA did not begin planning changes to amputee care until 2006, and the changes were not fully functional until 2010.[16]

The survey results showed greater use of prosthetic devices for the younger OEF/OIF group than for the older and less healthy Vietnam groups.[17] Satisfaction varied between the two groups, depending on the type of amputation.[18] Overall satisfaction with prostheses was significantly higher in the OIF/OEF cohort than in the Vietnam war cohort—on a scale from 0 (low) to 10 (high), 7.5 and 7.0, respectively (Reiber et al., 2010, p. 285).[19] However, the rate at which amputees were not able to use their

---

[16] Sigford, 2010, p. xvi, reports that,

> [b]ased on the work and recommendations of a task force chartered in 2006, the full proposal for the new amputation system of care was finalized early in 2008. It received approval and funding to begin rollout in 2009. Funding has been provided to hire new staff, and regional amputation centers and polytrauma amputation network sites were expected to be fully functional by the end of 2009. The ACT [amputation care team] and APOC [amputation point of contact] components were expected to be fully functional by the end of 2010.

[17] Specifically, for unilateral lower-limb loss, the utilization rates were 94 percent for OEF/OIF and 89 percent for Vietnam; for unilateral upper-limb loss, the utilization rates were 76 percent and 70 percent, respectively; and for multiple limb loss, the utilization rates were 92 percent and 69 percent, respectively (Berke et al., 2010, p. 367).

[18] Individual studies of satisfaction with prosthetics include McFarland et al., 2010, for unilateral upper-limb loss; Gailey et al., 2010, for unilateral lower-limb loss; and Dougherty et al., 2010, for multiple traumatic limb loss.

[19] Berke et al., 2010, notes that

> [a] number of possible reasons exist for the higher overall satisfaction ratings in participants from the OIF/OEF conflict. At the outset is the structure of the initial care and rehabilitation process from the battlefield to

prosthetic devices—the rejection rate—was higher in the OIF/OEF group than in the Vietnam cohort, possibly because of the "availability of new types of prosthetic devices and the higher expectations of OIF/OEF" amputees.[20] Nevertheless, the study noted that a remarkably higher percentage "of OIF/OEF participants with major limb loss returned to Active Duty given the opportunities afforded by the DOD and the rehabilitation paradigm shift" (Reiber et al., 2010, p. 287).

The Extremity Trauma and Amputation Center of Excellence

Partly in response to events at Walter Reed in 2009, Congress mandated the establishment of the Extremity Trauma and Amputation Center of Excellence collaborative organization to enhance partnerships between DoD and VA, institutions of higher education, and other appropriate public and private entities. As directed by Congress, the center undertakes activities to

> implement a comprehensive plan and strategy for the Department of Defense and the Department of Veterans Affairs . . . . To conduct research to develop scientific information aimed at saving injured extremities, avoiding amputations, and preserving and restoring the function of injured extremities. Such research . . . [is to] address military medical needs and include the full range of scientific inquiry encompassing basic, translational, and clinical research. . . . To carry out . . . other activities to improve and enhance the efforts of the Department of Defense and the Department of Veterans Affairs for the mitigation, treatment, and rehabilitation of traumatic extremity injuries and amputations. (Pub. L. 110–417, 2008, Sec. 723)

Of particular note is the activities of the Clinical Care Division, which involve analyzing and disseminating

> standards of care and evidence based practices and provid[ing] policy guidance for the treatment, management, and rehabilitation of extremity injuries and amputa-

---

rehabilitation care at DOD facilities. Also, expansion to multidisciplinary care may affect overall rehabilitation and prosthetic satisfaction. Our survey included OIF/OEF participants who were at least 1 year from limb loss. The factors identified by study participants included their involvement in prosthetic selection, training, and maintenance. A number of advancements to prosthetic materials and components are available to OIF/OEF servicemembers/veterans that were not initially available following the Vietnam era. These may not have been uniformly offered to Vietnam veterans. Additionally, it appears that providing multiple prostheses with different components and allowing each servicemember to meet his or her rehabilitation potential further stimulates involvement in former and new physical activities. The participants' ages and being greater than 1 year from amputation to survey may affect study findings.

[20] Specifically, Reiber et al., 2010, p. 291, observed that

the annual rejection rate for those with unilateral upper-limb loss is 19.7-fold higher, for unilateral lower-limb loss is 15.0-fold higher, and for multiple limb loss is 19.9-fold higher. The availability of new types of prosthetic devices and the higher expectations of OIF/OEF servicemembers and veterans may explain the higher rejection rates.

tions to mitigate co-morbidities and maximize the functional return of patients. Determining best practices, particularly in the field of prosthetics, can bring about significant cost savings as well as enhance readiness by allowing service members to return to full duty. (Extremity Trauma and Amputation Center of Excellence, undated)[21]

Prosthetics

An article in *U.S. News and World Report*—"New Prosthetics Keep Amputee Soldiers on Active Duty" (Koebler, 2012)—attributed much of the success in the Army's program to advances in the tenacity of the soldier and advancements in prosthetics. In fact, the Army has led in the development and employment of new prosthetics ever since the Civil War. Historically, wars have often been catalysts for rapid innovation; since 9/11, that has included rapid innovations in prosthetics (see Figure 8.5).[22] Today, research sponsored by DoD's Defense Advanced Research Projects Agency (DARPA),[23] the VA, and the National Institutes of Health and advances by private companies worldwide in the fields of microprocessors, robotics, and artificial intelligence make state-of-the-art prosthetics available to military amputees.

Figure 8.6 shows an example of how these advances have been incorporated into new prosthetics widely used by OEF/OIF military amputees: the microprocessor knee, the C-Leg. The C-Leg is able to "sense the conditions acting on the knee joint and . . . quickly make internal adjustments. . . . Valves open or close electronically to increase or decrease fluid flow through the knee's internal ports . . . to vary resistance to knee flexion or extension" (Kapp and Miller, 2009, p. 560). Results of a clinical trial study with 17 amputees "show a statistically significant improvement in subjects' ability to

---

[21] For instance, Rehabilitation of Lower Limb Amputation Working Group, 2007; VA Employee Education System, 2008; and Management of Upper Extremity Amputation Rehabilitation Working Group, 2014, address the guidelines for upper and lower amputation and rehabilitation.

[22] Kevin Carroll, vice president of Hanger, a prosthetics company that has been in existence since 1861, makes this point:

> Unfortunately, when you have war, you have casualties, but with that comes innovation. Artificial joints are getting better at approximating the knee, elbow, wrist, and ankle, and microprocessors embedded in prostheses are able to pick up and adjust for impacts from walking, running, jumping, and climbing.
>
> The person doesn't have to worry about the prosthetic device; they're worrying about the task in front of them . . . . If they want to go back to be with their troops, that's an option for many soldiers these days. (as quoted in Koebler, 2012)

[23] In 2006, DARPA started the Revolutionizing Prosthetics program with the goal of expanding prosthetic arm options for military amputees. The fully neutrally integrated upper-extremity prosthesis it funded incorporates sensors for touch, temperature, vibration, and proprioception; enough power for extended use; and mechanical components that provide strength and environmental tolerance to heat, cold, water, humidity, dust, etc. With this new prosthetic, an upper-extremity amputee would be able to feel and manipulate objects just like a person with a native hand. In December 2016, Walter Reed took delivery on the first two advanced Life Under Kinetic Evolution (LUKE) arms. See Sanchez, undated; Johns Hopkins Applied Physics Laboratory, undated; and Defense Advanced Research Projects Agency, 2016.

Figure 8.5
Advances in Prosthetics from the Civil War to Today

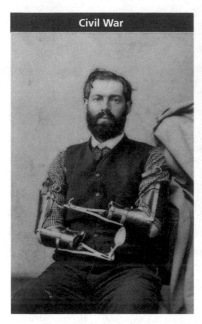

Civil War

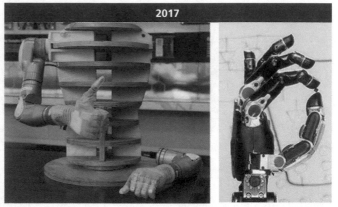

2017

DARPA's LUKE arm uses electrodes placed on the amputated limb to pick up electrical signals from the user's muscles. When the user tenses or flexes their arm, LUKE changes its position and grip. This is much more intuitive than basic prosthetics, which are generally controlled by switches or buttons or are adjusted manually by the wearer. The shoulder, elbow, and wrist are all individually powered, allowing the wearer to reach over their head and behind their back. Four independent motors in the hand offer the dexterity necessary to securely grip anything from a glass of water to a single egg. Force sensors in the fingers also give the wearer feedback on how hard they are gripping.

Samuel H. Decker devised his own prosthetics after amputation of both forearms following injuries when a gun exploded prematurely.

SOURCES: Historical photo (Civil War); DARPA, undated (black hand); DARPA, 2017 (wooden "chest").

descend stairs; time required to descend a slope; [and] sound-side step length while descending a hill" compared to a mechanical knee (Hafner et al., 2007, p. 216). While the C-Leg was traditionally given only to amputees that had proven their ability to walk, the Army Amputee Patient Care Program at Walter Reed was "the first facility in the world to utilized [sic] it as a rehabilitative knee unit" (Miller, 2004) by adjusting the microprocessor program as the patient progresses through rehabilitation.

The costs of advanced prosthetics are substantial; the C-Leg cost $58,000 in 2004; others cost as much as $87,000 (Scoville, 2004c).[24] Newer and more sophisticated prosthetics, such as LUKE, are estimated to cost at least $100,000 (Crotti, 2016).

More recent advances include the osseointegration of a transdermal prosthetic. Like a dental implant, a titanium implant is fused into the bone and left to heal:

---

[24] In 2007, Scoville, 2007b, reported that the average cost of prosthetic devices at Walter Reed was $115,000 per patient.

Figure 8.6
Microprocessor Knee

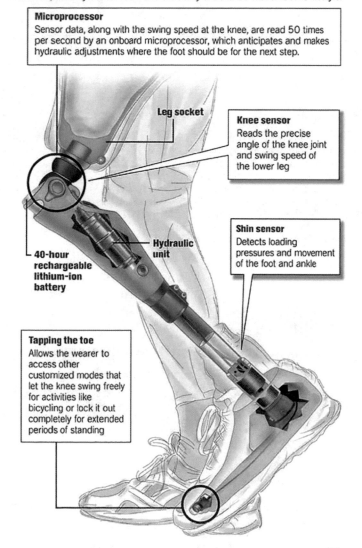

Getting out of the chair

The modern above-knee prosthesis, called the C-Leg, is a microprocessor-controlled marvel of metal and plastic. Introduced in the United States in 1999, this prosthesis is a vast improvement over earlier artificial legs, enhancing comfort, security and freedom and the ability to continue with an active lifestyle.

Microprocessor
Sensor data, along with the swing speed at the knee, are read 50 times per second by an onboard microprocessor, which anticipates and makes hydraulic adjustments where the foot should be for the next step.

Leg socket

Knee sensor
Reads the precise angle of the knee joint and swing speed of the lower leg

Shin sensor
Detects loading pressures and movement of the foot and ankle

40-hour rechargeable lithium-ion battery

Hydraulic unit

Tapping the toe
Allows the wearer to access other customized modes that let the knee swing freely for activities like bicycling or lock it out completely for extended periods of standing

SOURCE: Sisson Mobility Restoration Center, undated. Used with permission.

Three months later, that rod is pulled out through the soft tissues and skin and the prosthetic arm or leg latches directly to the implant, much like an artificial tooth is anchored into the jaw. . . .

By connecting the prosthesis to the bone, patients become more sensitive to surfaces, allowing them to touch and feel through their artificial limbs. (Gentzler, 2019)

Rehabilitation Facilities

Even as important and revolutionary as new prosthetics are, they are "one small but important aspect of the complex rehabilitation partnership between the veteran with limb loss" (Smith and Reiber, 2010, p. vii). The Army's program emphasizes holistic and comprehensive care, early rehabilitation, interdisciplinary teamwork, continual education, sports and recreational activities, and maintaining a therapeutic milieu in centers of excellence.[25] But this program could not fully accommodate the needs at the existing facilities at Walter Reed. Starting in 2003, plans were developed to provide additional capacity not only at Walter Reed but also at Brooke Army Medical Center in Texas and Naval Medical Center San Diego.

Brooke Army Medical Center and the Center for the Intrepid

In 2005, the Zachary and Elizabeth M. Fisher Armed Services Foundation/Intrepid Fallen Heroes Fund announced plans to raise $55 million for the construction of a world-class state-of-the-art physical rehabilitation facility at Brooke Army Medical Center in San Antonio, Texas, to be called the Center for the Intrepid (Intrepid Fallen Heroes Fund, undated; Scoville, 2005c). The Army Surgeon General agreed that Brooke, "as a Level 1 Trauma Center, Home of the ISR [Institute of Surgical Research] (Burn Center), and one of the two identified Military Amputee Patient Care Centers . . . [would be] an ideal location" (Scoville, 2005b) for such an advanced rehabilitation training facility for amputees. The Center for the Intrepid and a new Fisher House for military families were dedicated on January 29, 2007; the staff of 55 included active-duty Army medical staff, Department of the Army civilians, contract providers, and nine full-time VA employees (Hooper, 2007). In 2010, the Intrepid Fallen Heroes Fund constructed the National Intrepid Center of Excellence at Walter Reed, dedicated to research, diagnosis, and treatment of complex TBI and psychological health conditions of military personnel and veterans.

Comprehensive Combat and Complex Casualty Care Facility at Naval Medical Center San Diego.

While the facility at Walter Reed cared primarily for Army patients it also cared for Marines, Navy, Air Force, and DoD civilian amputees (Scoville, 2004b). During a

---

[25] Pasquina, 2010, summarizes the scope of the Army approach.

visit to Walter Reed, the Commandant of the Marine Corps asked why the Navy, which provided medical support for the Marine Corps, could not take care of the marines. Soon after, the Navy Surgeon General's Office began plans to establish a center for amputee care at the Naval Medical Center San Diego, permitting wounded marines the opportunity to receive the same level of care close to their home duty station (Cherry, 2005). The Navy's Comprehensive Combat and Complex Casualty Care facility at the Naval Medical Center San Diego, received its first patient in October 2006 and was fully operational by October 2007. This facility was designed to provide an aesthetic and medically advanced setting for prosthetic and rehabilitation services to military personnel stationed on the West Coast, particularly the Marines stationed in the San Diego area. It provides a "state of the art gait lab [that] includes a high resolution, accurate motion capture system to digitally acquire, analyze and display three-dimensional motion data [and] provide quantitative documentation of walking or running ability as well as identification of any underlying cause for gait deviations" (Navy Medical Center San Diego, undated).

Military Advanced Training Center at Walter Reed Army Medical Center

As noted earlier, it was clear by the end of 2003 that existing rehabilitation facilities at Walter Reed were inadequate. By November 2003, Walter Reed was caring for 48 soldiers with major limb loss, and more were coming.[26] A plan for short-term amputee patient care space requirements was initiated to alleviate the overcrowding, e.g., a temporary pod was leased and installed on the tennis court to house routine physical therapy care, but what was needed was a new, free-standing clinic extension.[27] In November 2003, Congress asked for "an infrastructure improvement plan for the United States Army Amputee Patient Care Program . . . based at Walter Reed Army Medical Center in Washington, D.C." (Office of the Surgeon General, Department of the Army, 2004, p. 1-1). On January 20, 2004, a report on the Infrastructure Improvement for the U.S. Army Amputee Patient Care Program was submitted to Congress (Office of the Surgeon General, Department of the Army, 2004). The report called for construction of the Military Amputee Training Center at Walter Reed.

The new center was projected to cost $10.9 million. The project was approved by Congress, and ground was broken for the new facility on November 19, 2004. Con-

---

[26] Scoville, 2003a, noted that, as of November 2003, "US Army facilities have cared for a total of 137 individuals who have sustained an amputation since Jan 2001[;] 80 involved one or more major limbs. Seventy-seven of these patients have been treated at WRAMC, including fifty-eight of the individuals with major limb amputation." As a point of comparison, by March 20, 2007,

> 570 service members [had] lost one or more major limbs as a direct result of Operation Iraqi Freedom and Operation Enduring Freedom (415 Army, 133 Marines, 15 Navy and 7 Air Force). Of these, approximately 80% sustained a single major limb amputation while 20% (113) have lost multiple limbs. Loss of an upper extremity occurred in 23% of the patients (132). Walter Reed has provided care for 438 and Brooke Army Medical Center 138 patients with limb loss. (Scoville, 2007b)

[27] Scoville, 2003g, reviewed the short-term options and alternatives.

struction was delayed, however, in part because the 2005 Defense Base Closure and Realignment Commission planned to close the Army facility. Eventually, the center was completed, in 2007, as a transitional medical facility, and in 2011, a new facility was opened at the joint Walter Reed National Military Medical Center in Bethesda (Scoville, 2005d; Scoville, 2006b; Scoville, 2006c; Scoville, 2007c).

Computer Assisted Rehabilitation Environment

The current facility—the Military Advanced Training Center—provides state-of-the-art care not only to combat amputees but also to "Wounded, Ill and Injured Service Members, Retirees and Family Members" using "sophisticated prosthetics and cutting-edge athletic equipment to confirm pre-injury capabilities as they restore their sense of selves" (WRAMC, undated). One prominent feature of the center is the Computer Assisted Rehab Environment, a treadmill gait-training system made up of an instrumented treadmill on a base platform with 6-degree-of-freedom motion and a large panoramic dome screen, on which a variety of scenes are projected (see Figure 8.7). (These systems have also installed at National Intrepid Center of Excellence, Center

Figure 8.7
Computer Assisted Rehabilitation Environment

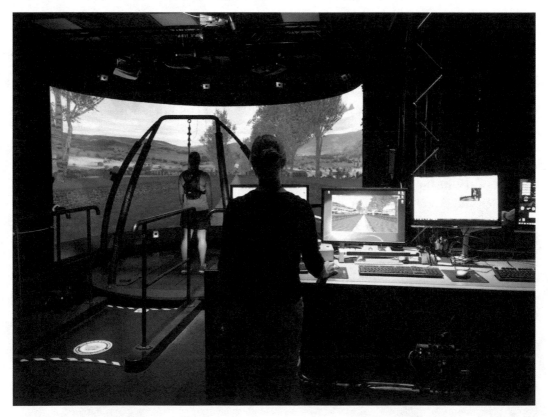

SOURCE: U.S. Navy photo/Regena Kowitz.

for the Intrepid for TBI, and the Naval Health Research Center in San Diego.) The system allows the operator to generate visual and physical perturbations that require the user to make dynamic responses to gait patterns as he or she walks through the scenes, which are synchronized with the movements of the platform and patient. A three-dimensional motion capture system collects data on movement as the patient moves on the platform. The system costs in excess of $1 million.

Ancillary Facilities

Conspicuously absent in the Army's request for additional facilities was any mention of the need for ancillary facilities to house and care for the patients during long stays at Walter Reed. The need should have been clear. In the early days of the program, in 2002, patients averaged 51 days before being transferred to the VA or home base. By early 2007, the program had not only grown in absolute numbers of patients being cared for concurrently, but patients spent "an average of 21 days as an in-patient and then have an average out-patient stay of 311 days" (Scoville, 2007b). Moreover, amputees were not the only outpatients Walter Reed was caring for, and housing was an issue. At the peak in 2005, nearly 900 outpatients were being housed in everything from old barracks to nearby hotels and apartments leased by the Army. Outpatients outnumbered inpatients 17 to 1 (Priest and Hull, 2007).

The medical program was intended to implement the concepts of "holistic/comprehensive care" and the "maintenance of a therapeutic milieu" (Pasquina, 2010). Physical and occupational therapy typically took place during two one-and-one-half–hour sessions daily. So, how did patients fare when they were not directly undergoing rehabilitation? The answer to that question came in the form of a headline of a *Washington Post* Pulitzer Prize–winning article from February 18, 2007: "Soldiers Face Neglect, Frustration at Army's Top Medical Facility" (Priest and Hull, 2007). The article documented living conditions at Walter Reed for those receiving outpatient care. As it turned out, this was not a new problem.[28] In fact, it was a Civil War lesson that had apparently not been learned (see Rostker, 2013, pp. 85–86). It was also not a problem unique to Walter Reed; a similar situation had been reported at Fort Stewart in 2003 (see Benjamin, 2003). The problem was pervasive and would result in a number of senior officials being fired,[29] the chartering of a cabinet-level task force on

---

[28] In September 2006, the Walter Reed garrison commander, Col. Peter Garibaldi, warned General Weightman, the medical center commander that "patient care services are at risk of mission failure" because of staff shortages brought on by the privatization of the hospital's support workforce (as reported in Abramowitz and Vogel, 2007).

[29] On March 1, 2007, MG George Weightman, WRAMC commander, was told that "the senior Army leadership had lost trust and confidence in the commander's leadership abilities to address needed solutions for soldier-outpatient care at Walter Reed Army Medical Center" (Vogel and Branigin, 2007). Secretary of the Army Francis Harvey appointed LTG Kevin Kiley, the Army Surgeon General, to temporary command of Walter Reed. Some immediately challenged his appointment because he had been "the facility's commander and . . . advocates have complained that he had long been aware of problems at Walter Reed and did nothing to improve its outpatient care" (Vogel and Branigin, 2007). Secretary of Defense Gates was "displeased" that Harvey had appointed Kiley

returning soldiers (Task Force on Returning Global War on Terror Heroes, 2007), an independent review for the Secretary of Defense (West et al., 2007), and a Presidential commission of inquiry (Dole-Shalala Commission, 2007a).

On March 30, 2007, President Bush made his 12th visit to Walter Reed (see Baker, 2007). On no previous visit had he visited the notorious Building 18, the barracks where outpatients were housed. He did not visit it on this trip because it had been closed. In remarks to the hospital staff he said,

> the problems recently uncovered at Walter Reed were not the problems of medical care. The Quality of care at this fantastic facility is great. And it needs to remain that way. . . . The problems at Walter Reed were caused by bureaucratic and administrative failures. The system failed you, and it failed our troops. And we're going to fix it. (Bush, 2007)

Medical Centers of Excellence

By 2007, "Congress realized that the Department of Defense had to do a better job preventing, diagnosing, mitigating, treating, and rehabilitating these injuries" (Davis, 2010, p. 23). Starting with the FY 2008 NDAA (Pub. L. 110-181, 2008), Congress mandated the establishment of a number of medical defense centers of excellence to coordinate, inspect, and oversee medical care in a number of specific areas, originally brain injuries, mental health problems, vision and hearing, and extremity injuries and amputations. The three pillars common to the centers are (1) identifying and proliferating best practices, (2) prioritizing the medical research agenda, and (3) enhancing patient-centered care. In November 2007, a number of centers were established to focus on psychological health and TBI, including the Defense and Veterans Brain Injury Center (DVBIC), the Deployment Health Clinical Center, and the National Center for Telehealth and Technology. In 2008 and 2009, the Hearing Center of Excellence was established under the leadership of the Air Force, the Vision Center of Excellence under the Navy, and the Traumatic Extremity Injuries and Amputations Center of Excellence under the Army. The centers are responsible for identifying strategies for preventing and mitigating injuries, directing research, and finding and communicating evidence-based best practices. In 2017, it was announced that the Defense Centers of Excellence would be merged into the Defense Health Agency and largely become part of Defense Health Agency J-9, the Research and Development Directorate (Defense Centers of Excellence for Psychological Health and Traumatic Brain Injury, 2017).

---

and immediately asked for Harvey's resignation, which he tendered. "Harvey said he offered Gates his resignation because he believed the Army let the wounded soldiers down. He said the furor has depressed the staff at Walter Reed, and he wanted to prevent any others from leaving or being fired" (Wolf, 2007).

Traumatic Brain Injuries

Since 2001, most casualties in Afghanistan and Iraq have been caused by explosive devices, predominantly IEDs. While IED attacks often result in the loss of a limb, a more frequent result is a traumatic injury to the brain. The blast creates

> a sudden increase in air pressure by heating and accelerating air molecules and, immediately thereafter, a sudden decrease in pressure that produces intense wind. These rapid pressure shifts can injure the brain directly, producing concussion or contusion. Air emboli can also form in blood vessels and travel to the brain, causing cerebral infarcts. In addition, blast waves and wind can propel fragments, bodies, or even vehicles with considerable force, causing head injuries by any of these mechanisms. Approximately 8 to 25 percent of persons with blast-related injuries die. (Okie, 2005, p. 2045)[30]

In some cases, shrapnel fragments from the blast penetrate the skull, with the primary brain injury resulting from

> the projectile passing through the brain, damaging neural, vascular, and support structures along its track. In addition to this damage, high-velocity supersonic projectiles can create a vacuum in their trail, giving rise to tissue cavitation. The rapid expansion and retraction of the vacuum cavity compresses and stretches neural and support structures, often tearing them. As the cavity may be many times larger than the projectile's track, injury is much more severe.
>
> The majority of military penetrating TBI occurs from penetrating fragment injuries and not from fired bullets. (Marshall et al., 2012, p. 361)

Symptoms of a mild TBI (mTBI) may not appear until days or weeks following the injury. These symptoms can be mild—such as headaches or neck pain, nausea, ringing in the ears, dizziness, and tiredness—or more severe—such as convulsions or seizures, slurred speech and weakness or numbness in the arms and legs. Those with penetrating and severe TBI may require hospitalization and rehabilitation to gain even partial recovery of cognitive, speech, and motor dexterity. The Army classifies TBI as severe or penetrating, moderate, or mild, as defined by the measures shown in Table 8.3.

---

[30] Burgess et al., 2010, provides a a more complete discussion of the basic mechanism of explosive injuries.

Table 8.3
DoD/VA Severity Stratification for Nonpenetrating TBI

Class of TBI	Imaging	Loss of Consciousness	Alteration of Consciousness or Mental State	Posttraumatic Amnesia	Glasgow Coma score
Mild	Normal	0–30 min	A moment up to 24 hours	0–1 day	13–15 points
Moderate	Normal or abnormal	>30 min and <24 hours	>24 hours; severity based on other criteria	>1 and <7 days	9–12 points
Severe	Normal or abnormal	>24 hours	>24 hours; severity based on other criteria	>7 days	3–8 points (coma)

SOURCE: Office of the Assistant Secretary of Defense for Health Affairs, 2007; Centers for Disease Control and Prevention et al., 2013, p. 18.

Prevalence of TBI

TBIs have gained a reputation as the signature wounds of the current conflicts.[31] However, only "severe and penetrating TBIs are recognized and triaged at the time of injury" (Centers for Disease Control and Prevention et al., 2013, p. 20). Those so injured

> receive immediate care on the battlefield and are then transported to military combat support hospitals, where they undergo brain imaging and are treated by neurosurgeons. Treatment may include the removal of foreign bodies, control of bleeding, or craniectomy to relieve pressure from swelling. Depending on their condition, these soldiers are eventually transferred to one of the DVBIC's eight participating U.S. hospitals for assessment and treatment. (Okie, 2005, p. 2045)

The vast majority of TBI cases are mild (mTBI), are closed-brain injuries, and are not diagnosed promptly; "mild TBI may go unnoticed if the individual walks away seemingly unharmed" (Bagalman, 2015, p. 7). These are not likely to be recorded as combat wounds (WIA). A survey of troops in 2012 and 2013 by the Mental Health Advisory Teams (MHATs) dispatched to Afghanistan and Iraq showed how often soldiers are

---

[31] As the IOM noted:

> TBI has been called the signature injury of OEF and OIF primarily due to blast exposure that is characteristic of this conflict. Exposure to blast might cause instant death, injuries with immediate manifestation of symptoms, or injuries with delayed manifestation. . . .

> That many returning veterans have TBI will likely mean long-term challenges for them and their family members. Veterans will need support systems at home and in their communities to assist them in coping with the long-term sequelae of their injuries. Further, many veterans will have undiagnosed brain injury because not all TBIs have immediately recognized effects or are easily diagnosed with neuroimaging techniques. (Committee on Gulf War and Health, 2009, p. xiii)

exposed to blast related events, the severity of the event, and the likelihood that the soldier would be evaluated by a medic or corpsman (see Table 8.4).[32]

There are three salient points about TBIs: First, most TBIs are classified as mild. Second, only a fraction of TBIs are recorded in military records, with many more being identified after the soldier leaves service through VA screening.[33] Third, TBIs are so prevalent in the general population that, even during periods of heightened troop deployments to Afghanistan and Iraq, the majority of TBI cases reported were among those troops not deployed (see Farmer et al., 2016, p. 1, and Chapman and Diaz-Arrasti, 2014). Figure 8.8 compares the numbers of mild, severe, and penetrating TBIs for the entire Army; note that severe and penetrating averaged only 2.7 percent of all TBIs.

Figure 8.9 shows the number of TBIs associated with a deployment. (It should be noted that, in some years, the number of deployment-associated TBIs actually exceeds

Table 8.4
Reports of Exposure to Blast-Related Events and of Being Evaluated by a Medic or Corpsman

Blast-Related Event During Deployment	2010 Exposed (%)	2010 Evaluated (%)	2011 Exposed (%)	2011 Evaluated (%)
Within 50 m of blast while dismounted	42.8	20.2	35.9	29.2
Physically moved or knocked over by explosion	20.2	40.0	15.6	55.7
Injury involving being dazed, confused, or "seeing stars"	9.2	62.5	10.6	63.4
Inside vehicle damaged in a blast	11.2	60.7	8.2	73.4
Knocked out (lost consciousness)	4.3	73.9	5.7	75.0
Injury involving losing consciousness	3.5	77.8	3.6	92.9

SOURCE: Office of the Surgeon General, U.S. Army Medical Command, 2013, p. 24.

---

[32] In 2012, DoD policy was changed to require that the unit's medic conduct a medical evaluation for TBI as soon as possible after a blast exposure occurs, unless the soldier has more serious injuries requiring immediate medical evacuation (DoD Instruction 6490.11, 2012; Office of the Surgeon General, U.S. Army Medical Command, 2013, p. 24).

[33] The Congressional Research Service reported to Congress:

As of September 2010, a total of 420,374 OEF/OIF veterans had been screened for TBI. Of those who were screened, 102,569 either reported a prior diagnosis of TBI or screened positive for possible TBI. A follow-up evaluation (which was not required for those who reported a prior diagnosis of TBI) was completed for 57,995 of those who screened positive for possible TBI, and a TBI diagnosis was confirmed in 18,280 of them. Note that the 18,280 represents only those OEF/OIF veterans with a TBI diagnosis confirmed by the VA's follow-up evaluation. It does not include OEF/OIF veterans who reported a prior diagnosis of TBI at the screening, nor does it include OEF/OIF veterans who do not receive VA health care. (Bagalman, 2011, p. 8)

**Figure 8.8
Traumatic Brain Injury, by Severity Stratification, CYs 2001–2016**

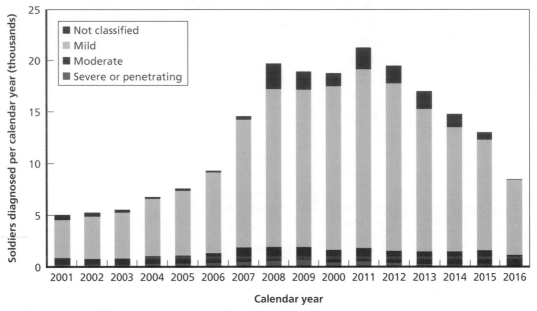

SOURCE: Carino, 2017a.

**Figure 8.9
Traumatic Brain Injury, by Deployment Status, CYs 2001–2016**

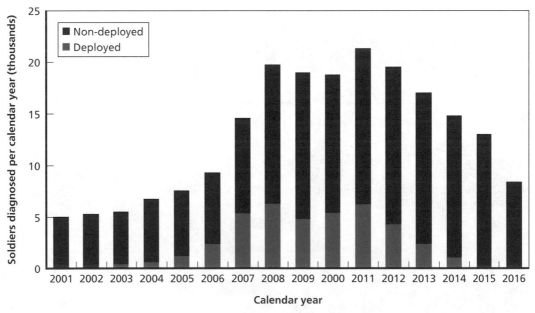

SOURCE: Carino, 2017b.

the reported number WIA, which means that many cases of TBI are not initially recorded.) However, 59 percent of the soldiers receiving medical care at WRAMC from January 2003 through February 2005 who had been exposed to blasts were found to have TBI; of those, 44 percent were classified as having mild TBI. One study noted that,

> [i]n many people who sustain mild TBI, the effects might not be immediately evident and might not be evident with conventional neuroimaging. That clearly presents a problem for VA with regard to preparation for the return of veterans from OEF and OIF with TBI that might not be apparent. (Committee on Gulf War and Health, 2009, p. 3)

Consequences of TBI

As one might have expected, the Committee on Gulf War and Health: Brain Injury in Veterans and Long-Term Health Outcomes found that, "the more severe the TBI, the more severe the outcome" (Committee on Gulf War and Health, 2009, p. 5).[34] Box 8.1 quotes the committee's findings.

In 2008, the Army reported that, of 2,525 infantry soldiers surveyed three to four months after returning from a year-long deployment to Iraq,

> 124 (4.9%) reported injuries with loss of consciousness, 260 (10.3%) reported injuries with altered mental status, and 435 (17.2%) reported other injuries during deployment. Of those reporting loss of consciousness, 43.9% met criteria for post-traumatic stress disorder . . . , as compared with 27.3% of those reporting altered mental status, 16.2% with other injuries, and 9.1% with no injury. (Hoge, McGurk, et al., 2008, p. 453)

The conclusion was that mTBI was "strongly associated with PTSD and physical health problems 3 to 4 months after the soldiers return home" (Hoge, McGurk, et al., 2008, p. 453).

In 2018, a large-cohort study of all 179,000 patients diagnosed with a TBI in the VHA health care system from October 1, 2001, to September 30, 2014, and a similar size propensity-matched comparison group found that "even mild TBI without loss of consciousness was associated with more than a 2-fold increase in the risk of dementia diagnosis" (Barnes et al., 2018).

Treatment of TBI

Treatment for TBI depends on its severity, the interval from injury to presentation, and the physical location where the injury occurs. Severe and penetrating TBIs are recognized and treated at the time of injury, often in ICUs and neurosurgical units

---

[34] See also Boyle et al., 2014.

Box 8.1
Findings of the Committee on Gulf War Health

Sufficient Evidence of an Association
- Penetrating TBI and decline in neurocognitive function associated with the region of the brain affected and the volume of brain tissue lost.
- Penetrating TBI and long-term unemployment.
- Severe TBI and neurocognitive deficits.
- Moderate or severe TBI and dementia of the Alzheimer type.
- Moderate or severe TBI and parkinsonism.
- Moderate or severe TBI and endocrine dysfunction, particularly hypopituitarism.
- Moderate or severe TBI and growth hormone insufficiency.
- Moderate to severe TBI and long-term adverse social-function outcomes, particularly unemployment and diminished social relationships.
- Moderate or severe TBI, in the subset of patients who are either admitted into or discharged from rehabilitation centers or receive disability support, and premature death.
- TBI and depression.
- TBI and aggressive behaviors.
- TBI and post concussion symptoms (such as memory problems, dizziness, and irritability).

Limited/Suggestive Evidence of an Association
- Moderate or severe TBI and psychosis.
- Moderate TBI and neurocognitive deficits.
- Mild TBI resulting in loss of consciousness or amnesia and unprovoked seizures.
- Mild TBI and ocular and visual motor deterioration.
- Mild TBI with loss of consciousness and dementia of the Alzheimer type.
- Mild TBI with loss of consciousness and parkinsonism.
- Mild TBI and posttraumatic stress disorder in Gulf War military populations.
- TBI and decreased alcohol and drug use in the 1–3 years after injury.
- TBI and completed suicide.

Inadequate/Insufficient Evidence to Determine Whether an Association Exists
- Moderate or severe TBI and brain tumor.
- Mild, moderate, or severe TBI that is survived for 6 months or more and premature death.
- Mild TBI and neurocognitive deficits.
- Mild TBI (without loss of consciousness) and dementia of the Alzheimer type.
- Mild TBI and posttraumatic stress disorder in civilian populations.
- Mild TBI and long-term adverse social functioning, including unemployment, diminished social relationships, and decrease in the ability to live independently.
- TBI and mania or bipolar disorder.
- TBI and attempted suicide.
- TBI and multiple sclerosis.
- TBI and amyotrophic lateral sclerosis.

SOURCE: Quoted from Committee on Gulf War and Health, 2009, pp. 10–12.

(Centers for Disease Control and Prevention et al., 2013, p. 20),[35] with long-term outcomes varying from full recovery to complete dependence on care providers. The vast majority of TBIs, however, are categorized as mild and are usually treated and released from emergency departments, where they are generally told to seek further medical

---

[35] Typical observable symptoms of moderate and severe TBI "include persistent headache, vomiting or nausea, convulsions or seizures, coma or vegetative state, dilation of one or both pupils, dysfunctional speech, weakness or numbness in the extremities, loss of coordination, and increased confusion, restlessness, or agitation" (Farmer et al., 2016, p. 2).

care if symptoms persist or worsen; "85–90 percent with mild TBI recover within three months" (Farmer et al., 2016, p. xii).

DoD policy (DoD Instruction 6490.11, 2012) requires that all soldiers "exposed to a potentially concussive event be screened for TBI using the Military Acute Concussion Evaluation . . . , and be required to rest for 24 hours regardless of results" (DVA and DoD, 2016, p. 23). To assist in the management of TBI, the Brain Trauma Foundation, in collaboration with the DVBIC, the Henry M. Jackson Foundation for the Advancement of Military Medicine, and USUHS, published the *Guidelines for the Field Management of Combat-Related Head Trauma* (Knuth et al., 2005). These guidelines included a decision tree to assist front-line providers with triage decisionmaking (Knuth et al., 2005, p. 95). In 2008 (and updated in 2016), DoD and the VA published *VA/DoD Clinical Practice Guideline for the Management of Concussion–Mild Traumatic Brain Injury*, "to provide . . . healthcare providers with a framework by which to evaluate, treat, and manage the individual needs and preferences of patients with a history of mild traumatic brain injury" (DVA and DoD, 2016, p. 5).

The evidence the Management of Concussion–Mild Traumatic Brain Injury Working Group reviewed as it created the guidelines suggested that

> the majority of individuals who sustain a single concussion recover within hours to days without residual deficits. Post-concussion symptoms are nonspecific (e.g., headache, nausea, dizziness, fatigue, irritability, concentration problems), which makes it very difficult to definitively attribute symptoms to the concussive injury, particularly as the time since the event lengthens. In addition, there is little evidence to suggest that treatment interventions should be different when symptoms are attributed to concussion versus a different etiology. Consequently, symptom-focused evaluation and treatment is recommended, particularly when the time since injury is greater than 30 days.
>
> The vast majority of patients who develop symptoms after concussion will do so immediately. In some cases, analogous to the acute trauma setting where initial events (e.g., life-threatening injury) may take precedence over other injuries (e.g., ankle sprain), patients may not notice some symptoms until later. However, with patients that are initially asymptomatic and develop new symptoms 30 days or more following concussion, these symptoms are unlikely to be the result of the concussion and the work-up and management should not focus on the initial concussion. (DVA and DoD, 2016, p. 26)

The working group also noted that "depression, anxiety and irritability are common co-occurring behavioral symptoms of mTBI" (DVA and DoD, 2016, p. 27) and should be treated in accordance with treatment and management recommendations for major depressive disorder, PTSD, substance use disorders, and patients at risk for suicide. They warned against attributing these conditions to TBI because this might bias providers who could miss important chronic or acute symptoms that may be more accurately associated with other conditions.

. . . Rather than reinforce mTBI as the "cause" of the patient's problems, the primary care provider should use an approach to care that is consistent with the treatment of chronic, multisymptom conditions. (DVA and DoD, 2016, p. 28)

Until recently, there has been little empirical evidence of service members receiving care for an mTBI diagnosis because of the difficulty of consistently identifying mTBI patients and the wide variety of treatments received. Accordingly, "DVBIC asked RAND to assess care provided to service members with an mTBI diagnosis," and RAND responded with "the first comprehensive analysis of the care delivered by the MHS to nondeployed active-duty service members who have experienced an mTBI" (Farmer et al., 2016, p. 3). RAND reported that the most prevalent treatments in the six months following an mTBI diagnosis were for behavioral health conditions, with adjustment disorders, anxiety disorders, depression, alcohol abuse or dependence, and PTSD the most common. Recovery was generally quick; in the cohort assessed, "(80–90 percent) received care for three months or less following their initial mTBI diagnosis, with most (75–80 percent) receiving care for four weeks or less" (Farmer et al., 2016, p. xvii).

Psychological Casualties and PTSD

In 2001, the U.S. Army went to war with a mental health model whose roots were firmly planted by Dr. Thomas Salmon during World War I. The focus of military psychiatry was maintaining the immediate combat capability of the unit, with the basic principles for battle fatigue captured in the PIES mnemonic.[36] The basic message was "You are neither sick nor a coward. You are just tired and will recover when rested" (Jones et al., 1995, p. 9). The lessons from Vietnam presented in *Military Psychiatry* (Jones et al., 1994) and *War Psychiatry* (Jones et al., 1995) were that PTSD was infrequent and could be accommodated through appropriate measures of combat and operational stress control (COSC), as the following excerpts from *War Psychiatry* suggest:

[Patients with] major depression and persistent schizophrenic-type psychotic disorders, who have a poor chance for rapid return to duty should be evacuated as soon as they can be stabilized and reliably distinguished from battle fatigue. Posttraumatic stress disorder (PTSD) should be prevented by routine unit (team)

---

[36] The claim that PIES reduced combat casualties was challenged; it was later claimed that "reported outcomes tended to exaggerate its effectiveness both as a treatment for acute stress reaction and as a prophylaxis for chronic disorders such as PTSD. It remains uncertain who is being served by the intervention: whether it is the individual soldier or the needs of the military" (Jones and Wessely, 2003, p. 411).

debriefings. The debriefings should be accomplished as soon after trauma as is tactically feasible, and again during homecoming. Deployed service members can tolerate high stress best when they know that the unit, the service, and the government are assuring that their families are well cared for and informed. (Jones et al., 1995, p. 246)[37]

[Most models] to reduce the incidence of PTSD and other acute psychiatric reactions . . . rely on the assumption that unit cohesion, training, and leadership are important in helping soldiers adapt to traumatic or adverse conditions. . . . Significant differences in the units highlight the role of trust toward the immediate commanders, unit identity, and professional soldiering knowledge. Moreover, the community support and effective integration of soldiers returning from battle into their units or homes appears to have the greatest influence on the development of long-term psychiatric sequelae. (Jones et al., 1995, p. 273)

A simple explanation of the facts concerning the prevention of PTSD and the helpfulness in maintaining unit cohesion in the face of trauma is usually all that is necessary. (Jones et al., 1995, p. 281)

[When] a group is allowed to ventilate fears, frustrations, and feelings about the event, and its individuals receive the support of their comrades, the likelihood of PTSD is decreased. (Jones et al., 1995, p. 289)

By 2011, when the next comprehensive review of combat psychiatry was published, the Army's view of PTSD had matured, as the Army Surgeon General noted in the foreword to *Combat and Operational Behavioral Health*:

One may think the diagnosis of posttraumatic stress disorder (PTSD) would be straightforward. On the contrary, it varies widely among different stakeholders. The more complex issues of the etiology of PTSD and traumatic brain injury, and effective treatments for these conditions, as well as their interaction with age, gender, and other medical issues, are far more daunting. (Ritchie, 2011, p. xxi)

In-Theater Psychiatric Support

After World War II, the psychiatric support for combat troops was provided by the division mental health activity, generally staffed by a psychiatrist, a psychologist, a social worker, and six mental health technicians, often augmented by a variety of combat

---

[37] The 2004 version of *VA/DoD Clinical Practice Guideline for the Management of Post-Traumatic Stress* noted:

The use of debriefings soon after exposure to traumatic events became part of military doctrine in the United States and elsewhere, as well as part of standards for early response to catastrophe for organizations, such as the Red Cross. (Management of Post-Traumatic Stress Working Group, 2004, p. 104)

Unfortunately, the technique appears to be of little help and may be harmful as prophylaxis for PTSD.

stress control (CSC) units.[38] As in so many other ways, operations after 9/11 were different from the doctrinal norm, which envisioned a linear battlefield with five echelons of care reflecting predictable positions relative to the forward line of troops. In Afghanistan and then Iraq, the battlefield was nonlinear; troops and the behavioral health resources that supported them were often scattered and residing in rustic installations called *firebases* or *forward operating bases* or rotating out from them. As the campaigns progressed and as the Army shifted from emphasizing the division to emphasizing the new, modular BCT, the provision of behavioral health care also changed. A brigade behavioral health officer (psychologist or social worker) and an enlisted mental health specialist were assigned to each BCT. This resulted in there being more providers and allowed for "projection of resources to commanders at lower levels (i.e., battalion and company)" (Warner, Appenzeller, et al., 2011, p. 90).

An assessment of the new system in 2007 found several advantages, including an increased ability to provide mental health services closer to the front line and the ability to interact with and regularly serve as consultants to lower levels of command (Warner, Appenzeller, et al., 2007; Warner, Breitbach, et al., 2007a; Warner, Breitbach, et al., 2007b). However, there were many problems, "including dispersed command and control, increased independence of each provider with decreased supervision, and an increased risk for provider burnout due to the smaller teams" (Warner, Appenzeller, et al., 2011, p. 92). Ideally, the senior psychiatrist assigned should be a field grade officer, with at least one tour after residency to gain experience as a practicing psychiatrist, and should be a graduate of the Captain's Career Course. However, this was seldom achieved in practice.[39]

---

[38] Warner, Appenzeller, et al., 2011, p. 92, notes that, as "Army mental healthcare evolved into the 1980s, it moved away from the roles of the divisional units and focused on the development of nonembedded combat stress control units."

[39] As noted in *Combat and Operational Behavioral Health*:

> The division psychiatrist position tends to be assigned to junior officers following completion of their psychiatric residency or fellowship. Many enter the position as a company-grade officer (captain) and are promoted to field grade (major) while in the position. For many incoming division psychiatrists, this is their first opportunity to practice independently. Furthermore, few of the incoming division psychiatrists are familiar with the operation and function of a division staff and most have not attended their branch-specific career course.

> Like the psychiatrist, the BCT BHO [behavioral health officer] position tends to be assigned to a junior to mid-level officer. Many enter the position as a company-grade officer and some will be promoted to field grade while in the position. In the past, the psychologists would likely have just completed their internship training and have not done any other operational tour. However, that has changed recently with requirements for licensure for deployability. Currently, most psychologists have completed a 1- or 2-year postinternship tour prior to arriving to the BCT. For social workers, most have completed one tour, generally at a medical center working with a senior social work officer, and then are assigned to an operational billet. For many incoming BCT BHOs, this is their first opportunity to practice without a senior supervisor in their discipline. Like psychiatrists, few of the incoming BCT BHOs are familiar with the operation and function of a brigade staff, and most have not attended their branch-specific career course. (Warner, Appenzeller, et al., 2011, p. 93)

Combat Stress Support Units

Besides the behavioral health personnel "organic" to the division and brigade, CSC units—companies and detachments—provided additional capabilities, including the following (see FM 4-02.51 [FM 8-51], 2006, pp. 2.1–2.9):

- *CSC companies* made up of six CSC preventive teams and four combat stress fitness (restoration) teams could be assigned to support a forward corps area or further to the rear. They supported the corps units behind two or three divisions, but the teams could be sent far forward to augment the division rear and even brigades in combat, as the CSC detachments do.
- *CSC detachments* supported one division or two to three separate brigades or regiments. They consisted of three four-person CSC preventive teams that move forward to brigade support areas when requested, and one 11-person combat stress fitness (restoration) team that could run a "combat fitness center" in the division support area or the corps forward area. The fitness team also provides preventive services to units in their vicinity and could go further forward. Detachments could be further broken down into preventive and fitness sections.
- *CSC teams* were small mobile teams sent out from CSC detachments or companies. They were tailored mixes of the five mental health disciplines, which might include psychiatric nursing and occupational therapy. The teams often had their own vehicles so that they could move forward to augment the tactical units or to support combat service support units over a wide area.

During the initial deployment to Afghanistan in late 2001, a pair of mental health technicians supported Kandahar, and a team of four (social worker, occupational therapist, and two technicians) were in Uzbekistan before relocating to Bagram Airfield in early 2002. A psychiatrist and social worker in Kuwait provided consultative services. These teams were small, but "[e]ffective screening and prevention programs, access to care in theater, and an underlying expectation of recovery [have] led to a return-to-duty rate in excess of 98 percent in recent years (Bacon, Barry, and Demer, 2011, pp. 771–772).

With the invasion of Iraq in 2003, the Army deployed five fitness teams and 14 prevention teams, but this deployment was less than what was doctrinally required, and the teams were manned at less than authorized strength. Generally, a fitness team was made up of three officers and seven enlisted personnel and cared for approximately 25 ambulatory patients. The combat fitness centers they set up were generally close to the CSH;[40] in essence, the CSC fitness center became the behavioral health clinic within the CSH. Initially, in 2003, the average daily census was between two and five patients, with a surge reaching nine to 12 patients. (Operation Iraqi Freedom Mental

---

[40] Forsten et al., 2011, pp. 754–759, offers a more complete discussion of the operations of the CSHs.

Health Advisory Team, 2003, pp. B-61 through B-63). It was CSH policy to evacuate any soldier admitted for more than seven days (Forsten et al., 2011, p. 757).

Psychotropic Medications

An increasingly important but often controversial issue in providing medical support to deployed combat soldiers, especially after Vietnam, was the use of psychotropic medications. In 2011, the Army noted:

> Until the mid-1990s, psychotropic medication use for the treatment of ongoing mental disorders during combat operations was uncommon. Stimulants and other psychotropic medications were used, at times, to enhance the vigilance and performance of fatigued service members. However, in the mid-1990s the introduction of medications with more favorable side-effect profiles—particularly the selective serotonin reuptake inhibitors (SSRIs)—revolutionized the role of medications in the practice of military operational psychiatry. The widespread incorporation of these medications into civilian and military garrison psychiatric practice has resulted in an evolution in operational practice such that medication use in combat operations now focuses on the capacity for soldiers with symptoms of psychiatric illness to return to their premorbid level of functioning, rather than on efforts to "enhance" baseline performance. (Schneider et al., 2011, p. 152)

The Army doctrine on the use of psychotropic medication evolved over past 20 years. Initially, it focused on triage and nonpharmacological interventions aimed at normalizing and minimizing combat stress. Little guidance was provided on the role and use of psychotropic medications. This changed in 2004, as the Army evaluated its experience during the initial year of OIF, leading to a revision in policy, formally published in 2006, that reflected "the gradual move towards acceptance of psychotropic medication usage in a combat zone" (Schneider et al., 2011, p. 154). That said, the Army provides little formal guidance except for the acute care of agitated patients.[41] The policy adhered to the PIES principles, providing patients with restorative care through a division mental health section or CSC detachment and, if warranted, movement to a CSH for stabilization, treatment, and determination for evacuation. In practice, the decisions regarding the treatment of other disorders, particularly bipolar II disorder and PTSD, depended on which medications were available, how significant the symptoms were, and how the patient initially responded to treatment. The decision of whether to treat attention-deficit hyperactivity disorder depended on whether the condition was previously diagnosed and how significantly the symptoms were interfering with assigned duties (see Schneider, Bradley, and Benedek, 2007, p. 682). In addition, psychiatrists treated a wide range of mood disorders—including major depressive disorder, dysthymic disorder, anxiety disorders, and other psychological symptoms (i.e., acute agitation, insomnia)—with a wide range of medications.

---

[41] See FM 4-02.51 (FM 8-51), 2006, Ch. 9, Combat and Operational Stress Control Stabilization.

The extent of medication use is indicated by responses to the MHAT survey question, "Have you taken any medication for a mental health or combat stress problem during this deployment?" During 2013, 2.6 percent of the soldiers indicated that they had taken medication for a mental health or combat stress problem during this deployment, compared to 1.8 percent in 2012, 3.5 percent in 2010, and 2.6 percent in 2009, a nonsignificant difference. As a point of reference, for a similar population, the civilian rates were 2.28 percent in 1996 and 4.59 percent in 2005. Thus, the values reported for soldiers fell within the national estimates for a similar demographic group (Office of the Surgeon General, U.S. Army Medical Command, 2013, p. 19).

The nature of the wars in Afghanistan and Iraq, their length, and the redeployment of combat veterans (often multiple times) presented a particularly difficult ethical dilemma for the Army, in which the use of medications played a role. For example,

> [i]f a soldier has a mood or anxiety disorder and a desire or duty to deploy to a combat zone, and a provider believes medication will help resolve the symptoms and contribute to success successful performance, then perhaps the ethical decision is to provide the treatment. . . . Modern psychotropic medications can clearly reduce psychiatric symptoms of many disorders in the combat theater. The extent to which medication and treatment may facilitate successful negotiation and processing of combat experience and thus reduce long long-term morbidity, however, remains an open question. (Schneider et al., 2011, p. 160)

Experience of Task Force Baghdad in Iraq: January 2005 to January 2006

A comprehensive example of how behavioral health services were provided in Iraq was presented in two articles published in the journal *Military Medicine* in 2007 describing the experience of Task Force Baghdad.[42]

Preparation for the deployment of the 3rd Infantry Division, the core element of Task Force Baghdad, started with multiple educational briefings designed to help decrease the stigma of seeking behavioral health care and to encourage soldiers to seek care and to maintain their readiness and effectiveness. Once in Iraq, Task Force Baghdad averaged 25,000 soldiers, peaking at 50,000 soldiers. For Task Force Baghdad, the 3rd Infantry Division mental health section consisted of one psychiatrist, two social workers, two psychologists, and six enlisted mental health specialists from the 3rd Infantry Division itself and two social workers and three mental health specialists from the 101st Airborne Division and 10th Mountain Division. The main division mental health clinic was located with the division support brigade, providing support to that brigade, the aviation brigade, and a single maneuver brigade, with a satellite behavioral health clinic located with a troop medical clinic. Each brigade ensured that resources were available to subordinate units at the multiple forward operating bases, establishing individual coverage plans.

---

[42] Warner, Breitbach, et al., 2007a, and Warner, Breitbach, et al., 2007b, describe the experience of Task Force Baghdad in Iraq from January 2005 to January 2006.

On average, there was one mental health provider per 3,100 soldiers in Task Force Baghdad. The majority of their time was spent delivering acute care and treatment, with the goal of returning as many soldiers as possible to duty, using the PIES principles.[43] During the 12-month deployment, division mental health recorded 5,542 clinic visits; 70.2 percent were for combat operational stress, and 29.8 percent were for psychiatric disorders, such as major depressive disorder or generalized anxiety disorder. "The top three factors accounting for combat operational stress were combat exposure (22.3%), peer/unit stressors (15.1%), and home-front stressors (35.2%)" (Warner, Breitbach, et al., 2007a, p. 909).

During the whole deployment, only 95 soldiers (0.4 percent) from Task Force Baghdad were deemed non–mission capable, were placed on unit rest/unit watch with duties restricted, or were sent to the restoration program or to the CSH. Of these 95 soldiers, 12 were eventually evacuated from theater. In all, there were 27 behavioral health evacuations from theater, a rate of 0.1 percent. Available data show that, for OEF (July 2002–October 2013) and OIF–New Dawn (March 2003–December 2011),

> the percentage of evacuations for behavioral health increased beginning in 2007, peaking at 18% in OEF (2012) and 21% in OIF-OND (2010).

> [Overall,] behavioral health ranked third for medical evacuations in both operations (18% to 21%), it ranked eighth for OEF hospitalizations (3.0%) and sixth for OIF-OND hospitalizations (6%). (Hauret et al., 2016, p. 17)

The Mental Health of the Deployed Force

Soon after troops were deployed to Afghanistan, the Surgeon General of the Army established a program in which MHATs would make periodic visits to Afghanistan and Iraq to "assess Soldier and Marine mental health and well-being, . . . examine the delivery of behavioral health care in Operation Iraqi Freedom (OIF), and . . . provide recommendations for sustainment and improvement to command" (Mental Health Advisory Team IV, 2006, p. 3). The MHAT assessed the mental health of the deployed force based on findings from anonymous surveys; on behavioral health, primary care, and unit ministry team surveys; on focus group interviews with soldiers and marines; on interviews and focus groups with Army and Navy behavioral health personnel; and on team members' personal observations. Figure 8.10 shows the percentage of the force deployed to Afghanistan and Iraq that met the criteria for acute stress, depression, or anxiety—all symptoms of PTSD.[44]

---

[43] Historically the Army had used the terms *proximity, immediacy, expectancy,* and *simplicity* (abbreviated as PIES) but began using BICEPS (brevity, immediacy, contact, expectancy, proximity, and simplicity) when it became the approved joint terminology (FM 4-02.51 [FM 8-51], 2006, p. 1-9).

[44] Soldiers' ratings of depression, generalized anxiety, and acute stress were assessed using standardized, validated scales, including the PTSD Checklist, Patient Health Questionnaire 9 (PHQ-9), and Generalized Anxiety Disorder 7 scale. These scales are not diagnostic but rather are standardized, validated scales that measure

Figure 8.10
Acute Stress, Depression, or Anxiety Mental Health Problems

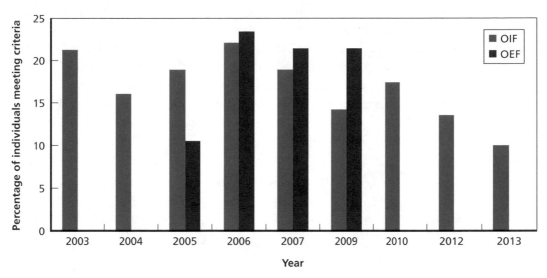

SOURCES: Thomas, 2010, pp. 6–7; Office of the Surgeon General, U.S. Army Medical Command, 2013, p. 16.
NOTE: Data unavailable for 2008 and 2011.

Several key findings from the various MHAT reports suggest (1) that there is a strong relationship between hours of sleep and psychological problems (see Figure 8.11) and (2) that the percentage of NCOs meeting the criteria for psychological problems, marital problems, and full PTSD was positively related to the number of deployments (see Figure 8.12). Specifically, NCOs on a third deployment were nearly twice as likely to report psychological problems and marital problems than NCOs on a first deployment. NCOs on a third deployment were also significantly more likely to have met the screening requirements for PTSD.

Soldiers also reported that there were significant barriers, such as unavailability of services, difficulty in getting an appointment, difficulty in getting time off from work for treatment, and difficulty in getting to the location were mental health specialist were available (Office of the Surgeon General, U.S. Army Medical Command, 2011, p. 34). Stigma associated with asking for help was also a significant barrier to receiving care. Soldiers felt embarrassed to be asking for help or thought that their leaders would hold it against them (see Figure 8.13).

---

whether a soldier reports symptoms consistent with the DSM-IV-TR criteria (American Psychiatric Association, 2000) for each diagnosis. Additionally, for depression and anxiety, soldiers must report impairment in their work or ability to get along with other people as being "very difficult." For acute stress, soldiers have to have a total score of at least 50 on the PTSD Checklist (Office of the Surgeon General, U.S. Army Medical Command, 2013, p. 17).

Figure 8.11
Relationship Between Sleep and Any Psychological Problem

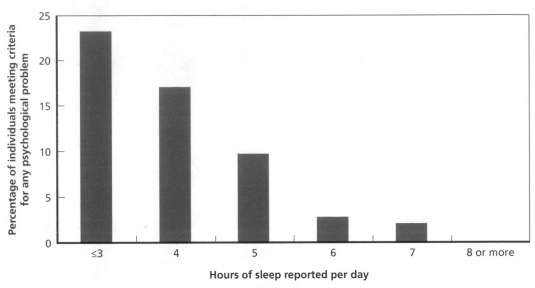

SOURCE: Office of the Surgeon General, U.S. Army Medical Command, 2013, p. 22.

Figure 8.12
Noncommissioned Officers with Psychological or Marital Problems or Who Screened Positive for PTSD, by Number of Deployments

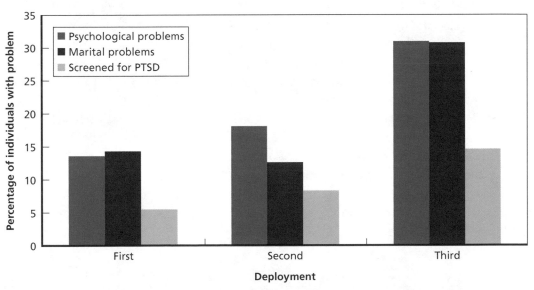

SOURCES: Thomas, 2010, p. 10; Office of the Surgeon General, U.S. Army Medical Command, 2013, p. 28.

Figure 8.13
Problems Soldiers Reported—Barriers to Care and Stigma Perceptions

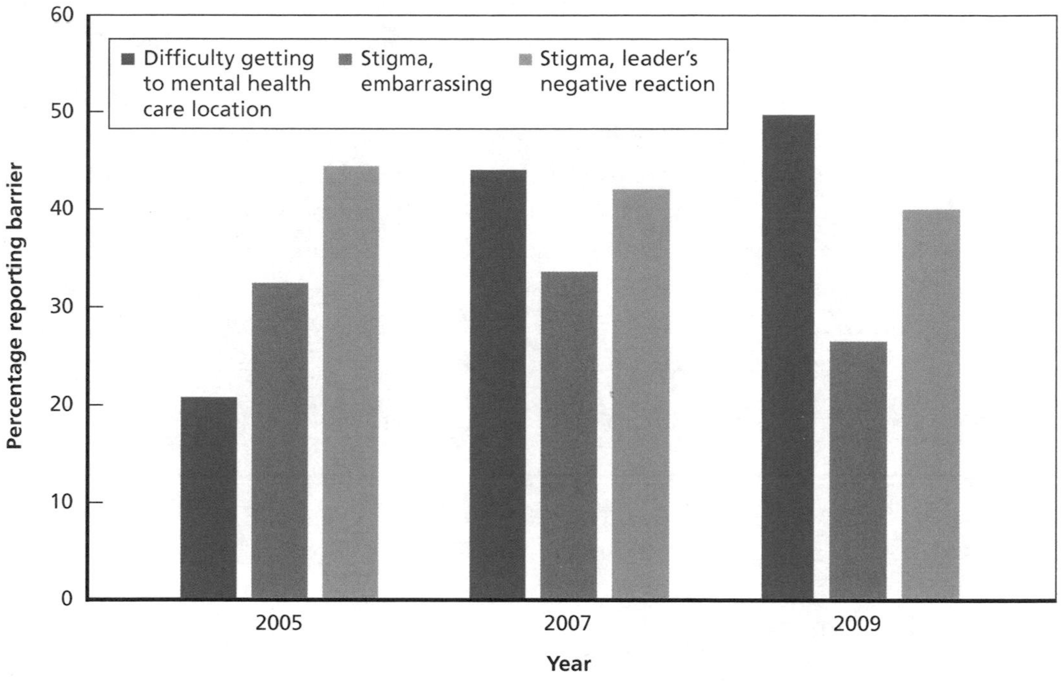

SOURCE: Thomas, 2010, p. 11.

Postdeployment Mental Health and PTSD
Prevalence of PTSD

As discussed earlier, the signs and symptoms of PTSD may occur either soon after the trauma or some time later and may present in an inconsistent pattern over time. PTSD may be apparent when a soldier is in theater, soon after returning home, or some time after the soldier has left the military. It may show up during a postdeployment Army screening or later, in a VA screening. Over time, the Army might provide some treatment, but most will probably be the responsibility of the VA. (Details of the VA program are discussed in Chapter Nine.) At the end of CY 2007, of the approximately 800,000 Army troops deployed to Afghanistan and Iraq (see Tanielian and Jaycox, 2008, p. 22), the Army reported only 28,000 cases of PTSD—3 percent.[45] This stands in stark contrast to the number of PTSD cases reported in the Post-Deployment Health Assessment (PDHA) and the Post-Deployment Health Reassessment

---

[45] The Army defines PTSD cases "as either two (2) outpatient encounters on different days with ICD9 [*International Classification of Diseases*, 9th revision (World Health Organization, 1978)] diagnostic code of 309.81; or inpatient encounter with ICD9 diagnostic code of 309.81. Incidence date is earliest encounter with diagnosis of PTSD (309.81), [and] deployment to OEF/OND/OIF lasting longer than 30 days, beginning prior to incident PTSD diagnosis" (Carino, 2017a, p. 3).

(PDHRA) of active-duty troops.[46] The Surgeon General's office recorded 5,005 cases of PTSD among soldiers deployed in CY 2005 and 8,511 among soldiers deployed during CY 2006, (Carino, 2017a, p. 3). The number also seems remarkably small compared with numbers reported by the VA and an independent survey of soldiers who had served in Afghanistan and Iraq.

Post-Deployment Health Assessment
In 2007, the Defense Health Board Task Force on Mental Health reported results from the PDHRA screening "indicate that 38 percent of Soldiers and 31 percent of Marines report psychological symptoms. Among members of the National Guard, the figure rises to 49 percent" (Defense Health BoardTask Force on Mental Health, 2007, p. ES-2).[47] The same year, the Division of Psychiatry and Neuroscience, Walter Reed Army Institute of Research, reported similar findings; specifically, of the 88,235 soldiers who had returned from deployment to Iraq between June 1, 2005, and December 31, 2006, and had completed both the PDHA and PDHRA, 24,944 were identified as having a clinician-identified mental health problem, including concerns about interpersonal conflict (active, 14.0 percent; reserve, 21.1 percent); other mental health concerns, including PTSD (active, 16.7 percent; reserve, 24.5 percent); depression (active, 10.3 percent); reserve, 13.0 percent); and overall mental health risk (active, 27.1 percent; reserve, 35.5 percent) (Milliken, Auchterlonie, and Hoge, 2007, pp. 2143–2144).

Department of Veterans Affairs
Higher numbers of returning soldiers with PTSD were also reported by the VA, as noted by the Defense Health Board Task Force on Mental Health in their report. The Task Force reported that, of

> the 686,306 OIF and OEF veterans separated from active duty service between 2002 and December 2006 who were eligible for DVA care, 229,015 veterans who accessed care since 2002, 83,889 (37%) received a diagnosis of or were evaluated

---

[46] One of the initiatives resulting from the Gulf War was mandatory postdeployment medical screening and the development of the process. That process involves returning service members answering mental and physical health screening questions and having a follow-up interview with a medical provider (e.g., not a mental health provider), who reviews the results and makes appropriate referrals. Initial assessment of data from the PDHA raised questions about the timing of screenings. While a majority of soldiers who initially reported PTSD symptoms later indicated that the symptoms remitted within a few months of returning home, another group of returning soldiers did not report PTSD symptoms until three to six months after deployment. To address this problem, DoD initiated a second screen in 2005. The PDHRA, administered 90 to 120 days after return from theater, focuses on mental health symptoms.

[47] The task force was stood up in response to Section 723 of the FY 2006 NDAA (Pub. L. 109-163, 2006), which had directed the Secretary of Defense to "establish within the Department of Defense a task force to examine matters relating to mental health and the Armed Forces" and produce "a report containing an assessment of, and recommendations for improving, the efficacy of mental health services provided to members of the Armed Forces by the Department of Defense." The task force was made up of seven military and seven civilian professionals with mental health expertise.

for a mental disorder, including PTSD (39,243 or 17%), non-dependent abuse of drugs (33,099 or 14%), and depressive disorder (27,023 or 12%). (Defense Health Board Task Force on Mental Health, 2007, p. 5)

Independent Estimates of Prevalence of PTSD

RAND provided a specific estimate of the prevalence of PTSD in a 2008 report, *Invisible Wounds of War: Psychological and Cognitive Injuries, Their Consequences, and Services to Assist Recovery* (Tanielian and Jaycox, 2008). In this research, originally commissioned by the California Community Foundation in 2006, RAND

> conducted a comprehensive study of the post-deployment health-related needs associated with post-traumatic stress disorder, major depression, and traumatic brain injury among OEF/OIF veterans, the health care system in place to meet those needs, gaps in the care system, and the costs associated with these conditions and with providing quality health care to all those in need. (Tanielian and Jaycox, 2008, p. iii)

To address the issues of prevalence, RAND created a "a broadly representative sample of the population of individuals who have been deployed as part of OEF/OIF" (Schell and Marshall, 2008, p. 88) and administered a telephone study of 1,965 individuals who had previously been deployed to Afghanistan and Iraq. The respondents reported

> substantial rates of mental health problems in the past 30 days, with 14 percent screening positive for PTSD and 14 percent for major depression. A similar number, 19 percent, reported a probable TBI during deployment.

> . . . [Of the] servicemembers who had been deployed for OEF/OIF as of October 2007, we estimate that approximately 300,000 individuals currently [2008] suffer from PTSD or major depression and that 320,000 individuals experienced a probable TBI during deployment. . . .

> . . . About half (53 percent) of those who met the criteria for current PTSD or major depression had sought help from a physician or mental health provider for a mental health problem in the past year. (Taniclian and Jaycox, 2008, p. xxi)

> . . . Of those who have a mental disorder and also sought medical care for that problem, just over half received a minimally adequate treatment. . . .

> Survey respondents identified many barriers that inhibit getting treatment for their mental health problems. (Tanielian and Jaycox, 2008, p. xxii)

Use of Mental Health Services

Given the potentially large number of returning soldiers whose responses met the screening criteria for major depression, generalized anxiety, or PTSD, a relatively small number actually sought mental health care. Of the approximately 25,000 soldiers who had completed both the PDHA and PDHRA on returning from Iraq and who had been identified to have a clinician-identified mental health problem, only one-fifth were receiving care for depression, PTSD, anger, suicide, or family conflict at the time of their screening. An earlier survey of combat infantry units reported similar results (see Table 8.5).

The pattern of not seeking help seems to be pervasive. It is consistent with data reported for veterans of World War II and for soldiers deployed to Afghanistan and Iraq in 2011.[48] In 2007, the Defense Health Board Task Force on Mental Health, citing reports from the MHAT that were "corroborated . . . from public testimony, comments

Table 8.5
Perceived Need for and Use of Mental Health Services Among Army Soldiers Whose Survey Responses Met the Screening Criteria for Major Depression, Generalized Anxiety, or Posttraumatic Stress Disorder

	After Deployment to	
Outcome	Afghanistan (%) (N = 220)	Iraq (%) (N = 151)
Need		
Acknowledged a problem	81	78
Interested in receiving help	38	43
Received professional help		
In past year		
Overall from any professional	23	40
From mental health professional	13	27
In past month		
Overall from any professional	17	32
From mental health professional	13	21

SOURCE: Adapted from Hoge et al., 2004, p. 20. Used with permission.

---

[48] In 1948, the National Research Council, in cooperation with the VA, the Army, and the Navy, undertook the largest postwar study of soldiers with psychological problems. Data were collected on 985 former soldiers admitted for psychoneurotic disorders during 1944. In addition, a control group of 397 Army enlisted men was randomly selected. Trained psychiatrists evaluated 67 percent of this sample. The remaining members of the sample filled out a questionnaire by mail. In all cases, VA claim folders were reviewed. Most of the clinical evaluations took place in the fifth or sixth year after first admission. The follow-up clinical examination of the men who were "definitely ill at separation" showed that 60 percent had some improvement in their conditions, although most were "not entirely free of psychiatric illness" (Brill and Beebe, 1955, p. 135). Of this group, only 36 percent had actually sought treatment, and "[t]here is no evidence that treatment played an important role in the general improvement which occurred between separation and follow-up" (Brill and Beebe, 1955, p. 135). The researchers also reported that, "treatment had been obtained through the VA by [only] 11 percent of the men, although about "40 percent . . . were drawing VA compensation for psychiatric disability" (Brill and Beebe, 1955, pp. 135–136).

from service members and their families, and discussions with mental health professionals, commanders, and chaplains obtained via site visits," found that the evidence of stigma in the military that often prevents individuals from seeking help for mental health problems was "overwhelming" (Defense Health Board Task Force on Mental Health, 2007, p. 15). As Table 8.6 illustrates, recent research shows that stigma was a barrier to seeking help and is strongest among individuals who screen positive for psychological problems (Hoge et al., 2004, pp. 13, 15; see also Hoge, Auchterlonie, and Milliken, 2006).[49]

The Defense Health Board Task Force on Mental Health noted three manifestations of stigma: self-stigma, public stigma, and structural stigma—how individuals perceive themselves, how they think they will be viewed by fellow soldiers and com-

Table 8.6
E1–E4 Soldiers in Iraq for Nine Months Who Screen Positive
and Not Positive for Any Mental Health Problems

	Agree or Strongly Agree (%)			
	MHAT VI OEF 2009		Joint MHAT 7 OEF 2010	
Factors That Affect Your Decision to Receive Mental Health Services	Screen Positive	Did Not Screen Positive	Screen Positive	Did Not Screen Positive
It would be too embarrassing	31.5	12.5	28.6	13.3
It would harm my career	34.6	13.7	29.2	15.4
Members of my unit might have less confidence in me	46.2	19.4	41.8	23.9
My unit leadership might treat me differently	48.3	22.2	46.0	23.7
My leaders would blame me for the problem	35.5	14.5	33.0	13.0
I would be seen as weak	49.2	24.0	48.9	25.8

SOURCE: Office of the Surgeon General, U.S. Army Medical Command, 2011, p. 33.

---

[49] Greene-Shortridge, Britt, and Castro, 2007, p. 159, makes the case that

> individuals who are experiencing mental health symptoms would be especially likely to consider the potential stigmatizing consequences of seeking mental health care because of the immediate relevance of the decision. Individuals who are not experiencing symptoms will likely not actively consider these consequences, leading to reduced reports of perceived stigma. This finding has important implications for interpreting the average perceived stigma of seeking care for a mental health problem among respondents. It is likely that such a value is an underestimate of the actual stigma felt by individuals actually possessing extensive mental health symptoms.

> Given findings from past research on societal and self-stigma, barriers to care, and the current statistics on rates of soldiers encountering traumatic events and experiencing symptoms of PTSD, it is not hard to see why soldiers would avoid seeking mental health care altogether.

manders, and the institutional policies or practices of the military itself. While having recommendations to combat all, the task force called particular attention to the cultural bias of the military.[50]

Structural Stigma and Cultural Bias

Recently, a number of studies have confirmed that "active duty servicemembers fear that visiting a mental health care provider will jeopardize their careers because of the military's long-standing policy of reporting these types of problems through the chain of command" (Committee on the Assessment of Readjustment Needs of Military Personnel, Veterans, and their Families, 2013, p. 9). Using data from the 2011 DoD Health Related Behaviors Survey (Barlas et al., 2013), GAO estimated that 37 percent of the active-duty force "thought that seeking counseling or mental health care treatment through the military would probably or definitely damage a person's military career" (see Table 8.7).

Unfortunately, there is ample justification for the fear that seeking mental health care will negatively affect a career. A 2014 RAND report identified 203 DoD policies that may contribute to stigma (Acosta et al., 2014, p. 82). For example, an Army policy requires careful vetting of "criminals, *persons with psychological issues*, insurgent ele-

Table 8.7
Survey Estimates Regarding Active Component Service Members' Perceived Effect of Seeking Mental Health Care on a Service Member's Career

	Percentages of Service Members Who					
	Believe seeking counseling or mental health care through the military would probably or definitely damage a person's military career			Have sought mental health care through the military and believe their career was affected somewhat negatively or very negatively		
	Total	Enlisted	Officer	Total	Enlisted	Officer
Army	37	38	35	21	21	18
Navy	42	42	42	24	25	21
Marine Corps	38	38	38	26	26	27
Air Force	34	34	37	18	18	19
All service members	37	37	38	22	22	20

SOURCES: Farrell, 2016a, p. 12. The GAO analysis is based on data from Barlas et al., 2013.

---

[50] The task force noted that, in the military,

> stigma represents a critical failure of the community that prevents service members and their families from getting the help they need just when they may need it most. Further, stigma is of particular concern in the military because of the degree to which military members may bear responsibility for lives beyond their own. Every military leader bears responsibility for addressing stigma; leaders who fail to do so reduce the effectiveness of the service members they lead. (Defense Health Board Task Force on Mental Health, 2007, p. 15)

ments, and many other categories of undesirable personnel [who] may attempt to gain employment within the police force" (Army Techniques Publication 3-39.10, 2015, p. 7-22; emphasis added).

The Army Struggles to Deal with the Realities of PTSD

Military traditions, attitudes, beliefs, practices, and policies that "engender pride, toughness, independence, and self-sufficiency . . . can also complicate the task of encouraging service members to seek help for psychological health concerns" (Meredith et al., 2011, p. 5). Acknowledging that military commanders have a "legitimate need to maintain discipline and enforce a strict code of conduct," the Defense Health Board Task Force on Mental Health also argued that commanders have a "clear responsibility to restore to full level of function a service member damaged in the line of duty, and to be cognizant of and attentive to the psychological aftermath of deployment, manifested in hidden injuries of the brain and mind" (Defense Health Board Task Force on Mental Health, 2007, p. 21). The authors highlighted what some have called the *invisible wounds of war*, such as PTSD and nonpenetrating concussive injuries resulting in mild to severe TBI, and that there was "significant variation in how behavioral symptoms are managed across the military" (Defense Health Board Task Force on Mental Health, 2007, p. 22).[51]

The concerns the Defense Health Board Task Force on Mental Health expressed were prophetic and have embroiled the Army in controversy for over a decade. In 2006, National Public Radio (NPR) reported the following:

> NPR found that soldiers who've come back from the war to Fort Carson in Colorado Springs, Colorado have had trouble getting the help they need, even when they are suicidal.
>
> The military's own studies show that tens of thousands of troops who've served in Iraq have symptoms of serious mental health problems. Those problems include depression, substance abuse and post-traumatic stress disorder, known as PTSD.

---

[51] Specifically, the task force noted that the

> Services vary in . . . [how] the behavioral symptoms that accompany these hidden injuries are taken into account during administrative, legal, or disciplinary action or adverse personnel actions (such as premature separations from service) attributable to disinhibitory behavior or declines in duty function. Two combatants with similar behavior may be handled in a markedly different manner depending on their unit of assignment or installation.

> The Task Force was also informed of instances in which returning service members were pressured by commanders and peers to accept an administrative discharge so they could be expeditiously cleared from the unit and replaced with a fully functional person. Such incidents may be attributed in part to the complex and often protracted Physical Evaluation Board (PEB) process. In sites such as Europe, where there are no units designated as Medical Holding Companies, the dilemma of balancing the legitimate treatment needs of injured service members with the needs for current unit combat readiness is even more challenging. (Defense Health Board Task Force on Mental Health, 2007, p. 22)

Administration officials have said, since the U.S. invaded Iraq, that they want to heal all the troops who've come home with emotional problems. But NPR found that the system at Fort Carson doesn't work the way it should, and for two main reasons. First, it's been overwhelmed by soldiers coming back from Iraq. It can take soldiers weeks to get appointments. And second, some officers at the base say they feel contempt for soldiers who have problems, like PTSD. They haze them. They punish them. They ridicule the soldiers in public. (Zwerdling, 2006b)

Similar reports were aired all throughout 2006 and 2007 (see Zwerdling, 2006a; Zwerdling, 2006d; Zwerdling, 2006c; Zwerdling, 2007a; and Zwerdling, 2007b), but the story did not end there:

- In 2009, Congress included a provision in the FY 2010 NDAA (Pub. L. 111–84, 2009, Section 512) requiring a medical examination before administrative separation of members diagnosed with or reasonably asserting PTSD or TBI.
- In 2012, the congressional requirements notwithstanding, the *Seattle Times* reported on an Army investigation of Madigan Army Medical Center (see Bernton, 2012a; Bernton, 2012b; Vogel, 2012), where a screening team reversed more than 300 PTSD diagnoses. Not only did the change disqualify the soldier from a 50-percent disability rating and a medical retirement that would include a pension and other benefits, but, in some cases, soldiers were labeled as possible malingerers and received bad conduct discharges, with a loss of VA benefits and services. As a result of the Madigan investigation, the Army reinstated the PTSD diagnoses to more than 100 service members, and the Secretary of the Army initiated a major review of PTSD and other behavioral-health diagnoses received by soldiers evaluated for medical retirement.
- In 2014, Defense Secretary Chuck Hagel, responding to petitions from Vietnam veterans to upgrade their discharges based on claims of unrecognized PTSD, directed the Boards for Correction of Military/Naval Records to ensure consistency in considering veterans' discharge upgrade requests related to PTSD (see Marshall, 2014).
- In 2013, the *Colorado Springs Gazette* ran a lengthy article detailing how "Psychological screenings [which were] supposed to be the last line of defense that protects troops with invisible wounds from being unfairly discharged for misconduct and stripped of benefits, . . . which are mandated by Congress, are not working" (Philipps, 2013).
- In 2015, Fort Carson was again the subject of an NPR story, this one recounting the case of an Army staff sergeant who had served two tours in Iraq who was fighting the Army's attempt to have him discharged for after a driving-under-the-influence conviction (see Zwerdling, 2015). When he claimed was suffering from PTSD, he was referred to a therapist who secretly recorded 20 hours of their meetings. Eventually, his case and the recordings were reviewed, and the Army

concluded that sergeant was "mistreated, and two of his therapists were subsequently reprimanded." His records were sent to Walter Reed, where he was diagnosed with PTSD and given a medical retirement, with honor and full benefits. Apparently, this was not an isolated case (see Table 8.8). Clearly, not all those dismissed with a mental health diagnosis had PTSD, but the number of misconduct discharges for those who served in Afghanistan and Iraq is troubling.

Table 8.8
Soldiers with Mental Health Disorders Who Were Dismissed for Misconduct, 2009–2015

Location	Iraq or Afghanistan Veterans	All Other Soldiers
Fort Hood	2,579	1,262
Fort Sill	1,768	1,362
Fort Bragg	1,865	1,123
Fort Bliss	1,332	1,182
Fort Lewis	1,559	950
Fort Carson	1,595	758
Fort Campbell	1,508	704
Fort Stewart	1,298	694
Europe	1,274	712
Fort Knox	796	903
Fort Riley	994	696
Fort Shafter	1,061	586
Fort Drum	924	544
Alaska	840	383
Fort Benning	657	419
Fort Polk	465	344
Korea	238	565

SOURCE: DoD, via Zwerdling, 2015.

NOTES: Includes soldiers with mental health conditions that were diagnosed within two years of separation date. Diagnoses include PTSD, TBI, adjustment disorder, anxiety disorder, and other conditions. Includes locations with more than 500 misconduct discharges.

- In 2016, the *New York Times* reported on a soldier who

  > was discharged from the Army at the height of the Iraq war because he was
  > not on a plane to Baghdad for his second deployment. Instead, he was in a
  > hospital after attempting suicide the night before. . . .
  >
  > Instead of screening [the soldier for PTSD], . . . the Army wrote him up
  > for missing his flight, then forced him out of the military with a less-than-
  > honorable discharge. When he petitioned the Army to upgrade his discharge,
  > arguing that he missed his flight because of undiagnosed PTSD, it rejected
  > his appeal. (Philipps, 2016)

  Army Board for Correction of Military Records rulings favorable to veterans surged to 45 percent from 4 percent, with a staff of 135 trying to process
  over 22,500 cases (Williamson, 2017). Just days after the *Times* report, the record
  review boards were told to waive any statutes of limitations that might bar considering a partition to upgrade, saying this: "Fairness and equity demand, in cases
  of such magnitude, that a Veteran's petition receive full and fair review, even if
  brought outside of the time limit" (Carson, 2016).

- In 2017, GAO reported to Congress that additional actions needed to ensure
  PTSD and TBI are considered in misconduct separations. GAO reported that
  91,764 service members had been separated for misconduct from FY 2011
  through FY 2015, with 16 percent (14,816) having been diagnosed with PTSD
  or TBI, some with both. Specifically, 8 percent had been diagnosed with PTSD,
  and 11 percent had been diagnosed with TBI, although other conditions, such as
  adjustment, alcohol-related, depressive, substance-abuse, and anxiety disorders,
  were more common (Williamson, 2017, pp. 12–13). Of the service members separated for misconduct and diagnosed with PTSD or TBI, 23 percent received
  an "other than honorable" characterization of service, and 71 percent received a
  "general" characterization of service. GAO reported that

  > [r]ecent Army audits have found that the Army did not have sufficient docu-
  > mentation to demonstrate that it was always considering whether PTSD or
  > TBI was a mitigating factor in servicemember's behavior prior to separating
  > them for misconduct. (Williamson, 2017, p. 28)
  >
  > As a result of policy inconsistencies and limited monitoring, DOD has little
  > assurance that certain servicemembers diagnosed with PTSD or TBI receive
  > the required screening and counseling prior to being separated for miscon-
  > duct. (Williamson, 2017, p. 31)

Treatment of PTSD

In 2008, the TBI, although other conditions undertook a study for the VA "to assess
the scientific evidence on treatment modalities for Posttraumatic Stress Disorder"
(Committee on Treatment of Posttraumatic Stress Disorder, 2008, p. ix). In reviewing
treatment modalities, the IOM highlighted Version 1.0 of *VA/DoD Clinical Practice*

Guideline for the Management of Post-Traumatic Stress (Management of Post-Traumatic Stress Working Group, 2004), noting that it recommended

> four psychotherapy treatments as being of significant benefit: cognitive therapy, exposure therapy, stress inoculation therapy, and EMDR [eye movement desensitization and reprocessing therapy]. Treatment modalities considered to offer some benefit include imagery rehearsal therapy, psychodynamic therapy, and PTSD patient education. The guidelines also identified two adjunctive treatments: dialectical behavioral therapy and hypnosis. Among the pharmacotherapy interventions, only one group, the SSRIs, was classified as being of significant benefit. Medications identified as having some benefit include TCAs [tricyclic antidepressants], MAOIs [monoamine oxidase inhibitors], sympatholytics, and novel antidepressants. Anticonvulsants, atypical antipsychotics, nonbenzodiazepine hypnotics, and the antianxiety drug buspirone were identified as having unknown benefit. Finally, drugs with no benefit or possible harm include benzodiazepines and typical antipsychotics. (Committee on Treatment of Posttraumatic Stress Disorder, 2008, p. 31)

However, the IOM concluded that there were "significant gaps in the evidence that made it impossible to reach conclusions establishing the efficacy of most treatment modalities" (Committee on Treatment of Posttraumatic Stress Disorder, 2008, p. ix). In 2010, DoD and the VA published a revised set of guidelines that incorporated the results of six years "of well-designed randomized controlled trials of pharmacological and psychotherapeutic interventions for post-traumatic stress" (Management of Post-Traumatic Stress Working Group, 2010, p. 3). These trials showed that "several types of cognitive behavioral therapies, counseling, and medications have been shown to be effective in treating PTSD" (Management of Post-Traumatic Stress Working Group, 2010, p. 4).

In addition to resources available through local military and VA facilities, treatment is available at the National Intrepid Center of Excellence at Walter Reed National Military Center for active-duty service members with TBI (mild to moderate) and psychological health conditions who have not responded to traditional treatment. In addition, the Center for Deployment Psychology at USUHS "trains military and civilian behavioral health professionals to provide high-quality, culturally sensitive, evidence-based behavioral health services to military personnel, veterans, and their families" ("Center for Deployment Psychology," undated). In 2012, President Obama signed *Improving Access to Mental Health Services for Veterans, Service Members, and Military Families* (EO 13625, 2012) to spur additional support to veterans and their families from the departments of Defense and Veterans Affairs (VA and DoD, undated). However, a 2015 article by RAND researchers noted that studies show that "less than half of military personnel and veterans who indicate need for mental health services actually receive such care" (Ramchand, Rudavsky, et al., 2015, p. 4).

Mental Health Care for U.S. Soldiers and Families: Challenges Remain

Compared with past conflicts, the efforts to mitigate the immediate and long-term psychological effects of the conflicts in Iraq and Afghanistan have been unparalleled. Since 9/11, the U.S. Army Medical Command has initiated a number of changes.[52] In addition, the DoD expanded postdeployment screening to include a second assessment three to six months after deployment. In theater, "[t]he number of mental health professionals directly assigned to combat brigades was increased, and combat-operational stress units were divided into smaller teams distributed throughout theater that could each provide the full range of services" (Hoge, Ivany, et al., 2016, p. 3). At home, the number of mental health providers across the Army increased from approximately 1,300 in 2007 to more than 3,000 in 2015, with licensed mental health professionals embedded within primary care clinics to provide "consultation to primary care providers, clinical assessments, triage, and brief cognitive-behavioral interventions" (Hoge, Ivany, et al., 2016, p. 5). In 2007, the Defense Health Board Task Force on Mental Health prepared an extensive report to Congress suggesting "A Way Forward" (Defense Health Board Task Force on Mental Health, 2007). As a result, "Congress appropriated nearly $1 billion in 2007 for PTSD and TBI research and enhancement of treatment capabilities. This decision was followed by sustainment of higher funding in subsequent years" (Hoge, Ivany, et al., 2016, p. 3). Nevertheless, a recent assessment found

> Although mental health efforts for service members have been unprecedented compared with those made during past conflicts, many challenges remain, including continued underutilization of mental health services, problems with treatment of substance use disorders, concerns with chronic pain and prescription opioid misuse, and lack of clarity on optimal strategies to address overlapping postdeployment physical and cognitive symptoms being attributed (or likely misattributed) to concussion. Studies in both the DOD and the VA show that despite improvements in screening and stigma perceptions, a large percentage of service members and veterans still do not seek mental health care when needed or do not receive an adequate number of treatment encounters for recovery. (Hoge, Ivany, et al., 2016, pp. 6–7)

---

[52] Programmatic changes by the Army Medical Command were designed to

ensure delivery of high-quality standardized mental health services, including centralized workload management; consolidation of psychiatry, psychology, psychiatric nursing, and social work services under integrated behavioral health departments; creation of satellite mental health clinics embedded within brigade work areas; incorporation of mental health providers into primary care; routine mental health screening throughout soldiers' careers; standardization of clinical outcome measures; and improved services for family members. (Hoge, Ivany, et al., 2016, p. 1)

CHAPTER NINE

Postconflict Care for the Casualties of War After 9/11

Chapters Six through Eight covered the events of and medical care during the recent conflicts in Afghanistan and Iraq. This chapter deals with the care the casualties of these conflicts receive after they return to the United States, specifically the interface between the departments of Defense and Veterans Affairs, and the changing role of the VA in providing long-term care for those who have served our country in the military.

As the operations in Afghanistan and Iraq continued, problems caring for war casualties developed on the home front because of the time-consuming administrative procedures for evaluating wounded service members to determine the most appropriate manner of discharge, the VA services needed to facilitate the transfer from the services to the VA, and the VA's provision of services to veterans after discharge.

Problems in Transitioning from Military to Veteran Status

In his memoir recounting his tenure as Secretary of Defense, Robert Gates said

> I was always convinced that the . . . [senior military leaders of the services] had been unaware of the bureaucratic and administrative nightmare that too often confronts our outpatient wounded. . . . During my entire tenure as secretary, I never saw the military services—across the board—bring to a problem as much zeal, passion, and urgency once they realized that these men and women who had sacrificed so much were not being treated properly after they left the hospital. (Gates, 2014, p. 135)

Medical Holding

The care and housing of significant numbers of soldiers who are not ready to return to their units or be discharged from the service has been a significant wartime problem since at least the Civil War. A report that could have been speaking of conditions at Fort Stewart in 2003 or WRAMC in 2007 described convalescent camps of the Civil War era:

[They were] neither Hospitals nor Camps, but partook of the nature of both, and formed a sort of halting-place for the soldier midway between them. They received men from the Hospitals who had so far recovered as no longer to need medical treatment, but who were yet not well enough for active service in the field. These men remained in the Convalescent camps until they regained their strength, or it became apparent that they were wholly incapable of further service, and then, as the case might be, were either sent to rejoin their regiments, or were discharged as disabled. (Stille, 1866, p. 301)[1]

The Civil War report went on to say that "these Convalescent Camps were always one of the most unsightly offshoots of the military system" (Stille, 1866, p. 302), a characterization that might also be applied to the medical holding unit at Fort Stewart, Georgia, in 2003.

Fort Stewart, 2003

On October 17, 2003, United Press International reported that, at Fort Stewart, Georgia, National Guard and Army Reserve soldiers,

including many who served in the Iraq war are languishing in hot cement barracks here while they wait—sometimes for months—to see doctors.

[These] soldiers are on what the Army calls "medical hold," while the Army decides how sick or disabled they are and what benefits—if any—they should get as a result. (Benjamin, 2003)

Acting Army Secretary Les Brownlee visited Fort Stewart on October 25, promising to make improvements and review other mobilization sites to determine whether the problems existed on other bases. He said that "[t]hose in medical status . . . should be in the improved level of billets, those that are air conditioned and have some of the other improvements, like indoor latrines" (as quoted in "Army Secretary Vows Improvements at Fort Stewart," 2003).

These reports captured the attention of members of Congress, particularly U.S. Senator Kit Bond (D-Missouri), cochair of the Senate National Guard Caucus, who called for hearings to investigate conditions in the medical holdover units ("Senator

---

[1] The report went on to say that the

vast number thus separated for a time at least, from their regular place in the army may be gathered from the statement that during the years 1863 and 1864, more than two hundred thousand such men passed through a single one of these convalescent camps, that in the rear of Alexandria. The proper management of such a place was an exceedingly difficult task. A permanent, effective, organization was almost impossible as the inmates were constantly changing, and as they belonged to nearly every Regiment in the service, and to all the staff departments of the Army. The consequence was that there could be no proper military duties regularly performed or steady discipline kept up, as the men were liable, from day to day, to be discharged. (Stille, 1866, pp. 301–302)

Credits UPI Report on Poor GI Care," 2003). On November 19, 2003, Brownlee and GEN Peter J. Schoomaker, Chief of Staff of the Army, testified before the Senate Armed Services Committee on current Army issues. They told the senators that

> [e]vents since the end of major combat operations in Iraq have differed from our expectations and have combined to cause problems for many soldiers—problems we have identified and are taking corrective actions to fix. For example, on October 30, we transferred 50 medical hold personnel from crowded conditions at Fort Stewart to the less-strained facilities at Fort Gordon. We are taking additional measures to resolve these problems, such as moving other medical hold personnel into climate-controlled buildings, seeking local civilian medical appointments, and increasing medical staff. (Brownlee, 2003, p. 13)

On January 20, 2004, the Army, issued Annex Q (Medical Holdover Operations) to Operating Order 04-01 (Howes, 2004), which provided policy and operational guidance and assigned responsibility for the management of individuals on medical hold or holdover status.[2] It established the Community Based Health Care Initiative, allowing reserve-component medical holdover soldiers to receive treatment and recuperate at or near their homes using local health care resources and tasked the Army Medical Command to maximize the throughput in MTFs by increasing staffing, shifting resources, or using additional resources to improve access and reduce the time soldiers spent on medical holdover status. It also charged the Installation Management Agency to ensure that soldiers with more than 30 days in medical holdover had suitable accommodations.

Despite these actions, the Army's policy of retaining amputees on active duty and providing extensive rehabilitation services meant that the number of patients on medical hold, particularly at Walter Reed, kept growing. By early 2006, the senior commander overseeing much of Walter Reed hospital's operation was asking his colleagues for ideas "of what might facilitate the flow of casualties through our treatment/ rehabilitation/discharge process . . . [to] reduce the number of MH/MHO [medical hold/medical holdover] before it bites us in the backside" (Deal, 2006). A year later, that senior commander was a central figure in the scandal that rocked Walter Reed (Vogel, 2007).

The Office of the Secretary of Defense Acts

The Army was not the only organization to respond to the reports from Fort Stewart. On October 29, 2003, the Under Secretary of Defense for Personnel and Readiness

---

[2] This policy defines a *medical holdover* as a "reserve component service member, pre-deployment or post-deployment, separated from his/her unit, in need of definitive health care based on medical conditions identified while in an active duty status, in support of the Global War on Terrorism." *Medical hold* is defined as "active or reserve component soldiers assigned or attached to military hospitals who are unable to perform even in a limited duty capacity" (Howes, 2004).

issued a policy memorandum to the secretaries of the military departments, requiring medical commanders to ensure that specialty care services be available for medical hold personnel (Chu, 2003). The policy also required the services to provide "uniform lodging in quality and type for the area where they were located." Concerned about providing housing equivalent to "visiting quarters, temporary lodging facilities, or . . . rental accommodations on the private economy typically provided to TDY [temporary duty] personnel," the under secretary made the point that reserve personnel on active duty should receive the same quality and type of lodging and support as other active-duty members. Finally, the policy required weekly reports from the military services through December 31, 2003, detailing the number of personnel on medical hold.

Concern for the welfare of casualties was not limited to heads of the military services. Throughout 2004, Deputy Secretary of Defense Paul Wolfowitz made regular visits to Walter Reed and the National Naval Hospital in Bethesda, Maryland. In addition, he frequently attended informal dinners organized by two Vietnam veterans and learned about the problems and issues wounded warriors confront. He gave them, or their families, his card and asked that they call him directly with any issues. Many did call, essentially setting up a wounded warrior care center run out of the Deputy Secretary's office. Eventually, on December 20, 2004, Secretary of Defense Rumsfeld directed the Under Secretary of Defense for Personnel and Readiness to establish a formal center within one month: *I think we ought to put together a team to see that the services take care of their troops after they're wounded, and when they return home and are discharged*" (as quoted in Julian, 2005; emphasis in the original).

Military Severely Injured Center

The Deputy Under Secretary of Defense for Military Community and Family Policy was given the operational responsibility to carry out Rumsfeld's mandate. Given the tight time line and the fact that DoD had recently established a successful call center, Military OneSource, to facilitate support for military personnel and their families, the call center model was quickly selected for the new Military Severely Injured Center (MSIC).[3] The existing contract for Military OneSource was modified to support the effort, e.g., office space was quickly secured through Military OneSource, and staff were detailed to the MSIC. The military services also provided staffing, as did the VA, the Department of Labor, and the Transportation Security Agency, which provided three people to help clear wounded warriors through airport security.

The MSIC opened on February 1, 2005, with initial remarks by Deputy Secretary of Defense Wolfowitz:

> Unfortunately, when our wounded veterans have to encounter the bureaucracy that deals with issues of medical disability, active duty status, family benefits, and all those kinds of issues, they encounter rules that often seem to be relics of the

---

[3]   The original name was Military Severely Injured Joint Operations Center.

last century—of World War II, when most of our wounded were young single men without families and when our ability to assist the severely wounded in rehabilitation was woefully much more limited. (Wolfowitz, 2005)

Under Secretary of Defense for Personnel and Readiness David S. C. Chu addressed the gathering at the center's opening (as quoted in Quigley, 2005):

"The purpose of the center is to bring things together to make sure no one falls through the cracks, make sure everyone has a single telephone number that they may call if they have a question, a problem, an issue that has not been properly resolved. . . .

"Our job may not be to resolve the issues; it may be to turn to the appropriate service provider . . . ."

Other times, the center staff members may need to take action themselves. . . .

The center's mission is not to replace government or military programs, Chu said. "It is to unify. It is to coordinate. It is to give every family member a place of recourse if they need it."

To carry out its mission, the MSIC refers callers to supporting governmental and nongovernmental organizations, including the American Legion, the National Association of State Directors of Veterans Affairs, and the National Guard Bureau's State Family Program Offices, which provide help in such areas as financial assistance, spouse employment, employment and internships with federal agencies, educational opportunities, and government, private sector, and nonprofit resources in states and local communities.

While senior leaders of the services and OSD might agree that the primary function of the MSIC would be "to facilitate a coordinated response" (Farmer, 2005), the MSIC, with Military OneSource as its model, was designed to be more proactive.[4] In October 2005, the Assistant Secretary of Defense for Health Affairs addressed the House Armed Service Committee:

A number of our severely injured Service members will . . . transition from the military and return to their hometowns or become new members of another civil-

---

[4] One service support organization, the National Military Family Association, described the MSIC as

a central Department of Defense (DoD) resource available to offer support services to seriously injured servicemembers and their families. The Center works with and compliments existing Service programs such as the U.S. Army's Wounded Warrior (AW2) Program, the Marine for Life Injured Support System, and Military OneSource. Support services are provided as long as seriously injured servicemembers and their families require quality of life support. Services are tailored to meet [the] individual's unique needs during recovery and rehabilitation. The Center offers counseling and resource referral in such areas as financial support, education, and employment assistance, information on VA benefits, family counseling, resources in local communities, and child care support. (National Military Family Association, 2006, pp. 5–6)

ian community. . . . [The MSIC] will ensure that during their rehabilitation we provide a "case management" approach to advocate for the Service member and his or her family. From the Joint Support Operations Center here in Arlington, Virginia, to their communities across America, we will be with them. This will continue through their transition to the Department of Veterans Affairs, and the many other agencies and organizations providing support to them. Our goal is to provide long term support to ensure that no injured Service member is left without assistance. (Winkenwerder, 2005, p. 10)

This level of direct OSD involvement in the operational delivery of services to wounded soldiers was unprecedented.[5] The military services, the traditional sole providers of services to the troops, were concerned from the beginning that the center would usurp their role in caring for wounded warriors. The services wanted injured service members to understand that they were still members of *their* services and were being supported by *their* service leaders and resources. In response to these concerns, the MSIC adjusted protocols referring callers to the appropriate service and acting as backup when necessary when caseload backlogs developed. Over time and in response to OSD's proactive creation of the MSIC, the services established their own new programs, expanded existing ones, and made it clear that they did not want OSD playing such a direct role in the providing services to *their* members. To some extent, this had been fought out when Military OneSource was established, but now it hit home, bringing into question the military services' ability to care for their wounded warriors.

In January 2006, Congress directed that, by June 1, 2006,

the Secretary of Defense shall prescribe a comprehensive policy for the Department of Defense on the provision of assistance to members of the Armed Forces who incur severe wounds or injuries in the line of duty. . . . (Pub. L. 109-163, 2006, Sec. 563(a)(1))

The policy shall include guidelines to be followed by the military departments . . . . The procedures and standards shall be uniform across the military departments except to the extent necessary to reflect the traditional practices or customs of a particular military department. . . . (Pub. L. 109-163, 2006, Sec. 563(a)(4))

The comprehensive policy . . . shall address . . . Coordination with the Severely Injured Joint Support Operations Center of the Department of Defense" (Pub. L. 109-163, 2006, Sec. 563(b)).

Through 2006, OSD and the services met to hash out the uniform policy. Despite efforts to accommodate the concerns of the military services, in the end, representatives to the policy working group from the Department of the Army and Department of the

---

[5]   The Navy developed the Safe Harbor Program; the Marine Corps set up the Wounded Warrior Regiment; and the Air Force created the Air Force Wounded Warrior Program.

Navy indicated that their departments disagreed with the overall policy. As a result, formal regulations were never published. In January 2007, the MSIC closed, transferring its remaining cases to the military services. Office space reverted to the Military OneSource program. Staff was reassigned to the Wounded Warrior Resource Center, which Congress had directed to be established in the FY 2008 NDAA (Pub. L. 110-181, 2008). This new center had a different focus, to "provide wounded warriors, their families, and their primary caregivers with a single point of contact for assistance with reporting deficiencies in covered military facilities, obtaining health care services, receiving benefits information, and any other difficulties encountered while supporting wounded warriors" (Pub. L. 110-181, 2008, Sec. 1616).

Walter Reed Army Medical Center, 2007

As it turned out, the January 2007 rollback of OSD's involvement in overseeing care for wounded soldiers was premature. Shortly after the MSIC began drawing down operations, the *Washington Post* published two stories decrying the living conditions in medical hold or medical holdover at WRAMC (Priest and Hull, 2007; Hull and Priest, 2007). The problem that the commander of hospital operations had highlighted at the beginning of 2006, and which he said had the potential to "bite us in the backside," did just that.

The majority of combat wounded returned to the United States had been admitted to Walter Reed. Either because of the severity of their injuries or because of the long waits for discharge determinations, they spent many months and sometimes a year or more on medical hold at Walter Reed before returning home or, if they remained on active duty, to a new duty station. As a result, the number of soldiers in medical hold at Walter Reed grew from a pre-9/11 level of 100 to 120 to as many as 874 during summer 2005. At the time of publication, the *Washington Post* noted that there were 700 soldiers and Marines in this status, outnumbering hospital patients 17 to 1. The average stay was 10 months, but some remained up to two years (Priest and Hull, 2007, p. 1). The Army used various facilities to house these patients, including the Mologne House, a nonappropriated fund hotel located on the Walter Reed campus, the Fisher Houses,[6] and contract hotel rooms. Some were assigned to live in what is known as Building 18, a former hotel in dire need of repair located across the street from the medical center.[7] Here is how a report from the *Washington Post* summarized the situation:

---

[6] Fischer Houses were established primarily to house the families of patients at military hospitals. They are donated by the Fischer House Foundation and are operated with donations. There is no charge to families.

[7] LTG Kevin C. Kiley, Surgeon General of the Army and former commander at Walter Reed, told the Senate Armed Service Committee on March 7, 2007 that:

> Upon reading the Washington Post articles, I personally inspected Building 18. As noted in the article, the elevator and security gate to the parking garage are not operational. Twenty-six rooms had one or more deficiencies, which require repair. Two of these rooms had mold growth on walls. Thirty outstanding work orders

While the hospital is a place of . . . daily miracles, with medical advances saving more soldiers than ever, the outpatients in the Other Walter Reed encounter a messy bureaucratic battlefield nearly as chaotic as the real battlefields they faced overseas.

On the worst days, soldiers say they feel like they are living a chapter of "Catch-22." The wounded manage other wounded. Soldiers dealing with psychological disorders of their own have been put in charge of others at risk of suicide. (Priest and Hull, 2007, p. 2)

The situation the *Washington Post* articles described "dismayed" and "mortified" leaders of DoD. The department did not dispute the findings. In fact, Secretary of Defense Robert Gates, who replaced Rumsfeld in December 2006, said he was "grateful to reporters for bringing this problem to our attention, but very disappointed we did not identify it ourselves" (West et al., 2007, p. B-3). The secretary moved quickly to address the needs of wounded warriors, and the President of the United States and Congress quickly followed his actions.

Secretary of Defense Takes Immediate Action

In response to the *Washington Post* stories on February 23, 2007, Gates announced he had created an independent review group to

inspect the current situation at Walter Reed here in Washington, the National Naval Medical Center in Bethesda and any other centers they choose to examine.

. . . [A]fter the facts are established, those responsible for having allowed this unacceptable situation to develop will indeed be held accountable. (West et al., 2007, p. B-3)

Not waiting for the findings of the independent review, Secretary of the Army Francis J. Harvey fired the commander of Walter Reed, MG George W. Weightman, on March 1, 2007, and assigned the Army Surgeon General, and former Walter Reed commander, LTG Kevin Kiley, as the interim commander of Walter Reed. Apparently, Secretary Gates was displeased that Harvey had chosen Kiley, whom critics had accused of long knowing about the problems. The following day, Harvey offered his resignation, reportedly at the request of the Secretary of Defense. His departure was

---

have been prioritized and our Base Operations contractor has already completed a number of repairs. We are also working closely with US Army Installation Management Command, the Army Corps of Engineers, and our Health Facility planners to replace the roof and renovate each room.

There are currently no signs of rodents or cockroaches in any rooms. In October 2006, the hospital started an aggressive campaign to deal with a mice infestation after complaints from Soldiers. Preventive medicine specialists inspected the building and found rooms with exposed food that attracted vermin. Removing the food sources and increased oversight by the chain of command has since brought this problem under control, although such problems require vigilant monitoring, which is on-going. (Kiley, 2007, pp. 4–6)

"announced on short notice by a visibly agitated Defense Secretary Robert Gates, . . . [who told reporters,] 'I am disappointed that some in the Army have not adequately appreciated the seriousness of the situation pertaining to outpatient care at Walter Reed'" (Wolf, 2007). On March 11, 2007, General Kiley submitted his own request to retire, "in the best interest of the Army" (DoD, 2007).

Secretary Gates then met with the Army Chief of Staff designate, GEN George Casey, and Army Vice Chief of Staff Dick Cody and told them "not to wait on the reviews or studies but to act right away to fix Walter Reed and look at the rest of the Army's treatment of wounded Warriors. . . . When in doubt, err on the side of the soldier" (Gates, 2014, p. 135). On April 17, 2007, DoD reported to Congress on the Army's Medical Action Plan, and that the Army had

> moved quickly to improve conditions and enhance services at Walter Reed [and] . . . . to control security, improve access, and complete repairs at identified facilities that provide for the health and welfare of our nation's heroes. On March 23, the Army opened its Soldier and Family Assistance Center—a one-stop shop that brings together case managers, family coordinators, personnel and finance experts, and representatives from key support and advocacy organizations in one location. The Soldier and Family Assistance Center reduces in-processing locations from seven to two. In addition, the Army's new Warrior Transition Brigade will be fully operational at Walter Reed on June 7th to assist soldiers assigned to medical holdover. This brigade will reduce cadre-to-Soldier ratios from 1:55 to 1:12. (Dominguez, 2007, p. 3)

Commission, Review Groups, and Task Forces

The fallout from the *Washington Post* articles was not limited to the firing of senior Army officials. The articles also set off a series of parallel investigations covering the whole administrative process of separating casualties and transferring them to the cognizance of the VA.[8] The first, established on February 23, 2007, was Secretary of Defense's Independent Review Group, cochaired by two former Secretaries of the Army, Togo West, Jr., and John Marsh (see West et al., 2007). This was followed less

---

[8] Even before the *Washington Post* articles, the Under Secretary of Defense for Personnel and Readiness, on March 10, 2005, had requested that the DoD IG review the transition process from DoD to VA, "including medical hold and medical holdover programs, . . . [to] help us improve the care we provide to Service members" (Inspectors General of the DoD and DVA, 2008, p. 11). The DoD IG reached out to the VA IG to form an integrated interagency team, which started its fieldwork in July 2006 and reported its findings on June 12, 2008. The interagency IG team identified areas for potential improvement and made observations about the process for transitioning service members and veterans. The observations addressed

- postdeployment integration, benefits, and mental health of injured service members
- benefits and support to families of injured service members
- data-sharing and case management among DoD, VA, and private-sector facilities.

than two weeks later, on March 6, 2007,[9] by the President's Commission on Care for America's Returning Wounded Warriors, cochaired by Senator Robert Dole and Secretary Donna Shalala, and the intergovernmental Task Force on Returning Global War on Terror Heroes, chaired by the Secretary of Veterans Affairs. The Dole-Shalala Commission had a broad charter to undertake a comprehensive look at the full life cycle of treatment for wounded veterans returning from the battlefield. The task force was charged with examining federal services provided to all returning Global War on Terror service members.[10]

The first to report was the West-Marsh Independent Review Group, on April 11, 2007. The commission and the task force delivered their reports to President Bush on July 30, 2007, and April 19, 2007, respectively. Generally, these reports commended the life-saving advancements in clinical care that had been made but agreed that the systems and processes to provide for the needs of the wounded, ill, and injured were outdated, cumbersome, and difficult for the service member and his or her family to navigate.

Administrative Actions by DoD and VA

On April 12, 2007, the Senate Armed Services Committee and the Senate Veterans Committee conducted a joint meeting to examine the disability rating systems the DoD and VA used and the transition of service members from DoD to the VA. The lead witness, Deputy Secretary of Defense Gordon R. England,[11] committed DoD to "work with the Commissions, the Congress, and partner agencies to clearly identify

---

[9]   On March 6, 2007, the President issued EO 13426 (Office of the Press Secretary, 2007).

[10]   The EO also directed the Secretary of Veterans Affairs to establish the Interagency Task Force on Returning Global War on Terror Heroes. This task force included representatives of the departments of Defense, Labor, Health and Human Services, Housing and Urban Development, and Education, as well as the Small Business Administration and the Office of Management and Budget. The EO set forth the task force's mission as follows:

> Sec. 9. Mission of the Task Force. The mission of the Task Force shall be to:
>
> (a) identify and examine existing Federal services that currently are provided to returning Global War on Terror service members;
>
> (b) identify existing gaps in such services;
>
> (c) seek recommendations from appropriate Federal agencies on ways to fill those gaps as effectively and expeditiously as possible using existing resources; and
>
> (d) (i) ensure that in providing services to these service members, appropriate Federal agencies are communicating and cooperating effectively, and (ii) facilitate the fostering of agency communications and cooperation through informal and formal means, as appropriate. (EO 13426, 2007)

This section of the EO opened the discussion to all returning service members. The task force was given 45 days to complete its work.

[11]   Other witnesses were, for DoD, David S. C. Chu, Under Secretary for Personnel and Readiness, and Preston M. Geren III, Acting Secretary of the Army, for the VA, Daniel L. Cooper, Under Secretary for Benefits, and Gerald Cross, Acting Principal Deputy Under Secretary for Health, VHA; and for the Veterans' Disability Benefits Commission, LTG James Terry Scott (U.S. Army, Ret.).

the problems and fix them" (England, 2007b, p. 2). On May 3, 2007, at the direction of Secretary Gates, Deputy Secretary England announced the establishment of the Wounded, Ill, and Injured Senior Oversight Committee (SOC)[12] to "ensure that the recommendations of the Independent Review Group, the President's Commission on Care for Returning Wounded Warriors, and the Interagency Task Force [on Returning Global War on Terror Heroes] are promptly and properly integrated and implemented, coordinated, and resourced" (England, 2007a). The SOC was to

> streamline, deconflict, and expedite the Department's efforts to improve the medical care process, disability processing, and transition activities to the Department of Veterans Affairs for all military personnel, but particularly to improve the support of an injured Service member's recovery, rehabilitation, and reintegration. (England, 2007a)

The SOC also assumed responsibility for developing and implementing policies designed to improve the care, management, and transition of recovering service members, as Congress had mandated in the FY 2008 NDAA (Pub. L. 110-181, 2008).[13]

The SOC was personally chaired by the deputy secretary and initially included the service secretaries, the chairman or vice chairman of the Joint Chiefs of Staff, the comptroller, the Under Secretary of Defense for Personnel and Readiness, the service chiefs or vice chiefs, the Assistant Secretary of Defense for Health Affairs, the DoD General Counsel, the Director of Administration and Management, and a senior representative from the VA. Later, the Office of Management and Budget was added, and White House representatives attended regularly. The SOC met weekly for more than one year. At the first meeting of the SOC, the Deputy Secretary of Veterans Affairs, Gordon Mansfield, accepted the invitation to cochair the committee, thus marking an unprecedented level of attention to the needs of wounded warriors on behalf of the senior leadership of both DoD and the VA. The SOC addressed a number of major focus areas, which the committee called *lines of action*: a disability evaluation system (DES); TBI and PTSD; case management; DoD/VA data sharing; facilities; a clean sheet review; legislation and public affairs; and personnel, pay, and financial support.

In 2009, GAO reported to Congress that DoD and the VA had "made substantial progress in jointly developing policies . . . in the areas of (1) care and management, (2) medical and disability evaluation, (3) return to active duty, and (4) transition of care and services received from DOD to VA" (Williamson, 2009b, p. i). The report

---

[12] Secretary Gates noted that the Wounded Warrior Task Force he had created, which Deputy Secretary England referred to as the SOC, dealt with the same "primary issues addressed by the West-Marsh independent review . . . and the presidential Dole-Shalala commission" (Gates, 2014, p. 136).

[13] Specifically, the 2008 NDAA directed DoD and the VA to develop and implement a policy covering each of the following: (1) care and management, (2) medical evaluation and disability evaluation, (3) the return of service members to active duty, and (4) the transition of recovering service members from DoD to VA (Pub. L. 110-181, Sec. 1611(a)(2), 2008).

highlighted the actions of the SOC to pilot a joint DES to improve the timeliness and resource use of its separate DESs and to establish the Federal Recovery Coordination Program in response to the report of the Dole-Shalala Commission. GAO commended the SOC for completing more than two-thirds of the required policies for the care and management of recovering service members, including the policies for transitioning recovering service members back to active duty or from DoD to the VA, and for developing the procedures, processes, and standards for improving the transition of policies to improve the medical and physical disability evaluation. The report highlighted areas that the SOC found particularly challenging, including increased support for family caregivers, improving TBI and PTSD screening and treatment, and release of psychological health treatment records to DoD by VA health care providers, particularly for members of the National Guard and Reserves (Williamson, 2009b, pp. 17–20). GAO also highlighted future challenges as a result of the SOC experiencing "turnover in leadership, reconfiguration in its organizational structure at DOD, and changes affecting policy development responsibilities" as well as "leadership changes caused by the turnover in presidential administrations as well as turnover in some of its key staff" (Williamson, 2009b, p. 20).

As the Bush administration drew to a close in 2008, it was clear that arrangements needed to be made to ensure the permanence of the wounded warrior support network, which had been established in an ad hoc manner, with borrowed manpower, through the SOC and its supporting structures. As a result, the Under Secretary of Defense for Personnel and Readiness established a new Deputy Under Secretary of Defense for Transition Policy and Care Coordination with supporting staff.[14] The position was to be a permanent liaison with the VA and assumed responsibility for the DES and policies overseeing the recovery care provided to wounded warriors and their families. This marks the first time that an organization at that senior a level was established in DoD with the full-time job of interfacing and coordinating with the VA.[15] Congress was also concerned about the survivability of the effort, particularly about DoD and VA coordination, and included a provision in the FY 2009 NDAA (Pub. L. 110–417, 2008) to continue the existence of the SOC through December 31, 2009; in the FY 2010 NDAA (Pub. L. 111–84, 2009), Congress directed DoD to establish a task force to assess the effectiveness of the policies and programs DoD developed and implemented (Pub. L. 111–84, 2009, Sec. 724).

On November 20, 2012, the Secretary of Defense established the DoD Task Force on the Care, Management, and Transition of Recovering Wounded, Ill, and

---

[14] This later became known as the Deputy Assistant Secretary of Defense for Wounded Warrior Care and Transition Policy but has now been dismantled into separate offices for wounded warrior care and transition policy.

[15] The Office of Strategic Planning and Performance Management was also established within the office of the Deputy Under Secretary of Defense for Plans; within it was an executive secretariat headed by a member of the Senior Executive Service to ensure interoperability of DoD and VA health information systems. It was staffed by DoD and VA employees and reported independently to the deputy secretaries of both agencies.

Injured Members of the Armed Forces (Recovering Warrior Task Force, 2012). At the recommendation of the task force, the SOC was consolidated in early 2012 with the more recently established interagency executive committee for coordination across the two departments, the Joint Executive Council.[16] Over its life, the SOC had won praise from GAO, but over time, GAO concluded that the SOC had

> lost many of the characteristics that had made it a strong decision making and oversight body . . . . What had originally made it strong were
>
> - high-level leadership participation without substitution of lower-ranking officials,
> - rapid policy development and quick decision making, and
> - rigorous monitoring to hold the military services and the two departments accountable for needed actions. (Williamson, 2012, p. 27)

GAO noted the "departure of [the committee's] cochairs, the Deputy Secretaries, as well as turnover in some of its key staff" (Williamson, 2012, p. 26) and disruptions due to "changing the organizational structure of the committee and realigning and incorporating the committee's staff and responsibilities into existing or newly created DOD and VA offices" (Williamson, 2012, p. 27).

Of particular interest was the transfer of responsibilities to line organizations within DoD. As noted, the Office of the Deputy Under Secretary of Defense for Transition Policy and Care Coordination was established in 2008. The office was renamed in 2009, as the Office of Wounded Warrior Care and Transition Policy, reporting to the Under Secretary of Defense for Personnel and Readiness. It was described as the

> single, centralized office for developing policy, coordinating interagency collaboration, and conducting outreach to address the broad set of issues confronted by wounded, ill and injured service members and their families. . . . [The office] also

---

[16] The task force found that there was

general agreement that a standing/ongoing joint DoD/VA coordinating body is needed to ensure that Service members and veterans are receiving care and services in a seamless manner. The SOC was an effective mechanism for sharing information between DoD and VA and for identifying obstacles and opportunities for coordination. However, the current role of the SOC is not well-defined . . . and there are questions about whether the SOC at this time is able to provide sustained attention at the highest levels to the issues facing RWs [Recovering Warriors] and to seek accountability across both departments. There has been no formal mechanism for assessing whether SOC initiatives and goals have been partially or formally implemented and met. . . . Duplication of effort by the SOC and the JEC [Joint Executive Council] addressing similar issues is not cost-effective and can lead to unnecessary competition for resources and direction.

Consolidation of the two bodies would continue to engage the power residing in the offices of the Deputy Secretary of Defense and the Deputy Secretary of VA. Those issues that are confined strictly to the RW population would be addressed within an appropriate working group or team within the consolidated council. (Green, Crockett-Jones, and Guice, 2011, pp. 23–24)

provided program oversight for the integrated disability evaluation system process and care coordination. (Williamson, 2012, p. 26)

In June 2012, it was again renamed, first as Warrior Care Policy in the Office of the Assistant Secretary of Defense for Health Affairs, and then on October 1, 2013, as the Defense Health Agency (DoD, undated).

Significant Issues

The various studies and commissions originally initiated to address the problems at Walter Reed ended up addressing a number of broader issues,[17] most notably (1) the creation of dedicated units to look after wounded soldiers while in outpatient status, (2) coordination between the DoD and VA in the management of cases, (3) the prioritization of services to facilitate treatment for those seriously wounded in combat, (4) support for their families, and (5) the reform of the medical and disability rating system to facilitate the transfer of responsibilities from DoD to the VA.

Warrior Transition Units

The Army's program to address the medical holding issues for enlisted personnel highlighted in the *Washington Post* articles was not limited to changes at Walter Reed. Across the Army, Warrior Transition Units (WTUs) were set up to provide an integrated continuum of care for soldiers who generally required more than six months of treatment or who had conditions that required them to go through the MEB process. The WTU was more than just a housing arrangement; it was designed as a system of supervised care for each soldier built around a triad of caregivers. The first caregiver was a primary care manager, usually a physician, to provide primary oversight and continuity of health care and ensure the quality of care. The second, a nurse case manager, was usually a registered nurse, who was to plan, implement, coordinate, monitor, and evaluate options and services. The final caregiver was an NCO squad leader, who was to build a relationship with the soldier to link him or her to the chain of command and, working alongside the other parts of the triad, ensure that the needs of the soldier and his or her family were met. The Army established 32 WTUs, one at every MTF with 35 or more eligible service members. The staffing ratios were "1:200 for primary care managers; 1:18 for nurse case managers at Army medical centers that normally see patients with more acute conditions and 1:36 for other types of Army medical treatment facilities; and 1:12 for squad leaders" (Bertoni and Pendleton, 2008, p. 6).[18]

---

[17] These fundamental issues were highlighted by Secretary Gates in his memoir (Gates, 2014, pp. 136–139).

[18] And as noted in Williamson, 2009a, pp. 9–11.

In February 2008, a year after the original *Washington Post* articles appeared, GAO reported on the progress the Army was making in implementing the WTU program; almost 75 percent of the required staff was onboard, and 21 of the 32 units were manned at 90 percent or more. However, about 20 percent of the staff had been borrowed from other parts of the MTF (Bertoni and Pendleton, 2008, p. 10).[19] In terms of soldiers served, 7,900 were assigned to WTUs (76 percent of the eligible population), but 2,500 soldiers going through the MEB process had not yet been assigned to WTUs.[20] By June 2008, the WTU population had reached 10,300 (Williamson, 2009a, p. 2). By late 2014. more than 64,000 soldiers had gone through WTUs, with 46 percent returned to active duty, and 53 percent separated from the Army (Tarrant, Friedman, and Parks, 2014a, p. 8).

Performance of WTUs Over Time

To monitor WTU performance and ensure feedback to installation leadership, the Army established the Wounded Soldier and Family Hotline and requires WTUs to hold monthly town hall meetings, initiate ombudsman programs, and conduct periodic program-satisfaction surveys on certain anniversary dates—30, 120, 280, and 410 days after entering the WTU. GAO, however, was concerned that the overall monthly response rates, which ranged between 13 and 35 percent, were sufficiently low to decrease

> the likelihood that the survey results accurately reflect the views and characteristics of the target population.

> Despite low response rates, the Army has not conducted additional analyses to determine whether its survey results are representative of the entire WTU servicemember population. (Williamson, 2009a, p. 17)

Prophetically, GAO concluded:

> Without representative information, the Army cannot reliably report servicemembers' satisfaction with the WTUs, and without such data Army officials could

---

[19] In July 2008, the Army told WTU commanders, MTF commanders, and senior installation commanders to fill 100 percent of WTU staff shortages, including those related to the triad of care. As of August 2008, Army data indicated that this goal had been met, with the exception of one position each at four locations.

[20] GAO noted that

> Army officials told us that the population of 2,500 servicemembers who had not been moved into a Warrior Transition Unit consisted of both servicemembers who had just recently been identified as eligible for a unit but had not yet been evaluated and servicemembers whose risk assessment determined that their care could be managed outside of a unit. Officials told us that servicemembers who needed their care managed more intensively through Warrior Transition Units had been identified through the risk assessment process and had been moved into such units. (Bertoni and Pendleton, 2008, p. 13)

potentially be unaware of serious deficiencies like those that were identified at Walter Reed in 2007. (Williamson, 2009a, p. 20)

Without such data, we continue to believe that the Army cannot reliably report servicemembers' satisfaction with the WTUs and that Army leadership could potentially be unaware of serious deficiencies in some of its WTUs. (Williamson, 2009a, p. 22)

On November 22, 2014, the *Dallas Morning News* and broadcast partner KXAS-TV published the first of a series of articles alleging mistreatment of soldiers assigned to WTUs at three bases in Texas: Fort Hood in Killeen, Fort Bliss in El Paso, and Fort Sam Houston in San Antonio. Their report noted that

[s]ome soldiers expressed satisfaction with their experience in the WTUs, but many others said they were frustrated and angry over their treatment.

Words like "harass," "belittle," "treated unfairly" and "insulting" come up frequently over the five-year period covered by the documents. The complaints included those made by soldiers to the Army Medical Command's ombudsman program as well as during town hall meetings and "sensing sessions" held within the WTUs. (Tarrant, Friedman, and Parks, 2014a, p. 3)

The heart of the problem seemed to be the "constant friction between military requirements and medical needs" (Tarrant, Friedman, and Parks, 2014a, p. 5), with soldiers complaining that a "drill sergeant–type culture exists within the WTUs that makes recovery harder, not easier, especially for soldiers dealing with mental health conditions such as PTSD" (Tarrant, Friedman, and Parks, 2014a, p. 4). For its part, the Army told the *Dallas Morning News* that it encourages soldiers to bring such issues forward through the chain of command or other official avenues, was aware of the complaints, but did not "see a pervasive problem out there when it comes down to treating our soldiers and family members with dignity and respect" (Col. Chris Toner, as quoted in Tarrant, Friedman and Parks, 2014b, p. 3). However, according to Dr. Stephen M. Stahl, a professor of psychiatry at the University of California, San Diego, who had been hired by the Army to improve Fort Hood's WTU program, much of the problem related to soldiers with PTSD. He found a "stunning lack of knowledge about PTSD. Many did not believe that PTSD was a real medical condition. . . . [T]he Army's warrior culture continues to hinder full acceptance of mental health conditions among soldiers" (Tarrant, Friedman, and Parks, 2014a, p. 8).

As it turned out, the issues the *Dallas Morning News* identified, particularly as they related to soldiers with PTSD, had been highlighted in several DoD IG reports as early as 2011. At Fort Drum, the DoD IG found that

[s]quad leaders also agreed that more training on TBI and PTSD would help them execute their Warrior support responsibilities because of the high number of War-

riors in the WTB [Warrior Transition Battalion] with one or both of these conditions. (Moorefield, 2011, p. 40)

During multiple group interviews, nurse case managers overwhelmingly agreed that they needed initial and ongoing training on behavioral health issues such as PTSD, substance abuse, and depression. They also recommended additional training on TBI, psychiatric medications, and Fort Drum–specific policies and procedures. (Moorefield, 2011, p. 41)

At Joint Base Lewis-McChord, the DoD IG reported,

WTB leadership commented that an estimated sixty percent of the Soldiers assigned to the JBLM [Joint Base Lewis-McChord] WTB had behavioral health issues, with an estimated forty percent of the Soldiers having PTSD or TBI. Given the prevalence of these conditions, WTB leadership and staff recognized the need for additional PTSD/TBI and behavioral health training opportunities. (Moorefield, 2013, p. 32)[21]

As a result of the articles in the *Dallas Morning News*, the House Armed Services Subcommittee on Military Personnel included a provision in the FY 2016 NDAA (Pub. L. 114–92, 2015) for GAO to review various aspects of the program (see Jahner, 2015; H.R. 1735, 2015).

While GAO did not directly address the issues raised by the *Dallas Morning News*, it did note in July 2016 that the original Army program was established when WTU soldiers' diagnoses were primarily for physical conditions (Farrell, 2016b).[22] Since then, the composition of diagnoses has changed significantly; during 2008, the first full year of the WTU program, 36 percent of WTU soldiers had behavioral health diagnoses; in 2015, about 52 percent had such diagnoses. As a result, social workers have been informally added to the WTUs' interdisciplinary team, often directly providing certain types of behavioral health care, such as therapy sessions, because obtaining appointments can be difficult otherwise. At one WTU GAO representatives

[21] The DoD IG also noted that a

Health Care Administrator from Madigan Army Medical Center (MAMC) reported that Soldiers in the WTB spent between 327 days and 455 days from start of MEB until the packages were forwarded for PEB. The established DoD standard for moving Soldiers through the MEB process was 100 calendar days. . . .

Subsequent to our visit, complaints were made by Soldiers and Soldiers' families to their congressional representatives about practices at MAMC which resulted in PTSD disability ratings being reversed by the forensic psychiatry team. Based on these complaints, on May 16, 2012, the Secretary of the Army and Army Chief of Staff announced a comprehensive, Army-wide review of Soldier behavioral health diagnoses and evaluations at all of its medical facilities since 2001. This effort, along with the already identified backlog of MEB cases placed an additional burden on MAMC resources. (Moorefield, 2013, p. 53)

[22] GAO noted that, because the WTU program "declined from a peak of 12,228 in 2008 to 2,628 in 2015," the Army "reduced the number of WTUs, from a high of 45 units in 2008 to the planned 14 by August 2016" (Farrell, 2016b, p. 1). Twelve additional community care units provide care through the TRICARE network.

visited, they noted that, "in addition to providing the social workers' therapy sessions, the unit borrows a psychiatrist from the local military treatment facility 2 days each week to provide behavioral health care" (Farrell, 2016b, p. 12). They also noted that, "[a]t the remaining WTU, the local military treatment facility contracted for a full-time psychiatrist to meet soldiers' need for behavioral health services" (Farrell, 2016b, p. 12). GAO did point out that these arrangements were ad hoc and had not been formally incorporated into the Army's staffing models. This is somewhat moot because the Army is having significant problems attracting and retaining mental health professionals. In fall 2015, the *Dallas Morning News* reported that "Fort Hood currently has four vacant psychiatrist positions, 11 vacant psychologist positions and 25 openings for social workers" (Tarrant, Friedman, and Parks, 2015).

Case Management—Coordination of Patient Clinical and Support Services

DoD and VA coordination of patient services has been a problem since the establishment of modern veterans' programs during World War I.[23] To improve coordination immediately after 9/11, the VA provided a vocational rehabilitation counselor to work with hospitalized patients at Walter Reed. Systemwide changes, however, remained problematic:

- In September 2003, the VA instructed its regional offices to work with DoD and to assign case managers and, in some cases, social workers and disability compensation benefits counselors to assist seriously injured service members returning from Afghanistan and Iraq.
- In spring 2004, VA submitted a draft memorandum of agreement to DoD's Office of the Assistant Secretary of Defense for Health Affairs proposing that DoD provide lists of all injured service members admitted to MTFs so that the VA might start to provide information and support to facilitate their eventual transition to the VA. The draft was not acted on.
- In 2005, GAO found that VA still lacked access to DoD data that would allow it to identify and locate all seriously injured servicemembers because DoD had "privacy concerns about the type of information that VA had requested and the time that VA wants it to be provided" (Bascetta, 2005b, p. 3).[24] In particular,

---

[23] The events are recounted in the Army's official history (Crane, 1927, p. 254):

> Application was made to the Surgeon General of the Army late in June, 1918, for permission to send representatives of the Federal Board for Vocational Education into Army hospitals to explain to disabled men the benefits of the new [Smith-Sears Act] law. The permission was not given until after the armistice began, on the grounds that the rehabilitated men would be needed in the Army for limited service and should not be brought into contact with civilians seeking their ultimate restoration to industrial life.

[24] GAO reported that the VA was

> challenged to reach injured servicemembers early for several reasons. First, determining the best time to approach recently injured servicemembers and gauge their personal receptivity to consider employment in the

DoD thought it premature for VA to begin working with injured service members who may, given advances in medicine and prosthetic devices, eventually remain on active duty. DoD officials told GAO that "information could be made available to VA 'upon separation' from military service, that is, when a servicemember enters the separation process" (Bascetta, 2005b, p. 16).

- On March 5, 2007, the Subcommittee on National Security and Foreign Affairs of the Committee on Oversight and Government Reform of the House of Representatives held its first congressional hearings to deal with conditions at Walter Reed. During those hearings, the issue of VA access came up with the Army Vice Chief of Staff, GEN Dick Cody. At the hearings, D.C. Representative Eleanor Holmes Norton said:

> it seems to me that one of the first orders of business would have been to get your two departments of the government so that they agree on a way to deal with these soldiers that reduces—considerably—not only the confusion, but the time spent in two systems trying to figure out which one is best for you.
>
> It's more than we ought to ask a soldier to do. ("Congressional Hearing on Walter Reed Army Medical Center," 2007, p. 119)

- In 2007, the Task Force on Returning Global War on Terror Heroes reported that

> [t]here are no formal agreements as to how active duty servicemembers will be co-managed when they receive health care and services from both DoD and VA. There are no agreements on the definition of case management, the functions of case managers, or how DoD and VA case managers transfer patients to one another to assure continuity of care. (Task Force on Returning Global War on Terror Heroes, 2007, p. 24)

- In January 2008, Congress enacted the FY 2008 NDAA (Pub. L. 110-181, 2008), which required DoD and the VA to jointly develop and implement a comprehensive policy on improvements to (1) care and management, (2) medical evaluation and disability evaluation, (3) the return of service members to active duty, and (4) the transition of recovering service members from DoD to VA. However, the

---

civilian sector is inherently difficult. The nature of the recovery process is highly individualized and requires professional judgment to determine the appropriate time to begin vocational rehabilitation. Further, because VA is trying to prepare servicemembers who are still on active duty for a transition to civilian life, DOD is concerned that VA's efforts may be working at cross purposes to the military's retention goals. Finally, because VA lacks systematic information from DOD on seriously injured servicemembers, VA cannot ensure that all servicemembers and veterans who could benefit from the VR&E [Vocational Rehabilitation and Employment] program have the opportunity to receive services at the appropriate time. (Bascetta, 2005b, p. 12)

DoD and VA were unable to resolve the issues of case management, leading to "confusion and the duplication of services" (Williamson, 2011, p. 20).[25]

- In March 2011, GAO noted that there were numerous problems in the coordination of the numerous, often overlapping programs. It identified seven programs that provided individual and separate recovery and nonclinical plans, five of which also developed their own clinical plans.[26] Moreover, it was common for soldiers to be enrolled in several programs at the same time. According to GAO,

> [i]n September 2010, approximately 84 percent of FRCP [Federal Recovery Coordination Program] enrollees were also enrolled in a military service wounded warrior program. According to one FRC, his enrollees have, on average, eight case managers who are affiliated with different programs. Individuals enrolled in multiple programs may have recovery plans or goals that have been developed by different programs. Moreover, some case managers of other programs consider themselves to be the single point of contact for their enrollees, even those enrolled in the FRCP. (Williamson, 2011, p. 22)

- In October 2011, GAO told Congress,

> DOD and VA have made little progress reaching agreement on options to better integrate the FRCP and RCP [Recovery Coordination Program], although they have made a number of attempts to address this issue. . . . This lack of progress illustrates DOD's and VA's continued difficulty in collaborating to resolve duplication and overlap between care coordination programs. (Draper, 2011, p. i)

When it last reported to Congress in November 2012, GAO found little had changed.[27]

---

[25] For example, GAO noted one case in which a federal recovery coordinator (FRC) and a wounded warrior program recovery care coordinator were each unaware that the other was involved, and each established conflicting recovery goals. The FRC advised the amputee to separate from the military to receive needed services from VA, while the recovery care coordinator set the goal of remaining on active duty. "These conflicting goals caused considerable confusion for this servicemember and his family" (Williamson, 2011, p. 24).

[26] See Table 4 in Williamson, 2011, pp. 21–22.

[27] The GAO report to Congress in 2012 has the following assessment:

> Since the inception of the RCP in 2008, the FRCP and RCP care coordination programs have conflicted with one another and with other case management programs that provide services to recovering servicemembers and veterans. Conflicting issues have arisen as to what populations they serve, the specific services each would provide, and when each program would get involved in the servicemembers' recovery process. Aligning and integrating these programs with one another—especially the FRCP with the RCP—has proven to be a major challenge for DOD and VA. While the departments are developing an interagency strategy for minimizing duplication between DOD's and VA's care coordination and case management programs, the success of this effort will depend upon achieving cooperation between the departments—which has been elusive for many years—as well as with the military services. (Williamson, 2012, pp. 37–38)

Priority Care for the Most Serious Casualties of Combat

One area that particularly frustrated Secretary of Defense Gates was the opposition he perceived from the military and civilian bureaucracies, which, he felt, "just could not or would not differentiate the wounded in combat from all others needing care" (Gates, 2014, p. 137). Gates thought "the number of troops wounded in combat . . . represented a small fraction of all those treated" (Gates, 2014, p. 139) who "should be dealt with as a group by themselves and be afforded . . . 'platinum' treatment in terms of priority for appointments, for housing, for administrative assistance, and for anything else" (Gates, 2014, p. 137).[28] Accordingly, on January 6, 2009, over the objection of the services, the Under Secretary of Defense for Personnel and Readiness promulgated a policy of expediting service members with "catastrophic conditions and combat-related causes" through the DES (Chu, 2009). The military services were doubtful about the use of this process, believing that the underlying message for the wounded would be that they were being pushed out of their services prematurely and acknowledging that most members preferred to remain on DoD rolls as long as possible, having greater trust in DoD benefits and services. While on DoD rolls, the person receives military pay. Even if retired at more than 30-percent pay (which these service members would be), the ultimate disability payment they would receive from the VA had yet to be determined, resulting in uncertainty and angst.[29]

Support for the Families of the Wounded

Essential for the recovery, rehabilitation, and reintegration of the severely wounded, ill, and injured are the families and friends who facilitate activities of daily living. Generally referred to as *military caregivers*, they help with daily activities, "such as bathing or dressing, help manage medications, provide transportation to medical appointments, help the disabled up and down stairs, and aid in other ways" (Ramchand, Tanielian, et al., 2014, p. 1). This enables some seriously injured veterans to live at home rather than in institutions. Most recipients of such care today are veterans, but active-duty service members make up about 20 percent of the total (Ramchand, Tanielian, et al.,

---

[28] Deputy Secretary England made a similar point in his testimony of April 17, 2007:

> Another problem with the transition from DoD to the DVA is that the disability ratings process is "one size fits all"—the same basic procedures are followed . . . for all individuals. The 11% of cases that are those wounded or severely wounded in war are funneled through exactly the same system as the other 89%, the career service members transitioning to retirement. (England, 2007b, p. 4)

He implicitly asked whether these 11 percent should be given special treatment and what that treatment should be.

[29] Gates's notion of tiering ran counter to the position historically taken by veteran service organizations and endorsed by the Veterans Disability Benefits Commission: that all wounded, ill, and injured service members should be accorded the same treatment and benefits, regardless of the timing and source of their infirmity. More frustrating for Secretary Gates, he wrote, was that he "would never succeed in cracking the obduracy and resistance to change of the department's personnel and health care bureaucracy, both military and civilian. It was one of my biggest failures as secretary" (Gates, 2014, p. 142).

2014, Table 2.1, p. 32). Caregivers are predominantly spouses, parents, friends, and neighbors (Ramchand, Tanielian, et al., 2014, Table 2.2, p. 34). The most prevalent medical conditions for which care has been provided are disabilities that impair physical movement (80.3 percent), mental health or substance abuse (64.0 percent), and hearing or vision problems (56.8 percent) (Ramchand, Tanielian, et al., 2014, Table 2.5, p. 48).

While on Active Duty

The rapidity with which severely injured service members are evacuated back to the United States and the relatively small number of casualties have allowed DoD to engage the families of the wounded in ways never before possible.[30] Throughout most of the conflicts in Afghanistan and Iraq, within hours of the decision to evacuate a wounded service member, a specially trained casualty assistance officer notifies the designated next of kin of the situation and arranges for up to three family members to receive Invitational Travel Orders to travel to the medical treatment facility to which the wounded service member will be taken. These orders, which are generally for two-week periods but can be extended, provide travel expenses, lodging, local transportation expenses, and an allowance for daily expenses. The local arrangements are handled through on-base Soldier and Family Assistance Centers. A survey by the Dole-Shalala Commission found that "most injured service members, especially active-duty personnel, have had family members join them soon after they are medically evacuated to the United States" (Dole-Shalala Commission, 2007b, p. 73), as shown in Figure 9.1; many relocate and give up jobs to provide care.

On average, family members stayed 45 days at bedside. A small number of the most severely injured underwent extensive periods of rehabilitation, often with family members in attendance. Until 2010, no explicit benefits were provided for caregiving supporting the wounded who are still on active duty. Starting in 2010, Congress authorized Special Compensation for Assistance with Activities of Daily Living for service members who incur permanent, catastrophic illnesses or injuries in the line of duty that require the services of a home health aide to provide nonmedical care, support, and assistance.

In addition to the normal resources DoD provides for the dependents of those on active duty, numerous military and community support organizations have supported the wounded and their families, as shown in Figure 9.2. The Fisher House Programs, which provide a temporary housing adjacent to MTFs, are of particular interest.[31] In 2016, 72 Fisher Houses were located on 24 military installations and at 29 VA medi-

---

[30] The families of the wounded have received an unprecedented level of support, but can this be sustained during a future conflict if the casualty rates and numbers are much higher, and if U.S. command of the air is less absolute, preventing AE to CONUS?

[31] The Fisher House Foundation also administers a program called Hero Miles that provides round-trip airfare to eligible wounded, injured, and ill service members and families. Service members who are not eligible for government-funded travel may be covered for visits home or to authorized events. Family or close friends may

Figure 9.1
Percentage of Returning Injured Service Members with Families in Attendance

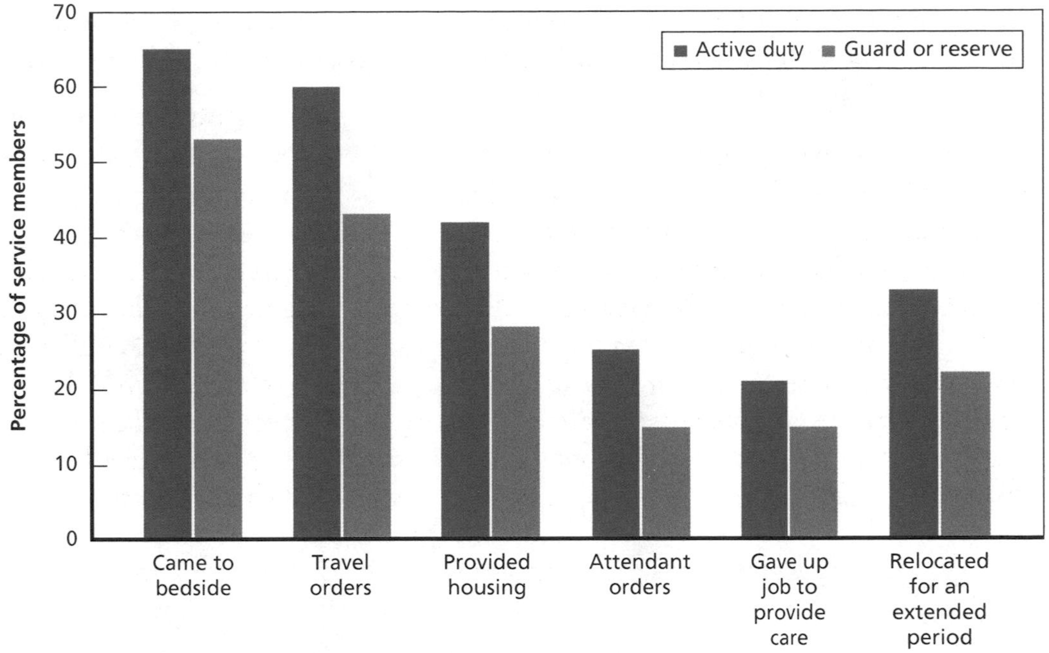

SOURCES: Dole-Shalala Commission, 2007a, p. 9; Dole-Shalala Commission, 2007b, pp. 74, 76.

cal centers, serving more than 28,000 families. The average stay lasts 10 days. These facilities have a daily capacity of 950 families.

Under the Auspices of the VA

Many casualties of war require continuing care after their initial hospitalization; this is often provided by professional caregivers but frequently by family members. There is a long history, going back to the Civil War, of the government financially support-ing disabled veterans by defraying the cost of long-term care, either by increasing vet-eran's pensions or by directly supporting caregivers through a variety of home-based programs.[32]

---

receive round-trip tickets to visit service members undergoing treatment at an authorized medical center. (See DVA, 2016d.)

[32] VA offers a variety of services through the Veterans with Family Caregivers program, including home-based primary care, home hospice care, homemaker and home health aides, home telehealth, respite care, and skilled home care (DVA, 2017c).

Figure 9.2
Percentage of Families Helped by Nonprofit Groups

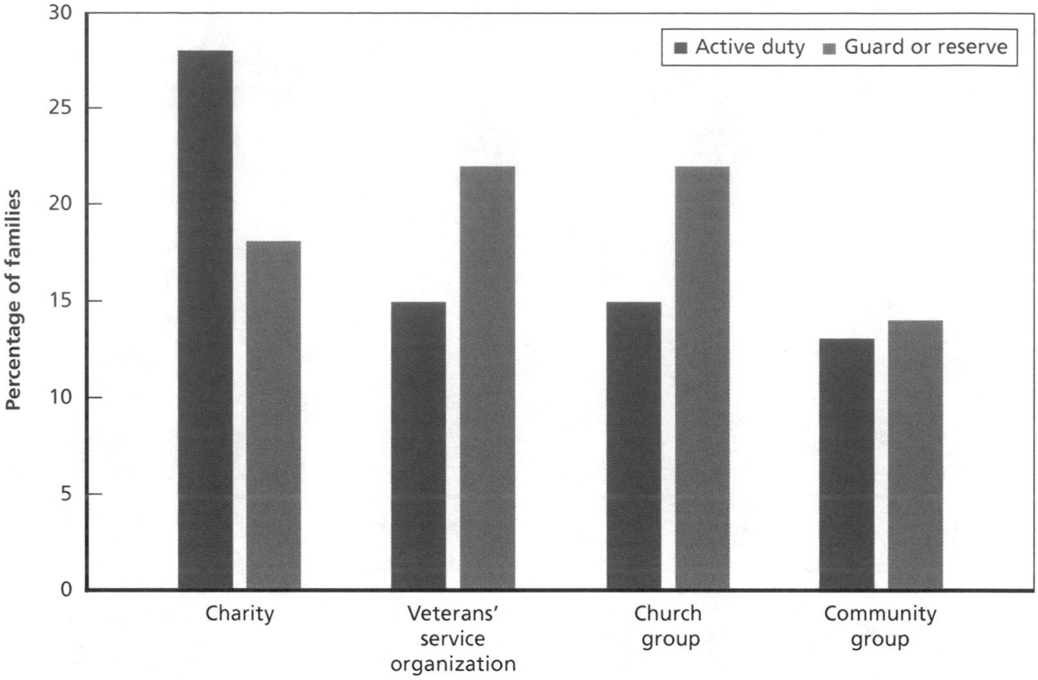

SOURCE: Dole-Shalala Commission, 2007b, p. 77.

Aid and Attendance and Housebound

Increased pensions for veterans suffering from certain service-connected disabilities who were "permanently and totally disabled as to render them utterly helpless, or so nearly so as to require the constant personal aid and attendance of another person," have been part of the veterans' pension system since the Civil War and were first initiated on June 6, 1866. The law was modified in 1873 to allow "the pension for a disability not permanent, equivalent in degree . . . during the continuance of the disability in such degree, at the same rate as that herein provided for a permanent disability of like degree."[33] Currently, veterans and survivors who are "eligible for a VA pension and require the aid and attendance of another person, or are housebound, may also be eligible for additional monetary payment" (DVA, 2015).[34]

---

[33] The approval of Pub. L. 66-190 on May 1, 1920, provided for payments "by reason of age and physical or mental disabilities, helpless or blind, or so nearly helpless or blind as to require the regular personal aid and attendance of another person" (Keener, 1994).

[34] In addition, monthly pension payments may be increased if a veteran meets one of the following conditions (DVA, 2015):

Program of Comprehensive Assistance for Family Caregivers

In May 2010, Congress passed the *Caregivers and Veterans Omnibus Health Services Act of 2010* (Pub. L. 111-163, 2010), which required the VA to establish a program to assist caregivers with the rigors of caring for seriously injured veterans. In May 2011, VHA established the Program of Comprehensive Assistance for Family Caregivers for post-9/11 veterans and the Program of General Caregiver Support Services for all other veterans, at each of its VA medical centers to provide financial stipend, access to health care insurance, mental health services and counseling, caregiver training, and respite care.[35] Caregivers were to be supervised by caregiver support coordinators at a planned coordinator-to-caregiver ratio of 1:34 to 1:167, depending on geographic dispersion.

To be eligible for the post-9/11 program, the veteran must have incurred or aggravated a serious injury, including TBI, psychological trauma, or other mental disorder, in the line of duty on or after 9/11. He or she requires another person—a caregiver—to assist with the management of personal care functions required in everyday living for a minimum of six continuous months at home. The caregiver must be at least 18 years of age and must be the veteran's spouse, son, daughter, parent, stepfamily member, extended family member, or someone who lives with the veteran full time. The VA provides the caregiver with either training (in the classroom, online, or through a self-study course), after which the caregiver must be able to demonstrate the ability to assist the veteran with personal care functions required in everyday living. While a veteran may have up to three approved caregivers at a time under the program, only the primary caregiver is eligible for the full range of services. A primary family caregiver will be designated who will receive a monthly stipend based on the veteran's level of need and required assistance. In addition, the primary family caregiver may also be eligible to receive his or her own medical care through the Civilian Health and Medical Program of the Department of Veterans Affairs (CHAMPVA) (DVA, 2017d),[36] the medical care insurance for family members of those who are totally disabled or who died of service-related causes. However, CHAMPVA limits eligibility to spouses, surviving spouses, and children. It does not extend to extended family members or others who might be caregivers and have given up their jobs and, thus, health insurance. GAO

- The veteran requires "the aid of another person in order to perform personal functions required in everyday living, such as bathing, feeding, dressing, attending to the wants of nature, adjusting prosthetic devices, or protecting" the veteran from the hazards of his or her "daily environment."
- The veteran is "bedridden, in that [the] disability or disabilities requires that [he/she] remain in bed apart from any prescribed course of convalescence or treatment."
- The veteran is a "patient in a nursing home due to mental or physical incapacity."
- His or her "eyesight is limited to a corrected 5/200 visual acuity or less in both eyes; or concentric contraction of the visual field to 5 degrees or less."

[35] These programs are administered by the National Caregiver Support Program Office in the VA's national headquarters; collectively, they are referred to as the Caregiver Support Program.

[36] CHAMPVA is a comprehensive health care benefits program in which the VA shares the cost of covered health care services and supplies with eligible beneficiaries.

reported that, "as of May 2014, about 15,600 caregivers were approved for the Family Caregiver Program, and the estimated obligations for FY 2014 are over $263 million" (Williamson, 2014, p. 3).

Demand for the program has been higher than initially expected. VHA officials originally estimated that approximately 4,000 caregivers would be approved for the program by the end of FY 2014, but by May 2014, almost 30,400 caregivers had applied, and about 15,600 had been approved (Williamson, 2014, p. 12),[37] with a caregiver support coordinator–to-caregiver ratio as high as 1 to 251.[38] In 2016, 24,555 primary family caregivers were approved for the program, with 5,250 also participating in CHAMPVA. The budget request for FY 2018 was $604 million, a 14-percent increase, to support more than 37,100 caregivers, an increase of 3,755 (10 percent) over the 2017 level (DVA, 2017a).

In 2016, a survey of enrollees in the VA health care program found that "28 percent of enrollees indicated that they needed assistance for some or all . . . activities. Among this group of enrollees, 97 percent of these enrollees indicated that their need resulted from a health condition related to active duty service" (Huang et al., 2017, p. 69). Care was provided by a spouse (59 percent of the time), followed by an adult son or daughter (26 percent), other family members (26 percent) or by a friend or neighbor (20 percent). Sixty-eight percent reported that their primary caregiver lived in the same household as themselves, and the majority (63.3 percent) spent 10 hours or less per week providing assistance. The vast majority of those responding to the survey (82.5 percent) indicated that those providing assistance did not receive support from any program, and only 5.8 percent reported that their caregiver was receiving support from a VA-sponsored program. However, "enrollees in Priority Groups 4–6, ages 65 years and older, and enrollees who make less than $35,000 annually reported greater likelihoods of receiving caregiver support ser-

---

[37] GAO also reported that,

> [a]s of May 2014, approximately 15,600 caregivers had been approved for the program. About 6,000 of these caregivers were assigned to Tier 3 (highest level) for their stipend payments, about 6,000 to Tier 2 (middle level), and 3,600 to Tier 1 (lowest level). The average monthly payments per tier were approximately $2,320 for Tier 3, $1,470 for Tier 2, and $600 for Tier 1. At this time, almost 8 out of 10 of the caregivers approved for the Family Caregiver Program were spouses, while other approved caregivers were parents, relatives, and friends. Most of these caregivers were assisting veterans with mental health diagnoses or brain injuries who may also have had other physical injuries or disabilities. Specifically, 92 percent of these veterans have a service-connected mental health condition, 63 percent have PTSD, and 26 percent have a TBI. (Williamson, 2014, p. 11)

[38] Caregiver support coordinators told GAO that

> follow-up home visits occur every 6 to 9 months, in contrast to the program's standard of every 90 days. Delays in home visits could be problematic because these visits provide medical staff with an opportunity to assess the welfare and environment of the caregiver and veteran—issues that may not be evident during clinic visits, such as whether special dietary needs are being met and whether medications are being properly administered. (Williamson, 2014, p. 18)

vices from both VA-sponsored and non–VA-sponsored programs for caregiver support services" (Huang et al., 2017, p. 74).

The Transition from DoD to the VA: The Medical and Disability Evaluation Systems

The President's Commission on Care for America's Returning Wounded Warriors—the Dole-Shalala Commission—concluded that

> [i]njured service members who received excellent medical care on the battlefield and in the acute care hospital setting sometimes find themselves in a maze of disability policies and procedures. (Dole-Shalala Commission, 2007b, p. 93)

The maze of policies and procedures, including medical and disability evaluations, starts with the fact that soldiers separating from the military usually deal with the administrative processes of both DoD and the VA. The DoD system focuses on the soldier's medical condition relative to his or her ability to continue doing his or her military job, a job that reflects his or her occupation, grade, and years of service. The VA system takes a broader view, considering how medical condition affects earning and well-being over a lifetime, regardless of the specifics of the veteran's former military career. As a result, the Dole-Shalala Commission noted that each system "provide(s) different amounts of compensation for the same injury, based on their different approaches to rating disabilities" (Dole-Shalala Commission, 2007b, p. 93). Adding to the confusion was the fact that, until relatively recently, each department administered its own medical evaluations; today, both departments use a single examination, resulting in a common assessment of a separating soldier's medical condition and rating. The following subsections describe the evaluation systems both departments employed at the time and the major changes since 2007, specifically, the development and adoption of the DoD/VA Integrated Disability Evaluation System (IDES).

DoD's Physical Disability Evaluation System

The system for disability determination dates to legislation in 1790 that allowed disabled military personnel to be placed on "the list of the invalids of the United States"; officers received up to one-half pay and enlisted personnel up to $5 a month for life.[39] The first comprehensive disability retirement system for all regular officers was established by Congress in August 1861.[40] An 1867 act was the first law to authorize disability retirement for enlisted personnel (but applied only to the Navy and Marine Corps).[41] Numerous changes followed during rest of the 19th century and first half of

---

[39] *An Act for Regulating the Military Establishment of the United States* was approved April 30, 1790. Between 1790 and 2019, the dollar experienced an average inflation rate of 1.45 percent per year. The purchasing power of $5 in 1790 equates to $136.54 as of early 2019 (Official Data Foundation/Alioth LLC, 2019).

[40] *An Act Providing for the Better Organization of the Military Establishment* was approved August 3, 1861.

[41] *An Act to Amend Certain Acts in Relation to the Navy* was approved March 2, 1867.

the 20th century. In June 1941, Congress passed the first legislation to extend disability retirement to Army enlisted personnel with 20 or more years of service, creating the disability retirement system employed during World War II (Pub. L. 77-140, 1941).[42]

The World War II system was widely criticized,[43] leading to the passage of the Career Compensation Act of 1949 (Pub. L. 81-351, 1949), which covered officer and enlisted personnel of both the regular and reserve components, and authorized temporary as well as permanent disability retirements. Since 1946, service members who are permanently unfit to perform their duties may be retired, providing that the disability is rated at 30 percent or more or that they have served at least 20 years. If the permanency of the disability cannot be determined, the service member may be placed on the TDRL, receiving the same retired pay but subject to periodic reevaluation.[44] Service members with fewer than 20 years of creditable service and a disability rating less than 30 percent receive a lump sum severance disability payment. Service members with service-connected disabilities would usually be eligible for VA disability compensation. Until recently, this military benefit was offset by any VA compensation received. However, the FY 2004 NDAA (Pub. L. 108-136, 2003) allowed some military retirees to concurrently receive VA and military benefits.[45] Generally, military disability retirement pay is taxable. Exceptions are (1) if the disability pay is for combat-related injuries

---

[42] For a more complete discussion of the early disability retirement systems, see Pleeter, 2005, pp. 736–745.

[43] Pleeter, 2005, p. 745, listed the following as the main complaints:

(1) the award of wholly tax-exempt retired pay of 75 percent of active duty pay to any officer retired for disability, regardless of its severity, was unduly generous and costly;

(2) the system, especially the Army "emergency officer" procedure, discriminated against non-regular officers as compared with regulars;

(3) the system discriminated against enlisted personnel as compared with officers; and

(4) the fact that retirement authority was limited to permanent disability tended to burden the active list with personnel retained solely for medical observation and evaluation of the permanency of a disability.

[44] According to Pleeter, 2005, pp. 749–750,

A member on TDRL has the same retired pay entitlement as a member permanently retired for disability, except that there is a 50 percent floor as well as a 75 percent ceiling on temporary disability retired pay. A member on the TDRL must be physically examined at least once every 18 months to determine whether there has been a change in his disability and whether the disability is permanent in nature. A final determination on permanency must be made within five years of the member's placement on TDRL. If a periodic or final physical examination shows that a member's disability is permanent and stable and is rated as 30 percent or more, or if he has at least 20 years of service, the member is permanently retired in a disability status. If it is determined that the member's disability is permanent but is rated as less than 30 percent and he has less than 20 years of service, the member is removed from TDRL, separated from the service, and given disability severance pay. If it is determined that he is physically fit to perform his duties, the member must be removed from TDRL, with a concomitant cessation of disability retired pay, after which, with his consent, he may be reappointed or reenlisted on the active list or permanently separated without entitlement to either disability, retired, or severance pays.

[45] For a discussion of the concurrent receipt issues, see Henning, 2006.

or (2) if the service member was in the military or was under a binding written commitment to become a member, on September 24, 1975.

How the System Works

Subject to the overall guidance from the Secretary of Defense, each military department is responsible for developing a physical DES that meets the unique demands of its service or services.[46] The system determines the fitness for duty of military members who have medical concerns. For those found unfit, the system assigns a *percentage of disability* for the unfitting conditions, which may determine lifelong compensation and access to military benefits. If a service member's disability is rated at 30 percent or higher, he or she is entitled to retire and thus receive the benefits that accrue to retirement without completing normal time in service to retirement. Among the more important benefits is lifetime access to military health care for the service member and his or her family. With a rating less than 30 percent, the individual would receive a disability severance payment equal to twice the number of years of service multiplied by monthly base pay. Higher ratings from the system are thus desirable, with retirement being the ultimate goal for many service members.

In the simplest terms, the DES is made up of four elements (see Figure 9.3): medical evaluation; physical disability evaluation, including appellate review; counseling; and final disposition.

In practice, however, the system is much more complex, as noted in Figure 9.4. In 2006, GAO found that

> the services were not achieving the DOD timeliness goals for processing disability cases and DOD was not monitoring achievement of these goals. . . . Our analysis . . . also suggests that outcomes for active duty and reserve component members of the military may not be consistent. (Bertoni, 2007, p. 2)

> [T]raining for MEB and PEB disability evaluation staff designed to produce timely and consistent decisions was lacking. (Bertoni, 2007, p. 3)

The Medical Evaluation Board

The MEB is the first step in the system for determining fitness for duty and, ultimately, a disability rating for a service member who has been wounded. After treatment at an MTF is considered complete, a MEB determines whether the member

---

[46] For a discussion of how the services implement the disability system differently, see Robertson, 2006, pp. 13–15:

> Specifically, the aspects of the system that differ among the services include: characteristics of the medical evaluation board (MEB) and physical evaluation board (PEB), the use of counselors to help service members navigate the system, and procedures to make line of duty determinations. (Robertson, 2006, p. 13)

Figure 9.3
Elements of the Disability Evaluation System

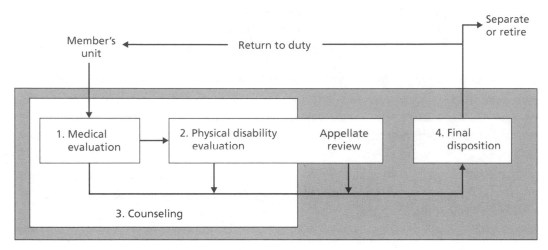

SOURCE: Marcum et al., 2002, p. 17.

meets the medical standard for retention, based on medical evidence,[47] DoD policy guidance, and military service regulations. The Army MEB generally consists of two or three physicians plus a reviewing authority. The board does not convene physically but passes the medical records among the designated members. Following Army regulations, the MEB documents the soldier's medical status and duty limitations based on the medical diagnosis and prognosis. The board then

> evaluates and reports on the (1) diagnosis; (2) prognosis for return to full duty; (3) plan for further treatment, rehabilitation, or convalescence; (4) estimated length of time the disabling condition will exist; and (5) medical recommendations for the disposition of the service member. (Marcum et al., 2002, p. 25)

> [It then determines] the service member's ability to meet medical retention standards only for his or her *current* military occupational specialty. (Marcum et al., 2002, p. 26)

The MEB may recommend either return to duty or referral to the Physical Disability Evaluation Board or may return the case for further medical evaluation, treatment, or clarification.

The Physical Evaluation Board

If the MEB determines that the soldier does not meet the medical standard, he or she is referred to the Army Physical Disability Evaluation Agency, the Adjutant General

---

[47] The medical evaluation is to determine whether "the service member meets the military's retention standards, according to each service's regulations" (Robertson, 2006, p. 8).

Figure 9.4
DoD Physical Disability Evaluation System

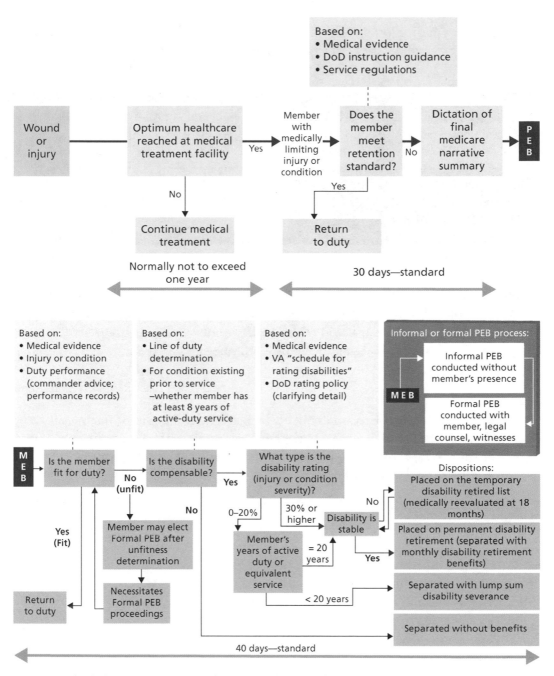

SOURCE: Dole-Shalala Commission, 2007b, p. 95.

Directorate of the Army Human Resources Command for evaluation by a PEB. It is the PEB that determines whether the soldier is fit for duty, that is, can perform the duties of their military specialty and their rank. There are two levels of adjudication: Informal PEB adjudication and Formal PEB adjudication. The Informal PEB reviews the soldier's records and issues findings and recommendations:

> The Informal PEB weighs the nature and degree of the service member's condition or impairment as presented in the medical board against the requirements and duties expected of the service member's office, grade, rank, or rating, and the commander's assessment of the service member's duty performance. (Marcum et al., 2002, p. 29)

If the soldier is found unfit, he or she may appeal the findings and recommendations and present his or her case in person with legal representation at the Formal PEB, which then issues findings and recommendations.

The PEB also determines whether dereliction of duty is involved; determines whether the injury is "compensable," that is, was incurred or permanently aggravated in the line of duty; and assigns a disability rating, based on the VA's Schedule for Rating Disabilities and DoD supplementary guidance. In addition, for those found unfit for further service, the PEB can recommend the type of discharge. For those whose conditions are "unstable," the PEB can recommend placement on TDRL if the disability is rated 30 percent or more or the member has more than 20 years of service and is eligible for retirement.

Appellate Review and Disposition Beyond the Physical Evaluation Board

The Formal PEB meets the requirement of the law for a full and fair hearing. In addition, the military departments provide the opportunity for additional appellate review; even after discharge, a final review is available by petitioning the Board of Correction of Military Records.

Performance of the DoD Disability Evaluation System

The DoD goal for the MED and PEB process was initially 70 days. GAO reported that, in 2005, the Army processed 9,322 active-duty and 4,426 RC soldiers. Figure 9.5 shows how the processing times changed between FY 2001 and FY 2005. In 2001, 43.5 percent of active-duty Army cases processed took more than 90 days overall. By 2005, the number of cases taking 91 days or more had fallen to 25.5 percent, while the number of cases completed in 30 days or less had risen from 1.6 percent to 16 percent. These improvements were accomplished as the overall active-duty caseload had increased from 6,627 in FY 2001 to 9,314 cases in FY 2005. Smaller improvements were also noted in the process of RC soldiers; the case load of National Guard and Army Reserve soldiers rose from 591, in FY 2001 to 4,426 in FY 2005.[48]

---

[48] Data in this paragraph derived from Robertson, 2006, pp. 11, 38.

Figure 9.5
Army Processing Time

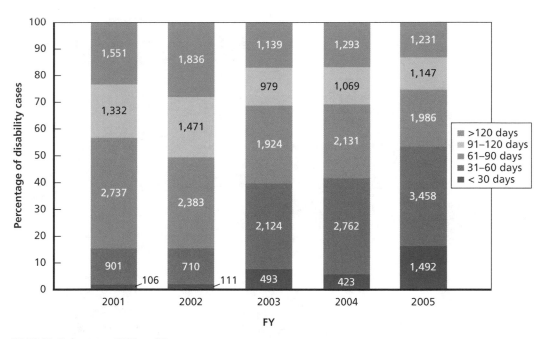

SOURCE: Robertson, 2006, p. 38.

VA's Disability Evaluation System

Before implementation of IDES, approximately 80 percent of all service members who went through DoD's Physical DES also filed a claim for VA disability compensation from the Veterans Benefits Administration. In addition, many more veterans who did not go through the DoD system but did receive a medical discharge apply for VA disability benefits. Figure 9.6 maps the VA process as it was for all applicants prior to the integrated system and continues to be followed for veterans who qualify only for VA disability. The administration assigns a service representative to obtain the relevant evidence, including a veteran's military service records, and a VA disability examination. Once all the necessary evidence has been gathered, a rating specialist determines whether the illness or injury is "service-connected" and, if it is, assigns a percentage severity rating based on the degree of disability. Unlike the DoD rating, which considers disability only determined to be unfitting for continued service, the VA rating considers disability arising from all medical conditions that arose or were aggravated during military service. Veterans who disagree can appeal to VA's Board of Veterans' Appeals and then to the U.S. federal courts. Veterans who have a single-disability rating of 60 percent or more, or a combined disability rating of 70 percent or more, and who are unable to work receive compensation at the 100-percent level (Scott et al.,

Figure 9.6
VA Disability Evaluation System

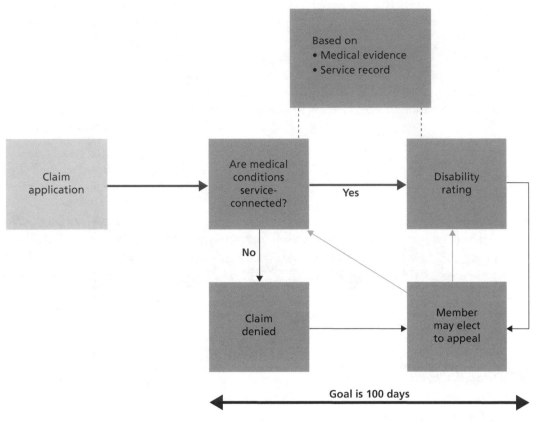

SOURCE: Dole-Shalala Commission, 2007b, p. 96.

2007, pp. 13–15). Additional compensation is awarded to veterans who have suffered certain losses, such as loss of eyesight or limb.

Problems with the System

The Independent Review Group, the Veterans Disability Benefit Commission,[49] the Dole-Shalala Commission, the Global War on Terrorism Task Force, and GAO documented problems with the DES.

Basis for Compensation Was Outdated

The Dole-Shalala Commission and the Veterans Benefits Disability Commission found that the basis for compensation was inadequate; consideration of lost earnings

---

[49] This commission "was established by the National Defense Authorization Act of 2004 . . . [to] provide recommendations to increase the efficiency and effectiveness of providing benefits and services to our veterans, their dependents, and survivors in a manner that reflects the dignity of their service" (U.S. House of Representatives, Committee on Veterans' Affairs, 2007, p. 2).

was a concept from the past, when service members returned to manual labor or their jobs on the farm. Today, more jobs are available that do not require physical exertion or the level of physical prowess required in the past. The Dole-Shalala report noted:

> In DoD, the objective of the disability payment system is not well-defined and, once again, it is governed by a complex set of rules and procedures. In part, DoD disability payments appear intended to compensate injured service members for the premature end to their military careers—in effect, a "retirement benefit" for those unable to reach actual retirement. The VA's system, as noted above, is intended to replace lost earnings capacity. A 21st century view acknowledges a disability's effects not just on earning, but also on social, family, and community participation. The current system touched on these issues indirectly, not by explicit policy. (Dole-Shalala Commission, 2007a, p. 23)

The guidelines used to determine disability were also outdated. The VA Schedule for Rating of Disabilities, which directs the percentages to be assigned for compensable conditions, had its origins in 1921. It was last comprehensive modification was done in 1945, and that modification formed the basis for the schedule used with the wounded warriors from the early years of OIF and OEF. All the groups that examined the system noted its deficiencies, particularly with regard to assigning ratings for TBI and PTSD, and called for reform.

Compensation for Mental Disabilities Was Generally Below Parity

The Veterans' Disability Benefits Commission contracted with the Center for Naval Analyses (CNA) for an assessment of the appropriateness of the VA disability and death benefits paid to veterans and their survivors. CNA found that

> VA compensation generally makes up for average lifetime earned income losses; however, . . . if a veteran enters [the VA system] early in life, VA compensation does not provide parity for the most severely disabled . . . .
>
> . . . Generally, those with a mental primary condition are below parity at the average first entry age. (Christensen et al., 2007, p. 62)

Lack of Transparency

The DES process was not transparent to the service member. The individual's service would conduct a physical to determine whether the individual met medical standards, and evaluators determined whether he or she was fit for duty and, if not found fit, set the disability percentage for the conditions causing unfitness. Following discharge, the VA conducted its own physical examination to determine all conditions related to an individual's military service. The VA's findings would therefore usually result in a higher disability rating than the military service involved had assigned. Naturally, this would lead the individual to wonder why this discrepancy existed. Explanations were often difficult.[50] Military leaders were unhappy with this process, which they believed pitted the service member against the military leadership.[51]

The system was also perceived to be unfair. There were discrepancies among the services with regard to the ratings assigned. The Independent Review Group noted:

> There is widespread variance in the application of regulatory guidelines within each Service and between Services. Variation continues at all levels of the disability process and into the Department of Veterans Affairs. This needlessly cumbersome and perceived adversarial process is the center of gravity in the disability evaluation system and must be completely overhauled.

> . . . It is almost as if a peacetime, draft-era program is being applied to an all-volunteer force engaged in war. (West et al., 2007, p. 28)

Process Seemed Endless

Finally, the time it took to adjudicate claims was considered unacceptably long. In 2006, GAO, reporting on the DoD system, found that "services were not achieving the DOD timeliness goals for processing disability cases and DOD was not monitoring achievement of these goals" (Bertoni, 2007, p. 2). While there had been some improvement over time, the DES process seemed endless to many, taking two years or more to complete, leaving some individuals in limbo and unable to get on with their lives.

---

[50] The Veterans Benefits Disability Commission was concerned about the consistency of disability ratings between DoD and VA (Veterans' Disability Benefits Commission, 2007, pp. 259–270). Accordingly, it contracted with CNA to compare DoD rating decisions with VA ratings and assess their consistency. The commission's conclusion was that the

> difference between DoD and VA combined or overall ratings is most likely due to variance in the number of conditions rated. VA rates 2.4 to 3.3 more conditions per person than do the services. The difference in the individual diagnosis ratings also contributes to the difference in the combined ratings. VA ratings for 8 of 13 individual diagnoses were higher by a statistically significant amount than ratings by the services for the same individuals. Finally, there appears to be some incentive on the part of the services to assign ratings less than 30 percent so that only separation pay is required and continuing family health care and other retirement benefits are not provided. This incentive is reflected in the DoD policy decision in 1986 to begin rating only the condition(s) found to be unfitting. (Veterans' Disability Benefits Commission, 2007, p. 267)

CNA found

> that roughly four-fifths of those who receive a DOD disability rating end up in the VA compensation system in less than 2 years. Hence, there is substantial overlap between the two systems. We also found on average that disabled veterans had substantially higher ratings from VA than from DOD. This is mainly because on average VA rates about three more conditions than DOD does. In addition, we found that even at the individual diagnosis level, VA gives higher ratings than DOD does on average. Last, while DOD and VA rate many of the same conditions, there are some systematic differences. There are some conditions that VA rates that are infrequently rated by DOD. (Christensen et al., 2007, p. 192)

[51] Title 16, Subtitle D of the 2008 NDAA (Pub. L. 110-181, 2008) contained a provision requiring DoD to establish a physical disability board of review to examine cases in which service members were separated with a disability rating of 20 percent or less. The act established time limits for these reviews, specifying those separated between September 11, 2001, and December 31, 2009. The Air Force became executive agent for this board.

Dole-Shalala Commission, 2007a, p. 22, noted that, if a service member chooses to appeal his or her rating, it took the VA an *average* of 657 days to resolve the case. The Independent Review Group found that, "during the transition from inpatient to out-patient and into the evaluation board system, the processes reverse their approach to the patient from one of advocacy and caring concern, to that of bureaucratic adversary" (West et al., 2007, p. 9).

In 2009, the GAO reported that, over the previous decade, "the total number of compensation claims decisions completed annually by VA and the average days compensation claims were pending improved, while the total number of claims pending at year end and the average days to complete a claim worsened" (Bertoni, 2009, p. 4). The peak number of backlogged cases was reached in early 2013, when first-time cases topped 610,000. The concerted efforts of top VA management brought the backlog down to 70,000 in October 2015, but it has since grown as resources and personnel have shifted to handle the appeal caseload (Shane, 2017).

Reform of the DES: The Integrated Disability Evaluation System

The Task Force on Returning Global War on Terror Heroes was the first of the commissions charged with addressing the problems at Walter Reed to report. This task force solicited comments on the delivery of federal benefits and services from stakeholders, including national veterans service organizations, and received more than 2,400 comments. The top three areas of concern were access to services and benefits (18 percent), case management (17 percent), and the disability processing system (14 percent) (Task Force on Returning Global War on Terror Heroes, 2007, p. 14). As a result, the task force recommended development of "a joint DoD/VA process for disability benefit determinations by establishing a cooperative Medical and Physical Evaluation Board process within the military service branches and VA" (Task Force on Returning Global War on Terror Heroes, 2007, p. 4).[52]

The West-Marsh Independent Review Group and the Dole-Shalala Commission reported essentially at the same time and were aware of each other's work. Both found

---

[52] As the Task Force on Returning Global War on Terror Heroes saw it,

[t]he development of a joint process whereby VA and DoD cooperate in the assignment of a disability evaluation that would be used in determining fitness for retention, level of disability for military retirement, and VA disability compensation would result in less discontent among servicemembers who believe they are assigned lower disability evaluations by DoD than by VA. This would also help VA provide better service to newly separated veterans by completing their claims in a timelier manner. There are, potentially, a number of provisions that could be undertaken to effect this recommendation, including providing Benefits Delivery at Discharge type service to those servicemembers undergoing the MEB/PEB process.

The impact of implementing this recommendation will be significant. In the near term, having DoD and VA work together to improve the VA disability claims process and the DoD MEB/PEB disability process should provide improvement across the services in consistency of decisions. In the longer term, having full cooperation in the disability claims process should provide improved service to servicemembers and veterans at a lower cost to the Government through increased efficiencies. (Task Force on Returning Global War on Terror Heroes, 2007, pp. 23–24)

the current system unacceptable. The Dole-Shalala Commission focused on a single medical examination and on rationalizing disability compensation so that DoD compensated for loss of military career opportunity. The VA instead compensated for long-term disability. DoD and VA went with the integrated process but did not address the purpose of and allocation of responsibility for compensation.

A Pilot Test of a New System

The SOC quickly focused its efforts on field testing an alternative DES.[53] To obtain the data for determining the pilot design, the DoD and VA conducted an intensive five-day tabletop exercise that simulated alternative approaches incorporating variations of (1) a single, comprehensive medical examination to be used by both DoD and VA; (2) a single disability rating for each medical problem identified during the examination, performed by VA; and (3) incorporating a DoD-level evaluation board for adjudicating fitness for duty.[54] Moving quickly, a full-scale test of the pilot was started at treatment centers in the Washington, D.C., area—WRAMC; the National Naval Medical Center in Bethesda, Maryland; and the Malcolm Grow Air Force Medical Center at Andrews AFB, Maryland—in November 2007. As fielded, the pilot had three key features (Bertoni, 2008, p. 9):

- a single physical examination conducted to VA standards as part of the MEB
- disability ratings prepared by VA for all disabilities found during the examination, for both DoD and VA use in determining individual overall disability ratings and associated benefits
- additional outreach and nonclinical case management provided by VA staff at the DoD pilot locations to explain VA results and processes to service members.

The goal of the pilot was to "implement a streamlined disability evaluation that has potential for reducing the time it takes to receive a decision from both agencies, improv-

---

[53] For example, the Veterans Benefits Disability Commission had called for a streamlined MEB/PEB structure in which would give

> each service member a single, objective rating that would apply to military disability retirement pay or severance pay as well as VA disability compensation. . . . The disability rating should be completed prior to discharge to maintain continuous financial support and health care for separating service members.

> Key to this realignment would be the development and implementation of a single, comprehensive medical examination protocol that would be used by both the services and VA. This protocol would require examining all conditions that were found on exam, and not be restricted to the "unfitting" conditions. Service members would not be subjected to multiple examinations. It might be appropriate for the examinations to be conducted by VA medical staff at some locations and by DoD staff at others. Training and certification of all examiners will be essential for consistent, high-quality examinations. (Veterans' Disability Benefits Commission, 2007, pp. 268–269)

[54] For a more complete discussion, see Bertoni and Pendleton, 2008, pp. 19–23.

ing consistency of evaluations for individual conditions, and simplifying the overall process for servicemembers and veterans" (Bertoni and Pendleton, 2008, p. 24).

In December 2010, GAO told Congress that the pilot, renamed IDES, had been expanded to 24 more facilities, and DoD and the VA were planning for an expansion worldwide by the end of FY 2011 (Gould and Stanley, 2010, p. 24). IDES had "achieved three key goals relative to the legacy process: increased servicemember satisfaction, improved case-processing time, and a reduction in servicemember appeal rates" (Bertoni, 2010, p. 11). GAO was concerned, however, because "case processing times have been steadily increasing as the caseload has increased" (Bertoni, 2010, p. 12). By the following May (2011), IDES had been deployed to 73 locations, covering 66 percent of all military disability cases. However, average case processing times "increased significantly, such that active component [AC] servicemembers' cases completed in March 2011 took an average of 394 days to complete—99 days more than the revised 295-day goal" (Bertoni, 2011, p. 2). GAO attributed this increase to a number of administrative and logistical problems.[55] The trend in increasing case process time continued into FY 2011, as IDES was deployed, as reported by GAO and shown in Table 9.1. The VA/DoD Joint Executive Committee reported a similar trend, as shown in Table 9.2.

Table 9.1
Time Lines for IDES Cases Resulting in Receipt of VA Benefits

	FY			
	2008	2009	2010	2011
Completed cases	154	956	3,878	6,312
Average process time (days)				
Active duty (goal = 295)	283	313	357	394
National Guard/Reserve (goal = 305)	297	316	370	420
Cases meeting goals (%)				
Active duty	63.4	50.2	31.6	18.8
National Guard/Reserve	65.0	51.7	37.2	18.0

SOURCES: Bertoni, 2012a, p. 9; Bertoni, 2012b, p. 6.

---

[55] GAO noted

> implementation challenges that . . . contributed to delays in the process. The most significant challenge was insufficient staffing by DOD and VA. Staffing shortages and process delays were particularly severe at two pilot sites we visited where the agencies did not anticipate caseload surges. The single exam posed other challenges that contributed to delays, such as disagreements between DOD and VA medical staff about diagnoses for servicemembers' medical conditions that often required further attention, adding time to the process. Pilot sites also experienced logistical challenges, such as incorporating VA staff at military facilities and housing and managing personnel going through the process. (Bertoni, 2011, p. 2)

Table 9.2
Timeliness of IDES Cases Resulting in Receipt of VA Benefits

	FY					
	2009[a]	2010[b]	2011[c]	2012[d]	2013[e]	2014[f]
Cases entering DES Pilot/IDES	4,822	14,207	32,804	62,763	95,058	124,701
Cases completed	687	3,401	11,805	29,254	59,409	90,768
Average process time (days)						
Active duty (goal = 295)	289	314	367	364[g]	374[g]	316[g]
National Guard/Reserve (goal = 305)	270	300	350	344[g]	404[g]	396[g]

[a] Gould and McGinn, 2009, p. 17.
[b] Gould and Stanley, 2010, p. 24.
[c] Gould and Rooney, 2011, p. 44.
[d] Gould and Wright, 2012, p. 45.
[e] Gibson and Wright, 2013, p. 48.
[f] Gibson and Junor, 2014, p. 45.
[g] Completed in the month of September of the FY.

On September 2, 2014, the congressionally mandated DoD Task Force on the Care, Management, and Transition of Recovering Wounded, Ill, and Injured Members of the Armed Forces published its fourth and final report. This task force noted that, over the previous three years, it had made 18 recommendations to improve both processes and equitable outcomes. It acknowledged that DoD and the VA had made many improvements but found that "inadequacies of the system remain, including such complexity as to make navigating the system a lengthy and mystifying ordeal" (Nathan and Crockett-Jones, 2014, p. 12). The task force's recommendations notwithstanding, IDES, as shown in Figure 9.7, remains the process in place as of this writing.

The VA in the Post-9/11 World

The Veterans Health Administration
VHA provides health care to eligible veterans through 23 Veterans Integrated Service Networks. Overall, in 2016, the VA maintained 168 medical centers and hospitals; 300 readjustment counseling centers (vet centers); 1,055 VA clinics; 11 VA residential and extended care sites; and 56 regional offices (DVA, 2016c, p. 7). It accomplished nearly 107 million outpatient visits; treated some 599,000 surgical and medicine and 152,000 mental health inpatients; and provided institutional long-term support and services for more than 115,000 patients at a cost of $70.6 billion (VHA, 2016b, p. 5). The VHA employed more than 25,000 physicians and 93,600 nurses (VHA, 2016b, pp. 5, 19). Congress funds the VHA annually. Unlike an entitlement program—in

Figure 9.7
Integrated Disability Evaluation System

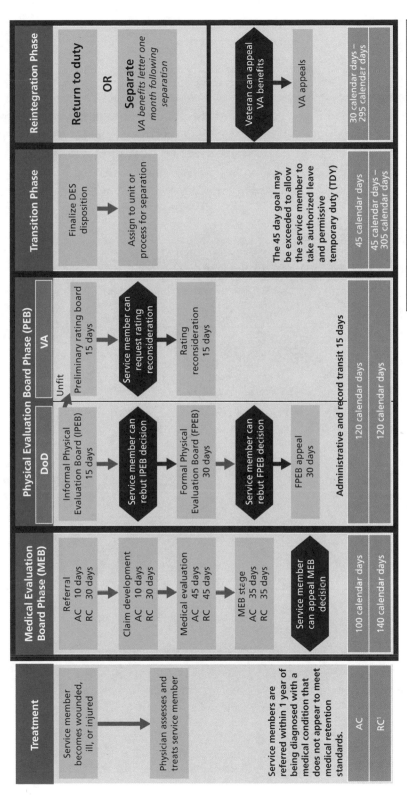

SOURCE: Adapted from U.S. Department of Defense Warrior Care, undated.
NOTES: FPED = formal physical evaluation board; IPED = informal physical evaluation board.

[1] Reserve component member entitlement to VA disability benefits begins upon release from active duty or separation.

which the government would be obligated to provide all the health care that enrolled veterans demanded—the VHA has restricted enrollment to keep its spending within its budget.[56]

Changing Demographics in the Post-9/11 Period

After years of sustained conflict, the VA and the population of veterans have changed significantly (see Table 9.3). In 2015, 93 percent of service-connected disabled veterans were enrolled in the VHA health care system, and 69 percent of enrollees used health care in 2015, up from 58 percent in ten years (National Center for Veterans Analysis and Statistics, 2016, p. 16). Moreover, not only had the likelihood of service-connected

Table 9.3
Selected Veterans Health Administration Characteristics, FYs 2002–2015

Fiscal Year	Total Enrollees (M)[a]	Outpatient Visits (M)[b]	Inpatient Admissions (000)
2002	6.8	46.5	564.7
2003	7.1	49.8	567.3
2004	7.3	54.0	589.8
2005	7.7	57.5	585.8
2006	7.9	59.1	568.9
2007	7.8	62.3	589.0
2008	7.8	67.7	641.4
2009	8.1	74.9	662.0
2010	8.3	80.2	682.3
2011	8.6	79.8	692.1
2012	8.8	83.6	703.5
2013	8.9	86.4	694.7
2014	9.1	92.4	707.4
2015	9.0	95.2	699.1

SOURCE: Data as of July 27, 2017 from Department of Veterans Affairs, Veteran Health Administration.

[a] Includes nonenrolled veteran patients.

[b] Includes fee visits.

---

[56] For a comparison of the costs of VA and private-sector health care, see Goldberg, 2015, and Bass, Ellis, and Golding, 2014.

disabled veterans seeking VA health care increased, but so had the average disability rating (see Figure 9.8). Overall, the number of veterans using VA benefits increased slightly in recent years despite a 14-percent decline in the total veteran population since 2006. The number of female veterans using VA benefits has grown by more than 37 percent since 2006, compared to overall growth in the total number of female veterans, which was less than 11 percent (see Figure 9.9). The VA projects that, by 2043, women will make up 16.3 of the living veteran population (Aponte et al., 2017, p. vii). A recent RAND analysis found the following:

- **The three-decade decline in the number of veterans will continue.** The total number of veterans is expected to decrease by 19 percent between 2014 and 2024, assuming no major policy changes or large-scale conflicts. The median age of this population will continue to increase, and veterans are projected to become more geographically concentrated over this period.
- **Veterans who use VA for health care are typically older and sicker than other veterans; however, veterans who *rely most* on VA care tend to be younger and poorer** and to live in rural areas and lack health care from other sources.

Figure 9.8
Service-Connected Disabled Veterans by Disability Rating Group, FYs 1986–2013

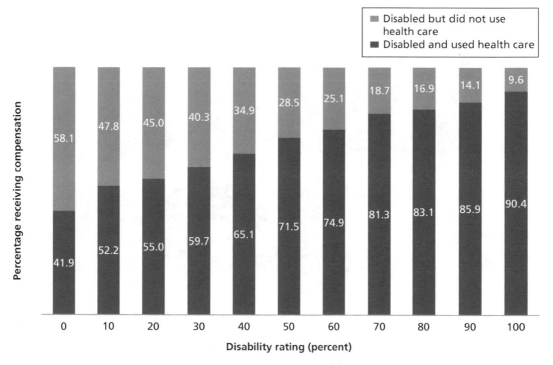

SOURCE: National Center for Veterans Analysis and Statistics, 2016, p. 17.

Figure 9.9
Benefits Used: Total and Female Veterans, 2006–2015

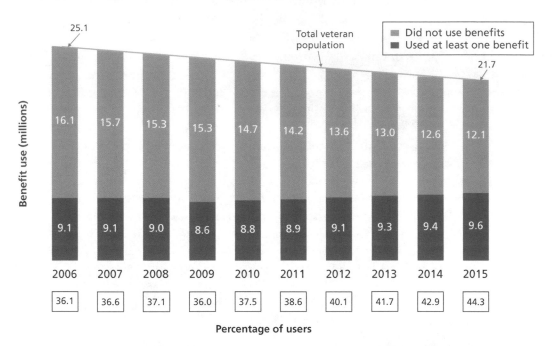

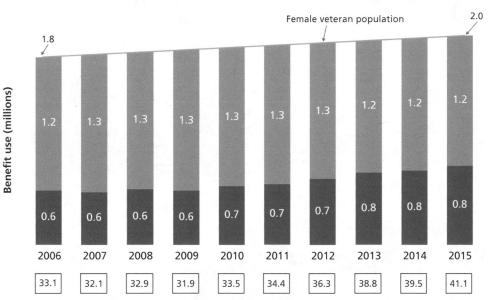

SOURCE: National Center for Veterans Analysis and Statistics, 2016, pp. 6–7.

- **Through 2019, the demand for VA services may outpace supply.** From 2020 and onward, demand for VA care will level off or decline, barring any major conflicts or changes in eligibility policy. (Farmer, Hosek, and Adamson, 2016, p. iii; emphasis in the original)

Care for Female Veterans

When GEN John W. Vessey, Jr., retired as Chairman of the Joint Chiefs of Staff in 1985, he was the nation's longest-serving active soldier, having served in uniform for 46 years. He lied about his age to enlist in the Minnesota National Guard in May 1939, was called to active duty in February 1941, and received a battlefield commission on the beach at Anzio on May 6, 1944. On February 2, 1984, General Vessey addressed the House Armed Services Committee:

The greatest change that has come about in the United States forces in the time that I've been in the military service has been the extensive use of women. That's even greater than nuclear weapons, I feel, as far as our own forces are concerned. (as quoted in "Gen. Vessey Sees Women as Biggest Military Change," 1984)

With the advent of the all-volunteer force and the end of conscription in 1973, the military began in earnest to recruit women to meet its manpower needs. When the draft ended, about 45,000 women were serving on active duty in the four services. By 1980, the number of women serving on active duty had increased to 171,000, about 8 percent of the active-duty force. Over the following decades, the role women play substantially expanded to include the final elimination of the so-called combat exclusion (see Figure 9.10).[57]

General Vessey's comment concerning the extensive use of women by the military notwithstanding, GAO found in 1982 that the

VA has not adequately focused on their needs. (Ahart, 1982, p. 1)

Although women have served in the military since at least World War I, they have not always received recognition as veterans and VA benefits equal to those given to male veterans. For example, women who served in the Womens Airforces Service Pilots (WASPs) during World War II were not legally eligible for VA benefits until 1979.

Even when women were recognized as veterans, they were not given the same benefits as male veterans. For example, until 1972, married female veterans received smaller education allowances under the GI bill than did married male veterans. In the 1960s, VA did not consider a woman's income equal to a man's for the purpose of qualifying for home loan guarantees.

---

[57] In January 2013, the Secretary of Defense and the Chairman of the Joint Chiefs of Staff directed the services to open all units, including those engaged in direct combat, and all positions to women, by January 1, 2016 (Farrell, 2015, p. 5).

Figure 9.10
Female Active-Duty Military Personnel, 1945–2015

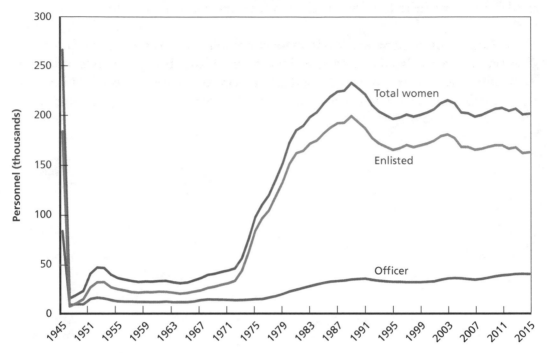

SOURCE: Aponte et al., 2017, p. 4.

> Although these inequities have been eliminated, VA health care programs have typically been oriented to male health care needs because most veterans are male. (Ahart, 1982, p. 2)[58]

> VA has not adequately considered the increasing female veteran population in long-range planning for construction and renovation projects or in designing facility renovations. (Ahart, 1982, p. 10)

In 2016, even as the female veteran population had grown from 2 to 10 percent—over 2 million female veterans—GAO found that the VA was still having problems meeting the health needs of female veterans. For example,

> [t]he fact that nearly 18 percent of VAMCs [VA medical centers] and outpatient clinics providing primary care lacked a women's health primary care provider in fiscal year 2015 suggests that VHA may face challenges ensuring that all women veterans have timely access to these providers, as required under VHA policy. (Williamson, 2016, p. 23)

---

[58] See also Willenz, 1983.

In 2015, the VA identified a number of barriers that were preventing women from receiving the full benefits of available care, and to "aid decision-makers in understanding how women interact with the current VA system and identify actionable opportunities for improvement" (Altarum Institute, 2015, p. 2). Since 1994, the Center for Women Veterans has been an advocate for women veterans within and outside the VA.[59]

Traumatic Brain Injury and PTSD

The signature wounds of the post-9/11 conflicts in Afghanistan and Iraq are traumatic brain injury and PTSD. According to the Veteran's Brain Injury Center, "22% of all combat casualties from these conflicts are brain injuries, compared to 12% of Vietnam related combat casualties. 60% to 80% of soldiers who have other blast injuries may also have traumatic brain injuries" (Summerall, 2017). Veterans of Iraq and Afghanistan exposed to blasts seem to experience postconcussive symptoms longer than the civilian population, with residual symptoms lasting 18 to 24 months after the injury. PTSD, chronic pain, and substance abuse are common and may complicate recovery.

TBI

The diagnosis of TBI is challenging because the

> brevity of the initial alteration of consciousness may cause the initial injury to go unnoticed and the patient may present some time after the original injury when details are unclear. Another factor is that these injuries can occur in chaotic circumstances, such as combat, and may be ignored in the heat of events. Clinicians may be presented with vague concerns and little relevant detail about the original injury. . . .
>
> . . . Because of the considerable symptom overlap between post-concussive symptoms and symptoms of many psychiatric and neurologic disorders, this process can be challenging. . . .
>
> . . . Patients with TBI often meet criteria for PTSD on screening instruments for TBI and vice versa. (Summerall, 2017)[60]

Since 2007, all veterans accessing VA care who have served in combat operations and separated from active duty service after 9/11 are screened for TBI.[61] The current

---

[59] Congress established the Center for Women Veterans through Pub. L. 103-446, 1994.

[60] The VA reported that, in FY 2009, of the 22,053 veterans diagnosed with TBI, 89 percent also had a mental health diagnosis, and 73 percent had a diagnosis of PTSD. Of the 305,335 veterans not diagnosed with TBI, 39 percent had a mental health diagnosis and 24 percent had a diagnosis of PTSD (Scholten and Bidelspach, 2016, p. 26). Of the 613,391 veterans the VA saw between FYs 2009 and 2011, 9.6 percent had a diagnosis of TBI, and 29.3 percent had a diagnosis of PTSD (Scholten and Bidelspach, 2016, p. 29).

[61] The VA reported that, from April 2007 to September 30, 2015, it had screened over 1 million veterans for possible mild TBI. Approximately 20 percent of veterans screen positive and are referred for comprehensive evalua-

VA screening tool is not definitive, and those who screen positive are referred for a comprehensive TBI evaluation. In 2014, the VA reported that "about half" of those who had screened positive and completed the evaluation were diagnosed with TBI as a result (VHA, 2014).

For those in need of rehabilitation services, the VA provides individualized comprehensive and specialized rehabilitation services at five regional centers, 23 network sites, and 86 local VA medical centers throughout the United States (see Figure 9.11). In addition, 39 polytrauma points of contact are located at VA facilities that are not affiliated with a regional center.

Figure 9.11
Veterans Health Administration Polytrauma TBI System of Care

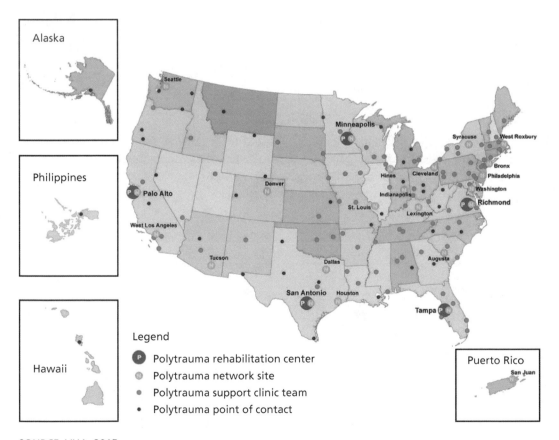

SOURCE: VHA, 2015.

---

tions; approximately 8.4 percent of the those screened receive TBI diagnoses; 137,810 completed comprehensive evaluation; and 82,468 received confirmed diagnosis of mild TBI (Scholten and Bidelspach, 2016, p. 9).

PTSD

Following the battles within the American Psychiatric Association and at the VA in the 1970s over what was then called Vietnam Syndrome (later PTSD), Congress mandated the establishment of the VA Special Committee on Post-Traumatic Stress Disorder (Bascetta, 2005a, p. 2). Established in 1985, the special committee focused on ways to improve VA's PTSD services. In 2005, GAO reported to Congress that "VA does not have sufficient capacity to meet the needs of new combat veterans while still providing for veterans of past wars" (Bascetta, 2005a, p. 4).[62] The VA objected to the GAO's conclusion, saying that it had

> provided PTSD services to approximately 6,400 OIF/OEF veterans to date. This is a small percentage of the total of more than 244,000 veterans treated for PTSD in the VA health care system, and indicates that VA does indeed have sufficient capacity to provide care to veterans with PTSD. (Bascetta, 2005a, p. 54)

The VA response, citing the number of OIF/OEF PTSD veterans it had served through 2005, was problematic, given that the number of new veterans it would see with PTSD would soon grow substantially. In 2003, the VA reported that only 1.1 percent of the OIF/OEF veterans using VA health care services had PTSD. The number of OIF/OEF veterans with PTSD grew from 230 in 2003 to 33,597 in 2007, which was 17 percent of the total that year. In 2012, the number of OIF/OEF PTSD patients reported were 119,482, or 23.6 percent of the total (Committee on the Assessment of Ongoing Efforts in the Treatment of Posttraumatic Stress Disorder et al., 2014, p. 40). More recently, the VA reported that, through June 30, 2015, "422,167 OEF/OIF/OND Veterans . . . [had been] seen for potential or provisional PTSD at VHA facilities following their return from Iraq or Afghanistan" (Epidemiology Program, Post-Deployment Health Group, 2017, p. 3). Even more impressive is the number of veterans receiving disability compensation for PTSD, and the severity of their disabilities, as indicated by the disability ratings reported. In 2014, the VBA reported to the IOM that,

> [i]n 2003, 196,641 OEF and OIF veterans had service-connected PTSD; however, as of 2013, 653,249 veterans had service-connected PTSD, or 17.5% of all veterans who were receiving compensation for service-connected health conditions in 2013. Of those, about 451,500 were adjudicated to be at least 50% disabled and so qualified for priority group 1 for VA care, and another 165,500 were at least 30% disabled but less than 50% and so qualified for priority group 2. PTSD is the third most common major service-connected disability, after hearing loss and tinnitus. (Committee on the Assessment of Ongoing Efforts in the Treatment of Posttraumatic Stress Disorder et al., 2014, p. 41)

---

[62] The GAO also found that most of the special committee's 24 outstanding recommendations had not been or had only partially been acted on, including recommendations first made more than a decade before, when the committee had been established (see Bascetta, 2005a, pp. 46–52).

VA PTSD Program

Following the call of the President's New Freedom Commission on Mental Health (2003, p. 5) for a transformed mental health system, the VA published its new five-year Mental Health Strategic Plan, which emphasizes mental health as an important part of veterans' overall health.[63] Money to implement the plan was provided for the first time in the FY 2005 budget.

The VA provides trauma-focused psychotherapies at general mental health clinics and primary care clinics with embedded mental health practitioners, and veterans may also receive counseling for PTSD symptoms in vet centers.[64] In addition, the VBA contracts with educational, vocational, and rehabilitation organizations or individual service providers for rehabilitation services for those who are substantially impaired by service-connected PTSD. Antidepressant medications can also be prescribed to treat PTSD symptoms.

In 2006, the VA asked RAND and the Altarum Institute to conduct an independent evaluation of the quality of the VA's mental health care system. RAND and Altarum found the following:

> Overall, the assessment of quality indicators suggests that in most instances the performance of VA care is as good as or better than that reported by other groups or shown by direct comparisons with other systems of care, but the level of performance often does not meet implicit VA expectations. (Watkins et al., 2011, p. 154)

> Overall, veterans' perceptions of VA services were favorable, although they did not perceive significant improvement in their conditions. (Watkins et al., 2011, p. 159)

In 2014, the IOM concluded that

> VA does not track the PTSD treatments a patient receives, other than medications, or any treatment outcomes in the electronic health record. This lack of performance measures makes it difficult to determine whether the psychotherapies or pharmacotherapies being used are effective and safe for treating PTSD and any comorbidities. The exceptions to the lack of data collection in the VA are the SOPPs [specialized outpatient PTSD programs] and SIPPs [specialized intensive PTSD programs], where PTSD symptoms are measured at intake but treatment outcome measures are collected only for the SIPPs at 4 months after veterans leave the programs. For several of the SIPPs, the difference in veterans' PTSD symptoms prior to and after treatment is not substantial, and it was not clear whether or how those outcome data are used to improve the programs. (Committee on the Assessment of Ongoing Efforts in the Treatment of Posttraumatic Stress Disorder et al., 2014, p. 87)

---

[63] Miller, 2012, pp. 107–111, discusses the development of the five-year plan and its link to the commission.

[64] Committee on the Assessment of Ongoing Efforts in the Treatment of Posttraumatic Stress Disorder et al., 2014, pp. 66–70, discusses the various options.

In 2016, the Warrior Care Network was launched as a partnership between the VA, the private Wounded Warrior Project, and four regional academic medical research hospitals: UCLA Health in Los Angeles, Emory Healthcare in Atlanta, Massachusetts General Hospital in Boston, and Rusch University Medical Center in Chicago (Wounded Warrior Project, 2016). Veterans and active-duty U.S. military with mental health disorders or injuries incurred during deployment on or after 9/11 are eligible; after appropriate screening, patients receive PTSD treatments at no cost.

Issue for the VA in the Post-9/11 Period

The essential issue for the VA in the post-9/11 period was access to health services—which veterans would receive what health services. It manifested the controversy over the implementation of the Veterans' Health Care Eligibility Reform Act of 1996 (Pub. L. 104-262, 1996); the reports in 2014 of excessive waiting times for appointments at VA medical centers that eventually resulted in the resignation of the Secretary of Veterans Affairs and the firing of a number of top executives and hospital administrators; the passage of the Veterans Access, Choice, and Accountability Act of 2014 (Pub. L. 113-146, 2014), which established new ways eligible veterans could have immediate access to needed health services; and expanded health services for female veterans.

Access Has Expanded Over Time

Congress established and directly funds the VA health care system to care for the medical needs of soldiers who were injured during wartime after they leave military service and veterans permanently incapacitated as a result of their service. Over time, however, veterans' health care has evolved to provide care for veterans other than those with service-connected disabilities—for example, a lower-income vet with a non–service-connected disability—and has "become increasingly complex and a source of frustration to veterans who are often uncertain about which services they are eligible to receive and to VA physicians and administrators who find them difficult to administer" (Baine, 1996b, p. 3).

Immediately after the end of World War II, the VA hospital system grew tremendously. By 1947, however, the VA again had excess hospital capacity; in 1947, Congress created a presumption that a diagnosis of a chronic psychiatric condition within two years of discharge would be regarded as service-connected. In 1962, the definition of a service-connected disability was changed to include "any condition traceable to a period of military service, regardless of the cause or circumstances of its occurrence" (Baine, 1996b, p. 27)—prior to that, designation as a service-connected condition was not assured unless the condition was incurred or aggravated during wartime service. In 1966, Congress expanded eligibility for hospital care to peacetime veterans (in service after January 1955). Eligibility for non–service-connected disabilities was extended to peacetime veterans who could not afford the cost of care in 1973. In 1976, Congress authorized hospital care for treating a non–service-connected condition of any veteran 65 or older without regard for ability to pay and authorized outpatient care for any disability to any veteran 50 percent or more service-connected disabled. Congress also directed the VA to give priority to service-connected veterans and others receiving benefits because of a need for aid and attendance benefits, or those permanently housebound. In 1986, the higher-income veterans with non–service-connected disabilities became eligible if they agreed to contribute toward their care.

Outpatient care was authorized in 1960. Further changes were made in 1973, 1976, and 1986. In 1988,

> veterans with (1) service-connected disabilities rated at 30 or 40 percent or (2) with incomes below the maximum pension rate were placed in the mandatory care category for outpatient treatment for prehospital and posthospital care and for care that would obviate the need for hospital care. (Baine, 1996b, p. 28)

Figure 9.12 shows the eligibility criteria for outpatient care in effect until Congress passed the Veterans' Health Care Eligibility Reform Act of 1996 (Pub. L. 104-262, 1996), which put inpatient and outpatient care on the same statutory footing. This enabled the VA to provide care in the most medically appropriate setting, subject only to the degree to which there were appropriated funds to pay for such care, clearly indicating that veterans' health care is not an entitlement.

Figure 9.12
Eligibility Criteria for Outpatient Care Prior to Eligibility Reform

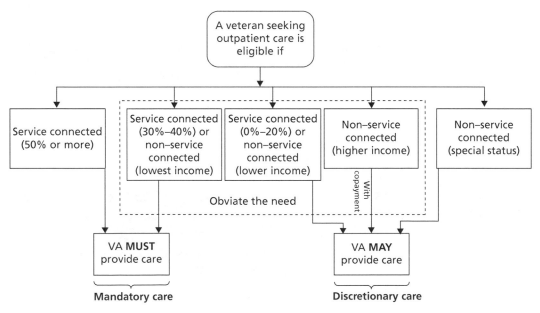

SOURCE: Adapted from Panangala, 2006, p. CRS-9.

Veterans' Health Care Eligibility Reform Act of 1996

The Veterans' Health Care Eligibility Reform Act of 1996 reflected the fact that the VA had

> evolved and expanded since World War II. Congress has enlarged the scope of the Department's health care mission and . . . extended to additional categories of veterans eligibility for the many levels of care the VA now provides. No longer a health care system targeted just to the service-connected veteran, the VA has also become a "safety net" for the many lower-income veterans who have come to depend upon it. . . . Budget considerations have been a frequent brake on such legislative initiatives. The resulting body of VA health care eligibility law is one which many view as more of a patchwork than a rational, comprehensive system.

> The longstanding call for "eligibility reform" reflects frustration with provisions of current law which are widely regarded as complex, confusing, and in some respects, inconsistent with sound medical practice. (House Committee on Veterans' Affairs, 1996, p. 3)

> The reported bill would revise provisions . . . governing eligibility for VA hospital and outpatient care . . . . It would substitute a single uniform eligibility standard for the complex array of standards governing access to VA hospital and outpatient care. . . . [I]t would employ a clinically appropriate "need for care" test, thereby ensuring that medical judgment rather than legal criteria will determine when care will be provided and the level at which that care will be furnished. (House Committee on Veterans' Affairs, 1996, p. 4)

The Veterans' Health Care Eligibility Reform Act of 1996 (Pub. L. 104-262, 1996) established a patient enrollment system with priority categories, allowing the VA to manage access when the VA did not have the capacity to serve all veterans (see Box 9.1). Thereafter, veterans had to register with the VA to receive health services. On registering, the veteran is assigned to one of eight priority groups reflecting his or her service-connected disability rating, civilian income, and other factors (see Box 9.1). Once registered, however, all veterans, regardless of their priority group, had equal access to available medical services.

When the law was enacted, it was envisioned that the VA would use the priority enrollment system to balance the demand for medical services with the available funding from Congress. However, this was not the case. Demand was adjusted through the priority system only once, in 2003, when enrollments of high-income category 8 veterans were curtailed. However, in 2009, the Obama administration eased those restrictions somewhat.[65] Today, only veterans in subgroups 8e and 8g are excluded. If these restrictions were removed, one estimate is that 4.8 million additional veterans

---

[65] Under that policy, veterans whose gross household income exceeds VA's current geographic income limit by 10 percent or less may enroll for VA care, subject to cost-sharing requirements (Philpott, 2009).

Box 9.1
VA Priority Groups for Enrollment

Priority Group	Definition
1	• Veterans with VA-rated service-connected disabilities 50% or more disabling • Veterans determined by VA to be unemployable due to service-connected conditions
2	• Veterans with VA-rated service-connected disabilities 30% or 40% disabling
3	• Veterans who are Former POWs • Veterans awarded a Purple Heart medal • Veterans whose discharge was for a disability that was incurred or aggravated in the line of duty • Veterans with VA-rated service-connected disabilities 10% or 20% disabling • Veterans awarded special eligibility classification under 38 U.S.C. § 1151, "benefits for individuals disabled by treatment or vocational rehabilitation" • Veterans awarded the Medal of Honor
4	• Veterans who are receiving aid and attendance or housebound benefits from VA • Veterans who have been determined by VA to be catastrophically disabled
5	• Nonservice-connected Veterans and noncompensable service-connected Veterans rated 0% disabled by VA with annual income below the VA's and geographically (based on your resident zip code) adjusted income limits • Veterans receiving VA pension benefits • Veterans eligible for Medicaid programs
6	• Compensable 0% service-connected Veterans • Veterans exposed to ionizing radiation during atmospheric testing or during the occupation of Hiroshima and Nagasaki • Project 112 Shipboard Hazard and Defense participants • Veterans who served in the Republic of Vietnam between January 9, 1962, and May 7, 1975 • Veterans of the Persian Gulf War who served between August 2, 1990, and November 11, 1998 • Veterans who served on active duty at Camp Lejeune for at least 30 days between August 1, 1953, and December 31, 1987 • Currently enrolled Veterans and new enrollees who served in a theater of combat operations after November 11, 1998 and those who were discharged from active duty on or after January 28, 2003, are eligible for the enhanced benefits for five years post discharge Note: At the end of this enhanced enrollment priority group placement time period, Veterans will be assigned to the highest PG their eligibility status at that time qualifies for.
7	• Veterans with gross household income below the geographically-adjusted income limits for their resident location and who agree to pay copays

Box 9.1—Continued

Priority Group	Definition
8	• Veterans with gross household income above the VA and the geographically-adjusted income limit for their resident location, and who agree to pay copays

Veterans eligible for enrollment

Noncompensable 0% service-connected and:

• Subpriority a: Enrolled as of January 16, 2003, and who have remained enrolled since that date and/or placed in this sub priority due to changed eligibility status
• Subpriority b: Enrolled on or after June 15, 2009 whose income exceeds the current VA or geographic income limits by 10% or less

Nonservice-connected and:

• Subpriority c: Enrolled as of January 16, 2003, and who have remained enrolled since that date and/or placed in this sub priority due to changed eligibility status
• Subpriority d: Enrolled on or after June 15, 2009, whose income exceeds the current VA or geographic income limits by 10% or less

Veterans not eligible for enrollment

Veterans not meeting the criteria above:

• Subpriority e: Noncompensable 0% service-connected (eligible for care of their SC condition only)
• Subpriority g: Non–service-connected

SOURCE: Veterans Health Administration, 2016a.

would enroll, and the VA patient population would increase by 35.1 percent (Eibner and Krull, 2015, p. 125).

Enhanced Eligibility for Combat Veterans

In 2008, Congress provided for an "enhanced eligibility period" of five years after leaving active service during which recent combat veterans who were "discharged under other than dishonorable conditions" (DVA, 2017b), including activated reservists and members of the National Guard, could enroll in the VA health care system. They would, without disclosing their income, be placed in Priority Group 6, unless eligible for enrollment in a higher-priority group. This meant that combat veterans of the post-9/11 conflicts who had separated on or after January 28, 2003, would have, at least for the first five years after separation, free medical care and medications for any condition related to their service in the combat theater. For conditions not related to service in the combat theater, a small medical care or prescription drug copayment might be charged. According to the VA,

> Veterans who enroll with VA under this authority will continue to be enrolled even after their enhanced eligibility period ends. At the end of their enhanced eligibility period, Veterans enrolled in Priority Group 6 may be shifted to a lower priority group depending on their income level, and required to make applicable copays. (DVA, 2017a)

VA Enrollment 2016

In 2016, the VA estimated that there were 20.4 million living veterans (National Center for Veterans Analysis and Statistics, 2018, Table 2L), of whom 8.4 million were enrolled for health care (see Figure 9.13).

In the recent past, there has been a steady growth in the proportion of enrollees in Priority Groups 1 and 2, those veterans with service-connected disabilities, and a decrease in Priority Group 5, those with non–service-connected disabilities whose annual incomes are below the established VA means test threshold. In addition, the number of Veterans in Priority Group 7/8, those with a non–service-connected disability who have annual incomes above the threshold have decreased through natural attrition as veterans in this category are currently not being enrolled.

Waiting Times

The effects of the 1996 reforms were profound. Over a period of nearly 20 years, the number of unique veterans receiving medical care grew from 3.2 million in FY 1999 to 4.8 million in FY 2005 (Panangala, 2006, p. CRS-11), then to 5.9 million in FY 2014 (Eibner and Krull, 2015, p. 9), an increase of 84 percent. While the budget of the VA has been substantially increased since 1996 (see Scott, 2012), it is worth asking whether the increases have been sufficient to ensure maintenance of the quality of the system. One measure of the adequacy of the budget is access to the system, particularly the time it takes for a patient to get an initial appointment, which is tied to the length of the waiting list for new appointments. The Veterans' Health Care Eligibility

Figure 9.13
Enrollees by Priority Group

Priority group	Number of enrollees	Percentage of enrollees
1	1,979,847	23.6
2	711,684	8.5
3	1,192,474	14.2
4	180,350	2.1
5	1,866,340	22.2
6	550,595	6.6
7–8	1,920,263	22.9
Total	8,401,553	

SOURCE: Huang et al., 2017, p. 13.
NOTE: Numbers may not sum to 100 due to rounding.

Reform Act of 1996 (Pub. L. 104-262, 1996) set a number of outpatient care goals. Patients were to

> (1) receive an initial, nonurgent appointments [sic] with their primary care or other appropriate provider within 30 days of requesting one; (2) receive specialty appointments within 30 days when referred by a primary care provider; and (3) be seen within 20 minutes of their scheduled appointments. VA refers to these goals as the "30-30-20" goals. (Bascetta, 2000, p. 5)[66]

Knowing whether the VA is meeting this goal, however, depends on having accurate waiting time data,[67] which both GAO and the VA's own IG found to be a problem:

- In 2000, GAO told Congress that the VA lacked reliable national waiting time data, which "limits its ability to identify which facilities and clinics have the longest waiting times, . . . [and thus did not] know whether waiting time problems are systemwide or isolated to particular facilities" (Bascetta, 2000, p. 15).
- In 2005, the VA's IG audited outpatient scheduling procedures to determine the accuracy of the reported veterans' waiting times and found that schedulers did not follow established procedures and that actual waiting times were understated. The IG estimated that as many as 25,000 service-connected veterans nationwide

---

[66] In 2005, the VA IG set forth the background for the goals:

Two VHA policies set requirements for priority access to medical care for veterans with service-connected disabilities. The policies require that veterans with service-connected ratings of 50 percent or greater and veterans requiring care for service-connected disabilities must be scheduled for care within 30 days of the desired appointment dates. If an appointment cannot be scheduled within the 30-day time frame, VA must arrange for the veteran to receive care at another VHA medical facility or fee basis care from a non-VA provider at VA expense.

A third VHA policy establishes a goal of scheduling appointments within 30 days of the desired appointment date but not more than 4 months beyond the desired appointment date. The policy requires that all appointment requests must be acted on by the medical facility within 7 business days of the request, including consult referrals to a specialist. Acting on the request involves either scheduling the requested care or placing the patient on the electronic waiting list. VHA implemented the electronic waiting list in December 2002 to provide VHA medical facilities a standard tool to capture and track information about veterans waiting for clinic appointments and primary care panel assignments. (Staley, 2005, p. 1)

[67] An alternative to examining waiting lists would be to ask veterans themselves about their experience in getting appointments at the VA. In March 2016, 173,000 of the 8.4 million enrollees in the VA health program were invited to participate in a survey, and "46,571 enrollees submitted or returned a completed survey" (Huang et al., 2017, p. iv). Overall, their responses sharply contrasted with the waiting list stories reported; "a large majority responded favorably about their experiences with scheduling appointments and accessibility on the day of their visit to the VA or VA-approved facility," (Huang et al., 2017, p. 98). As reported, for those partaking in the 2016 survey, "about 80 percent indicated that they were able to find appointments at convenient times and days 'most of the time' or 'always/nearly always.' Seventy-three percent were able to get appointments within a reasonable time, and 88 percent indicated that their appointments took place as scheduled" (Huang et al., 2017, pp. 98–99).

waited longer than 30 days for their first appointment (Staley, 2005, p. ii).[68] Two years later, the IG found that "[s]chedulers were still not following established procedures for making and recording medical appointments. . . . As a result, the accuracy of VHA's reported waiting times could not be relied on" (Finn, 2007, p. ii). At the request of the chairman of the Senate Committee on Veterans' Affairs, the IG further considered whether waiting list data had purposely misrepresented patient waiting times to positively affect the performance measures used to support management bonuses. The IG found "no evidence that officials willfully manipulated waiting time information" (Finn, 2008, p. ii) but did conclude that "data used to make the SES [Senior Executive Service] bonus decision for the waiting time measure could not be relied upon" (Finn, 2008, p. ii).

The tone of the inquiries into VA waiting lists took an ominous turn when it was alleged that the failure to schedule medical appointments had resulted in the deaths of a number of patients. On April 9, 2014, the chairman of the House Committee on Veterans' Affairs announced that "shortly before this public hearing, VA provided evidence that a total of 23 veterans have died due to delays in care at VA medical centers" (U.S. House of Representatives, Committee on Veterans' Affairs, 2014). The chairman was followed by other members and a number of witnesses who also reported multiple deaths. This was soon followed by a report from CNN: "At least 40 U.S. veterans died waiting for appointments at the Phoenix Veterans Affairs Health Care system, many of whom were placed on a secret waiting list" (Bronstein and Griffin, 2014). The following month, the VA IG issued a report that concluded that, while its review documented "poor quality of care, we are unable to conclusively assert that the absence of timely quality care caused the deaths of these veterans" (Griffin, 2014, p. ii).

While the VA IG could not conclusively corroborate that veterans had died because of delays in getting appointments, he pointed to serious managerial, ethical, and potentially legal shortcomings, which were well known to VA leadership. The IG highlighted an April 2010 memorandum by the Deputy Under Secretary for Health for Operations and Management that said, "to improve scores on assorted access measures, certain facilities have adopted use of inappropriate scheduling practices sometimes referred to as 'gaming strategies'" (Schoenhard, 2010). He called for "immediate action . . . to review current scheduling practices to identify and eliminate all inappropriate practices" (Schoenhard, 2010). The failure to curtail these practices soon came

---

[68] The IG also reported that

> 7 percent of the nationwide survey respondents reported that their managers or supervisors directed or encouraged them to schedule appointments contrary to written guidance or directives. . . .

> VHA uses the percentage of next available appointments scheduled within 30 days as one of its measures for evaluating medical facility director performance. The VHA goal is that at least 90 percent of all next available appointments are scheduled within 30 days. (Staley, 2005, p. 6)

to light as whistleblowers came forward (Gardella, Reynolds, and Blankstein, 2014). On May 30, 2014, President Obama accepted Secretary Eric Shinseki's resignation (see Obama, 2014). On June 27, 2014, Rob Nabors, the White House deputy chief of staff, reported to President Obama that the VHA had "a 'corrosive culture' that affects employee performance and patient care [and that had] 'impeded appropriate management, supervision and oversight'" (Nelson and Kesling, 2014). The White House review found the following:

- The 14-day scheduling standard is arbitrary, ill-defined, and misunderstood. . . . It is a poor indicator of either patient satisfaction or quality of care and should be replaced with a more insightful measure.
- The Veterans Health Administration (VHA) needs to be restructured and reformed. It currently acts with little transparency or accountability with regard to its management of the VA medical structure. The VHA Leadership structure is marked by a lack of responsiveness and an inability to effectively manage or communicate to employees or Veterans.
- A corrosive culture has led to personnel problems across the Department that are seriously impacting morale and, by extension, the timeliness of health care. The problems . . . are exacerbated by poor management and communication structures, distrust between some VA employees and management, a history of retaliation toward employees raising issues, and a lack of accountability across all grade levels.
- The Department's failures have generated a high level of oversight. . . .
- The technology underlying the basic scheduling system used by VA medical facilities is cumbersome and outdated. . . .
- Many of the resource issues VA faces are endemic to the health care field . . . . VA has also demonstrated an inability to clearly articulate budgetary needs and to tie budgetary needs to specific outcomes.
- VA needs to better plan and invest now for anticipated changes . . . . (Office of the Press Secretary, 2014)

Veterans' Access to Care Through Choice, Accountability, and Transparency Act of 2014

In response to the waiting list scandal, President Obama signed what is commonly called the Veterans' Access, Choice, and Accountability Act of 2014 (Pub. L. 113-146, 2014) into law on August 7, 2014 (DVA, undated a; Panangala, 2017). This act expanded access to VA-purchased medical care from private providers, granted the Secretary of Veterans Affairs additional power to fire senior executives, provided for an independent assessment of the VA health care delivery systems, and established the Commission on Care to "examine the access of veterans to health care from the DVA and strategically examine how best to organize the VHA, locate health care resources, and deliver health care to veterans during the 20-year period" (Commission on Care, 2016, p. 265).

Independent Assessment of the VA Health Care Delivery Systems

The independent assessment of the VA's health care delivery systems was carried out by the MITRE Corporation, McKinsey & Company, RAND Corporation, Grant Thornton LLP, the IOM, and numerous smaller companies and consultants. A final integrated report building on 12 major assessment reports provided information and data for four systemic findings concerning the VA's ability to execute its mission:[69]

- a disconnect in the alignment of demand, resources, and authorities
- uneven bureaucratic operations and processes
- nonintegrated variations in clinical and business data and tools
- leaders not fully empowered due to a lack of clear authority, priorities, and goals.

The last three of the four systemic findings are business oriented; the first, however, is unique to the VA and requires a fundamental rethinking of the way medical care is provided to veterans in line with the Commission on Care's call for a far-reaching organizational transformation of the whole VA health care system.

Commission on Care: Redesigning the Veterans' Health Care Delivery System

The veterans' health care delivery system was originally designed to be hospital based and to focus on treating veterans with service-connected disabilities in government-owned and -operated hospitals. Over time, it has morphed into a broad-based system that aspires to provide a full range of medical services to veterans with service-connected disabilities and lower incomes. Ensuring access to this promised care has not always been possible.[70] According to the commission,

> [d]ue to changing veteran demographics, increasing demand for VHA care in some markets, and declining demand in other markets, more veterans being adjudicated as having service-connected conditions, aging facilities, provider shortages and vacancies, and other factors, VHA faces a misalignment of capacity and demand that threatens to become worse over time. Some facilities and services have low volumes of care that can create quality concerns, and in high demand areas, VHA often lacks the capacity to avoid lengthy wait times and other access issues. (Commission on Care, 2016, p. 3)

---

[69] CMS Alliance to Modernize Healthcare, 2015, pp. xiii–xx, summarizes the four systemic findings together with recommendations.

[70] In 2016, the then Under Secretary of Veterans Affairs for Health, Dr. David J. Shulkin, noted,

> In the nearly 2 years since unacceptable VA waiting times came to light, it's become apparent that the VA alone cannot meet all the health care needs of U.S. veterans. The VA's mission and scope are not comparable to those of other U.S. health systems. Few other systems enroll patients in areas where they have no facilities for delivering care. Fewer still provide comprehensive medical, behavioral, and social services to a defined population of patients, establishing lifelong relationships with them. These realities, combined with the wait-time crisis, have led the VA to reexamine its approach to care delivery. (Shulkin, 2016, p. 1004)

. . . Providing veterans timely care remains a challenge today, notwithstanding establishment of the *Choice Program* and VHA leadership's focus on improving access. Access is not a problem for VHA alone: Delivering timely care is challenging for many providers and health systems, in part due to the unavailability of providers in some communities and national shortages of some categories of health professionals.

. . . [P]roviding timely access to care is not simply a matter of increasing staffing, modernizing IT systems, installing new leadership, or any other single effort, although all of these changes are needed. (Commission on Care, 2016, p. 18; emphasis in the original).

The Veterans Choice Program

With the passage of the Veterans' Access, Choice, and Accountability Act of 2014 (Pub. L. 113-146, 2014), Congress tasked VHA with creating the temporary Veterans Choice Program (VCP) to alleviate access issues by allowing greater use of community care for enrolled veterans who meet the law's wait-time or distance-to-a-VHA-facility requirements. The act supplemented existing authorities that enable the VA to purchase care for certain veterans in the private sector and was both time and resource limited.[71] The program would terminate when expended funds reached the cumulative statutory limit of $10 billion, or on August 7, 2017, whichever came first. However, the time limit was extended on April 19, 2017, and additional funds were appropriated. Figure 9.14 illustrates the process for obtaining care through the VCP.

The law establishing the VCP also called for a "comprehensive independent assessment of VHA care delivery and management systems" and the establishment of a "commission to review that assessment, examine access to care, and look more expansively at how veterans' care should be organized and delivered during the next 2 decades" (Commission on Care, 2016, p. 21). The resulting Commission on Care found that "both the design and implementation of the law have proven to be flawed. VHA must instead establish high-performing, integrated, community-based health care networks, to be known as the VHA Care System" (Commission on Care, 2016, p. 24).

Transformation of the VHA Care System into Integrated, Community-Based Health Care Networks

The Commission on Care called for a fundamental transformation of the current system. The commission made it clear that

> merely clarifying and simplifying the rules for purchased care . . . is not sufficient to achieve that goal. VHA must replace the arbitrary eligibility requirements and

---

[71] Veterans who live more than 40 miles away from the nearest VA health clinic or who are unable to get an appointment in a reasonable time would be able to receive "choice cards" allowing them to seek treatment providers that accept Medicare or TRICARE or at facilities run by DoD.

Figure 9.14
Eligibility Process to Access Care Through the Veterans Choice Program

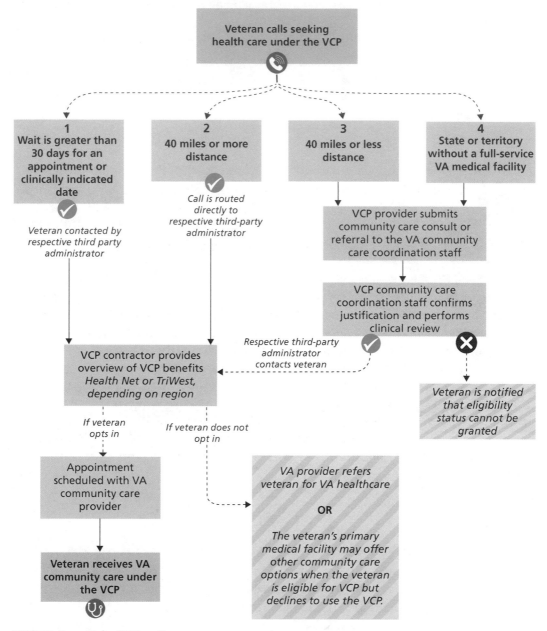

SOURCE: Panangala, 2017, p. 5.

unworkable clinical and administrative restrictions of current purchased programs with the new VHA Care System, available to all enrolled veterans. (Commission on Care, 2016, p. 26)

Among the commission's recommendations were the following:

- [That] integrated, community-based health care networks [be developed], including VHA providers and facilities, Department of Defense and other federally-funded providers and facilities, and VHA-credentialed community providers and facilities. (Commission on Care, 2016, p. 3)
- [That these] networks be developed with local VHA leadership input and knowledge to ensure their composition is reflective of local needs and veterans' preferences.
- Veterans choose a primary care provider from all credentialed primary care providers in the VHA Care System.
- Veterans choose their specialty care providers from all credentialed specialty care providers in the VHA Care System with a referral from their primary care provider. (Commission on Care, 2016, p. 4)

VA Under the Trump Administration

Midmorning on March 28, 2018, Secretary of Veterans Affairs, David Shulkin received a phone call from the White House Chief of Staff, telling him that he was being fired by President Trump. Shulkin's removal from the VA was widely expected. Secretary Shulkin had recently been the subject of a "scathing" report about a business trip he took to Britain and Denmark in 2017, a report he called "inaccurate and biased" (Davis, 2018). By most accounts, his dismissal was the result of "an increasingly contentious debate over whether to give veterans the option of using the benefits they earned through military service to see private doctors rather than going to government hospitals and clinics" (Fandos, 2018).[72] The move to privatize the VA reportedly was being pressed by the Concerned Veterans for America, a group backed by Charles G. Koch and David H. Koch, and was

> part of a long-running battle over how to deliver health care to the nation's veterans. . . . Some conservatives, including some advisers to the White House, favor gradually dismantling that system and allowing veterans to choose to receive taxpayer-subsidized care from private doctors instead. (Philipps and Fandos, 2018)

The stage was set for confrontation when "Trump appointed a VA secretary who wants to preserve the fundamental structure of government-provided health care; the president also installed a handful of senior aides who are committed to a dramatically different philosophy" (Arnsdorf, 2018, p. 3). In July 2016, candidate Trump embraced a vision for the VA, endorsed by the Koch brothers–backed Concerned Veterans for America, that emphasized private-sector alternatives. "Veterans should be guaranteed

---

[72] A senior White House official told the *New York Times* that Dr. Shulkin's firing that was "based more on a damaging report . . . [of his] use of government funds on a trip to Europe released last month than on a dispute over policy" (Fandos, 2018).

the right to choose their doctor and clinics, whether at a VA facility or at a private medical center" (as quoted in Arnsdorf, 2018, p. 4). After the election, this line faced united opposition from major veterans groups, which were firm against privatizing the VA,[73] and privatization received little support from Secretary Shulkin, who would argue that "privatization is a political issue aimed at rewarding select people and companies with profits, even if it undermines care for veterans" (Shulkin, 2018). Ultimately, Congress will determine the future of the VA.

Transformation of the VA

The transformation of the VA started in 2014, with the passage during the Obama administration of the Veterans Access, Choice, and Accountability Act and expanded with the passage of the VA Maintaining Internal Systems and Strengthening Integrated Outside Networks Act of 2018 (VA MISSION Act; Pub. L. 115-182, 2018). The path forward, however, has not been without difficulties. The GAO reported that

> numerous factors adversely affected veterans' timely access to care through the Choice Program. These factors included (1) administrative burden caused by complexities of referral and appointment scheduling processes; (2) poor communication between VA and its medical facilities; and (3) inadequacies in the networks of community providers established by the TPAs [third-party administrators], including an insufficient number, mix, or geographic distribution of community providers. (Silas, 2019, summary)

These shortcomings notwithstanding, the Trump administration sponsored and passed the VA MISSION Act, which created the Veterans Community Care Program. Under this program, "a veteran can seek care in the community if he or she needs a service that is unavailable at the VA, resides in a state with no full-service VA medical facility, meets certain access standards for drive- or wait-time, qualifies under standards for previous programs, or if it is in the best medical interest of the veteran" (Panangala and Sussman, 2019). Even as officials reported that "more than a million veterans have consulted the VA about going to a private doctor in the first three months," the VHA head Richard Stone said that "VA is not privatizing, and veterans are choosing VA" (quoted in Sisk, 2019). Nevertheless, with an increase from 8 percent of veterans eligible for private community-based care under the old VCP to an estimated 40 percent now eligible under the Veterans Community Care Program, the eventual effects of a community care option on the VA have yet to be seen. (See Sisk, 2019, p. 2).

---

[73] Arnsdorf, 2018, and Gordon, 2017, recount the behind-the-scenes fighting over the future of the VA.

Legacy

The 9/11 attacks ushered in the longest sustained period of armed conflict in the history of the United States and, over the past 18 years, have brought to the fore a number of issues that had not been adequately resolved in the past. Unfortunately, as often happens, it takes a much-publicized failure of the system to be the catalyst for change. Two of the most notable system failures in the post-9/11 period highlighted in this chapter were (1) the poor conditions of the medical holding barracks at the Army's Walter Reed Medical Center and (2) the fraudulent VA appointment waiting lists at VA hospitals.

In the first case, the *Washington Post* articles concerning the troop-holding facilities at Walter Reed not only resulted in the firing of the Secretary of the Army but were the catalyst for the Army to set up new military transition units. In addition, the review groups, task forces, and commissions established by Secretary of Defense Gates and President Bush went beyond the immediate problems. These groups examined a broader set of underlying problems, including the coordination of patient care by DoD and the VA and the military discharge process, which eventually lead to the creation of IDES to facilitate the transfer of wounded soldiers from DoD to the VA.

In the second case, the "scandal" of veterans waiting for an appointment at the VA eventually resulted in the resignation of the Secretary of Veterans Affairs and raised the issue of access to VA services, bringing into question the very premise on which the VA was built. Originally, the federal government supported only disabled veterans, compensating them for physical disabilities that prevented them from working, usually loss of sight or limb. If the veteran was indigent, the government paid for a place in an asylum, usually a state veterans' home. During and after World War I, care for veterans expanded to include rehabilitation and hospitalization for those with medical problems related to their time in service. In 1924, this was extended to hospitalization of indigent veterans. In the 1970s, the VA started to focus on outpatient services and providing comprehensive care, which was not limited to the care associated with the primary service-connected medical problem. The Veterans' Health Care Eligibility Reform Act of 1996 (Pub. L. 104-262, 1996) instituted

> a single uniform eligibility standard for the complex array of standards governing access to VA hospital and outpatient care. . . . [The standard] would employ a clinically appropriate "need for care" test, thereby ensuring that medical judgment rather than legal criteria will determine when care will be provided and the level at which that care will be furnished. (House Committee on Veterans' Affairs, 1996, p. 4)

The waiting-list crisis directly resulted in the establishment of the VCP and the Commission on Care, which called for the replacement of the current VA with a new "integrated, community-based health care" system. It remains to be seen whether the final legacy of the waiting list scandal will be a new VA health system, in whole or in part.

CHAPTER TEN

Summary: What Happened?—What Have We Learned?—How Did We Get Here?

This summary reprises the last chapter of the first volume of *Providing for the Casualties of War* (Rostker, 2013), which examined the evolution of care from ancient times through World War II, and extends the discussion into the current period, incorporating the post–World War II conflicts in Korea, Vietnam, and the Middle East.

The accounts in these two volumes tell us that the care today's casualties of war receive is relatively new in human history, dating back less than a century. From the time of the Greeks to World War I, just being a soldier was an open invitation to death from the countless communicable diseases that were the scourge of military camps. For those who were wounded, the inability to control infections meant that simple wounds often turned into festering sores, often with deadly results. Moreover, the difficulties of organizing medical services and evacuating the wounded from the battlefield added to the misery and undoubtedly increased the loss of life. Care for surviving, disabled veterans was at best no more than some cash compensation—payments to U.S. veterans have been very generous compared to those of other nations—and, as a last resort, a place in a veterans' asylum for the indigent. World War I changed all this, with the introduction of widely available rehabilitative services.

The changes brought about during World War I were remarkable both because they were built so firmly on the steady evolution of medical care soldiers had received through time and, at the same time, because they broke with what had gone before in significant ways. Over time, the role the state played in the care of sick and wounded soldiers and disabled veterans had steadily increased, but little had suggested the range of services the state would provide to veterans by the end of the war and afterward. Starting in World War I, society has changed how it views the disabled, and rehabilitative services are now being provided along with education and training for both disabled and nondisabled veterans to ease the transition back to civilian life and to care for them in their old age.

This chapter explores four broad themes, evident throughout history, that define the quality of care a wounded soldier would receive: (1) the ability to react to the changing nature of combat itself, the kinds of wounds received, the state of medical science, and the ability of physicians and surgeons to deal with disease and the consequence of wounds; (2) the ability to deliver medical services on and, later, off the battlefield; (3) the increasing role of national governments in providing care—financial, domestic, and rehabilitative—to veterans after the battle; and (4) finally, the capacity to address the psychological and cognitive injuries—the invisible wounds of war—that transcend the immediate battle. These trends began in antiquity and have followed through to the present.

Nature of Combat, the Wounds Received, and the Ability of Physicians and Surgeons to Deal with Disease and the Consequences of Wounds

The first broad theme from history is the interplay between the nature of combat itself, the kinds of wounds received, and the ability of physicians and surgeons to deal with disease and the consequences of wounds (bleeding, shock, and infection). Prior to the Renaissance, military combat involved men fighting each other at close quarters with rocks, knives, swords, and arrows. Wounds were generally inflicted as one soldier crushed, cut, or slashed at another. It was a period that the military historian Trevor Dupuy called "the Age of Muscle" (Dupuy, 1980). The mass casualties of later wars were unknown, awaiting the introduction of gunpowder during the late Middle Ages.

The Ancient World

In ancient times, with the exception of the expeditionary armies of Alexander the Great (356–323 B.C.) and Rome during the later years of the Republic and the Imperial period (3rd century B.C.–4th century A.D.), battles were most often fought close to home by citizen soldiers pressed into military service for the defense of the community or to engage in limited offensive actions for short periods. Their skills as soldiers were limited, and the damage that could be done was also limited, unless panic set in, with those who fled being left to the mercy of the winning side. Given the poor state of medical knowledge, most wounds from spears and swords were fatal. An analysis of the ancient text of the *Iliad* shows that only arrow wounds had a mortality rate of less than 50 percent. As a result, those who could extract an arrow with skill were much valued.

In the most ancient of times, care for wounded soldiers was the purview of priests, who tried to explain the mysteries of sickness and death as matters in the hands of the gods. If the soldier survived, friends and family provided his care. It was the Greeks, and later the Romans, who freed medicine from religious restrictions and allowed empirical medicine to develop. Unfortunately, without knowledge of anatomy and basic science, their reasoning often led down disastrous paths, as was the case with their misunderstanding of the healing process and the use of bleeding and purging. The Greeks and Romans had the lethally wrong notion of the value of infection and of "laudable pus" as an indication of natural healing. After the fall of Rome, the care of wounded soldiers regressed as the Catholic Church dictated medical doctrine. Empirically based medical care would not again take hold until the rise of the nation-state in the 17th century, when military medicine could again achieve the level of sophistication and quality of care imperial Rome provided its soldiers.

The zenith of medical care in the ancient world came during the Roman Empire. While the Greeks invented the tourniquet to stop bleeding, it was the Romans who finally learned how to control bleeding once the tourniquet was removed. While neither the Greeks nor the Romans knew how to control infections, they both washed wounds with wine and vinegar, which contained natural bactericides and were more-effective antiseptics than what Joseph Lister used in 1865. In total, however, the legacy from the ancient world was not positive. Acceptance of the teachings of the Roman physician Galen about the cause and treatment of infection caused countless deaths. These teachings dominated modalities for wounds until the end of the 19th century.

After Rome

After the fall of Rome, Western Europe receded from the well-ordered structure and discipline of the Romans, replacing it with the feudal system of obligations between the lord and vassal. The care a soldier received was equal to his station in life; feudal lords cared for their knights, and monasteries cared for the poor and ordinary soldier.

One historian summed it up this way: The common soldier

> received little medical attention in war—"he was brought to be sacrificed, he was used while in health and when sick or wounded left to die." . . . The scope of the military surgeon was limited by the policy of discharging soldiers who were unfit rather than treating them . . . [and was] based upon the cynical though economic fact that it cost more to cure a soldier than levy a recruit. What medical attention there was available was devoted to the treatment of the nobles and knights. (Cantlie, 1974, p. 10)

The Crusades, starting in 1096, have been described as "undisciplined caravans," rather than coherent military forces. The tactics used and the wounds and care a soldier received could easily be described in Homeric terms. Unsanitary conditions allowed dysentery, fever, and typhus to run wild, with most soldiers dying even before they entered battle. At best, the treatment of wounds was reminiscent of Roman times: pressure on the wound, cauterization of arteries, and washing with wine and vinegar. By the late Middle Ages, however, some dared to challenge the orthodoxies of the Church. Theories were put forth suggesting that pus was not essential for the healing of wounds, but these notions were generally ignored. The laudable pus theory persisted to the great detriment of the wounded until Louis Pasteur finally debunked it in the later part of the 19th century, some six centuries later—less than 150 years ago.

The Renaissance profoundly changed the nature of war. First, it saw the rise of nation-states and the professionalization of armies. Second, the introduction of gunpowder allowed the use of small arms and artillery and the development of new tactics—all of which increased the severity of battle injuries. Devastatingly gruesome gunshot wounds, often resulting in shattered and compound fractures and amputations, replaced simple, clean cuts. It became common practice to cauterize all wounds, although the ligature of arteries and the use of turpentine, which had antiseptic properties, were also used. An early version of the modern hemostat made the amputation of the larger limbs a more acceptable procedure. The signature wound of this "age of gunpowder" became an amputated limb. With other wounds, a soldier either got better or died. Improved survival through amputation, however, meant that a steady stream of crippled veterans who were largely unemployable became a legacy of war long after the battles were over.

In America
Revolution
In the British colonies of North America, the medical treatment and care the wounded received reflected the English practices of the time. A series of wars with France, starting in 1688 and carried to the colonies during the French and Indian War (1756–1763), made North America the training ground for colonial officers who took up arms against the mother country in 1775. However, the tactics used on the frontier proved of little value in set battles against formations of British regulars during the Revolution. Suffering defeat after defeat in New York and Pennsylvania in 1776 and 1777, it was during the harsh winter at Valley Forge (1777–1778) that Baron Von Steuben, a Prussian, finally taught the Continental Army the art of 18th-century warfare.

The tactics of the era sought to blast opponents off the battlefield with concentrated musket fire from files of troops. It was not the individual soldier who mattered but the integrity of the line and how well the line stood after receiving a volley. But holding the line in the face of musket volleys was only part of what made for a disciplined force; the ability to withstand an assault by an enemy with the "terror weapon" of the 18th century, the bayonet, was critical, and it was not until 1779 that American units demonstrated that capability.

During the Revolution, actual battles were short and relatively infrequent, and soldiers spent most of their time in camp or maneuvering from one location to another. The American soldier had more to fear from camp life or being captured by the British than from the wounds of battle. Poor camp sanitation and the resulting disease accounted for 90 percent of all deaths, but things were not much better in the British camps, where 84 percent of deaths resulted from such diseases as typhus, typhoid fever, and malaria. Smallpox, which the Virginia Governor, Patrick Henry, described as "more destructive to an Army in the Natural way, than the Enemy's Swords" (as quoted in Gillett, 1981, p. 75), was largely controlled on the American side by a program of inoculation in 1777 and 1778 that General Washington had ordered.

Despite the enlightened inoculation program, the care given soldiers was largely ineffective. According to the leading medical authorities of the time, the standard care for all kinds of ailments was bloodletting, sweating, emetics, laxatives, and enemata. Surgeons took the lack of swelling and the absence of pus as bad signs that a wound was not healing. Given such medical treatments, it is no wonder that gunshot wounds to the torso most often got infected, leading to death, and that wounds to the extremities and fractures, particularly compound fractures, usually resulted in amputation, with mortality rates as high as 65 percent. Those who survived the loss of a limb were disabled for life and were dealt with accordingly.

Mexican War

As deadly as disease had been during the Revolution, the Mexican War, fought between 1846 and 1848, was the deadliest ever fought by an American army. While the Regular Army did most of the fighting and sustained battle casualties twice as high as the volunteers, the death rate from disease was twice as high for the volunteers as for the Regular Army. The volunteer camps were described as "sink-holes of filth and squalor" (Irey, 1972, p. 286), with many dying from malaria, measles, mumps, dysentery, and diarrhea. That description could have also been used to describe the conditions in the Union camps outside Washington in the early days of the Civil War.

Civil War

The American Civil War (1861–1865) was the first total war of the industrial age, and conflict became deadlier. On the eve of the war, the Regular Army numbered about 15,000 officers and men. By the time the war was over, 2.3 million men had served the Union, and as many as 1 million men wore the gray uniforms of the Confederacy. It has been estimated that one in ten Union soldiers died or were incapacitated, one in four for the Confederacy. During the Revolution, 90 percent of all deaths were from disease, compared with only 61 percent during the Civil War. These statistics do not reflect a sudden improvement in the treatment of disease, although there was a new focus on camp sanitation, so much as the nature of the conflict. During the Civil War, the mortality rate from disease in the Union Army was twice that of a similar group of men during peacetime. Some have argued that the high casualties were the direct result of using tactics most suitable for smoothbore muskets even though the armies had shifted to the more-deadly rifled muskets, breach-loading rifles, and machine (Gatling) guns. Others point to the different scale of operations, in which steamships and railroads made long-range, wide-scale campaigns possible and in which the soldiers fought in battles that were often only days apart.

The use of chloroform and ether to provide "pain-free" surgery was widespread, but surgeons still could not control infection and were ignorant of how it spread in hospitals. The vast majority of wounds Union soldiers suffered were from the Minié ball, which shattered bone and crushed soft tissues, carrying bacteria-laden bits of clothing and other debris into the wound. The death rate from wounds to the chest or abdomen was as high as 87 percent. But the most common wounds were to the extremities, often resulting in amputations—the hallmark wound of the Civil War. The average mortality rate for amputations of the lower extremities was 40 percent, but almost 21,000 amputees survived the war—12.1 percent of all wounded Union soldiers were amputation survivors. In 1862, Congress authorized the Army Medical Department to issue artificial limbs, making America the world leader in the field of prosthetics. Up until then, the provision of a prosthetic was a private matter, with surgeons selecting the particular amputation technique based upon the economic status of the patient. The amputation a poor person got was appropriate for the peg leg he or his family could afford. A rich person's amputation was appropriate for the articulated prosthesis he or his family could buy.

Union Surgeon General William A. Hammond once noted that the Civil War was fought at the "end of the medical middle ages" (Faust, 2008, p. 4). Just two years after the war's end, Joseph Lister demonstrated the benefits of carbolic acid spray as an antiseptic, yielding a corresponding two-thirds reduction in the death rate from amputations. However, it would be another 50 years before the use of antiseptics would become standard practice in the U.S. Army.

Spanish-American War

The official postwar assessment after the Spanish-American War was that, when the war started in 1898, the Army's Medical Department had lacked the plans, personnel, equipment, and effective doctrine necessary to support an army in the field. As a result, disease ravaged the troops in the United States and overseas. Actual casualty rates were low, with more soldiers dying from nonbattle causes than the total battle casualties, combat dead and wounded combined. This war, however, provided the impetus for major change.

World War I

When the United States entered World War I in 1916, the war had been going on for almost three very bloody years of stalemate. During those years, observers were dispatched who returned with lessons from the European experience. Together with the national preparedness movement, these lessons meant that the Army's medical establishment was better prepared for this war than for any in our history. And preparations came none too soon, because the lethality of the modern battlefield greatly increased during World War I, resulting in millions of casualties. By the beginning of the 20th century, many new inventions had revolutionized military communication, transportation, and combat vehicles. The new terror weapon was the machine gun. The increased lethality of artillery made the linear tactics of the 19th century obsolete. This was also a war of stalemate. Despite the advances in technology, neither side could gain an advantage as casualties mounted. What the Americans brought to the war in

1917 was not new technology or new tactics or great generalship but fresh troops, and that proved to turn the tide of battle.

Between April 1917 and Armistice Day, November 11, 1918, the Army increased from fewer than 200,000 to over 3.5 million men. The first troops arrived in Europe in July 1917; by the time hostilities ceased, almost 2 million men were overseas. What is generally not appreciated is that most American casualties occurred over about 100 days, between August 1918 and November 1918. Reflecting the mobility of American troops during the final campaign, most American battle injuries resulted from gunshots, not gas or artillery, which was very different from the experiences of the other allies, who had fought years of trench warfare.

As late as the Spanish-American War of 1898, nonbattle deaths had far exceeded combat casualties or deaths at the hands of the enemy. During World War I, the survival rate rose sharply as those WIA received medical care that limited infections. The Army's vaccination program had largely eliminated typhus. If it were not for the great influenza epidemic of 1918, World War I would stand out as the first great conflict in which noncombat deaths lagged substantially behind battlefield deaths and casualties.

World War II

For the United States, the story of World War I is the story of a European conflict. By contrast, World War II was a truly global conflict of enormous magnitude. Where the U.S. Army of World War I grew to about 3.5 million men, the U.S. Army of World War II peaked at over 8 million men, with an additional 4 million in the other armed services. In total, 16 million Americans served during World War II. This was total mobilization, with over 60 percent of the men of military age—those between 18 and 36 years of age—in uniform. After the initial defeats of American forces in the Philippines and on a handful of Pacific Islands, American forces were generally on the offensive, and combat centered on small infantry units supported by armor, artillery, and effective close air support.

For the American medical establishment, World War II required a new way of doing business; decentralization was the guiding principle for the organization of military medicine. World War II was fought with the lowest overall death rate in the history of the U.S. Army, although this statement hides the lethality of combat. For those in combat units, casualty rates remained high and would have been higher if not for the advances in medical care made during the war, such as the use of blood plasma and whole blood, antibiotics (sulfa drugs and penicillin), and improvements in the chain of evacuation that standardized care and moved patients quickly to higher echelons so that they might receive the best care possible. As a result, the death rate for those wounded who reached hospitals was half that of World War I. World War II also produced five times the neuropsychiatric casualties of World War I, foretelling issues for later wars.

Korean War

As the seeds of World War II were sown by the flawed peace following World War I, so the seeds of America's next two wars were sown by the unstable divisions of two countries in Asia that had been occupied by Japan: Korea and Vietnam. For the United States, the failure of the joint Soviet-American commission and then of the UN Temporary Commission on Korea precipitated North Korea's invasion of South Korea on June 25, 1950.

For the Army, the Korean War was really five wars in one, each very different from the others in terms of combat and the medical support provided. First, there was the defensive war in summer 1950, as American troops and their support were rushed to Korea to stop the advancing North Koreans. During this period, medical support was chaotic. Second, that September brought the rapid advance of UN and U.S. forces after the Inchon landing and the breakout from the Pusan Perimeter. Third, the subsequent harsh winter conditions led to retreat and withdrawal from North Korea. Fourth, was the counterattack during the spring offensive of 1951. Fifth and finally, there was a long period of static warfare that was reminiscent of the trench warfare of World War I. During each of these periods, the tactical situation rapidly changed, and medical support adapted to new situations fundamentally changing how care was provided.

During the first period, when American combat units were being thrown into the breach to stem the North Korean advance, the medical infrastructure was struggling to take hold, and almost as many American soldiers were KIA as WIA, far exceeding the normal WIA-to-KIA ratio of 4.1 to 1. During the second phase of the war, after the Inchon landing and the breakout from the Pusan, American forces advanced rapidly, and medical units struggled to keep up. The third was a period of retreat and withdrawal under pressure from the newly introduced Chinese forces, but more soldiers were taken off the line because of cold-weather injuries than were killed or wounded in battle. During this period, medical support was overwhelmed—with hundreds of wounded, operating in below zero temperatures, and with medical personnel themselves among the casualties—and was stretched to the breaking point. Eventually, a stable line was established and cease-fire negotiations started, ushering in a period of static or trench warfare and routinized medical support that lasted until 1953.

Overall, the rate of battle casualties in Korea was somewhat lower than that of World War II. The volatility of the conflict and the widespread use of modern ballistic body armor contributed to the overall reduction in casualties in Korea as compared with World War II. The KIA rate was highest in July 1950, as troops were sent into battle to blunt the North Korean advance and establish a defensive perimeter around the port city of Pusan, and was lowest after negotiations started, only to rise for relatively short periods as both sides mounted local attacks to gain tactical advantage along what would become the final cease-fire line.

Overall, the number of battle deaths per 1,000 average annual strength was 43.2 in Korea, compared with 51.9 in the European Theater of Operations from June 1944 to May 1945. The infantry comprised only 20 percent of total Army strength but suffered about 70 percent of the total casualties. In general, shell fragments caused the greatest number of wounds, but small-arms bullets caused the greatest number of deaths. In Korea, 21.8 percent of those who had been hit died, compared to 25.1 for those hit in the European theater and 28.8 percent for all of World War II. In World War II, the WIA/KIA ratio was 3.9 for all theaters; in Korea, that ratio was 4.1. Of those admitted to medical treatment facilities, 2.5 percent died, compared with 4.5 percent for World War II.

Since the Civil War, the frequency of combat amputations has steadily decreased, and survival rates have steadily increased, but during and after World War II, the Army's approach to treatment of acute injuries of major arteries remained a problem. The policy of the Army Medical Department at the start of the Korean War was to tie off or ligate all vascular wounds, a procedure that had not changed much since the time Roman legions held the field. This changed in Korea as arterial surgery became almost commonplace, and the amputation rate from injured arteries fell from 49 percent during World War II to approximately 7 to 13 percent during Korea.

Vietnam

America's second post–World War II conflict did not really start in 1966, when the Marines first deployed to South Vietnam, but at the Potsdam Conference in July 1945, when the allied powers decided to return all of Indochina—Vietnam, Laos, and Cambodia—to France. By 1946, there was open warfare between the Viet Minh and the French, which finally ended with the French defeat at Dien Bien Phu in 1954. The international peace conference that followed formally ended the war with what was to be a temporary division of Vietnam, but by 1959, communist forces, both indigenous and from the north, were fighting in South Vietnam. By 1961—the end of the first year of the Kennedy administration—more than 4,000 American military personnel were on the ground in South Vietnam. In March 1965, President Johnson ordered U.S. Marines to South Vietnam to protect the large airfield at Da Nang. Soon, offensive operations were approved, and by the end of 1965, 185,000 troops were on the ground. The firepower and mobility America brought to the battle, however, were never decisive because the Viet Cong responded by infiltrating more troops from North Vietnam. By 1968, it was clear that neither side could achieve a strategic advantage.

The Viet Cong's Tet offensive in early 1968 changed the whole tenor of the war. While the Viet Cong lost a great many troops and did not permanently take control of any cities, Tet shook the confidence of American political leaders that the war could be won. It also unleashed a wave of antiwar protests that divided the nation. Soon, there was new emphasis on negotiations, Vietnamization, and withdrawal. In July 1973, the parties agreed to stop fighting, to the withdrawal of American troops, and to the eventual reunification of Vietnam "through peaceful means." With the United States out of the way, there was little to prevent resumption of the war; by the end of April 1975, Vietnam was united under the communists.

Vietnam was a "dirty" war in terms of enemy tactics, types of wounds sustained, and the terrain over which it was fought. Vietnam was a mainly a guerrilla war, more reminiscent of the Philippine insurrection than any of the other wars the United States fought in the 20th century. Most casualties were caused by small arms fire, booby traps, and mines, rather than by the conventional artillery and other explosive fragments that had previously been so dominant. The Viet Cong's use of crude punji-stick booby traps seldom resulted in death but frequently resulted in infected wounds. Even with the use of use of modern antibiotics, whole-blood transfusions, and advanced surgical techniques, infection due to the dirt and debris from mines and to punji-stick wounds was a problem.

In Vietnam overall, the number of American deaths was relatively low, reflecting the tempo of battle. The number of nonbattle deaths from illnesses was negligible, and the rate of hospitalization for disease was more than 25 percent lower than that for Korea and less than one-half that for the European theater of operations during combat operations in World War II. However, the wounds from booby traps and mines were devastating, making the proportion of limb-threatening wounds greater. Despite rapid evacuation by air ambulance and even as arterial surgery become relatively common, amputations were more prevalent in Vietnam than in any war since the Civil War. Moreover, the care received in Army CONUS hospitals was quite inconsistent, with some amputees being transferred to the VA even before their wounds had closed. It was not until the wars in Iraq and Afghanistan that the Army addressed the continuity of treatment and rehabilitation as indistinguishable parts of the healing process and implemented a policy that retained amputees through rehabilitation.

Middle East Wars: Persian Gulf War, Afghanistan, and Iraq

In retrospect, the post–World War II period can be divided into two parts. The first is the Cold War against international communism, with its not-so-cold flare-ups in Korea and Vietnam. The second is the wars in the Middle East, whose root cause is the geographic accident that placed a significant portion of the world's supply of oil in an unstable region of artificial states created from the remnants of the Ottoman Empire after World War I. The first of these more-recent conflicts, the Persian Gulf War of 1991–1992, was actually two designated military operations, Operation Desert Shield and Operation Desert Storm, which initially promised to be a formidable test of the American military rebuilt after Vietnam.

The Iraqi military that the United States and its coalition partners faced in fall 1991 comprised more than 50 well-equipped divisions, with more than 700 combat aircraft. American military planners expected a sizable number of combat casualties, ordered over 16,000 body bags, and deployed 65 major triservice hospitals and more than 41,000 medical support personnel. When the ground war commenced on January 17, 1991, more than 18,000 hospital beds were available in theater. An additional 5,500 hospital beds were ready in Germany, backed up by 22,000 beds in CONUS. The war, however, was over in a little more than 100 hours and produced far fewer casualties than expected: 148 battle deaths, 145 nonbattle deaths, and 470 WIA.

While the war hardly stressed or tested the medical support system, it was clear enough from the tempo of operations that the Army's MASHs and CSHs lacked the mobility and surgical capabilities needed to keep up with a rapidly changing tactical situation. After operations Desert Shield and Desert Storm, a rethinking of battlefield medicine resulted in the closure of MASH units, the establishment of small FSTs, a new emphasis on training for the immediate treatment of combat trauma, on the rapid evacuation of combat casualties from the theater of operations, and on the quality of en route medical care as patients were flown back to the United States.

In Afghanistan and Iraq, the new system allowed battle casualties to be treated almost immediately after being wounded, moving to an Echelon II FST within minutes, then heading on to an Echelon III CSH within hours. When medevac flights were short, casualties were taken directly to a CSH, skipping over the FST echelon. For the most crucial casualties, transferring out of the combat zone to an Echelon IV facility could now take as little as 12 hours. For those returning to the United States, the stay at the Echelon IV facility at Landstuhl, Germany, routinely lasted no longer than two or three days. A process that had taken 45 days during the Vietnam War could now take three days or less.

With the exception of the first three weeks of OIF, combat in both Afghanistan and Iraq was highly unconventional, as the weapons used and the wounds they caused clearly showed. Over time, the prevalence of gunshot wounds decreased, while blast wounds from rocket-propelled grenades; mortars; mines; bombs; grenades; and, especially, IEDs increased sharply. By 2017, IEDs accounted for 54 percent of wounds in Afghanistan and 31 percent of combat casualties in Iraq. The lethality and devastating effects of the high-explosive blast injuries from IEDs and land mines resulted in severe limb injuries and a high mortality rate for penetrating head injuries among troops both on foot and in armored vehicles.

Overall, a larger proportion of wounded personnel in Iraq and Afghanistan survived than in any previous American conflict, largely because of improved body armor; the development of MRAPs; an increased focus on prehospital TCCC training; improvements in hemorrhage control, for example, through widespread use of tourniquets; and rapid evacuation from the battlefield, within the golden hour.

Given the prevalence of IEDs and land mines and their devastating effects, it is a tribute to battlefield medicine that the overall rate of amputations remained low. Since the beginning of combat in 2001, more than 1.3 million Army soldiers have deployed to Afghanistan and Iraq. In that time, the Army has reported more than 3,900 hostile deaths and more than 36,000 WIA but only 1,098 major limb amputations and 179 minor limb amputations. Fewer of the wounded were amputees, at 3.5 percent, than in

Vietnam. However, increasing numbers of multilimb amputations indicate increasing wound severity. In Afghanistan, 39 percent of amputations were multilimb; in Iraq, the number was 24 percent in Iraq. Both percentages are much higher than the 2 to 20 percent reported for World War I, World War II, the Korean War, and the Vietnam War.

When the United States was attacked on 9/11, the Army and the entire DoD were unprepared to provide rehabilitation services to combat amputees. From its review of Russian experiences in Afghanistan during the 1980s, however, the U.S. Army knew it would likely face a significant number of blast casualties, including traumatic amputations. Within a matter of days, the Surgeon General had his staff working to reestablish an Army amputee center. In a marked departure from policy during Vietnam, the Army took the position that the loss of a limb was not necessarily a career-ending injury. If amputees had been discharged and transferred to the VA in the past, now the Surgeon General thought the Army should provide state-of-the-art rehabilitation and restoration care, with the goal of providing amputees the option to remain on active duty to complete their military careers. The Army's support for amputees did not stop there. As the Army saw it, it had a role in the continued care of amputees even after they had left the service. Amputees were generally medically retired and, therefore, would have access to the military health care system, if they chose to use it, for the rest of their lives. In 2004, the Army established the Disabled Soldier Support System program—later renamed the U.S. Army Wounded Warrior Program—to help disabled soldiers, largely amputees, cut through red tape to facilitate remaining on active duty or, if they chose to leave, to obtain a medical retirement.

Initial plans for an amputee center were approved within days of the first U.S. SF entering Afghanistan. By the end of summer 2002, the Chief of Staff of the Army had approved funds to establish the amputation center at WRAMC.

The impact of the Army's new program was almost immediately clear. Of the first 53 soldiers who had sustained major amputations in Afghanistan, 11 had lost more than one limb, and 47 were treated at Walter Reed. One-quarter also received some VA care. A 2010 survey showed that 39 percent of amputees from Afghanistan and Iraq had received prosthetics from the military; during Vietnam, that number was less than 1 percent. Moreover, the Army's long-term retention of amputees was significant: Seven years after the amputations, 14 percent of all amputees, 17 percent of amputees who had lost one limb, and 5 percent of amputees who had lost more than one limb were still on active duty. Much of the success of the Army's efforts to keep amputees on active duty can be attributed to new prosthetics that incorporate advanced microprocessors and to the Army's rehabilitation program, which adjusts the microprocessors to the progress of the patient.

Some unexpected and negative consequences were, however, associated with the Army's new amputee program. Previously, amputees averaged 51 days at Walter Reed before being transferred to the VA. In 2007, with the new program in place, amputees were spending an average of 21 days as inpatients and an average of 311 days as outpatients. At the program's peak in 2005, nearly 900 outpatients at Walter Reed were being housed in old barracks, nearby hotels, and leased apartments, and outpatients outnumbered inpatients 17 to 1. In spring 2007, problems in these temporary living arrangements were highlighted in a series of *Washington Post* articles, which eventually resulted in the dismissal of Walter Reed's commander, the Surgeon General of the Army, and the Secretary of the Army, as well as a number of high-level commissions and changes to the process for discharging soldiers from the military and moving them to the VA.

The extensive use of IEDs in Afghanistan and Iraq did not result only in limb loss. A more frequent result was TBI, which has been called the signature wound of the wars in Afghanistan and Iraq. The symptoms of TBI can be mild—such as headaches or neck pain, nausea, ringing in the ears, dizziness, and tiredness—or more severe—such as convulsions or seizures, slurred speech, and weakness or numbness in the arms and legs. However, only severe and penetrating TBIs are recognized and triaged at the time of injury, and these usually require hospitalization and rehabilitation. The vast majority of TBI cases are mild, are closed-brain injuries, are not diagnosed promptly, and are not likely to be recorded as combat wounds (WIA). Moreover, even at the height of combat, most TBIs reported were among troops not deployed to Afghanistan and Iraq. However, the IOM has found sufficient evidence of an association between TBI and a long list of chronic neurocognitive and behavioral symptoms, including PTSD.

Organization of Medical Services on and off the Battlefield

The second broad theme from history is the effectiveness of medical logistics, both the organization of medical services within the military and care provided to soldiers on the battlefield. What started as rather haphazard organization of medical care for the military has grown into military medical departments as sophisticated as any civilian health care organization.

The Ancient World

The most detailed recounting of medical logistics in the early Grecian period is from Homer's *Iliad*. Whether real or legend, the tales rang true and were accepted in the ancient world. The care of the wounded depicted suggests that care was not provided by the state but left in the hands of individual warriors and their servants, a pattern that has been repeated throughout history. More generally, campaigns between city-states were usually fought near home, and care from family and friends was readily available. The campaigns of Alexander the Great stand in sharp contrast. They were fought thousands of miles from home, making it particularly difficult to replace Greek soldiers lost to disease or in battle. That placed a premium on keeping the army as healthy as possible and caring for the sick and wounded so that they could return to the ranks. Alexander used wagons as ambulances, and some have credited him with organizing the first military medical corps in any Western army, albeit small by today's standards or even the standards of the Imperial Roman army, only three centuries later.

Originally, the Roman army was a citizen force on the model of the Greeks. The care of wounded had not progressed beyond the care Homer described. On the march, Roman armies customarily took their wounded with them, and it was a generally accepted obligation of the wealthy to open their homes to care for the wounded. A professional army started to take hold with Roman expansion, starting in the 3rd century B.C. However, the individual armies' politician-commanders raised had no medical corps per se, and medical care was haphazard, depending greatly on the largess of the general. Informally, a de facto medical service developed when soldiers started specializing in the healing arts.

Augustus established the first unified Roman army and, with it, a formal medical corps. The army provided a range of medical capabilities that were unique in the ancient world. It established its own medical training program and standardized care based on its own medical manuals. The medical unit included animals and vehicles for transporting patients and supplies. Roman military forts had hospitals for the treatment and recuperation of sick and wounded soldiers and were designed to accommodate upwards of 10 percent of the legion's personnel, with remote hospitals on the frontier being larger.

The care a Roman soldier received was strikingly different from that available to the average Roman citizen. A number of scholars have concluded that the quality and effectiveness of Roman military medicine were generally not surpassed until at least the 17th century—some would say 18th century—and in some areas, the same care a soldier received during World War I can be found in Roman medical guides of the 1st century A.D. The general competency of military medical staff is suggested by the surgical instruments excavated from the ruins of Roman military hospitals and the fact that, after leaving the army, they were valued as civilian physicians.

After Rome

During the early Middle Ages, care on and off the battlefield most often fell to the clergy, where the imposition of religious doctrine impeded the quality of care received. The sharp division of the medical profession into the domains of physicians and surgeons can be traced to the 12th century, when the Catholic Church forbade the clergy to shed blood. Priests and monks continued to practice medicine, and surgery was relegated to their former lay assistants, whose primary duty was shaving the monks' heads with sharp blades—thus arose the lower-status profession of the barber-surgeon. During the First Crusade (1096–1099), there is no evidence that the armies systematically provided for their wounded, but it is likely the wounded were taken to the nearest friendly town for care. After the fall of Jerusalem in 1098, various knightly orders established hospices to care for sick and wounded soldiers, as well as for pilgrims destined for the Holy Land. These were the forerunners of today's modern hospitals.

As power in Europe became centralized under a few national leaders, armies developed, and attention was given to the care of the troops, particularly the valuable professional troops. The first account of a mobile hospital set up in tents dates to 1180. During the Third Crusade (1189–1192), Emperor Frederick of Germany provided transportation for the sick. The chronicler of the battle of Alona in Spain in 1484 tells us that Queen Isabella established the Queen's Hospital: "six large tents and their furniture, together with physicians, surgeons, medicines and attendants; and commanded that they should charge nothing, for she would pay for all" (Garrison, 1922, p. 95). Charles V, her grandson, carried through her benevolent care for his soldiers; surgeons who were "skilled, experienced, and trained" were assigned to each troop (Lynch, Weed, and McAfee, 1923, p. 27).

In France in 1550, Henri II created "ambulant hospitals" (from which the word *ambulance* is derived), which followed the movements of troops and triaged the wounded to fixed hospitals. In 1708, Louis XIV (1638–1715) established the French Medical Corps, with 200 physicians and surgeons, and constructed 51 military hospitals across France. Later, in 1794, military teaching hospitals were created to provide medical personnel to the army. Pierre-Francois Percy and Dominique-Jean Larrey, senior medical officers in Napoleon's army, made significant improvements in how war casualties were cared for on the battlefield, particularly by introducing a mobile ambulance corps for evacuating the wounded.

The English Army, during the reign of Henry VIII (1509–1547), regularly employed surgeons to care for the wounded. Some of these were provided by a guild known as the Company of Barber-Surgeons of London as a condition of its royal charter. Captains of troop companies were also authorized to recruit their own surgeons. However, the critical evacuation problem was not addressed, which increased the loss of life and depleted the ranks of fighting men as they carried their comrades to safety. A century later, during the English Civil War, the Royalists left their wounded on the battlefield in the hope that they would receive "humane treatment" at the hands of their enemies. In contrast, the New Model Army of the Commonwealth included a physician general, a surgeon general, and an apothecary general, and one surgeon was authorized for each company of troops. While Parliament provided some medicines, the surgeons provided the liniments, ointments, and battle dressings, with the troops themselves ultimately bearing the cost. In addition, given the large number of wounded, central hospitals were established in London and Dublin and in Scotland to relieve the burden on regimental hospitals.

By the end of the 17th century, military medicine had become a definite function of government, with two competing views of how to care for the wounded. These centered on the roles of general and regimental hospitals—a conflict that carried over to America and was not resolved until the Civil War. Peacetime general hospitals were built in central locations. During a war, as the army increased in size and deployed overseas, the general hospitals provided the staff to form new central hospitals that accompanied the troops to large garrison towns. The general hospitals were staffed with elite physicians who had trained at Oxford or Cambridge but who frequently lacked military experience.

Routine care and the immediate care of battle casualties were the responsibilities of the regimental surgeon and hospitals. The medical officers assigned to each regiment were generally not university graduates, having apprenticed with a physician or surgeon, and received commensurately low pay. They were often poorly treated because, while they held a commission from the King, they did not hold the social position usually associated with such commissions. Medical mates who supported the regimental surgeons had even less training and received lower pay. Efforts to improve the qualifications of regimental medical staff were frustrated by the poor rates of pay, which, by one account, were only one-quarter of what a civilian physician might make. It was at this time that care from professional female attendants, not "camp followers," was routinized.

Conditions along this medical chain or echelon were variable and uncertain. The policy was to evacuate the sick to general hospitals as soon as possible, which often led to overcrowding and the spread of epidemic disease. The alternative of keeping the wounded in regimental hospitals fared little better because these were often nothing more than sheds or barns. Moreover, transporting the wounded from the battlefield was always a problem, even for the winning side. As a result, in 1743, Britain and her allies concluded a treaty with France to regulate the care of the wounded that foreshadowed the Geneva Conventions of the next century.

No country entered the 19th century with an adequate military medical system, but most were transformed by the end of the century. The impetus for change was the horrid performance of the French and British military medical systems during the Crimean War and the advances of the Americans during the Civil War and of the Germans during the Franco-Prussian War of 1870.

In Britain, while the army largely ignored the age of reform (1780–1850), important changes to the provision of medical care did occur, including commissioning physicians from a wider range of British universities; making promotions on the basis of knowledge and ability, rather than seniority or patronage; establishing fixed time-in-grade requirements for promotion; increasing pay; recognizing the military nature of medical service by awarding military decorations to medical officers; and establishing a system of medical reporting that provided data for a study of the mortality of soldiers living in military barracks. These data, which showed a mortality rate for soldiers higher than that for the general population, were used to convince the government that money spent in bettering the soldiers' health could save lives. Even with these advances, the army's Medical Department was unprepared for the realities of modern warfare, which came in 1854 with the Crimean War. Following an all-too-familiar trend, disease accounted for more than 90 percent of all deaths. Progress, however, was made with the dispatch of a corps of female nurses under the direction of Florence Nightingale and the establishment of the civilian Sanitary Commission, which had the authority to impose changes on the military.

Finally, in 1873—a decade after the American Civil War and three years after the Franco-Prussian War—the regimental hospital was abolished, and a modern organization of battlefield care was developed that provided bearer companies, movable field hospitals, stationary hospitals, general hospitals, sanitary detachments, depot medical stores, and hospital ships. In 1877, medical officers were finally given the power to command their own staff and patients. In 1878, the pay, privileges, and ranks of medical officers were brought into line with the rest of the army. In 1879, a medical reserve corps was established. The new system was tested and adjusted during the first and second Boer Wars (1880–1881 and 1899–1902) in South Africa. With the exception of the failure to fully appreciate the value of inoculation against disease and the need to vaccinate the force, these changes provided an efficient medical organization that was in place at the outbreak of World War I.

The last of the great powers to reform, and then only partially so, was France. It was not until 1889 that France established an autonomous military medical service, but even then, the medical staff was not seen as a core component of a war-fighting staff. In the early days of World War I, the chief surgeon of the French Army complained of a lack of personnel, the poor technical competence of the staff, and his inability to coordinate with the general staff during the flow of battle.

In America
Revolution

During the Revolutionary War, wounded soldiers were cared for by an evolving array of treatment facilities that were often in open conflict with one another, usually over bureaucratic issues, particularly the tension between general and regimental hospitals. The argument in favor of the general hospital was the need to address the often-poor qualifications of regimental surgeons and their mates and the observation that a single general hospital was cheaper to run than a collection of regimental hospitals. The argument in favor of the regimental hospital was that it kept patients close to their comrades and, because such hospitals were dispersed, lessened the effects of epidemics, which infected more in larger hospitals.

The pattern of conflict after the Revolution followed a common path. During crises, the small Regular Army was augmented by equally ill-prepared volunteers and militias from the states. The medical establishment that supported the Regular Army in peacetime, now responsible for medical care of its own force and what was needed to support the regimental surgeons of the volunteers and militia, was equally unprepared. At the start of the War of 1812, nine months elapsed before Congress even reestablished the posts of Physician and Surgeon General and Apothecary General. Quite predictably, there was friction between the regimental surgeons and the medical staff of the Regular Army.

Mexican War

Even with the establishment of a permanent peacetime Medical Department in 1818, the Army was unprepared to support the initial medical needs at the onset of the Mexican War in 1848, resulting in great loss of life, mainly to disease.

Civil War

While some improvements followed the Mexican War, the Medical Department still could not cope with the evacuation of the wounded from the battlefield, and no plans existed for the care of mass casualties. Unprepared even for a minor war, the Army Medical Department was overwhelmed in the earliest months of the Civil War. The names of the Surgeon General, Dr. William A. Hammond; the Medical Director of the Army of the Potomac, Dr. Jonathan Letterman; and the Sanitary Commission will forever be linked to the innovations that transformed military medicine during the Civil War. Medical advances were made steadily over the course of the war; as a result, by the end of hostilities, the new system of battlefield care and evacuation by ambulances, trains, and ships had become the prototype for battlefield medicine for the great wars of the 20th century. The focus of care shifted from the regimental hospitals to large-scale military hospitals constructed in major cities and accessible by rail. By the end of the war, the Union operated 192 general hospitals with a total capacity of over 118,000 beds, some with more than 3,000 beds. Notable was the increase in trained women nurses, who transformed the delivery of care both during the war and after. Their value had become so indispensable that, within a decade, a permanent nursing school was established in New York City.

Convalescent Camps were also established to receive men from the hospital who no longer needed medical treatment but who were not well enough to return to their units for active service. Soldiers remained in these camps until they regained their strength or were discharged from the service. Today, the Army's WTUs perform essentially the same function that the Convalescent Camps performed during the Civil War.

Spanish-American War

Unfortunately, many of the advances made during the Civil War were short lived in the American Army. Following the war, the general hospitals and the Hospital Transports and Ambulance Corps were dispensed with, and the medical supplies were sold. After Reconstruction, the Regular Army's strength decreased to 25,000 soldiers, who mainly served at small posts in the west. Despite the quiescence of the period, there were several notable advances, including establishment of the Hospital Corps (1887) and the Army Medical School (1893).

These changes were significant, serving as a basis for the professionalization of the Medical Department, but when the Spanish-American War started, the Army Medical

Department lacked the plans, personnel, equipment, and doctrine necessary to support an army in the field. After the war, the Dodge Commission, appointed by President McKinley, investigated the conduct of the war, concluding that the performance of the Army Medical Department had been a fiasco.

Reforms by Secretary of War Elihu Root followed, including creation of the Nurse Corps in 1901; new regulations in 1904 that addressed the assignment of medical personnel and the allocation of ambulance companies and field hospitals; and new medical manuals that laid out a system to move the casualties from the battlefield, to battalion aid stations, to field hospitals, and then to permanent hospitals. The new system was tested in field maneuvers in 1910 and 1913. In 1916, the deployment of medical units to support General Pershing's campaign along the Mexican border was a precursor of the deployments to Europe that were to come.

The Medical Department was reorganized in 1908, and Congress authorized the Medical Reserve Corps, the forerunner of the entire Army Reserve System. When war came in 1916, the Reserve and National Guard provided a mechanism for commissioning applicants without resorting to contract surgeons, as had been necessary in the Spanish-American War. A separate reserve corps for nurses was organized in 1912, as the American Red Cross Nursing Service. On the eve of World War I, 8,000 had registered. Eventually, the Red Cross provided the Army with more than 20,000 nurses. The final transformation of the Army Medical Department took place with the National Defense Act of 1916.

World War I

At the start of World War I, the Medical Department dispatched observers to Europe. When the United States finally entered the war, important lessons had already been learned concerning military hospitals, care for the neuropsychiatrically wounded, amputations, and rehabilitation, making the Army Medical Department better prepared than it had been for any previous war. Nevertheless, to meet this challenge, it had to grow very quickly. While the Army increased in size by a factor of 19, the medical services increased 131-fold. In March 1917, the Army had approximately 3,000 medical personnel; by November 1917, that number had grown to 394,000. At the time of the Armistice, 27 percent of all physicians in America were in uniform.

On the battlefield during World War I, the wounded benefited from two innovations in the movement of casualties: the motorized ambulance and the widespread use of hospital trains. The care the wounded received incorporated new advances in medicine and new battlefield techniques for limiting infections and took place in well-staffed general and specialized hospitals. The centerpiece of medical support was the division hospital. The average time it took to evacuate the wounded to a field hospital now was measured in hours, not days.

To care for returning war wounded, the Army built hospitals at debarkation points and in local draft districts. Special facilities were fashioned for patients with tuberculosis; psychiatric conditions; and orthopedic, oral, and plastic surgery, as well as physical and occupational therapists and other rehabilitative services. When the war ended, the Army had 92 large hospitals in the United States, with a combined capacity of over 120,000 beds. The sick and wounded were moved through the system on hospital trains. In addition to psychiatric programs, considerable emphasis was placed on physical reconstruction and the rehabilitation of wounded soldiers prior to discharge.

World War II

Both World Wars had one thing in common. The conflicts started years before the entry of the United States, giving the Medical Department time to prepare. In 1939, when war began in Europe, the Army Medical Department was geared to serve a garrison army. The almost 13,000 officers and men of the Medical Department operated seven general and 119 station hospitals in the United States, Hawaii, the Philippines, and the Panama Canal Zone. By June 1940, six months before the United States entered the war, the Medical Department employed 18,000 people. Six months after Pearl Harbor, the Medical Department numbered 118,000. By the end of the war, the Medical Department employed about 664,000 officers and soldiers. Importantly, the Medical Department now included more than just physicians and nurses: Dietitians, physical therapists, pharmacists, and even medical administrators were now permanent fixtures.

World War II was very different from previous wars. This was truly a world war. It was fought around the globe in several theaters of operation, with commands that largely controlled their own assets, including medical units. In Washington, the Department of War reorganization of March 1942 changed historic reporting relationships, and only decisions about the professional standards of care would remain in the purview of the Surgeon General; operational control of medical units was left to the theater commanders and their chief medical officers.

One reason for the low mortality rate during World War II was the rapidity with which seriously wounded soldiers could travel through the five echelons of evacuation to receive the specialized care they needed. The speed actually increased as the war went on and stood in sharp contrast to what had been possible only 25 years earlier in World War I. Medevacs by air, which had averaged only 272 per month in 1943, hit a peak in July 1945, with 12,326 patients debarking from aircraft. The increased role aircraft were playing in these evacuations by war's end foretold the revolution in military medical care that was to take place in the latter half of the 20th century.

Medical care for those wounded in combat centered on general, specialized general, and convalescent hospitals. By the fall of 1943, convalescent patients accounted for approximately 75 percent of the patient load of general hospitals. Unfortunately, convalescent centers often lacked the essential personnel and facilities that were considered essential for rehabilitation programs.

One reason convalescent centers were considered necessary was the inability of the VA to care for returning veterans. The situation was so critical that, on December 4, 1944, President Roosevelt ordered the Secretary of War *not* to discharge overseas casualties from the service until they had received "the maximum benefits of hospitalization and convalescent facilities," including "physical and psychological rehabilitation, vocational guidance, prevocational training and resocialization" (Roosevelt, 1944). After the close of World War II, the Army Medical Department demobilized along with the rest of the Army, transferring these convalescent centers to a newly revitalized VA under the direction of Army General Omar Bradley.

Korean War

Just five years passed between the end of World War II and the start of the Korean War, but the changes in the interim for the Army Medical Department and the medical support to the troops were enormous. Before World War II, the majority of Army physicians were general practitioners, with only a few specialists. During the war, the ranks swelled with all kinds of health professionals. The challenge after the war was to incorporate these changes and to remake the permanent medical department into a modern, specialty-oriented medical system without compromising the medical support needed for combat. Unfortunately, when the Korean War started, that goal had not yet been achieved. The Army was unprepared to provide the medical support combat forces required. During the first critical months of the war, medical personnel could only be drawn from those available in the Far East and those the Army could immediately reassign from the United States and Europe. Eventually, new physicians were conscripted, but the tension between working with what the draft provided and while rotating personnel to "share the burden" meant that there was a constant need to train newcomers. As a result, most battlefield care was provided by physicians with no military training, limited surgical training, and even less training in treating trauma casualties.

Throughout history, the central issue for forward medical support for battlefield casualties has been where on the battlefield to provide medical care for the critically wounded. How close to the fighting can medical or surgical units be without unduly risking their safety, yet still meet the medical needs of the wounded? What the Army wanted was an Echelon III capability in an Echelon II environment. As always, this involves the interplay of tactics, terrain, and technology.

Experience gained during World War II led the Army to finalize the design for the MASH in 1945. This 60-bed, self-contained, and mobile hospital was staffed with surgical and medical personnel and was equipped to provide definitive, life-saving surgery and postoperative care for patients until it was safe to transport them to a rear-area hospital. As designed, the MASH could be disassembled and be ready to depart within six hours and, on arriving at a new location, could be operational within four hours.

In Korea, the key to the success of the MASHs was the employment of two World War II technologies: the jeep ambulance and the helicopter. Helicopters and MASH units will always be linked in the minds of the American public, thanks to the television show *M*A*S*H*. But in the mountains of Korea, the workhorse was the jeep ambulance, with helicopters reportedly flying fewer than one-half of all true surgical cases. Nevertheless, over the course of the war, helicopters carried 18,000 patients, many of whom would not have survived without a smooth ride and the patients' rapid arrival at a clearing station, MASH, or hospital.

As was true during World War II, most patients were initially evacuated from Korea by ship. By the end of the war, however, over 300,000 intratheater patient trips were recorded, and 95.4 percent of the soldiers evacuated from the Far East (Korea and Japan) to CONUS arrived by air transport. In less than a decade after the end of World War II, the whole system of casualty evacuation had radically changed. Starting with helicopters and extending to long-range transport aircraft, the period from wounding to definitive care in the United States had been dramatically reduced, with more to come.

Vietnam

Medical support in Vietnam was very different from that of any previous war. The deployed combat units of divisions and separate brigades originally planned to follow the well-established doctrinal lines of the five-echelon medical support model. However, in Vietnam, the geography of the country; the fluidity of combat operations; and, particularly, changing technology resulted in far-reaching modifications of the traditional linear model. While the Korean War saw the introduction of the helicopter as a combat air ambulance, its use matured in Vietnam, fundamentally changing the way medical care is provided on the battlefield.

Some units, like the 1st Cavalry Division (Airmobile), had their own extensive fleets of aircraft and were able to adhere to the traditional evacuation model, in which most casualties were first evacuated to one of its clearing stations and then, if warranted, sent on to a surgical hospital. Those who could not tolerate this two-stage process, the most severely wounded, were evacuated directly from the battle to a surgical, evacuation, or field hospital. The divisions that did not have their own organic air ambulance units followed a different model and evacuated their wounded directly to surgical hospitals using helicopters assigned to and operating from the hospitals. These Dust Off helicopters belonged to the echelons above division—to the corps or logistic command or to the Army medical brigade or medical command—and transported the wounded outside the division's area of operations. When this happened, divisional medical companies were often assigned to the receiving hospitals to provide additional resources, and the traditional functions of division clearing stations and hospitals merged. In practice, the critical role the chain of evacuation from battalion aid station to division clearing station had played in past wars gave way to the direct evacuation of the wounded to a surgical, evacuation, or field hospital well to the rear of the division's area of operations. This was a radical change in the doctrine of forward surgical support. By 1970, the paradigm of care had shifted from one that emphasized bringing the surgeons to the wounded to one of bringing the wounded to the surgeons and giving immediate care in a more-pristine facility. Accordingly, numbers of physicians in the division decreased from 34 to 12, and one-half of the divisional wheeled ambulances were eliminated.

Middle East Wars: Persian Gulf War, Afghanistan, and Iraq

The medical scheme employed in Afghanistan and Iraq was substantially different from the one that had deployed to the Persian Gulf a decade before. Since the age of Napoleon, there have been competing schemes for caring for battle casualties by moving the surgeons as far forward as possible and/or rapidly removing the wounded to a well-staffed and -equipped rear-area hospital. Efforts to move the surgeons forward faltered as MASH units became larger and less mobile. The advent of helicopters to transport the most critically wounded off the battlefield was a great step forward but had a reverse effect, with MASH units being set up farther from the front lines and tending to become more permanent.

In Afghanistan and Iraq, the focus shifted to the treatment of trauma. Surgeons were moved far forward in small FSTs—each with 20 personnel, two operating room tables, and no beds—designed to provide immediate care to the estimated 10 to 15 percent of wounded who required surgical intervention to control hemorrhage and/or be stabilized to survive the trip to the CSH in the rear.

There was also a new emphasis on trauma training. In 2001, just in time for the wars in the Middle East, the Army established a trauma training center at the Miller School of Medicine of the University of Miami to provide predeployment refresher training and to teach new concepts, skills, and teamwork unique to combat trauma. Not every deployed FST received such training, and many of the deployed surgeons felt they were not adequately prepared to operate in the combat environment. However, between 2002 and 2015, 112 FSTs did complete the program.

A further change in the system of casualty care put in place after the Gulf War and ready by the time forces deployed to Afghanistan was a unified, or *joint*, system for rapid intertheater evacuation of patients to the United States. After Operation Desert Storm, there was a new focus on achieving a smaller theater footprint and rapidly evacuating patients to the United States for definitive treatment. To accomplish this, the Air Force designed the new CCATT, with advanced emergency room skills, and changed the policy from transporting only *stable* patients to transporting *stabilized* patients—patients with assured airways, stabilized fractures, all hemorrhage controlled, and fluid resuscitation begun. The new long-range C-17 aircraft was ideal for the new mission and became a flying ICU as it provided evacuations from the combat theater to CONUS.

Even after troops were deployed to Afghanistan and Iraq, changes in battlefield prehospital care—hemorrhage control and rapid intratheater evacuation—were made that further reduced the loss of life. Research during and after Vietnam showed that as many as 8 percent of KIAs were preventable, with the leading cause of these deaths being severe loss of blood from extremity wounds. This eventually led to a new set of guidelines for combat first aid, the reintroduction of the tourniquet, and the use of new hemostatic agents to promote clotting and stem the loss of blood.

The use of helicopters reduced the time between wounding and arrival at a medical facility in Korea and Vietnam. The average time from wounding to initial surgical treatment had been 10.5 hours during World War II but was 6.3 hours during the Korean War and 2.8 hours in Vietnam. By the time troops were deployed to Afghanistan, it was widely held that morbidity and mortality increase significantly after the first hour. However, the geography and tactical geometry in Afghanistan made the one-hour standard infeasible. Nevertheless, in 2009, Secretary of Defense Robert Gates directed that one hour—the golden hour—would be the goal and ordered a 25-percent increase in the number of helicopters assigned to medevac. This substantially improved mission performance, with an increase from 25 percent to 75 percent of all missions achieving the one-hour goal. Casualty statistics improved correspondingly.

Role of the State in Caring for Veterans

The third broad theme from history is the increased involvement of states in taking care of veterans in general and of disabled veterans in particular. Prior to World War I, programs for veterans centered on pensions and "soldiers homes," where the aged and disabled could live. After World War I, *rehabilitation* became an important third element of veteran care. This new emphasis ultimately gave rise to the VA and a vast array of programs designed to help disabled veterans become productive members of society.

The Ancient World

In the ancient world, care for the wounded was generally a private affair, rather than a state responsibility. When a citizen soldier was wounded, his care usually fell to his family and friends. After the war, the citizen-soldiers, now veterans, returned to their families and their farms. They had fulfilled their obligations as citizens, earned the adulation of their neighbors, and sometimes gained a portion of the spoils. The city-states of classical Greece, however, are noteworthy because they were the first governments to take *some* responsibility for wounded soldiers, widows, and orphans. As early as 594 B.C. in Athens, a maimed soldier was to be "maintained at the public charge" (as quoted in Snyder, Gawdiak, and Worden, 1991, p. 2). A generation later, in his famous funeral eulogy, Pericles pledged public support for the children of those killed in battle. The phrase "to the victors belong the spoils" had particular meaning in ancient times because plunder was shared among the victorious troops, providing wealth in lieu of salaries or pensions. In the conquering armies of Alexander the Great (356–323 B.C.), which fought far from home, soldiers unfit for further service were usually discharged in place and granted land, becoming colonists who would thus help Hellenize the conquered territories.

The picture we have of the Roman army comes into focus after the civil wars and with the founding of the empire by Augustus in 27 B.C. For the first time, soldiers paid military allegiance ultimately to the emperor, not to the commanders of their legions. In turn, Augustus regulated everything, from their pay, the period of their enlistment, and the money and benefits they would receive when they retired, generally at 25 years of service. Soldiers who served to retirement were granted citizenship, if they were not already citizens; allotments of land; a substantial payment equal to 14 times their annual salaries; and exemption from taxes and certain duties other citizens were required to carry out. By one account, half of those recruited into service lived through to retirement.

There were also provisions for those disabled from wounds or disease. If the disabled had served for at least 20 years, he received the same as any other honorably discharged soldier. For lesser periods of service, he received a reduced pension based on his years of service.

For the Romans, the issues of widows and children were less straightforward. The ordinary soldier was not allowed to marry, a policy many armies, including our own, continued until recent times. As a result, Roman soldiers joined burial societies, which paid out substantial sums on the retirement or death of a member. Payments were also made if a soldier left service because of wounds or illness. It should be noted that this notion that soldiers should give up part of their pay for the promise of future care is repeated throughout history. It lies behind today's Servicemembers' Group Life Insurance program, the Chatham Chest of the British Navy of the 17th century, and the deductions made from the pay of American sailors for the upkeep of the Navy Home in Biloxi, Mississippi.

After Rome

We have little to learn from the way soldiers and veterans were treated in Europe during the Middle Ages, except perhaps that advances in care and enlightened treatment could be transitory. In the early Middle Ages, it fell to the feudal lord to care for the knights in his service or to the monasteries to care for ordinary soldiers. Disabled and chronically ill veterans were either taken care of by family or friends or treated like any other indigent poor person, with no special consideration for how the disability came about or for the years of loyal service. Only gradually, with the rise of the nation-state, would this change.

The move to the nation-state reduced the reliance on mercenaries, whose loyalty went to the highest bidder, in favor of the citizen soldier, whose loyalty was to the sovereign. To encourage voluntary enlistments, the monarchs of the day had to improve the living conditions of their soldiers and provide both medical care and veterans' programs. While medical care for the sick and wounded soldier could be justified on the grounds that it returned a soldier to the fight, care for a veteran was more problematic. Monarchs often resented that they had to spend money on people who no longer were of value to them. Some saw a cheap way out by directing others to provide for veterans in their stead. A common way was to direct the church to take on this responsibility and, during Louis IX's reign in France, each monastery was given a quota. In a supreme act of audacity, the king required monasteries that could not take care of their quotas to provide their charges with cash pensions, so that they might take care of themselves. Not only did the church object, this system did not serve the veterans well. Few took to the monastic life, and what money they received went quickly, with the result that former soldiers often became beggars. Accordingly, French monarchs were increasingly forced to take on the responsibility for their disabled and elderly veterans.

Soldier's homes began to emerge in the late 1500s. Henry IV (1589–1610) established a royal home for destitute and disabled soldiers, later extended to the widows and orphans of soldiers killed in battle. Cardinal Richelieu, during the reign of Louis XIII (1610–1643), started work on a home for old and disabled soldiers. The work was continued under Louis XIV, and l'Hôtel des Invalides, a hospital for aged and disabled soldiers, opened in 1670. For its upkeep, the government provided funds equal to a fixed proportion of the total military budget. However, this was never adequate; built for 4,000 pensioners, more than 15,000 applied for residency between 1676 and 1704.

Louis XV found the large numbers of crippled veterans still begging on the streets of Paris repugnant. His remedy was to issue an edict making begging a crime under penalty of death. Eventually, he introduced a pension system for disabled soldiers and assigned the less disabled to garrisons in frontier towns, the *compagnies détachés d'invalides*. By 1763, there were 150 such units, with 15,000 troops. A census taken at the time of the French Revolution found 3,000 men actually living in Les Invalides in Paris, with approximately 26,000 pensioned soldiers living outside the capital.

Britain, insulated by the English Channel, never had a large standing army; however, after the Thirty Years War with Spain, as many as 80,000 returning soldiers faced severe problems reintegrating into civilian life. In earlier times, the church would have taken up their plight, but the church-based system of local care was disbanded when Henry VIII brought the Protestant Reformation to England. For his daughter, Queen Elizabeth I, these returning veterans, with their war-honed skills in arms, posed a threat that could not be ignored.

Queen Elizabeth found spending money on veterans particularly vexing and tried to pass the responsibilities on to local counties by act of the Privy Council. When this did not work, she got Parliament to act, setting off a struggle between a miserly national government and reluctant local governments, the echoes of which can still be heard. The Acte for the Relief of Souldiours of 1593 provided both a rationale for pensions, *compassion* and *practicality*, and a mechanism for providing state support for a decentralized system of local care. While the national law specified that disabled veterans were entitled to life pensions and even gave the local authorities specific authority to raise taxes *on themselves* to pay for the pensions, local authorities chose to grant pensions only to those they determined were unable to work and were otherwise destitute. Eventually, in 1647, Parliament gave in and took over the responsibility for pensions but, realizing their cost, made inability to work the only basis for determining whether someone was eligible for a disability pension.

Disabled seamen were treated separately from disabled soldiers. England was a seafaring nation, and the problem of disabled seamen was less episodic and long term. In 1590, at the request of sailors, a mutual fund was established and held in a box at Chatham; the fund itself became known as the Chatham Chest. The fund was originally financed by members' contributions, which were deducted from their pay, along with funds later provided by the government. Pensions were granted on a fixed scale, with different rates, say, for the loss of a limb or for the loss of both arms.

During the English Civil Wars (1642–1651) and immediately after, Parliament again attempted to push the burden of issuing pensions to local communities with no better success. Eventually, royal hospitals were established that were modeled after the French Les Invalides, but like the Chatham Chest, they were financed by deductions from the pay of soldiers and sailors. The rise of the royal hospitals was the final nationalization of the care of disabled veterans. It put an end to the county scheme, but not necessarily to the benefit of the disabled. Rather than being maintained by tax revenues, the hospitals were royal charities paid for principally by deductions from soldiers' and sailors' own pay and were later assigned a proportion of the spoils of war and fines levied on the soldiers for minor infractions of the rules. Levied fines are also used today to support the Armed Forces Retirement Home in the United States.

In Britain, care for veterans, war widows, and orphans has always been problematic. For the wealthy and privileged of the officer class, little was required. For the common soldier, whom the Duke of Wellington once described as "the scum of the earth" (Coss, 2010, p. 29), little was given. It eventually fell to concerned citizens to augment the funds the government provided veterans. As distinct from the purely religious hospices run by the charitable orders of the past, these civilian organizations were essentially secular, even as they often saw their mission as part of a "Christian duty" to care for the ill and disabled. The appeal for private funds was so pervasive that Parliament established the Royal Patriotic Fund Corporation to coordinate and oversee such private contributions. After the Boer War, the Soldiers and Sailors Help Society even established workshops to teach useful trades to men discharged as medically unfit and disabled. These, together with similar programs established in France and Belgium, were the forerunners of the government programs established after World War I.

In America

Revolution

While the American system of care was originally based on the British model, it stands in sharp contrast in how it has treated veterans in general and the disabled, widows, and orphans in particular. Where Britain was niggardly, America was generous, even from its earliest days. The English law of 1593, the Acte for the Relief of Souldiours, set the standard for the American colonies but was implemented more generously. In 1636, the Plymouth Colony (Massachusetts) was the first to provide care for those who survived battle wounds, and soldiers sent outside the colony if "maimed or hurt" were maintained completely by the colony during their lives. By the time the Declaration of Independence was signed in 1776, 11 of the 13 colonies had made arrangements for the maintenance of "hurt or maimed" soldiers.

Initially, the Continental Congress left the issue of disability pensions in the hands of the individual colonies—providing a national standard for the states to follow that promised half pay for life for a disabled officer, soldier, or sailor and with proportional relief for those only partially disabled. Congress also provided that pensioned officers, soldiers, and sailors capable of limited duty were to be formed into a *Corps of Invalids* to provide limited service. The same year, Congress resurrected a practice dating to the Romans: To encourage men to join and stay in the Army, Congress authorized grants of land for those who served for the duration of the war. The grants ranged from 100 acres of land for enlisted men to 1,100 acres for a major general.

Congress next turned to the issue of nondisability or service pensions. After much debate and at the insistence of General Washington, Congress voted half pay for life, or five years at full pay, for officers and one year's pay as a discharge bonus for rank-and-file soldiers. The government, under the Articles of Confederation, failed to provide for payment of this obligation, and many veterans, thinking them worthless, sold them for pennies on the dollar, only to see speculators get rich when the new government of President Washington, under the Constitution, agreed to pay them in full. Finally, in 1828, Congress redressed the grievances of the surviving 850 Revolutionary War officers and soldiers with a grant of full pay for life.

In 1780, Congress also partially addressed the needs of widows and orphans. It provided for delivery of half pay to the widows and orphans of officers for seven years. No provision was made for the widows and orphans of the other ranks until 1836. When the Continental Army was disbanded on November 3, 1783, Congress established a schedule of disability pensions to be administered by the states. The standard for total disability was half pay for officers and $5 per month for enlisted men, with partial payments for a partial disability. In 1790, with an uneven and inconsistent record of state payment, Congress took over payment of invalid pensions. In 1792, the rolls listed 1,500 invalid pensioners. What followed was a long series of Revolutionary War pension laws, which became more and more generous over time.

Following the European model, disabled veterans were generally helped through cash payments, with hospitals and domiciles being established for acute medical care and for indigent veterans. In 1798, following the British tradition of the Chatham Chest, Congress provided for the relief of sick and disabled merchant seamen by imposing a special tax on any American ship coming from a foreign port and garnishing a portion of each seaman's wages. The following year, Congress authorized the U.S. Navy Asylum, later renamed the U.S. Naval Home, for "disabled and decrepit navy officers, seamen, and marines" (as cited in McCarl and Ginn, 1925, p. 1006) to be paid for by the same 20 cents a month garnishment imposed on merchant seamen the year before. A similar institution for the Army opened in 1851; it continues today as the U.S. Soldiers Home. In 1855, St. Elizabeth's Hospital in Washington, D.C., opened for the treatment of the mentally ill of the Army and Navy. For those who had fought for the Union, the Civil War saw a continuation of the American pattern of providing substantial care for the disabled and generous financial benefits for nondisabled veterans.

Civil War

The General Law of 1862 applied to all those who served the Union in the Army or Navy, including regulars, volunteers, militia, and Marines, and without further acts of Congress, all future wars (Glasson, 1900). It authorized compensation for disabilities incurred as a direct consequence of performing military service and for subsequent deaths from injuries received or disease contracted as a *direct consequence of the performance of a soldier's military duty.* The law was particularly generous when it came to widows, orphans, and other dependents and later expanded to include surviving mothers, sisters, fathers, and brothers. They were to receive pensions equivalent to the rate the deceased family member would have received for a total disability. The law also established a medical screening system for rating disabilities and, with subsequent amendments, increased the level of compensation for specific disabilities, such as loss of limbs or eyesight or deafness. The law was later amended to address the issue of caregivers. After 1866, the law provided for additional payments to be given to the disabled who required regular or even partial "aid and attendance" in an amount greater than the payments for a "total disability in both feet" or "the incapacity to perform manual labor."

For the 20,000 amputees who survived the war, the pensions were not adequate to cover the cost of artificial limbs, and the economic situation of the wounded even weighed on surgeons' decisions about which type of amputation to perform. In 1862, Congress addressed this by authorizing the Army Medical Department to issue artificial limbs. By the end of 1867, over 6,000 artificial limbs had been issued, and a program was started to replace them every five years. This program was the first large-scale attempt of any government to systematically address the issue of rehabilitation, soon to be one of the major pillars of a modern program for the care of veterans.

In his Second Inaugural Address, President Lincoln promised, "to care for him who shall have borne the battle and for his widow and his orphan." As the war was drawing to a close, Congress chartered the national homes to provide long-term care for veterans of the Union Army, splitting the costs with the states that had not seceded in 1861. The states set up their own homes, and by 1865, over 9,000 veterans were receiving care in 33 state homes in 28 states. Twenty states provided "haven for veterans' wives, widows and mothers."

After the war, such organized Union veterans groups as the Grand Army of the Republic pressured the Republican-controlled Congress to vote increasingly generous pensions, which soon became the largest cost item in the federal budget. In 1864, 1866, and 1873, Congress increased the maximum compensation and expanded pensions for those who had contracted diseases during their service. By 1888, 64 percent of all pensions were for diseases and other nonbattlefield injuries, rather than from battle wounds. The Arrears Act of 1879 allowed soldiers with newly discovered war-related disabilities to receive a single payment equal to all the pension payments they would have received if they had made the claim at the time of the war. Finally, the Dependent and Disability Pension Act of 1890 provided that veterans incapable of *manual labor* would receive a pension even if the cause were not service connected.

The Civil War pension became an "old-age and survivors' benefit program" almost 50 years before the enactment of Social Security. Death benefits under the 1890 act were paid to the current widows and children without regard to the cause of the veteran's death or his marital status at the time of his service. In 1893, 41.5 percent of the federal budget went toward Civil War pensions. By 1906, simply reaching the age of 62 was enough for the pension to start. In 1914, of the nearly 500,000 Civil War pensioners, only 12 percent were disabled.

The Civil War pension was, however, one that not all Americans shared equally. Those of the old South who had fought against the Union received nothing, even though they paid taxes to the federal government, in the form of high tariffs designed to protect business in the northern states, the businesses of their old enemies. The care of disabled veterans who had fought against the Union was left solely to their states of the Old Confederacy, and payments were only a fraction of what a similarly wounded Union veteran received.

World War I

At the beginning of World War I, and following the Civil War model, everyone thought of *disabled* in terms of amputations and blindness, and care for the disabled meant a pension and, possibly, a place in a soldiers' home. Soon, in keeping with other Progressive Era reforms, there was a new commitment—not only to heal the wounded but also to return the disabled to productive lives, a commitment that continues to this day.

The three organizations responsible for caring for the disabled veterans of World War I were the Bureau of War Risk Insurance, which provided the funds; the Federal Board for Vocational Education, which provided vocational reeducation; and the U.S. Public Health Service, which provided health care. The triad of agencies proved unwieldy. Eventually, Congress created the Veterans' Bureau, as an independent agency reporting directly to the President, to take over the veterans programs from the three agencies.

In 1924, the hospitals of the Veterans' Bureau had almost 10,000 vacant beds, and Congress expanded veterans' access to health care by opening the system to "veterans of all wars needing . . . care" regardless of service connection. As time went on, service-connected admissions dropped, but non–service-connected admissions grew steadily, accounting for 92 percent of all admissions in 1940.

In 1930, as the country moved into the Great Depression, the Veterans' Bureau joined with the National Homes for Disabled Volunteer Soldiers and the Bureau of Pensions to form the VA. In 1933, the Roosevelt administration severely cut back on veterans' programs. In a move reminiscent of the Elizabethan Privy Council of 1593, President Roosevelt took the radical position that state and local governments should have primary responsibility for the care of veterans whose disabilities are not connected to their military service. In 1934, Congress overrode the President's veto and restored almost all the benefits curtailed the previous year, including access to VA facilities for veterans whose needs and disabilities were not connected to their military service.

During the 1930s, Congress authorized the VA to acquire only enough hospital beds to meet the needs of neuropsychiatric and tuberculosis patients; veterans with other non–service-connected disabilities were to be served on a space-available basis. Between 1931 and 1941, however, the number of VA hospitals increased by half, and bed capacity doubled. Unfortunately, with the shift in the kinds of care the VA provided, the institution began to appear to be a warehouse for the mentally ill and indigent and as a backwater of the medical profession. It was this system that faced the influx of millions of World War II veterans.

World War II

Before the war, the physical rehabilitation of those injured or disabled would be the province of the VA, not the Army or Navy. However, once war came, a shortage of critical personnel and a lack of facilities severely limited the VA's ability to receive patients. In fact, the VA played a relatively minor role in the care of American service members discharged during World War II, continuing to serve mainly its prewar constituency.

During the early years of the war (1942–1943), less than 10 percent of VA hospital admissions were discharged soldiers. On June 30, 1945, there were 21,000 World War II veterans in VA hospitals, compared with 58,000 in Army convalescent hospitals and 153,000 in Army general hospitals. After the war, many Army facilities were transferred to the VA, but some disabled service members were kept on active duty to receive additional rehabilitation services, rather than being transferred to the VA.

Programs for World War II veterans came in two stages. The first, the Disabled Veterans' Rehabilitation Act of 1943, provided for indigent care on a space-available basis and authorized vocational training for the disabled. The second, best known as the GI Bill, was signed into law in 1944, providing for college or vocational education for returning veterans, as well as various loan programs for purchasing homes or starting small businesses for all veterans, even those without disabilities.

In the months immediately following the end of the war, the VA underwent nothing short of a revolution. The task of building a modern VA fell to LTG Omar N. Bradley. Bradley made major changes, including decentralizing VA decisionmaking, creating a professional medical corps independent of Civil Service regulations, and hiring thousands of new physicians. He established VA hospital affiliations with medical schools, organized physician-training programs at VA hospitals, established prestigious advisory boards, and put a new emphasis on rehabilitation. The increase in the government's role in caring for veterans of World War II can be seen in the increase in the employment at the VA from 65,000 in 1945 to a peak of 200,000 in 1948 and in the 13-fold increase in its budget.

Korean War

Even before the start of war in Korea, the VA was having serious problems. In 1950, President Truman appointed a special committee to report on the veterans' hospitalization program and the needs of disabled veterans. The committee focused on four endemic problems that resonate to this day: the inability of the VA to appropriately staff its facilities, waiting times to gain access to VA hospitals, the transfer of disabled service members from DoD to the VA, and the care of veterans whose medical needs were not related to their military service. In 1950, 51.2 percent of patients in VA hospitals were receiving care for service-connected disabilities; 16.4 percent were service-connected cases being treated for non–service-connected disabilities; and 32.4 percent were non–service-connected patients.

In January 1955, President Eisenhower, noting the New Deal expansion of social services available to all citizens, regardless of veteran status, asked General Bradley, the former Chairman of the Joint Chiefs of Staff and former head of the VA, for a systematic assessment of the structure, scope, philosophy, and administration of pension, compensation, and benefits veterans and their families receive. Bradley's report endorsed service-connected and postservice readjustment benefits but questioned non–service-connected benefits. According to the Bradley Commission, the

> justification [for non–service-connected benefits] is weak and their basic philosophy is backward looking rather than constructive. Our society has developed more equitable means of meeting most of the same needs and big strides are being made in closing remaining gaps. The non-service-connected benefits should be limited to a minimum level and retained only as a reserve line of honorable protection for veterans whose means are shown to be inadequate and who fail to qualify for basic

protection under the general Old-Age and Survivors Insurance system. (Bradley Commission, 1956a, p. 138)

In 1959, in a move reminiscent of actions taken at the end of the 19th century concerning Civil War veterans and their families, Congress reaffirmed its commitment to all disabled veterans—those with service-connected disabilities and those whose disabilities did not arise from military service—by defining old age as a disabling condition. Congress provided that, in the future, disability pensions would be available to all unemployed veterans who had reached the age of 65 and who had a disabling condition of 10 percent or more—a rating most elderly could meet—even if the disabling condition was not related to military service. The amount of the benefits, however, would depend on dependent status and the levels and types of other income received.

Vietnam

American troops were first deployed to Vietnam in March 1965, but in the annual reports the VA sent to Congress in January 1966 and 1967, the administrator did not mention Vietnam or that the VA's workload might increase. It seemed official Washington did not want to make long-run plans for a war everyone hoped would be over quickly. When it was over, one-third of all living war veterans had served during the Vietnam era, one-quarter of whom had actually been deployed to Vietnam. As had occurred at the start of World War II, little was being done to prepare for the millions of veterans who would demand services. When it was over, Vietnam veterans made up 26 percent of all veterans. On average, they were almost one-half the age of the World War II veterans. The VA now had to deal with two very large, distinct veteran populations, and it was not just their age that was different. In 1971, the VA administrator told Congress VA psychologists viewed the Vietnam-era veteran as "a major challenge":

> Several important factors contribute to this challenge: the general psychosocial characteristics of this generation of veterans; the accelerated pace of technological and social changes in the American society; the prolonged and inconclusive nature of the Vietnam conflict; and the fact that a greater portion have sustained, and survived serious physical disabilities and emotional trauma from combat experience. (Administrator of Veterans Affairs, 1971, p. 16)

Not only did the VA seem frustrated with Vietnam veterans, but those who were receiving services were frustrated with the VA. A large number were asking for age-segregated wards, and about one-third expressed dissatisfaction with VA programs. Spurning old-line veteran service organizations, such as the American Legion, the Veterans of Foreign Wars, and the Disabled Veterans of America, Vietnam veterans founded an advocacy organization devoted to their own needs in 1978, the Vietnam Veterans of America. Soon it and other grassroots advocacy groups were pressing the VA hard for special programs to help with what was first called Vietnam syndrome and later became known as PTSD and to provide treatment for the illnesses veterans argued were caused by exposure to the herbicide Agent Orange.

In one important way, how Vietnam veterans affected the VA is hard to discern because it took place just as the VA was changing the way it was delivering services. Between 1964 and 1976, the number of veterans grew by 20 percent, but the average daily patient load at VA hospitals decreased by 29 percent, and outpatient visits increased by 166 percent. During this period, both the VA and entities across the civilian sector were making concerted efforts to move chronically ill patients, particularly psychiatric patients, out of hospitals and instead emphasize outpatient care. For many veterans, however, outpatient care is problematic because it puts the burden on them to have the discipline to take their medicines and keep appointments.

Middle East Wars: Persian Gulf War, Afghanistan, and Iraq

Today, the VA runs the nation's largest health delivery system, with 168 medical centers and hospitals; 300 readjustment counseling centers (vet centers); 1,055 VA clinics; 11 VA residential and extended-care sites; and 56 regional offices. As of this writing, it has accomplished 106 million outpatient visits; treated 599,000 surgical and medicine and 152,000 mental health inpatients; and provided institutional long-term support and services for 115,000 patients. The more than $70 billion dollars per year appropriated by Congress provide care for veterans who have applied for VA health care and received it according to a priority system established in 1996. There is one exception, however: At least for the first five years after separation, today's veterans are eligible for free medical care and medications for any condition related to their service in the combat theater. For conditions not related to service in the combat theater, small copayments might be expected for medical care or prescription drugs. Today, only higher-income veterans with noncompensable 0-percent service-connected or non–service-connected disabilities are ineligible to enroll.

In 2015, 93 percent of service-connected disabled veterans were enrolled in the VHA health care system, most—69 percent—using available VA services. This was an increase in the utilization rate of enrolled service-connected disabled veterans of 11 percentage points in the previous ten years. Overall, 44.3 percent of all veterans use at least one veteran's benefit. Even with the growing popularity of the VA health programs, the VA still faced three challenges: the lengthy bureaucratic discharge review process, the need to provide services to female veterans, and long waiting lists.

The first challenge was to reduce the lengthy bureaucratic process of transferring disabled service members from the armed forces to the VA. The maze of policies and procedures starts with the fact that soldiers separating from the military must deal with the administrative processes of both DoD and the VA. The DoD system focuses on the soldier's medical condition relative to his or her ability to continue doing his or her military job—a job that reflects occupation, grade, and years of service—while the VA system takes a broader view considers the impact of his or her medical condition on earnings and well-being over a lifetime, regardless of the specifics of former military career. Ultimately, DoD and the VA agreed to develop a new system—IDES—incorporating a single physical examination conducted to VA standards, a VA-prepared disability rating system for both DoD and VA to use to determine individual and overall disability ratings, and VA case-management staff assigned to DoD facilities to explain the processes to service members. While the new system was an improvement, a congressionally mandated independent task force judged the system to be complex and noted that navigating it remained "a lengthy and mystifying ordeal" (Nathan and Crockett-Jones, 2014, p. 12).

The second challenge was to provide services to female veterans. Their numbers have increased sharply since the end of conscription and the advent of the all-volunteer force in 1973. In 2016, female veterans accounted for 10 percent of the veteran population, and the VA was still having difficulty meeting their health needs because many outpatient clinics still lacked a women's health primary care provider. In 2015, the VA identified a number of barriers to women veterans' access to care in an effort to focus investments and resources to improve services for women veterans. The Center for Women Veterans, established in 1994, remains the central advocate for woman's issues within the VA.

The third challenge was to reduce what were reported to be very long waiting periods for initial, nonurgent appointments with primary care providers. In 2014, there had been reports of excessive waiting times and fraudulent waiting lists. The excessive waiting times were not substantiated, but fraudulent waiting lists were uncovered at some VA facilities. This led to the resignation of the VA secretary on May 30, 2014, and to the firing of a number of top executives and hospital administrators. It also led to the passage of the Veterans Access, Choice, and Accountability Act of 2014 (Pub. L. 113-146, 2014), which enhanced the VA's ability to purchase care for certain veterans in the private sector. This legislation also called for independent assessment of the existing system and a fresh look at how veterans' health care might be delivered in the future.

The resulting Commission on Care challenged the very foundation of the veterans care system established after World War I, calling for a fundamental transformation of the current system. The commission made it clear that

> merely clarifying and simplifying the rules for purchased care, . . . is not sufficient to achieve that goal. VHA must replace the arbitrary eligibility requirements and unworkable clinical and administrative restrictions of current purchased programs with the new VHA Care System, available to all enrolled veterans. (Commission on Care, 2016, p. 26)

The commission envisioned

- [That] integrated, community-based health care networks [be developed], including VHA providers and facilities, Department of Defense and other federally-funded providers and facilities, and VHA-credentialed community providers and facilities. (Commission on Care, 2016, p. 3)
- [That these] networks be developed with local VHA leadership input and knowledge to ensure their composition is reflective of local needs and veterans' preferences.
- Veterans choose a primary care provider from all credentialed primary care providers in the VHA Care System.
- Veterans choose their specialty care providers from all credentialed specialty care providers in the VHA Care System with a referral from their primary care provider. (Commission on Care, 2016, p. 4)

In essence, this would fundamentally change the system and move the VA from a direct provider of health care services consistent with congressional funding to an entitlement system for all eligible and enrolled veterans, with the VA maintaining facilities and providing services not available from the private sector.

Recent Awareness of Psychological and Cognitive Injuries: The Invisible Wounds That Transcend the Immediate Battle

The fourth broad theme from history is the relatively recent awareness of the psychological and cognitive consequences of war. While some have claimed that psychiatric impairment, such as PTSD, is a result of modern warfare, a strong case can be made that such conditions have been with us all along. Jonathan Shay, for example, examined the Homeric tales and found accounts of both physical and psychological combat wounds (Shay, 1994; Shay, 2002). Nevertheless, it was not until the Civil War that psychiatric casualties were even recognized and not until World War I that treatments were developed.

The Civil War Through World War II

During the Civil War, neuropsychiatric casualties were reported after major battles. By one account, after the battle of Antietam, upwards of one-third of the Confederate Army of Northern Virginia was classified as "sulkers" or "stragglers." Many seemed to get better with rest, and those seriously impaired were simply dismissed and left to find their own way. World War I was the first war in which neuropsychiatric casualties became significant. The term *shell shock* is most readily associated with World War I, but it was a term that the man who coined it soon wished would go away. The original assumption was that being too close to an exploding shell caused dysfunctional behaviors. But a soldier displaying neuropsychiatric symptoms yet showing no physical signs could be accused of cowardice and sentenced to death as a warning to other "malingerers." (During the war, 17 British soldiers were executed for cowardice.) It soon became clear that immediate proximity to an exploding shell was not necessarily the only reason for soldiers to display neuropsychiatric symptoms. Rather, these symptoms were a psychological or emotional response to the strains of terrifying and overwhelming battle experiences. Nevertheless, a sharp divide remained between those who believed that war neurosis was a physical condition and those who believed that the primary cause was emotional.

The significance of psychiatry in general during World War I cannot be over stressed. The Army's official history notes:

> Whereas mental illness had been almost wholly ignored and the medical advances before the war dealt almost exclusively with physical diseases, the wide prevalence of neuroses among soldiers was apparently leading to a revision of the medical and popular attitude toward mental and functional nervous diseases, and stimulating widespread interest in their observation and study. (Bailey, Williams, and Komora, 1929, p. 8)

At the start of World War II, the Army was convinced that it could effectively screen out those predisposed to neuropsychiatric problems before they joined. While more than 1.25 million men were rejected because of perceived mental and emotional abnormalities—the largest single cause for rejection, at 12 percent of all those examined—screening did not achieve its goal. The number of neuropsychiatric disorders during the war was to be two to three times higher than during World War I.

Because the Army relied solely on screening, it was unprepared to deal with the neuropsychiatric casualties that overseas deployments and combat brought. In the field, the goal was to return a soldier to his unit as quickly as possible. While the exact number of neuropsychiatric cases will never be known, the best estimate is that the number far exceeded admissions for battle wounds. Between January 1943 and December 1945, 18.8 percent of all soldiers returning to the United States were neuropsychiatric patients—a number equivalent to 12 combat divisions. Army policy emphasized discharging these soldiers rather than treating them, until treatment was authorized in March 1945. Once treatment was authorized, such "shortcut" treatments as therapeutic hypnosis and drugs, along with group therapy, were often pursued because of the shortage of mental health professionals.

After the war, the services and the VA undertook a large study of former soldiers admitted for neuropsychiatric disorders. The follow-up clinical examination of the men who were "definitely ill at separation" showed that only 36 percent had actually sought treatment, and there was "no evidence that treatment played an important role in the general improvement which occurred between separation and follow-up" (Brill and Beebe, 1955, p. 135). It should also be noted that, while the VA treated only a small number of the subjects of the study or the total number receiving payments for neuro-psychiatric disabilities, it had all that it could handle treating those who did seek help. After the war, 30 percent of all disability awards were for neuropsychiatric problems, and psychotic and other neuropsychiatric patients occupied more than half of the beds at VA hospitals. On the eve of the Korean War, care for the neuropsychiatric casualties of World War II remained problematic.

Korea

The unquestioned goal of military psychiatry in Korea was to keep as many fighting men on the line as possible by applying the PIES principles (proximity, immediacy, expectancy, and simplicity). The neuropsychiatric casualties and psychiatric services mirrored the operational situation on the ground. During the initial chaotic period around Pusan, there were no dedicated psychiatric services, but psychiatric casualties were low because men concentrated on fighting for survival. As things stabilized, psychiatric casualties increased, with most evacuated to Japan. The recovery rate was low—few returned to their units. After the landing at Inchon and the breakout from the Pusan Perimeter, the tenets of PIES were more rigorously applied, and the recovery rate increased. Later, when the line stabilized during the period of extended negotia-tions, the rotation system took hold, and new psychiatric problems appeared, ones that foreshadowed problems that would become very prominent in Vietnam.

In terms of the psychiatric condition of the force, Korea is best known for the plight of the American POWs. According to interviews with returning POWs at the time, some had collaborated with the enemy, and others had turned on their own. As these stories began to circulate, some charged that POWs had been brainwashed, play-ing into the anticommunist hysteria of the day. Others saw the alleged behavior POWs as proof of a growing decadence in American society. That charge would be heard again to describe many returning from Vietnam.

Vietnam

The story of the psychiatric casualties of the Vietnam War is a tale of three wars—the one that ended with Tet Offensive in January 1968; the one of the initial post-Tet period, from late 1968 to 1970; and the one that began with the final withdrawal of American troops ending in 1973. The aftermath of combat itself brought a new under-standing of PTSD. Before the Tet Offensive, Army psychiatrists were complimenting themselves that the incidence of psychiatric impairment was much lower than it had been during World War II. They attributed this to the 12-month rotation policy and fact that most combat was brief, if intense, coming sporadically amid periods of relative calm. This all changed after Tet, as opposition to the war increased both at home and among the troops in Vietnam and as the behavior of soldiers deteriorated. AWOLs, less-than-honorable discharges, desertions, and illicit drug use rates all increased. Army psychiatrists were prepared to deal with traditional combat stress but not with the increase in psychiatric cases seen throughout the Army but especially in Vietnam. The unprecedented rise in "psychosocial casualties" of Vietnam foretold the rise in the number of veterans who reported problems adjusting to civilian life after the war.

As early as 1969, it was clear that returning soldiers were having problems dealing with the psychological consequences of their experiences in Vietnam. Some of what was being reported was undoubtedly common to returning soldiers of previous wars, but other issues, such as depression over doubts about the legitimacy and worth of this war, seemed unique to Vietnam. As a result, Vietnam veterans were not finding a sympathetic ear or much of a helping hand at the VA, which was built around the heroic legends of World War II. The lingering effects of fear of an often-unseen enemy and guilt for partaking in what was increasingly being thought of as an unjust and worthless war were not something that the psychotherapists at the VA had been trained to handle.

Even the DSM did not have diagnostic nomenclature that recognized or legitimized Vietnam-related trauma. This would slowly change after the ground-breaking expositions of a Yale psychiatrist, Dr. Robert Jay Lifton, and the challenge to psychiatric orthodoxy of a New York University professor, Dr. Chaim F. Shatan. It would culminate in 1978 with the American Psychiatric Association's agreement that the forthcoming revision to the DSM would include PTSD. The following year, the Vietnam Veterans' Outreach Program and the first vet centers were established to help veterans make a satisfying postwar readjustment to civilian life. Importantly, veterans did not need a formal determination of service-connected disability to receive counseling or psychotherapy at these centers. Originally set up to serve only those who had served in Vietnam, the mission of the centers was expanded in 1991 to combat veterans who fought in Lebanon, Grenada, Panama, the Persian Gulf, and Somalia. By 1996, when Congress extended the eligibility to include World War II and Korean combat veterans, there were 205 such centers. In 2003, eligibility was extended to veterans of OEF, OIF, and subsequent veterans of the Global War on Terrorism. While the original focus was on PTSD, services were expanded to include assistance not only for PTSD but also for sexual trauma, alcohol and drug assessment, and suicide prevention. In 2015, there were 300 vet centers.

Middle East Wars: Persian Gulf War, Afghanistan, and Iraq

When the U.S. Army went to war in 2001, it deployed a mental health model firmly rooted in World War I. The basic message, captured in the mnemonic PIES, was this: "You are neither sick nor a coward. You are just tired and will recover when rested." The lesson learned from Vietnam was that PTSD was infrequent and could be accommodated through appropriate measures of combat and operational stress control. By 2011, when the first comprehensive review of combat psychiatry covering the deployments to Afghanistan and Iraq was published, (Ritchie, 2011) the Army's view of PTSD had matured and become nuanced.

Reports from Afghanistan and Iraq showed that, at the height of combat operations in 2006, more than 20 percent of the deployed force met the criteria for acute stress, depression, or anxiety—all symptoms of PTSD (Thomas, 2010, pp. 6–7; Office of the Surgeon General, U.S. Army Medical Command, 2013, p. 16). Furthermore, there was a strong relationship between hours of sleep and psychological problems, and the percentage of NCOs surveyed with psychological problems, marital problems, and PTSD positively related to the number of deployments. Specifically, NCOs on a third deployment were nearly twice as likely to report psychological problems, marital problems, and PTSD as NCOs on their first deployment. Soldiers also reported that there were significant barriers to receiving mental health treatment, especially because of the stigma associated with asking for help.

By 2001, it was well accepted that the signs and symptoms of PTSD could occur soon after the trauma or some time later and could present in an inconsistent pattern over time. That might explain why, of the approximately 800,000 Army troops who had been deployed to Afghanistan and Iraq, the Army reported only 28,000 cases of PTSD (3 percent) at the end of CY 2007. The Army's report (Carino, 2016) stands in stark contrast to the number of PTSD cases reported by the PDHA, the Post-Deployment Health Re-Assessment, the VA, and an independent survey of those who had served in Afghanistan and Iraq (Tanielian and Jaycox, 2008). Typically, these showed that between 10 and 20 percent of the force screened positive for PTSD, with a smaller number, perhaps 20 percent, receiving care for PTSD and other mental health problems.

For today's career-oriented Army, the fact that a significant portion of the career force may suffer from PTSD and other serious mental health problems brought on by multiple combat deployments is very unsettling, especially because the behaviors associated with these conditions are so antithetical to the military's traditions, attitudes, beliefs, practices, and policies. Even with the Defense Health Board Task Force on Mental Health's call for commanders to discharge their "clear responsibility to restore to full level of function a service member damaged in the line of duty, and to be cognizant of and attentive to the psychological aftermath of deployment, manifested in hidden injuries of the brain and mind" (DoD Task Force on Mental Health, 2007, pp. 21–22), there is significant variation in how behavioral symptoms are considered in administrative, legal, or disciplinary proceedings. In 2014, Secretary of Defense Chuck Hagel ordered a review of previously issued less-than-honorable discharges. It appears that thousands of discharges will eventually be upgraded because a diagnosis of PTSD or a TBI event was not properly considered. However, in 2020 ,Congress found it necessary to direct that,

> [f]or [discharge review] cases based in whole or in part on PTSD or TBI related to combat, a BCMR [Board of Military Records] or DRB [Discharge Review Board] is [will now be] required to seek advice and counsel from a psychiatrist, psycholo-

gist, or social worker with training in PTSD, TBI, or other trauma treatment. (Mendez et al., 2020, p. 16)

Given that signs and symptoms of PTSD often do not manifest themselves until after the soldier has left the service, the responsibility for caring for those with PTSD and TBIs falls most heavily on the VA. This was certainly true for the veterans of Afghanistan and Iraq. In 2003, the VA reported that only 230 (1.1 percent) of the new veterans they were seeing had PTSD. By 2007, the number had grown to 33,597, or 17 percent of the total that year. In 2012, the number of reported PTSD patients had grown further, to 119,482, or 23.6 percent of the total. Even more impressive is the number of veterans receiving disability compensation for PTSD and the severity of their disabilities. In 2014, the Veterans Benefits Administration reported that 653,249 veterans had service-connected PTSD—17.5 percent of all veterans who were receiving compensation for a service-connected health condition. Of those, about 451,500 had a disability rating of least 50 percent, and another 165,500 had rating of least 30 percent. PTSD is the third most common major service-connected disability, after hearing loss and tinnitus.

As of this writing, the DoD and the VA believe that a number of cognitive behavioral therapies, counseling, and medications seem to be effective for treating PTSD. In addition, resources and treatment are available at the National Intrepid Center of Excellence at Walter Reed National Military Center to augment what is available through local military and VA facilities for those who have not responded to traditional treatment.

Themes

The two volumes of *Providing for the Casualties of War* present the broad themes that influenced the care that has been provided throughout history. Although these major developments are described as four discrete areas, they are in fact interrelated. Advances in one complement another and sometimes counter changes in a third. For example, advances in medical science have been matched with improvements in how the wounded are cared for on the battlefield, even as technology has worked to increase the lethality of new systems. This occurred, for example, when gunpowder was introduced and again during World War I. The overall reduction of battlefield mortality since World War II suggests that advances in medicine and medical support have won out, at least temporarily, over the increased lethality of new technologies. The demons of war, however, may yet have the final say, as the number of neuropsychiatric casualties increases in current wars and as our ability to provide care lags.

Neuropsychiatric casualties notwithstanding, today's soldiers are the beneficiaries of the most advanced medical care ever provided. Today's professional volunteer Army is made up of the highest quality soldiers—physically and mentally—of any force fielded. They are equipped with the most advanced military equipment in the world, including protective gear and protective vehicles. If wounded, soldiers receive lifesaving medical care immediately and are transported off the battlefield and back to the United States with speed and continuity of care that could only be imagined a few years earlier. After returning home, patients receive care from career medical professionals in world-class facilities, and a record number of soldiers remain on active duty. For those who leave service, the American system for caring for veterans provides not only for those with service-connected disabilities but also for poorer veterans who may not have the means to fully participate in our civilian fee-for-service medical system. Today, new programs that utilize private-sector medical care when VA services are not fully available are designed to address delivery problems when the VA system of clinics and hospitals is unable to reach those in need of care. Soldiering is still a deadly occupation. However, even though the Army has been at war since 2001, it has not had to rely on conscription to fill its ranks. Today's soldiers know that, if wounded, they will receive the most advanced medical care available possible while in service and after as a veteran.

History of the Mobile Army Surgical Hospital: Not a New Concept

In concept, the idea of a mobile surgical hospital was not new when the Korean conflict began but dates at least to the 17th century.

Marching and Flying Hospitals

In 1689, William III of England employed a MASH-type unit, the *marching hospital*, during his campaign in Ireland. Cantlie recounts,

> The Marching Hospital, as its name implies, was designed to move with the army, and possessed its own wagons and tentage. Its task was to open up as close to the regimental hospitals [aid stations] as the tactical situation allowed, receive and treat their sick and wounded, and either keep them until recovery or evacuate them back to the Fixed Hospital in the rear. As the range of cannon fire was at this period limited the hospital could be sited within a mile of the front line. (Cantlie, 1974, p. 45)

The staff of the marching hospitals included female nurses (*tenders*) recruited from civilian institutions and, eventually, male orderlies to do the heavy work. The wives of soldiers were employed to do the washing, cooking, and feeding of the sick. The design of the hospital was flexible but generally provided 300 beds. Originally, bedrolls were carried, but later, wooden bedsteads were introduced "for the greater comfort of the patients" (Cantlie, 1974, p. 49). Tentage and general ward supplies, such as bedpans and urinals, were carried in the hospital's own wagons. The system carried over into the 18th century, albeit with a change in name: The marching hospital became the flying hospital.

The proximity of the hospital to the front notwithstanding, it was usual for a wounded soldier to be left on the battlefield until the end of the battle and then be collected by fellow soldiers and carried to a medical facility somewhere to the rear.[1] This changed during the Napoleonic wars under French barons Dominique-Jean Larrey and F. P. Percy. Larrey is noted not only for his insistence on immediate amputation of wounded limbs and a system of priority that gave care to the most seriously wounded first but also for placing surgical teams near the front lines—medical officers carried their instruments in their saddlebags—and the use of specially designed horse-drawn "flying ambulances" to rapidly transport the more critically injured away from the battlefield" (Oritz, 1998, p. 21) accompanied by an "early version of emergency medical technicians" (Manring et al., 2009, p. 2169). Percy's competing system transported surgeons and their equipment close to the battle and relied on stretcher-bearers to bring the wounded to them. At the time, Larrey's system was judged to be safer, more mobile, and more flexible; was "more effective and expedient in proving effective care to the wounded foot soldier than Percy's system"; and "became the standard medical evacuation for Napoleon's armies" (Oritz, 1998, pp. 22–23). Nevertheless, Percy's idea of a semimobile field hospital—bringing the wounded to the hospital rather than medical care to the wounded—became the norm prior to World War I.

Triage

Before proceeding, we should note that Larrey's preference for treating the most badly wounded first without regard to the chance of survival runs counter the more general goal of saving the maximum number of lives. For the British, this changed in 1846, when,

> to make their efforts most effective, surgeons . . . [began to] focus on those patients who need immediate treatment and for whom treatment is likely to be successful, deferring treatment for those whose wounds are less severe and those whose wounds are probably fatal with or without immediate intervention. (Iserson and Moskop, 2007, p. 277)

During World War I, the term *triage* came into common use. It was taken from the French word *trier*, to sort, and soldiers with critical but less-complicated wounds given

---

[1]   In his memoirs, Larrey notes:

> I now first discovered the inconveniences to which we were subjected in moving our *ambulances*, or military hospitals. The military regulations required that they should always be one league distant from the army. The wounded were left on the field, until after the engagement, and were then collected at a convenient spot, to which the *ambulances* repaired as speedily as possible; but the number of wagons interposed between them and the army, and many other difficulties so retarded their progress, that they never arrived in less than twenty-four or thirty-six hours, so that most of the wounded died for want of assistance. . . . This suggested to me the idea of constructing an *ambulance* in such a manner that it might afford a ready conveyance for the wounded during the battle. (Larrey, 1814; emphasis in the original)

preference over the most badly injured. Now, the rule would be the greatest good for the greatest number, e.g.,

> a critical and treatable patient should not be given priority for treatment if the time required to provide that treatment would prevent treatment for other patients with critical but less complicated injuries. This approach explicitly recognizes that, when resources are limited, some patients who could be saved may be allowed to die to save others. (Iserson and Moskop, 2007, p. 277)

Others went even further in recognizing the principle of conservation of force. A British manual listed the goals of triage as, first, conservation of manpower, and second, the interests of the wounded (Manring et al., 2009, p. 2170). NATO's military handbook from 1958 describes the following triage categories: "(1) those who are slightly injured and can return to service, (2) those who are more seriously injured and in need of immediate resuscitation or surgery, and (3) the 'hopelessly wounded' or dead on arrival" (Iserson and Moskop, 2007, p. 277).

World War I

Before World War I, armies continued to envision war as a series of episodic battles; the "wounded could be collected after the fighting, and evacuation would be rapid since hostile fire would not be slowing ambulances, which would speed patients to well-equipped rear-area hospitals" (Marble, 2012, p. 4). The American system, prior to 1914, is a clear example:

> The American medical structure of 1914 was typical of armies. Small medical detachments in the battalions collected casualties and ran aid stations. Ambulance companies evacuated casualties to hospitals and supplemented the aid stations. Field hospitals (with negligible surgical capacity and no nursing capability) would keep the combat units of each division mobile by taking patients, but would themselves stay mobile by channeling patients farther back, to evacuation hospitals. These in turn would evacuate patients as soon as possible to base hospitals, where most surgery would be performed. These stages had different names in different countries, but the outline was very similar. Military aspects dominated medical ones: effects on patients of prolonged bouncing in ambulances were secondary to keeping combat units mobile. (Marble, 2012, p. 4)

By 1915, the British and French had come to the conclusion that the seriously wounded needed forward surgery. The system that "compels the most severely wounded to travel farthest" (Cowdrey, 1985, p. 5) was not working. What was needed was "surgeons near the front to stabilize the worst cases for their long journey to the rear" (Cowdrey, 1985, p. 5). The French response was the Ambulance Chirurgical

Automobile (or *autochir*),[2] a stripped-down mobile surgical hospital that could work 4 to 12 miles behind the front, within artillery range. Such mobile hospitals were not on the American Army's Tables of Organization, but as American forces completed their training in France and faced the prospects of combat, the chief surgeon of the American Expeditionary Force (AEF) came to the conclusion that the accepted practices had to change.[3] With the approval of GEN John Pershing, the AEF commander, the Army bought 20 mobile hospitals from the French.

The new arrangement called for one mobile and one evacuation hospital per division, rather than two evacuations per division. The mobile hospital was to treat the desperately wounded who needed treatment immediately and could not tolerate further transportation. The new units would consist of 12 officers, 80 enlisted men, and 22 nurses divided into six surgical teams. They were authorized two trucks each to carry a sterilizer, X-ray machine, and electric generator. Figure A.1 shows radiology and sterilizer trucks of the Army Mobile Hospital No. 39, set up at Aulnois-sur-Vestuzy, France. When they needed to move, additional trucks were to be temporarily assigned to carry "a light frame operating room, tentage, hospital material sufficient to establish a surgical hospital of 120 beds."[4]

At first, when the front was stable, the mobile hospitals were attached to evacuation hospitals, but starting in September 1918, with the Battle of Saint-Mihiel,[5] they generally moved forward close to the divisional triage hospital. Marble notes:

> Having the MH [mobile hospital] alongside the divisional *triage* hospital worked extremely well; the other field hospitals could handle gas patients, the sick, and neuropsychiatric patients, then bandage and treat the lesser surgical patients who would go back to the evacuation hospital for treatment. All this meant that the MH got only the urgent surgical patients. (Marble, 2012, p. 11; emphasis in the original)

The urgent patients specifically were those with "sucking chest wounds, perforated abdomens, severe hemorrhage, and shock" (Marble, 2012, p. 12).

There were, however, problems that would resonate in further incarnations of these mobile hospitals, all concerning the issue of mobility. In particular, while pared

---

[2] For a discussion of the French mobile hospitals, see Lynch, Ford, and Weed, 1925, pp. 185–186.

[3] Marble, 2012, p. 8, reports that, in the Weekly War Diary for January 26, 1918, the AEF's chief surgeon stated that the Army's organizational structure was "defective in that it was never designed to furnish first class surgical facilities close to the front. This has become he accepted principle of surgical procedure."

[4] From General Order 70, General Headquarters, AEF, May 6, 1918, as reproduced in Lynch, Ford, and Weed, 1925, p. 187.

[5] The Battle of Saint-Mihiel, September 12–19, 1918, was the first battle in which the AEF participated independently. The AEF, led by General Pershing, attacked German troops who were retreating from the Saint-Mihiel salient to the Hindenburg Line.

Figure A.1
Radiology and Sterilizer Trucks of the Army Mobile
Hospital No. 39, Aulnois-sur-Vestuzy, France

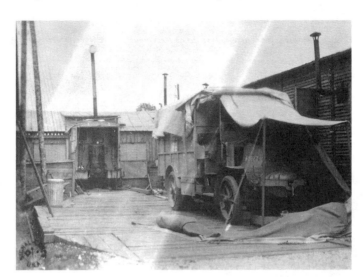

SOURCE: National Library of Medicine: Record Unit 101400381.

down, the weight of the unit was still substantial; it lacked its own trucks; and terrain, weather, and road congestion would slow ambulances bringing and evacuating patients from the hospital. Nevertheless, Jaffin concluded:

> The successes and the problems from World War I served as the basis for medical doctrine after the war and the Medical Department up to the present. Some names have changed, but the functions remain unchanged from World War I. Mobile hospitals became mobile army surgical hospitals . . . , field hospitals became divisional clearing companies, and base hospitals became general and station hospitals. The flow of patients from the front back through the medical system differs today [1990] only through more efficient means of evacuation. (Jaffin, 1990, p. 184)

World War II

The Army started World War II with an organizational model for medical support based on a concept of linear warfare better suited for the plains of Europe than for the island-hopping of the Pacific, where "battalions and regiments [operated] independently on small islands or in dense jungle" (Marble, 2012, p. 19).

War in the Pacific

In the Pacific, to meet the needs of performing surgery forward, the portable surgical hospital was developed. It could be attached to task forces to provide early front-line surgical care in amphibious operations. In theory, with a capacity of 25 beds, its equipment and supplies could be carried on the backs of the 33 soldiers and four officers who formed the unit. It could work alongside a medical battalion's collecting company or collecting station to stabilize the seriously wounded for evacuation, as well as alongside a clearing company or clearing station, but "only those who require immediate surgery or who are non-transportable . . . [were to] be admitted" (FM 8-5, 1942, Change 2, p. 3). Figure A.2 shows a portable surgical hospital in New Guinea during the fighting in early 1944.

The portable surgical hospital, in the words of one division surgeon,

> proved to be of tremendous value. It would be hard to give an exact estimate of the number of lives that were definitely saved by their emergency surgery and heroic work performed near the front lines. They have proven that they have a definite place with combat troops in this type of warfare. (as quoted in Condon-Rall and Cowdrey, 1998, p. 135)

The following account of medical support during the fighting in New Guinea in 1942 well illustrates the role the portable surgical hospital played:

> Aiding the wounded entailed considerable risk. On Papua the Red Cross gave no protection. The 17th Portable Surgical Hospital "never displayed the Red Cross

**Figure A.2
Wounded of the 186th Infantry Regiment, 41st Division,
Being Carried into the 12th Portable Surgical Hospital,
Hollandia, Dutch New Guinea**

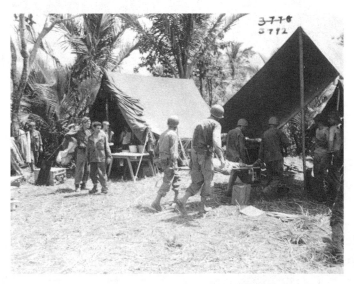

SOURCE: U.S. Army Photo. National Library of Medicine: Record
Unit 101442958.

and our men never wore the arm brassard." Hospitals were bombed unmercifully, and medics were shot while carrying litters . . . .

From the battalion aid stations, relay teams carried the wounded 800 to 1,200 yards back over twisting trails to collecting stations and portable surgical hospitals, often housed in shelters of leaves cut from the jungle, where they received additional treatment. . . .

. . . The four officers and twenty-five enlisted men of the Third Portable Surgical Hospital . . . carried their 1,250 pounds of equipment in pack frames to the front. Here they set up close to the regimental collecting station, forward of the command post and only about 300 yards from the Japanese. . . .

[D]uring a single week—its first on the line—the tiny hospital performed sixty-seven major surgical procedures, including amputations, resections of the bowel, and serious chest operations. (Condon-Rall and Cowdrey, 1998, pp. 133–134)

While the portable surgical hospital proved effective during the jungle campaigns on the more conventional battlefield on Luzon in late 1944 and 1945, the compromises that made them man-portable became clear. Without dedicated transportation, the portable surgical hospitals could not keep up with the troops they were supporting, which were moving by truck (Marble, 2009).[6] Moreover, these hospitals lacked standard surgical equipment because the trade-off of surgical capability for mobility cut deeply into what could be done for patients.[7] Experience in the Pacific proved the value of forward surgery but would not be the model for how forward surgery should be organized for the more-conventional linear battlefields of the European theater.

War in Europe: North Africa, Italy, Northern France, Southern France, Germany
The fighting in Europe was nothing like the jungle fighting in the Pacific, except for the need for forward surgery to tend to the roughly 6 percent of casualties who could not be transported without immediate surgical care. To handle these cases, the Army in North Africa established auxiliary surgical groups made up of specialists who would augment other units wherever needed, e.g., forward to clearing stations or to evacu-

---

[6]   See also Condon-Rall and Cowdrey, 1998, p. 347.

[7]   Greenwood, 2013, states that

> From the very first, the portable surgical hospital was a compromise solution to meet a dire need. While it had many strengths, the hospital also had numerous weaknesses. The most important of their shortcomings could be grouped into four major areas: (1) they lacked much of the equipment needed for definitive surgery, especially in the area of anesthesia, due to the weight limitations that were imposed to maintain their portability; (2) they lacked the bed capacity to hold and care for postoperative patients, especially for abdominal cases, prior to evacuation, which the tactical situation dictated more often than the patients' medical status; (3) the skills and experience of the assigned surgeons, especially after the first year or so, were often insufficient to meet the heavy surgical demands placed on the units; and (4) they were really never entirely self-sufficient and had to operate with larger units for adequate logistical support.

ation hospitals. However, when employed forward, they could not provide adequate postoperative care. Moreover, the surgical hospitals, employed during the initial phases of the North African campaign (November 1942 to May 1943), could provide such care but failed because they "could not keep up with the clearing station [they supported] and . . . could not be broken up into small, independent units" (Graves, 1950, p. 71). The command surgeon thought that the best answer was "a platoon of the field hospital, with its most complete surgical equipment would be most suitable with the attachment of surgical and shock teams as required" (Marble, 2012, p. 25), and that system took hold.[8] Figure A.3 shows such a field hospital platoon.

For the rest of the war in Europe—from Sicily in 1943, to Normandy in 1944, and to the final assault on Germany in 1945—the standard practice was to divide field hospitals into smaller mobile units augmented by surgical teams, which had their own transportation to carry tentage, instruments, and the supplies they needed. The surgical team would set up near clearing stations, and the field hospital platoons "arrived last and took over the job of holding and caring for the wounded as the surgical team finished with them" (Cosmas and Cowdrey, 1992, p. 531). Eventually, the personnel and equipment of an Army collecting company were added to each field hospital platoon. This allowed the field hospital platoon to move forward, leaving nontrans-

Figure A.3
Initial Stage of the Establishment of a Field Hospital Platoon

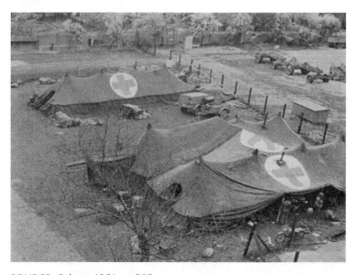

SOURCE: Odom, 1961, p. 305.

---

[8]   Field hospitals were designed to be able to split into 100-bed platoons and "had many capabilities the clearing companies lacked, and it was mobile enough. Surgical and shock teams from an ASG [auxiliary surgical group] could provide the necessary personnel" (Marble, 2012, p. 25).

portable patients in the care of elements of the collecting company. The patients were evacuated as soon as they became transportable, after which the elements of collecting company left behind would rejoin the field hospital platoon.[9] While the system generally worked well, there were problems that were finally addressed when the concept was formalized in the design of a new unit.[10] Figure A.3 shows Third Army Field Hospital Platoon set up near a division clearing station.

As well as the match-up of augmented field hospital platoons, auxiliary surgical groups, and elements of divisional clearing and collecting worked, this arrangement was still an improvisation, and some sought a more permanent solution. The Third Army command surgeon proposed a new unit made up of two platoons that would combine the elements that had previously been lashed together, with the platoons leapfrogging one another as the front moved forward (Cosmas and Cowdrey, 1992, p. 531). The Chief Surgeon for Army Field Forces, BG Frederick Blesse, proposed a 60-bed surgical hospital, with surgeons assigned rather than attached and with nurses, X-ray capabilities, and its own trucks for full mobility. The consulting surgeons—the civilian surgeons temporarily in service for the duration of the war— strongly opposed the plan, preferring the ad hoc arrangement of augmentation teams that allowed "elite" surgeons to go where the action was and not waste their talents (Marble, 2012, pp. 31–32). On August 23, 1945, the Surgeon General's office published Table of Organization and Equipment 8-571, which set forth requirements for the new, 60-bed mobile surgical hospital—the MASH—as a self-contained, mobile hospital unit to handle definitive surgery immediately behind the front lines. It was to be "truly mobile, fully staffed with the surgical and medical personnel, and equipped to provide definitive, life-saving surgery and postoperative care for non-transportable patients" (Greenwood, 2013).[11] As designed, the MASH was made up of headquarters elements and

> a preoperative and shock treatment section, an operating section, a postoperative section, a pharmacy, an X-ray section, and a holding ward. Fourteen medical offi-

---

[9] As described in Odom, 1961, p. 306.

[10] Wiltse, 1965, p. 170, notes that

> In the Sicily Campaign organization and facilities for front-line surgery were greatly improved over those of the Tunisia Campaign. The most important single development was the use of field hospital platoons, with attached surgical teams, for treatment of nontransportable casualties in the division area. [However,] . . . [f]ield hospital commanders were reluctant to undertake dispersed operation by platoons, and were generally unfamiliar with the technique of functioning in that manner. There was also some resistance to accepting the attachment of surgical teams, as implying some degree of reflection on the competence of the regular hospital staff.

[11] According to Marble, 2012, p. 32, "The new unit would have six surgeons, five physicians for the wards, a radiologist, two anesthetists, twelve nurses, three administrative officers, and ninety-five enlisted men. It would have ten 2.5-ton trucks, one jeep, and a three-quarter-ton truck; there were ten trailers to carry more gear" needed to support its 60 beds.

cers, twelve nurses, two Medical Service Corps officers, one warrant officer, and ninety-seven enlisted men formed the complement. (Cowdrey, 1987, p. 70)

The TO&E provided tents and trucks with the expectation that a MASH could be "disassembled, loaded onto vehicles, and ready to depart on 6 hours notice. After arrival at its new location, it was to be operational be operational within 4 hours" (Baker, 2012, p. 424).

Korea

On the eve of the Korean War, the Army had formally established five MASHs, but none were effectively fielded, and none were in the Far East. The first to see combat, the 8055th MASH, was hastily organized on July 1, with "ten medical officers, 95 enlisted men and 12 nurses assigned" (Cowdrey, 1985, p. 5) by stripping available personnel from other units in Japan. By July 10, it was at work in Taejon, Korea alongside the clearing company of the 24th Infantry Division. It operated as designed, providing forward surgery for those who could not stand a journey by ambulance to the 8054th Evacuation Hospital in Pusan or by air to Japan or to a Navy hospital ship off the coast. However, the realities of war in Korean broke the very design of the MASH.

To be effective, this small, 60-bed surgical hospital was designed to fit into a medevac scheme (Table 3.1), to provide an Echelon III capability in an Echelon II environment, and to serve the so-called "nontransportable" close to the front. However, the lack of transportation due to an inadequate road and rail network and the volatile tactical situation soon overwhelmed the MASHs—even with the later-deployed 8063rd and 8076th MASHs. In November 1950, the 8055th and the other MASH units expanded to 150 beds, eventually to 200 beds.[12] Moreover, without deployed field hospitals, the MASHs soon became more than surgical hospitals, seeing nonsurgical patients as well. As the chief surgeon of the 8076th MASH noted, "[w]e had to improvise in our treatment. . . . The MASH units were responsible for treatment of all the wounded who were brought to its tents" (Apel and Apel, 1998, p. 63). Figure A.4 shows a deployed MASH.

The key to keeping the MASHs mobile, even as their postoperative capacity grew, was rapid transportation. With the arrival of their own helicopter detachments, they could transport the most critically wounded from the front, so there was less need for them to be so far forward. The MASH could therefore, for example, stand back at a relatively safe distance while still meeting the needs of the most critical nontransportable casualties. Soon, MASH units were even specializing in surgical treatment, transferring patients among themselves (Apel and Apel, 1998, p. 80). As the front stabilized,

---

[12] It was not until February 1952 that their TO&E was changed back to 60-bed status, they continued to function as 200-bed semi–evacuation hospitals throughout 1952 (Lindsey, 1954, p. 84).

Figure A.4
Deployed Mobile Army Surgical Hospital

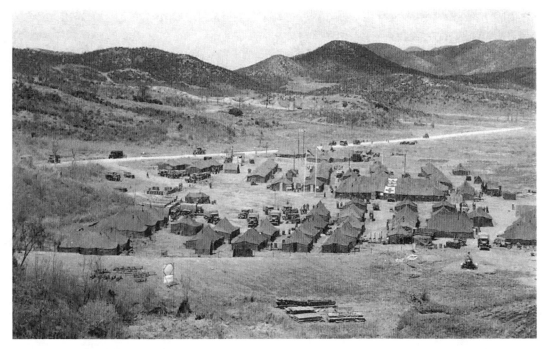

SOURCE: Ginn, 1997, p. 240.

they moved into more permanent facilities well behind the division clearing station, in "central locations from which they could normally support any division sector with the corps" (Lindsey, 1954, p. 84).[13]

---

[13] Lindsey, 1954, p. 85, also notes that, despite the "heavy investment" the MASH units made "in comfort and luxury construction" in their semifixed facilities, e.g., "buildings, walkways and clubs and fancy quarters," these units were still able to demonstrate, through "realistic training exercises," their ability to "load up the tentage, and go."

Transportation of the Wounded: Jeep Ambulances and Helicopters

Transportation of the wounded from the place of wounding to a medical facility is the first critical link in caring for war casualties. During the Revolution, Congress stipulated that the Quartermaster General provide "a suitable number of covered and other wagons, litters, and other necessaries for removing the sick and wounded" (Brown, 1873, p. 36). Larrey and Percy understood the importance of transportation and provided especially constructed ambulances (as discussed in Appendix A). A half-century after the Napoleonic Wars, however, during the initial months of the Civil War, Americans were still completely unprepared to transport casualties from the battlefield. It would fall to the Surgeon of the Army of the Potomac, MAJ Jonathan Letterman, to build the first ambulance corps—the forerunner of the hierarchical approach to the treatment of the wounded that finally took hold in the 20th century. Still, even with advances in motorized ambulances, the wounded could not be moved fast enough to the rear, so the capabilities of the rear had to be moved to them. It was the so-called nontransportable patients who drove the need for the MASH and its predecessors. The basic requirement for forward surgery came from the poor condition of these wounded and their inability to withstand the journey to a third-echelon facility. How close surgeons needed to be to the fighting was very much determined by how difficult it was to transport patients to the clearing stations. The more difficult, the closer the surgical team needed to get. The nature and size of the forward surgeries also reflected the rigors of transporting postoperative patients to field and evacuation hospitals. The driving factors were terrain and road conditions, and in Korea, the transports of choice, highlighted in the introduction to the TV show *M*A*S*H*, were the jeep ambulance and helicopters. While the helicopters were critical in saving the lives of the few who would not survive being transported over land, the jeep ambulance developed during World War II was the workhorse in the mountains of Korea.

The Jeep Ambulance

One of the most significant advances in the care a wounded soldier received during World War II was the development of the jeep ambulance (see Figure B.1).[1] As late as 1935, the role of horse-drawn ambulances was still being debated (Shambora, 1935, p. 28). It was not until July 1940 that the Army formally asked American automobile manufacturers to submit designs for "a general purpose, personnel, or cargo carrier especially adaptable for reconnaissance or command, and designated as 1/4-ton 4x4 Truck" (Technical Manual 9-803, 1944, p. 2-3). As conditions permitted, medevac was soon motorized, with the jeep playing an important role. In the European theater,

> the divisions, by late 1944, in effect had motorized their entire chain of evacuation. . . . By late autumn they routinely extended motor transport forward of the aid stations as well, whenever possible right to the place where casualties lay on the battlefield. Medics now used jeeps, belonging to battalion aid stations and collect-

Figure B.1
Litter-Jeep Ambulance Evacuation

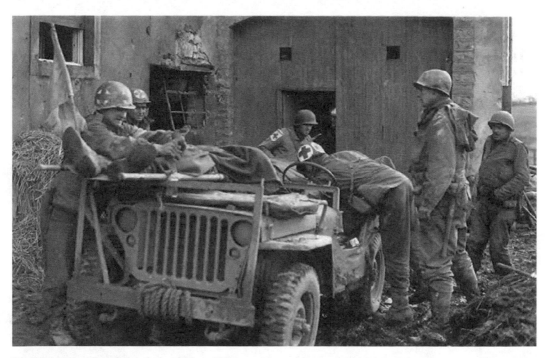

SOURCE: Cosmas and Cowdrey, 1992, p. 532.

---

[1]   American Society of Mechanical Engineers, 1991, p. 3, states that "General George C. Marshall called the Jeep vehicle 'America's greatest contribution to modern warfare.' The Jeep MB model served in every World War II theater as a litter bearer, machine-gun firing mount, reconnaissance vehicle, pickup truck, front-line limousine, ammo bearer, wire layer, and taxi."

ing companies, in preference to litter bearers, for moving wounded in the forward areas. Fitted with brackets for carrying litters, these small sturdy vehicles could go most places men on foot could; they could accommodate two or three litters each, and as many ambulatory patients as ingenious drivers could crowd on board. (Cosmas and Cowdrey, 1992, p. 364)

In Korea, the litter jeep proved itself again, "not merely as a field expedient to replace unavailable ambulances but as a preferred vehicle because its low profile made it a less inviting target" (Cowdrey, 1987, p. 150). The use of the jeep ambulance is highlighted in this report from May 19, 1951:

Normally, litter jeeps from our medical company collecting station pick up their patients at the battalion aid station. In this operation, however, the litter jeeps passed the aid station and came up the road to a point only fifty yards from the base of the mountain on which the battalion was fighting. . . .

A man wounded on the firing line was immediately treated then he was carried down the mountain by a five-man litter team. The trip took an hour and a half.

Once the patient reached the jeep evacuation point his bandages were checked and adjusted, and his general condition observed. Seriously wounded were loaded two to a jeep; lightly wounded were often loaded seven to a vehicle—one in the front seat, four in the back, two on the hood.

The jeeps bypassed the battalion aid station and took the patients to the advanced clearing station. Here the seriously wounded were evacuated by helicopter. (Sarka, 1955, pp. 110–111)

Helicopter

If the jeep revolutionized medevac during World War II, the helicopter did the same during the Korean War. Evacuation of the wounded through the air had been the dream of the Army's Medical Corps from the earliest days of military aviation.

World War I

Soon after the Wright Brothers flew at Kitty Hawk, two U.S. Army medical officers designed an airplane for transporting patients. But CPT George H. R. Gosman and Lieutenant A. L. Rhodes were unable to obtain official backing (Vanderburg, 2003). During World War I, a French medical officer, Dr. Eugene Chaissang, modified two French military planes and used them to evacuate wounded personnel from Flanders on April 18, 1918. The fuselages of the planes were too narrow to hold stretchers, so patients were inserted through the side of the fuselage, behind the pilot's cockpit. The planes had enough space for two wounded soldiers. The first successful air ambulance in the United States was created by Army CPT William C. Oaker and MAJ William E. Driver in 1918 by modifying a Jenny biplane, including removing the rear cockpit and rearranging equipment so a standard Army stretcher would fit.[2]

World War II

For all practical purposes, helicopters came too late to see any real service during World War II. The first flight of Igor Sikorsky's experimental XR-4 took place a little more than a month after the attack on Pearl Harbor. The U.S. Army Air Force ordered 30 YR-4s for "service testing and flight training" ("R-4 Sikorsky Helicopter," undated). One was sent to the China-Burma-India theater and, in late April 1944, executed the first recovery of wounded personnel from a downed Stinson L-1 aircraft carrying wounded British soldiers ("WW II Helicopter Evacuation," undated).[3] In May 1945, in the Philippines, helicopters were used to evacuate "sick and wounded from inaccessible mountain positions" (Smith, 1993, p. 421). Despite these successes, the main focus of the helicopter's development and early deployment after the war was on searching for and recovering downed pilots. Figure B.2 shows the Coast Guard testing the use of a helicopter during World War II.

The Key West Agreement

Further Army consideration of helicopters was sidetracked when the National Security Act of 1947 (Pub. L. 80-253, 1947) established the U.S. Air Force as a separate service, leaving the Army with only a few hundred light planes. Friction between the services resulted in several high-level conferences on future "roles and missions." The most important was in early March 1948, in Key West, Florida. While the Key West Agreement "allowed the Military Services to continue to possess assets that might otherwise belong to the primary role of another Service" (Eilon and Lyon, 2010, p. 8), Army aviation was restricted to "observation, reconnaissance, local messenger and courier service, and emergency wire laying and evacuation" (Kitchens, 2003, p. 2). At the start of the Korean War, the Army had no medevac helicopters. It was almost by accident that helicopters were pressed into service—a service made all the more critical by the "nature of the Korean conflict and of the Korean countryside" (Cowdrey, 1987, p. 95).

---

[2]   See Clingman, 1989, pp. 4–5, and Vanderburg, 2003, pp. 6–7.

[3]   The American Helicopter Society History Committee provided an account of the first use of helicopters for medical evacuation:

> Apr 23–May 4, 1944: Lt. Carter Harman evacuates 21 wounded and injured personnel in Burma with a Sikorsky YR-4B during a service test with the 1st Air Commando Group. This allows the Army Air Force to continue the ramping up of helicopter production and begin to commit helicopters into official tables of equipment of combat units. In addition to highlighting the promise of helicopters in unimproved regions, the experiment also showcases the limited durability and poor maintainability of 1st generation helicopters. (AHS Helicopter History Committee, 2007)

Figure B.2
The Coast Guard Tests the Navy's First Helicopter, HNS-1
(Army R-4 Sikorsky), for Air-Sea Rescue During
World War II

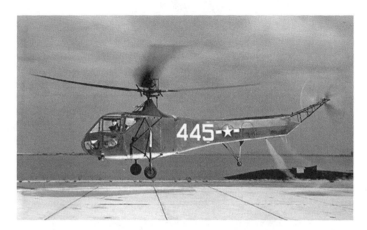

SOURCE: U.S. Coast Guard viaCoast Guard Aviation Association, undated.

Korea

In summer 1950, the Air Force 3rd Rescue Squadron, which had been sent to Korea to rescue downed pilots, found that it had little to do, since the North Korean air force had largely been eliminated by American airpower, and few allied planes were being shot down. Soon, however, the squadron's commander began receiving calls from Army units to evacuate wounded soldiers. On August 3, on the first of what would be many flights, an Air Force H-5 flew patients from the 8055th MASH to the evacuation hospital in Pusan, 100 km away. The H-5, however, was limited because it was not equipped to fly nonambulatory patients. When that was required, a litter was pressed into service, and "the rear right-hand window had to be removed and the stretcher case loaded head first through the window and across the passenger compartment. During the flight, the patient's feet remained outside the helicopter" (Parker and Batha, 1982, p. 14). Figure B.3 shows a Marine Corps H-5 with the litter patient sticking out of the passenger compartment window. Eventually, external litter pods were added.

In fall 1950, the Air Force continued to fly medevac missions. In October 1950, the Army Surgeon General visited Korea and became convinced of the need for the Army to have its own air ambulance helicopters. Within a month of his return to Washington, the two services had agreed that the Army would provide front-line evacuation and that the Air Force would evacuate patients outside the combat zone. In January 1951, new Army medical helicopter detachments started to arrive:

> Each detachment had four helicopters; two had Bell H-13s, and two had Hiller
> H-23s. Each helicopter had one pilot and was rigged with two exterior pods for

Figure B.3
Marine Corps HO3S-1 [H-5] Helicopter Evacuating a Casualty

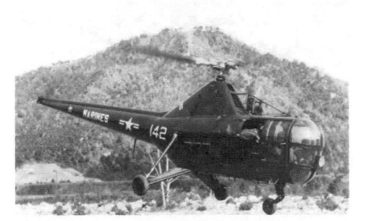

SOURCE: Parker and Batha, 1982, p. 14.

litter patients; one ambulatory patient could be carried at the same time under ideal conditions. (Ginn, 1997, p. 244)[4]

Medevac by helicopter was new, and both the pilots and ground personnel had to learn the limits of front-line evacuation, as an officer assigned to Eighth Army Headquarters noted:

> In the popular conception, helicopters landed on mountain peaks, lifted straight up into the air, and operated in all types of weather. It was necessary to understand that helicopters could not fly at night, operate in bad weather, or land on sloping terrain. They needed takeoff space; they could not fly in heavy winds; they had limitations of range and altitude. They also had less lifting power in the thin, warm air of summer.

> Ground troops had to understand the importance of reporting accurate coordinates to locate the patient. They had to be taught the necessity of marking the landing site with panels and of using colored smoke grenades to indicate proper location and wind direction. (Blumenson, 1955, p. 112)

The new units, with four H-13 Sioux helicopters each, were placed under the operational control of the Eighth U.S. Army command surgeon, who assigned them to the MASH units at the front.[5] While the three detachments had at most 11 aircraft,

---

[4] For a discussion of the activation of these detachments, see Driscoll, 2001, p. 291.

[5] Each unit consisted of four helicopters, four pilots, and four mechanics (Blumenson, 1955, p. 211).

these "evacuated about 17,000 casualties" (Dorland and Nanney, 1982, p. 11).[6] It has been reported that "[o]ne pilot evacuated 922 casualties and logged 545 missions in 700 hours over a 14-month period" (U.S. Army Transportation Museum, undated). Figure B.4 shows an H-13 with the two skid-mounted cocoons.

While the H-13s had been procured explicitly for the medevac mission, they were no more suited for that mission than the H-5s had been (Driscoll, 2001, p. 292). Like the H-5s, they lacked litter platforms, but detachments "quickly received permission to fit platforms on the skid assemblies so that litters could be mounted on either side of the fuselage" (Dorland and Nanney, 1982, p. 15), again using the Navy's Stokes litter. Being on the skids presented its own problem: The patients had to be protected from the elements, including the dust kicked up by the helicopter itself. As shown

Figure B.4
Medics Carry a Wounded Soldier Toward an H-13 Helicopter

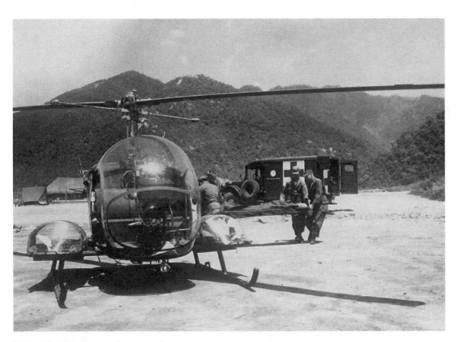

SOURCE: U.S. Army photo.

---

[6] Driscoll, 2001, p. 295, reports that

> From January 2, 1951, three helicopter detachments (with a total of 11 aircraft) evacuated 5,040 patients to rear areas during the first 12 months of operations, consuming a total of 4,421 hours of flying time. Helicopter evacuations in 1952 surpassed the number in 1951 by 2,883, for a total of 7,923. The last 7 months of the war, in 1953, increased the rate of evacuations, with the monthly totals reaching record highs of more than 1,000 during heavy fighting in June and July in the "Pork Chop" area. . . .

> Between January 1, 1951, and the cessation of active hostilities on July 27, 1953, helicopter detachments under the control of the Army Medical Service evacuated a total of 17,690 patients.

in Figure B.5, a Plexiglas hood was fashioned to cover the patient's upper body, with fabric for the lower body. A system to keep the patients warm was jerry-rigged to duct warm air off the engine manifolds onto the litter. They also "devised a way for en route transfusions of plasma or whole blood" (Dorland and Nanney, 1982, p. 16). It would be a full six months before new litter mounts that could accommodate standard Army litters finally arrived in Korea.

As envisioned, medevac helicopters were to stay clear of enemy fire, but that dictum was often violated. Without radios to properly direct them to where they were most needed, pilots "began the practice of siting their aircraft in the fields at clearing stations near the tactical headquarters just behind the front lines" (Dorland and Nanney, 1982, p. 13). Moreover, given the reach of the helicopters and their ability to transport the most critically wounded, the MASHs were able to stand back from the front lines farther than they might have been able to if only ground transportation had been available.

While medevac helicopters were a great innovation, as ambulances had been during the Civil War, some things never seem to change. On June 23, 1951, the Eighth U.S. Army command surgeon had to remind commanders that helicopters were to be used "only to provide immediate evacuation of non-transportable and critically ill or injured patients who needed surgical or medical care not available at forward facilities" because "ground commanders sometimes requested helicopters more as a convenience than as a necessity" (Dorland and Nanney, 1982, p. 17). This admonition had a famil-

Figure B.5
Modifications Made to the H-13 to Improve Patient Comfort

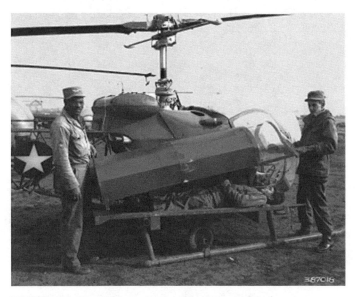

SOURCE: U.S. Army Transportation Museum, undated.

iar ring. Early in the Civil War, it was common for ambulances to be commandeered as baggage carts for officers. In 1862, responsibility for ambulances was taken from the Quartermaster Department and given to the Medical Department, and, by order of the commanding general, "officers offending [were to be placed] in arrest for trial for disobedience of orders" (McClellan, 1862). Nevertheless, resupply became a critical secondary mission for helicopters, as one MASH surgeon recalled: "[E]ach time a helicopter evacuated soldiers to a field hospital, it would return with supplies" (Apel and Apel, 1998, p. 83).

Throughout the war, requests for air evacuation had to be tightly controlled, and the service was available only to the most seriously wounded:

> The request for air evacuation went over to the corps surgeon. The corps surgeon's air operation officer acted much like a dispatcher. Each MASH supported at least one corps level unit. The corps surgeon's air operations office would task the MASH helicopter detachment supporting that corps to send a copter. . . .

> . . . As the helicopter approached the battalion aid station to pick up the wounded, it was an easy target. . . .

> . . . As soon as the helicopter hit the ground, the medics carried the wounded on a litter, placed the litter on the helicopter just above the skids, and strapped it down. . . . All this had to be done as quickly as possible and was often done under direct enemy fire. . . .

> Helicopter evacuation required much closer selection of evacuees than did evacuation by field ambulances or litter. The battalion surgeon or the medic on scene decided quickly who was to be evacuated based upon several criteria: the extent of the wound itself, the availability of aircraft, the number of casualties, and other means of evacuation available. (Apel and Apel, 1998, pp. 76–77)

In retrospect, the use of helicopters for medevac was an outstanding achievement during the Korean War and foretold more-extensive use a decade later in Vietnam. Generally, there was "sufficient lift for the worst [surgical cases] . . . except during a few periods of unusual activity. . . . [However,] roughly speaking, something less than half of the true surgical . . . [cases were] moved by helicopter" (Lindsey, 1954, p. 80). The numbers were still significant, especially for those critically wounded.[7]

---

[7] Blumenson, reports:

> Helicopters in Korea had evacuated eight thousand casualties by 1 November 1951. Many of these men would not have survived without this transportation. The smooth ride and the rapid arrival at a clearing station or hospital possibly caused a lower rate of shock fatalities than in World War II. The treatment of head injuries was expedited because helicopters carried patients swiftly to neurosurgical teams. (Blumenson, 1955, p. 113)

References

Abramowitz, Michael, and Steve Vogel, "Army Secretary Ousted," *Washington Post*, March 3, 2007.

Abt Associates, "Initial Findings: National Vietnam Veteran Study Reveals Long-Term Course of PTSD and Link to Chronic Health Conditions," press release, Cambridge, Mass., August 8, 2014.

Acosta, Joie D., Amariah Becker, Jennifer L. Cerully, Michael P. Fisher, Laurie T. Martin, Raffaele Vardavas, Mary Ellen Slaughter, and Terry L. Schell, *Mental Health Stigma in the Military*, Santa Monica, Calif.: RAND Corporation, RR-426-OSD, 2014.

Adkins, Robinson E., *Medical Care of Veterans*, Washington, D.C.: U.S. Government Printing Office, 1967.

Administrator of Veterans Affairs, *Annual Report for the Fiscal Year Ended June 30, 1940*, Washington, D.C.: U.S. Government Printing Office, January 3, 1941.

———, *Annual Report for Fiscal Year Ending June 30, 1951*, Washington, D.C.: U.S. Government Printing Office, 1952.

———, *Annual Report for Fiscal Year Ending June 30, 1952*, Washington, D.C.: U.S. Government Printing Office, 1953.

———, *Annual Report for Fiscal Year Ending June 30, 1953*, Washington, D.C.: U.S. Government Printing Office, 1954.

———, *Annual Report for Fiscal Year Ending June 30, 1954*, Washington, D.C.: U.S. Government Printing Office, 1955.

———, *Annual Report for Fiscal Year Ending June 30, 1955*, Washington, D.C.: U.S. Government Printing Office, 1956.

———, *Annual Report for Fiscal Year Ending June 30, 1956*, Washington, D.C.: U.S. Government Printing Office, 1957.

———, *Annual Report for Fiscal Year Ending June 30, 1957*, Washington, D.C.: U.S. Government Printing Office, 1958.

———, *Annual Report: Administrator of Veterans Affairs, 1958*, Washington, D.C.: U.S. Government Printing Office, 1959.

———, *Annual Report: Administrator of Veterans Affairs, 1959*, Washington, D.C.: U.S. Government Printing Office, 1960.

———, *Annual Report: Administrator of Veterans Affairs, 1960*, Washington, D.C.: U.S. Government Printing Office, 1961.

———, *Annual Report: Administrator of Veterans Affairs, 1961*, Washington, D.C.: U.S. Government Printing Office, 1962.

————, *Annual Report: Administrator of Veterans Affairs, 1964*, Washington, D.C.: U.S. Government Printing Office, 1965.

————, *Annual Report: Administrator of Veterans Affairs, 1965*, Washington, D.C.: U.S. Government Printing Office, 1966a.

————, *Annual Report: Administrator of Veterans Affairs, 1966*, Washington, D.C.: U.S. Government Printing Office, 1966b.

————, *Annual Report: Administrator of Veterans Affairs, 1967*, Washington, D.C.: U.S. Government Printing Office, 1968.

————, *Annual Report: Administrator of Veterans Affairs, 1968*, Washington, D.C.: U.S. Government Printing Office, 1969.

————, *Annual Report: Administrator of Veterans Affairs, 1969*, Washington, D.C.: U.S. Government Printing Office, 1970.

————, *Annual Report: Administrator of Veterans Affairs, 1970*, Washington, D.C.: U.S. Government Printing Office, 1971.

————, *Annual Report: Administrator of Veterans Affairs, 1971*, Washington, D.C.: U.S. Government Printing Office, 1972.

————, *Annual Report: Administrator of Veterans Affairs, 1972*, Washington, D.C.: U.S. Government Printing Office, 1973.

————, *Annual Report: Administrator of Veterans Affairs, 1976*, Washington, D.C.: U.S. Government Printing Office, 1977.

————, *Annual Report: Administrator of Veterans Affairs, 1977*, Washington, D.C.: U.S. Government Printing Office, 1978.

————, *Annual Report: Administrator of Veterans Affairs, 1978*, Washington, D.C.: U.S. Government Printing Office, 1979.

————, *Annual Report: Administrator of Veterans Affairs, 1979*, Washington, D.C.: U.S. Government Printing Office, 1980.

————, *Veteran's Administration 1980 Annual Report: Our 50th Anniversary*, Washington, D.C.: U.S. Government Printing Office, 1981.

————, *Veterans Administration Annual Report 1981*, Washington, D.C.: U.S. Government Printing Office, 1982.

Ahart, George J., "Actions Needed to Insure That Female Veterans Have Equal Access to VA Benefits," memorandum to Daniel K. Inouye, Washington, D.C.: U.S. General Accounting Office, September 24, 1982.

AHS Helicopter History Committee, "1941–1945: Born of War," 2007.

Allen, Casey J., Richard J. Straker, Clark R. Murray, William M. Hannay, Mena M. Hanna, Jonathan P. Meizoso, Ronald J. Manning, Carl I. Schulman, Jason M. Seery, and Kenneth G. Proctor, "Recent Advances in Forward Surgical Team Training at the U.S. Army Trauma Training Department," *Military Medicine*, Vol. 181, No. 6, June 2016, pp. 553–559.

"Allied Troop Levels—Vietnam, 1960 to 1973," table, American War Library website, 2008.

Altarum Institute, *Study of Barriers for Women Veterans to VA Health Care: Final Report*, Washington, D.C.: U.S. Department of Veterans Affairs, Women's Health Services, April 2015.

American Psychiatric Association, *Diagnostic and Statistical Manual of Mental Disorders*, various editions, 1952–2013.

American Society of Mechanical Engineers, "The JEEPMB: An International Historic Mechanical Engineering Landmark," Toledo, Ohio, July 23, 1991.

An Act for Regulating the Military Establishment of the United States, 1st Cong., 2nd Sess., April 30, 1790

An Act Providing for the Better Organization of the Military Establishment, 37th Cong., 1st Sess., August 3, 1861.

An Act to Amend Certain Acts in Relation to the Navy, 39th Cong., 2nd Sess., March 2, 1867.

An Acte for the Relief of Souldiours, 1593.

Anderson, Scott, "Fractured Lands: How the Arab World Came Apart," *New York Times*, August 11, 2016.

Apel, Otto F., Jr., and Pat Apel, *MASH: An Army Surgeon in Korea*, Lexington, Ky.: University Press of Kentucky, 1998.

Aponte, Maribel, Florinda Balfour, Tom Garin, Dorothy Glasgow, Eddie Thomas, and Kayla Williams, *America's Women Veterans: Military Service History and VA Benefit Utilization Statistics*, Washington, D.C.: Office of Data Governance and Analytics, National Center for Veterans Analysis and Statistics, Department of Veterans Affairs, February 2017.

Appleman, Roy E., *South to the Naktong, North to the Yalu (June–November 1950)*, Washington, D.C.: U.S. Army Center of Military History, 1960.

———, *Escaping the Trap: The US Army X Corps in Northeast Korea, 1950*, College Station, Tex.: Texas A&M University Press, 1990.

Army Dismounted Complex Blast Injury Task Force, *Dismounted Complex Blast Injury*, Fort Sam Houston, Tex.: Office of the Surgeon General, Department of the Army, June 18, 2011.

Army Institute of Professional Development, *Combat Lifesaver Course: Student Self-Study, Interschool Subcourse 0871*, Fort Sam Houston, Tex.: U.S. Army Medical Department Center and School, Department of Combat Medic Training, 2012.

"Army Manpower Draft Expected to End in June" *New York Times*, August 5, 1949, p. 3.

Army Quartermaster Museum, *Armored Vest Fact Sheet*, Washington, D.C.: Office of the Quartermaster General, December 23, 1952.

Army Regulation 40-501, *Standards of Medical Fitness*, Washington, D.C.: Headquarters, Department of the Army, August 4, 2011.

"Army Secretary Vows Improvements at Fort Stewart," CNN, October 25, 2003.

Army Techniques Publication 3-39.10, *Police Operations*, Washington, D.C.: Headquarters, Department of the Army, January 2015.

Army Wounded Warrior Program, *5th Anniversary Report, 2004–2009*, Alexandria, Va., 2009.

Arnold, Arthur L., "Inpatient Treatment of Viet Nam Veterans with Post-Traumatic Stress Disorder," in Stephen M. Sonnenberg, Arthur S. Blank, Jr., and John A. Talbott, eds., *The Trauma of War: Stress and Recovery in Vietnam Veterans*, Washington, D.C.: American Psychiatric Press, 1985.

Arnold, James R., ed., *Health Under Fire: Medical Care During America's Wars*, Santa Barbara, Calif.: Greenwood, 2015.

Arnsdorf, Isaac, "Inside the Trump Administration's Internal War Over the VA," *Politico*, February 16, 2018.

Association of the U.S. Army, "The U.S. Army Between World War II and the Korean War," AUSA Background Brief No. 40, March 1992.

Atkinson, Rick, "The IED Problem Is Getting Out of Control. We've Got to Stop the Bleeding," *Washington Post*, September 30, 2007.

Bachkosky, Jack, "Lightening the Load," briefing slides, Washington, D.C.: Naval Research Advisory Committee, September 2007.

Bacon, Bryan L., Matthew J. Barry, and James Demer, "Operational Psychiatry in Operation Enduring Freedom," in Elspeth Cameron Ritchie, ed., *Combat and Operational Behavioral Health*, Washington, D.C.: Borden Institute, Walter Reed Army Medical Center, 2011.

Bagalman, Erin, *Traumatic Brain Injury Among Veterans*, Washington, D.C.: Congressional Research Service, R40941, May 5, 2011.

———, *Health Care for Veterans: Traumatic Brain Injury*, Washington, D.C.: Congressional Research Service, R40941, March 9, 2015.

Bailey, Jeffrey, Mary Ann Spott, George P. Costanzo, James Dunne, Warren Dorlac, and Brian Eastridge, eds., *Joint Trauma System: Development, Conceptual Framework, and Optimal Elements*, Fort Sam Houston, Tex.: U.S. Army Institute of Surgical Research, 2012.

Bailey, Pearce, Frankwood E. Williams, and Paul O. Komora, *The Medical Department of the United States Army in the World War*, Vol. X: *Neuropsychiatry in the United States*," Washington, D.C.: Office of the Surgeon General, Department of War, 1929.

Bailey, Sue, *Medical Readiness Strategic Plan (MRSP) 1998–2004*, Washington, D.C.: Office of the Assistant Secretary of Defense for Health Affairs, DoD 5136.1-P, August 1998.

Baine, David P., *Agent Orange: VA Needs to Further Improve Its Examination and Registry Program*, Washington, D.C.: U.S. General Accounting Office, GAO/HRD 86-7, January 1986.

———, *Military Physicians: DOD's Medical School and Scholarship Program*, Washington, D.C.: U.S. General Accounting Office, GAO/HEHS-95-244, September 1995.

———, *Readjustment Counseling Service: Vet Centers Address Multiple Client Problems, but Improvement Is Needed*, Washington, D.C.: U.S. General Accounting Office, GAO/HEHS-96-113, July 1996a.

———, *VA Health Care: Issues Affecting Eligibility Reform Efforts*, Washington, D.C.: U.S. General Accounting Office, GAO-HEHS-96-160, September 1996b.

Baker, Michael S., "Military Medical Advances Resulting from the Conflict in Korea, Part I: Systems Advances That Enhanced Patient Survival," *Military Medicine*, Vol. 177, No. 4, April 2012, pp. 423–429.

———, "Lead, Follow, or Get out of the Way: How Bold Young Surgeons Brought Vascular Surgery into Clinical Practice from the Korean War Battlefield," *Annals of Vascular Surgery*, Vol. 33, No. 5, May 2016, pp. 258–262.

Baker, Peter, "At Walter Reed, Bush Offers an Apology," *Washington Post*, March 31, 2007.

———, "Inside the Situation Room: How a War Plan Evolved," *New York Times*, December 6, 2009.

Barlas, Frances M., William Bryan Higgins, Jacqueline C. Pflieger, and Kelly Diecker, *2011 Health Related Behaviors Survey of Active Duty Military Personnel*, Fairfax, Va.: ICF International, February 2013.

Barnes, Deborah E., Amy L. Byers, Raquel C. Gardner, Karen H. Seal, W. John Boscardin, and Kristine Yaffe, "Association of Mild Traumatic Brain Injury With and Without Loss of Consciousness with Dementia in US Military Veterans," *JAMA Neurology*, Volume 75, No. 9, September 1, 2018, pp. 1055–1061.

Barrett, George, "Portrait of the Korean Veteran," *New York Times*, August 9, 1953.

Bascetta, Cynthia A., *Veterans' Health Care: VA Needs Better Data on Extent and Causes of Waiting Times*, Washington, D.C.: U.S. General Accounting Office, GAO/HEHS-00-90, May 2000.

———, *VA Health Care: VA Should Expedite the Implementation of Recommendations Needed to Improve Post-Traumatic Stress Disorder Services*, Washington, D.C.: U.S. Government Accountability Office, GAO-05-287, February 2005a.

———, *Vocational Rehabilitation: More VA and DOD Collaboration Needed to Expedite Services for Seriously Injured Servicemembers*, Washington, D.C.: U.S. Government Accountability Office, GAO-05-167, January 2005b.

Baskir, Lawrence M., and William A. Strauss, *Chance and Circumstance: The Draft, the War, and the Vietnam Generation*, New York: Alfred A. Knopf, 1978.

Bass, Elizabeth, Philip Ellis, and Heidi Golding, *Comparing the Costs of the Veterans' Health Care System with Private-Sector Costs*, Washington, D.C.: Congressional Budget Office, December 2014.

Beard, Jeanne L., "Albert Deutsch: The Historian as Social Reformer," Journal of the History of Medicine and Allied Sciences, Vol. 18, No. 2, 1963, excerpted in "Albert Deutsch (1905–1961) Papers Archives Finding Aid," Washington, D.C.: American Psychiatric Association Foundation, Melvin Sabshin, M.D., Library and Archives, April 12, 1985.

Beebe, Gilbert W., and Michael E. DeBakey, *Battle Casualties: Incidence, Mortality, and Logistics Considerations*, Springfield, Ill.: Charles C. Thomas, Publisher, 1952.

Beekley, Alec C., Harold Bohman, and Danielle Schindler, "Modern Warfare," in Eric Savitsky and Brian Eastridge, eds., *Combat Casualty Care: Lessons Learned from OEF and OIF*, Falls Church, Va.: Office of the Surgeon General, Department of the Army, 2012.

Beekley, Alec C., and David M. Watts, "Combat Trauma Experience with the United States Army 102nd Forward Surgical Team in Afghanistan," *American Journal of Surgery*, Vol. 187, No. 5, May 2004, pp. 652–654.

Begnoche, Paul O., *Bioterrorism: An Assessment of Medical Response Capabilities at Ben Taub General Hospital, Houston, Texas*, thesis, Houston, Tex.: U.S. Army Medical Department Center and School, 2001.

Beitler, Alan L., Glenn W. Wortmann, Luke J. Hofmann, and James M. Goff, Jr., "Operation Enduring Freedom: The 48th Combat Support Hospital in Afghanistan," *Military Medicine*, Vol. 171, No. 3, March 2006, pp. 189–193.

Belasco, Amy, *Troop Levels in the Afghan and Iraq Wars, FY 2001–FY 2012: Cost and Other Potential Issues*, Washington, D.C.: Congressional Research Service, R40682, July 2, 2009.

———, *The Cost of Iraq, Afghanistan, and Other Global War on Terror Operations Since 9/11*, Washington, D.C.: Congressional Research Service, RL33110, December 8, 2014.

Bellamy, Ronald F., "The Causes of Death in Conventional Land Warfare: Implications for Combat Casualty Care Research," *Military Medicine*, Vol. 49, No. 2, February 1984, pp. 55–61.

Bellows, Henry W., *Provision Required for the Relief and Support of Disabled Soldiers and Sailors and Their Dependents*, New York: U.S. Sanitary Commission, December 15, 1865.

Beninati, William, Michael T. Meyer, and Todd E. Carter, "The Critical Care Air Transport Program," *Critical Care Medicine*, Vol. 36, No. 7 Supplement, July 2008, pp. S370–S376.

Benjamin, Mark, "Sick, Wounded U.S. Troops Held in Squalor," United Press International, October 17, 2003.

Berke, Gary M., John Fergason, John R. Milani, John Hattingh, Martin McDowell, Viet Nguyen, and Gayle E. Reiber, "Comparison of Satisfaction with Current Prosthetic Care in Veterans and Servicemembers from Vietnam and OIF/OEF Conflicts with Major Traumatic Limb Loss," *Journal of Rehabilitation Research & Development*, Vol. 47, No. 4, 2010, pp. 361–371.

Berlien, Ivan C., and Raymond W. Waggoner, "Selection and Induction," in Albert J. Glass and Robert J. Bernucci, eds., *Neuropsychiatry in World War II*, Vol. I: *Zone of Interior*, Washington, D.C.: U.S. Government Printing Office, 1966.

Bernton, Hal, "40% of PTSD Diagnoses at Madigan Were Reversed," *Seattle Times*, March 21, 2012a.

———, "Army Opens Wide Review of PTSD-Diagnosis System," *Seattle Times*, March 17, 2012b.

Berry, Frank B., "The Story of 'The Berry Plan'," *Bulletin of the New York Academy of Medicine*, Vol. 53, No. 2, March–April 1976, pp. 278–282.

Berry, Marie L., *Improving Interface Between Aeromedical Evacuation and En Route Systems*, thesis, Maxwell Air Force Base, Ala.: Air Command and Staff College, Air University, 2002.

Bertoni, Daniel, *GAO Findings and Recommendations Regarding DOD and VA Disability Systems*, Washington, D.C.: U.S. Government Accountability Office, GAO-07-906R, May 25, 2007.

———, *Military Disability System: Increased Supports for Servicemembers and Better Pilot Planning Could Improve the Disability Evaluation Process*, Washington, D.C.: U.S. Government Accountability Office, GAO-08-1137, September 2008.

———, *Veterans' Disability Benefits: Preliminary Findings on Claims Processing Trends and Improvement Efforts*, Washington, D.C.: U.S. Government Accountability Office, GAO-09-910T, July 29, 2009.

———, *Military and Veterans Disability System: Pilot Has Achieved Some Goals, but Further Planning and Monitoring Needed*, Washington, D.C.: U.S. Government Accountability Office, GAO-11-69, December 2010.

———, *Military and Veterans Disability System: Worldwide Deployment of Integrated System Warrants Careful Monitoring*, Washington, D.C.: U.S. Government Accountability Office, GAO-11-633T, May 4, 2011.

———, *Military and Veterans Disability System: Improved Monitoring Needed to Better Track and Manage Performance*, Washington, D.C.: U.S. Government Accountability Office, GAO-12-676, August 2012a.

———, *Military Disability System: Preliminary Observations on Efforts to Improve Performance*, Washington, D.C.: U.S. Government Accountability Office, GAO-12-718T, May 23, 2012b.

Bertoni, Daniel, and John H. Pendleton, *DoD and VA: Preliminary Observations on Efforts to Improve Care Management and Disability Evaluations for Servicemembers*, Washington, D.C.: U.S. Government Accountability Office, GAO-08-514T, February 27, 2008.

Berwick, Donald, Autumn Downey, and Elizabeth Cornett, eds., *A National Trauma Care System: Integrating Military and Civilian Trauma Systems to Achieve Zero Preventable Deaths After Injury*, Washington, D.C.: National Academies Press, 2016.

Biderman, Albert D., "Dangers of Negative Patriotism," *Harvard Business Review*, Vol. 40, No. 6, November/December 1962, pp. 93–99.

———, *March to Calumny: The Story of American POW's in the Korean War*, New York: Macmillan Company, 1963.

bin Laden, Osama, "Declaration of War Against the Americans Occupying the Land of the Two Holy Places: Al Qaeda's First Fatwa," *PBS News Hour* website, 1996.

Birtle, Andrew J., *The Korean War: Years of Stalemate, July 1951–July 1953*, Washington, D.C.: U.S. Army Center of Military History, 2006.

Blackbourne, Lorne H., David G. Baer, Brian J. Eastridge, Frank K. Butler, Joseph C. Wenke, Robert G. Hale, Russel S. Kotwal, Laura R. Brosch, Vikhyat Bebarta, M. Margaret Knudson, James R. Ficke, Donald Jenkins, and John B. Holcomb, "Military Medical Revolution: Military Trauma System," *Journal of Trauma and Acute Care Surgery*, Vol. 73, No. 6, Supplement 5, December 2012, pp. S388–S394.

Blair, Clay, *The Forgotten War: America in Korea 1950–1953*, New York: Times Books, 1987.

Blanck, Ronald R., and William H. Bell, "Medical Aspects of the Persian Gulf War: Medical Support for American Troops in the Persian Gulf," *New England Journal of Medicine*, Vol. 324, No. 12, March 21, 1991, pp. 857–859.

Blank, Arthur S., Jr., "The Veterans Administration's Viet Nam Veterans Outreach and Counseling Centers," in Stephen M. Sonnenberg, Arthur S. Blank, Jr., and John A. Talbott, eds., *The Trauma of War: Stress and Recovery in Vietnam Veterans*, Washington, D.C.: American Psychiatric Press, 1985.

Blough, David K., Sharon Hubbard, Lynne V. McFarland, Douglas G. Smith, Jeffrey M. Gambel, and Gayle E. Reiber, "Prosthetic Cost Projections for Servicemembers with Major Limb Loss from Vietnam and OIF/OEF," *Journal of Rehabilitation Research & Development*, Vol. 47, No. 4, 2010, pp. 387–402.

Blumenson, Martin, "Helicopter Evacuation," in John G. Westover, ed., *Combat Support in Korea*, Part V: *Medical Support*, Washington, D.C.: U.S. Army Center of Military History, 1955 (online version of 1987, 1990 reprint).

Bonds, Timothy M., Dave Baiocchi, and Laurie L. McDonald, *Army Deployments to OIF and OEF*, Santa Monica, Calif.: RAND Corporation, DB-587-A, 2010.

Booth, John E., "Veterans: Our Biggest Privileged Class," *Harper's Magazine*, July 1958, pp. 19–25.

Boulanger, Ghislaine, "Post-Traumatic Stress Disorder: An Old Problem with a New Name," in Stephen M. Sonnenberg, Arthur S. Blank, Jr., and John A. Talbott, eds., *The Trauma of War: Stress and Recovery in Vietnam Veterans*, Washington, D.C.: American Psychiatric Press, 1985.

Boulton, Mark, *Failing Our Veterans: The G.I. Bill and the Vietnam Generation*, New York: New York University Press, 2014.

Bourne, Peter G., "Military Psychiatry and the Vietnam Experience," *American Journal of Psychiatry*, Vol. 127, No. 4, October 1970, pp. 481–492.

———, "The Viet Nam Veteran: Psychosocial Casualties," *Psychiatry in Medicine*, Vol. 3, No. 1, March 1972, pp. 23–27.

Bowman, Tom, "172,000 New Tourniquets Ordered for U.S. Soldiers," *Baltimore Sun*, March 18, 2005.

Bowsher, Charles A., *Agent Orange: VA Needs to Further Improve Its Examination and Registry Program*, Washington, D.C.: U.S. General Accounting Office, GAO/HRD-86-7, January 1986.

Boyle, Eleanor, Carol Cancelliere, Jan Hartvigsen, Linda J. Carroll, Lena W. Holm, and J. David Cassidy, "Systematic Review of Prognosis After Mild Traumatic Brain Injury in the Military: Results of the International Collaboration on Mild Traumatic Brain Injury Prognosis," *Archives of Physical Medicine and Rehabilitation*, Vol. 95, No. 3, Supp. 2, 2014, pp. S230–S237.

Bradley Commission—*See* President's Commission on Veterans' Pensions.

Bradley, Omar N., *Annual Report of the Administrator of Veterans' Affairs for the Fiscal Year Ended June 30, 1945*, Washington, D.C.: U.S. Government Printing Office, 1946.

Bradley, Omar N., Clarence G. Adam, William J. Donovan, Paul R. Hawley, Martin D. Jenkins, Theodor S. Petersen, and John S. Thompson, "Letter of Transmittal from the Commission on Veterans' Pensions," to the President of the United States, Washington, D.C., April 23, 1956.

Bradley, Omar N., and Clay Blair, *A General's Life: An Autobiography by General of the Army Omar N. Bradley*, London: Sidwick & Jackson, 1983.

Brevard, Sidney B., Howard Champion, and Dan Katz, "Weapons Effects," in Eric Savitsky and Brian Eastridge, eds., *Combat Casualty Care Lessons Learned from OEF and OIF*, Falls Church, Va.: Office of the Surgeon General, Department of the Army, 2012.

Brill, Norman Q., "Hospitalization and Disposition," in Albert J. Glass and Robert J. Bernucci, eds., *Neuropsychiatry in World War II*, Vol. I: *Zone of Interior*, Washington, D.C.: U.S. Government Printing Office, 1966, pp. 195–253.

———, testimony before the Subcommittee on Veterans Affairs of the Committee on Labor and Public Welfare, U.S. Senate, 91st Cong., 1st and 2nd Sess., hearing on the Examination of the Problems of the Veterans Wounded in Vietnam, Washington, D.C.: U.S. Government Printing Office, 1970.

Brill, Norman Q., and Gilbert W. Beebe, *A Follow-Up Study of War Neuroses*, Washington, D.C.: U.S. Government Printing Office, 1955.

Brill, Norman Q., and Herbert I. Kupper, "Problems of Adjustment in Return to Civilian Life," in Albert J. Glass and Robert J. Bernucci, eds., *Neuropsychiatry in World War II*, Vol. I: *Zone of Interior*, Washington, D.C.: U.S. Government Printing Office, 1966a, pp. 721–727.

———, "The Psychiatric Patient After Discharge," in Albert J. Glass and Robert J. Bernucci, eds., *Neuropsychiatry in World War II*, Vol. I: *Zone of Interior*, Washington, D.C.: U.S. Government Printing Office, 1966b, pp. 729–733.

Brill, Norman Q., Mildred C. Tate, and William C. Menninger, "Enlisted Men Discharged from the Army Because of Psychoneuroses: Follow-Up Study," *Journal of the American Medical Association*, Vol. 128, No. 9, 1945, pp. 933–637.

Bronstein, Scott, and Drew Griffin, "Hospital's Secret List," CNN, April 23, 2014.

Brook, Tom Vanden, "Armored Trucks Cut IED Deaths Among Allied Troops," *USA Today*, September 7, 2010.

Brown, Harvey E., ed., *The Medical Department of the United States Army from 1775 to 1873*, online reprint, Washington, D.C.: U.S. Army Medical Department, Office of Medical History, 1873.

Brown, John Sloan, *Kevlar Legions: The Transformation of the U.S. Army, 1989–2005*, Washington, D.C.: U.S. Army Center of Military History, 2011.

Brown, Paul W., "Rehabilitation of the Combat-Wounded Amputee," in William E. Burkhalter, ed., *Orthopedic Surgery in Vietnam*, Washington, D.C.: Office of the Surgeon General, Department of the Army, and U.S. Army Center of Military History, 1994, pp. 189–209.

Brownlee, Les, "Current Army Issues," testimony before the U.S. Senate Committee on Armed Services, Washington, D.C.: U.S. Government Printing Office, November 19, 2003.

Broyles, Thomas E., *A Comparative Analysis of the Medical Support in the Combat Operations in the Falklands Campaign and the Grenada Expedition*, thesis, Fort Leavenworth, Kan.: U.S. Army Command and General Staff College, 1987.

Buckenmaier, Chester, and Lisa Bleckner, *Military Advanced Regional Anesthesia and Analgesia Handbook*, Washington, D.C.: Borden Institute, Walter Reed Army Medical Center, 2008.

Bundy, McGeorge, "National Security Action Memorandum N3. 273," to Secretary of State, Secretary of Defense, Director of Central Intelligence, Administrator of AID, and Director of USIA, Washington, D.C., November 26, 1963.

Burgess, Paula, Ernest E. Sullivent, Scott M. Sasser, Marlena M. Wald, Eric Ossmann, and Vikas Kapil, "Managing Traumatic Brain Injury Secondary to Explosions," *Journal of Emergencies, Trauma, and Shock*, Vol. 3, No. 2, April–June 2010, pp. 164–172.

"Bush a Convert to Nation Building," *Washington Times*, April 7, 2008.

Bush, George H. W., "Remarks at the Aspen Institute Symposium in Aspen, Colorado," Houston, Tex.: The Museum at the George Bush Presidential Library, August 2, 1990.

Bush, George W., "Speech on Defense Strategy," Charleston, S.C.: The Citadel, 1999.

———, "Commencement Address at the United States Naval Academy in Annapolis, Maryland," Washington, D.C.: The American Presidency Project, May 25, 2001.

———, "Text: Bush Calls for End to Terrorism," *Washington Post*, April 17, 2002.

———, "Remarks to Medical Personnel at Walter Reed Army Medical Center," press release, Washington, D.C.: The White House, December 18, 2003.

———, "President Bush Visits Troops at Walter Reed Army Medical Center," press release, Washington, D.C.: The White House, March 30, 2007.

———, *Decision Points*, New York: Crown Publishers, 2010.

Butler, Frank K., and Lorne H. Blackbourne, "Battlefield Trauma Care Then and Now: A Decade of Tactical Combat Casualty Care," *Journal of Trauma and Acute Care Surgery*, Vol. 73, No. 6, Supplement 5, 2012, pp. S395–S402.

Butler, Frank K., Jr., John Haymann, and E. George Butler, "Tactical Combat Casualty Care in Special Operations," *Military Medicine*, Vol. 161, Supplement 1, August 1996, pp. 3–16.

Butler, Frank K., David J. Smith, and Richard H. Carmona, "Implementing and Preserving the Advances in Combat Casualty Care from Iraq and Afghanistan Throughout the US Military," *Journal of Trauma and Acute Care Surgery*, Vol. 79, No. 2, 2015, pp. 321–326.

Byrd, Harry F., *Veterans' Pension Act of 1959*, report to accompany H.R. 7650, U.S. Senate, Committee on Finance, 80th Cong., 1st Sess., Report No. 666, August 12, 1959.

Camp, Norman M., "The Vietnam War and the Ethics of Combat Psychiatry," *American Journal of Psychiatry*, Vol. 150, No. 7, July 1993, pp. 1000–1010.

———, "US Army Psychiatry Legacies of the Vietnam War," in Elspeth Cameron Ritchie, ed., *Combat and Operational Behavioral Health*, Washington, D.C.: Borden Institute, Walter Reed Army Medical Center, 2011.

———, *US Army Psychiatry in the Vietnam War: New Challenges in Extended Counterinsurgency Warfare*, Fort Sam Houston, Tex.: Borden Institute and the U.S. Army Medical Department Center and School, 2015.

Cantlie, Neil, *A History of the Army Medical Department*, Vol. I, London: Churchill Livingstone, 1974.

Carey, Michael E., "Learning from Traditional Combat Mortality and Morbidity Data Used in the Evaluation of Combat Medical Care," *Military Medicine*, Vol. 152, No. 1, January 1987, pp. 6–13.

Carino, Michael, *Army Casualty: Summary Statistics*, briefing slides, Falls Church, Va.: Office of the Surgeon General, Department of the Army, Program Analysis & Evaluation Office, February 12, 2017a.

———, "Army TBI Diagnoses: All Severity Types by Deployment Status: CY 2000–CY 2015, Q2," briefing slide, Falls Church, Va.: Program Analysis & Evaluation Office, Office of the Surgeon General of the Army, May 1, 2017b.

———, "Cause of Injuries," briefing slide, Falls Church, Va.: Office of the Surgeon General, Department of the Army, Program Analysis & Evaluation Office, May 25, 2017c.

Carino, Michael J., *Army Casualty: Summary Statistics Overview—Update*, Falls Church, Va.: Office of the Surgeon General, Department of the Army, March 2016.

Carlton, Paul K., "Foreword," in William W. Hurd and John G. Jernigan, eds., *Aeromedical Evacuation: Management of Acute and Stabilized Patients*, New York: Springer-Verlag, 2003.

Carson, Brad, "Consideration of Discharge Upgrade Requests Pursuant to Supplemental Guidance to Military Boards for Correction of Military/Naval Records (BCMRs/BCNR) by Veterans Claiming Post Traumatic Stress Disorder (PTSD) or Traumatic Brain Injury (TBI)," memorandum to Secretaries of the Military Departments, Washington, D.C., February 24, 2016.

"Center for Deployment Psychology," Psychological Health Center of Excellence website, undated.

Centers for Disease Control and Prevention, National Institutes of Health, Department of Defense, and Veterans Administration Leadership Panel, *Report to Congress on Traumatic Brain Injury in the United States: Understanding the Public Health Problem Among Current and Former Military Personnel*, Washington, D.C., June 2013.

Central Intelligence Agency, Historical Staff, *Overview of the Office of Medical Services, 1947–1972*, Langley, Va., OMS-6, February 1973.

Chapman, Julie C., and Ramon Diaz-Arrastia, "Military Traumatic Brain Injury: A Review," *Alzheimer's & Dementia*, Vol. 10, No. 3 supp., 2014, pp. S97–S104.

Cherry, Bobby, "Amputee Center Cost," memorandum to Robert Granville, Navy Medical Center San Diego, May 17, 2005.

Christensen, Eric, Joyce McMahon, Elizabeth Schaefer, Ted Jaditz, and Dan Harris, *Final Report for the Veterans' Disability Benefits Commission: Compensation, Survey Results, and Selected Topics*, Alexandria, Va.: CNA Corporation, August 2007.

Chu, David S. C., "Personnel on Medical Hold," memorandum to Secretaries of the Army, Navy, and Air Force, Washington, D.C.: Office of the Under Secretary of Defense for Personnel and Readiness, October 29, 2003.

———, *Expedited DES Process for Members with Catastrophic Conditions and Combat-Related Causes*, Washington, D.C.: Office of the Under Secretary of Defense (Personnel and Readiness), January 9, 2009.

CIA—*See* Central Intelligence Agency.

Citizens Commission on Graduate Medical Education, *The Graduate Education of Physicians*, Chicago: Council on Medical Education, American Medical Association, 1966.

"Clamp: Potts' c.," *Stedman's Medical Dictionary*, 26th ed., Baltimore and Philadelphia: Williams & Wilkins, 1995, p. 348.

Clarke, Jonathan E., and Peter R. Davis, "Medical Evacuation and Triage of Combat Casualties in Helmand Province, Afghanistan: October 2010–April 2011," *Military Medicine*, Vol. 177, No. 11, November 2012, pp. 1261–1266.

Clasper, Jon, and Arul Ramasamy, "Traumatic Amputations," *British Journal of Pain*, Vol. 7, No. 2, 2013, pp. 67–73.

Cleland, Max, testimony before the Subcommittee on Veterans Affairs of the Committee on Labor and Public Welfare, U.S. Senate, 91st Cong., 1st and 2nd Sess., hearing on the Examination of the Problems of the Veterans Wounded in Vietnam, Washington, D.C.: U.S. Government Printing Office, 1970.

———, "Potential Exposure of Veterans to Chemical Defoliants During the Vietnam War," memorandum to Directors of VA Hospitals, et al., Washington, D.C., May 18, 1978.

———, testimony before the House Committee on Veterans Affairs, Subcommittee on Medical Facilities and Benefits, 96th Cong., 2nd Sess., hearing on Agent Orange, Washington, D.C., February 25, 1980.

———, *Strong at the Broken Places*, Atlanta, Ga.: Longstreet Press, 2000.

Clingman, Fred M., *Analysis of Aeromedical Evacuation in the Korean War and Vietnam War*, thesis, Wright-Patterson Air Force Base, Ohio: Air Force Institute of Technology, Air University, 1989.

Clinton, William J., "Remarks to the Veterans of Foreign Wars Conference," Washington, D.C.: The White House, March 6, 1995.

CMS Alliance to Modernize Healthcare, *Independent Assessment of the Health Care Delivery Systems and Management Processes of the Department of Veterans Affairs*, Vol. I: *Integrated Report*, McLean, Va.: MITRE Corporation, September 1, 2015.

Coast Guard Aviation Association, "Sikorsky HNS-1 'Hoverfly,'" U.S. Coast Guard Aviation History website, undated.

Colbach, Edward M., "Ethical Issues in Combat Psychiatry," *Military Medicine*, Vol. 150, May 1985, pp. 256–265.

Cole, Ronald H., *Operation Urgent Fury: The Planning and Execution of Joint Operations in Grenada, 12 October–2 November 1983*, Washington, D.C.: Joint History Office, Office of the Chairman of the Joint Chiefs of Staff, 1997.

Collins, J. Lawton, *War in Peacetime: The History and Lessons of Korea*, Boston: Houghton Mifflin Company, 1969.

Commander, Walter Reed Army Medical Center, "Charter of the Board of Directors, U.S. Army Amputee Patient Care Program," Washington, D.C., October 14, 2003.

Commission on Care, *Final Report of the Commission on Care*, Washington, D.C., June 30, 2016.

Committee on Gulf War and Health, *Gulf War and Health*, Vol. 4: *Health Effects of Serving in the Gulf War*, Washington, D.C.: National Academies Press, 2005.

———, *Gulf War and Health*, Vol. 7: *Long-Term Consequences of Traumatic Brain Injury*, Washington, D.C.: National Academies Press, 2009.

———, *Gulf War and Health*, Vol. 8: *Update of Health Effects of Serving in the Gulf War*, 2009 update, Washington, D.C.: National Academies Press, 2010.

———, *Gulf War and Health*, Vol. 10: *Update of Health Effects of Serving in the Gulf War*, Washington, D.C.: National Academies Press, 2016.

Committee on the Assessment of Ongoing Efforts in the Treatment of Posttraumatic Stress Disorder, Board on the Health of Select Populations, Institute of Medicine, *Treatment for Posttraumatic Stress Disorder in Military and Veteran Populations: Final Assessment*, Washington, D.C.: National Academies Press, 2014.

Committee on the Assessment of Readjustment Needs of Military Personnel, Veterans, and their Families, *Returning Home from Iraq and Afghanistan: Assessment of Readjustment Needs of Veterans, Service Members, and Their Families*, Washington, D.C.: National Academies Press, 2013.

Committee on the Effects of Herbicides in Vietnam, *The Effects of Herbicides in South Vietnam*, Part A: *Summary and Conclusions*, Washington, D.C.: National Academy of Sciences, 1974.

Committee on Trauma and Committee on Shock, *Accidental Death and Disability: The Neglected Disease of Modern Society*, Washington, D.C.: National Academy of Sciences and National Research Council, 1966.

Committee on Treatment of Posttraumatic Stress Disorder, *Treatment of Posttraumatic Stress Disorder: An Assessment of the Evidence*, Washington, D.C.: National Academies Press, 2008.

Committee to Review the Health Effects in Vietnam Veterans of Exposure to Herbicides, *Veterans and Agent Orange: Health Effects of Herbicides Used in Vietnam*, Washington, D.C.: National Academy Press, 1994.

———, *Veterans and Agent Orange: Update 2012*, 9th Biennial Update, Washington, D.C.: National Academies Press, 2014.

Comptroller General of the United States, *U.S. Ground Troops in South Vietnam Were in Areas Sprayed with Herbicide Orange*, Washington, D.C.: U.S. General Accounting Office, FPCD-80-23, November 16, 1979.

———, *VA's Agent Orange Examination Program: Actions Needed to More Effectively Address Veterans' Health Concerns*, Washington, D.C.: U.S. General Accounting Office, GAO/HRD-83-6, October 25, 1982.

Condon-Rall, Mary Ellen, and Albert E. Cowdrey, *The Medical Department: Medical Service in the War Against Japan*, United States Army in World War II: The Technical Services, Washington, D.C.: U.S. Army Center of Military History, 1998.

"Congressional Hearing on Walter Reed Army Medical Center: House Committee on Oversight and Government Reform, Subcommittee on National Security and Foreign Affairs," *Washington Post*, transcript via CQ Transcripts Wire, March 5, 2007.

Congressional Budget Office, *The All-Volunteer Military: Issues and Performance*, Washington, D.C., July 2007.

Cordesman, Anthony H., Charles Loi, and Vivek Kocharlakota, "IED Metrics for Iraq: June 2003– September 2010," briefing slides, Washington, D.C.: Center for Strategic & International Studies, November 11, 2010.

Cosmas, Graham A., and Albert E. Cowdrey, *The Medical Department: Medical Service in the European Theater of Operations*, Washington, D.C.: U.S. Army Center of Military History, 1992.

Coss, Edward J., *All for the King's Shilling: The British Soldier Under Wellington, 1801–1814*, Norman, Okla.: University of Oklahoma Press, 2010.

Costanzo, George, and Mary Ann Spott, *Joint Theater Trauma System (JTTS)/Joint Theater Trauma Registry (JTTR)*, briefing slides, Fort Sam Houston, Tex.: U.S. Army Institute of Surgical Research July 10, 2010.

Cowdrey, Albert E., "MASH vs M*A*S*H: The Army Mobile Surgical Hospital," *Medical Heritage*, January/February 1985.

———, *United States Army in the Korean War*, Vol. IV: *The Medic's War*, Washington, D.C.: U.S. Army Center of Military History, 1987.

Cowley, R. Adams, "A Total Emergency Medical System for the State of Maryland," *Maryland State Medical Journal*, Vol. 27, No. 7, July 1975, pp. 36–45.

Crane, A. G., *The Medical Department of the United States Army in the World War*, Vol. XII, Part One: *Physical Reconstruction and Vocational Education*, Washington, D.C.: U.S. Government Printing Office, 1927.

Critical Care Air Transport Team, "Who We Are," webpage, July 21, 2016.

Crotti, Nancy, "Futuristic LUKE Arm to Go on Sale," Qmed website, July 12, 2016.

Cubano, Miguel A., and Martha K. Lenhart, eds., *Emergency War Surgery*, 4th ed., Fort Sam Houston, Tex.: Office of the Surgeon General, Borden Institute, 2013.

Dao, James, "A Nation Challenged: The President; Bush Sets Role for U.S. in Afghan Rebuilding," *New York Times*, April 18, 2002.

DARPA—*See* Defense Advanced Research Projects Agency.

Datel, William E., *A Summary of Source Data in Military Psychiatric Epidemiology*, Washington, D.C.: Walter Reed Army Institute of Research, December 1975.

Datel, William E., and Arnold W. Johnson, Jr., *Psychotropic Prescription Medication in Vietnam*, Washington, D.C.: Office of the Surgeon General, Department of the Army, May 1978.

Davidson, Ellen Breslin, *Restructuring Military Medical Care*, Washington, D.C.: Congressional Budget Office, July 1995.

Davis, Jessica, "Watchdog Says VA Secretary David Shulkin Misused Federal Funds," *Healthcare IT News*, February 14, 2018, p. 1.

Davis, Susan A., "Department of Defense Medical Centers of Excellence," testimony before the Military Personnel Subcommittee of the Committee on Armed Services, U.S. House of Representatives, 111th Cong., 2nd Sess., Washington, D.C.: U.S. Government Printing Office, 2010, pp. 23–25.

Deal, Virgil T., "Med Hold Way Ahead," email forwarded to multiple recipients, Washington, D.C.: Walter Reed Army Medical Center, January 17, 2006.

Dean, Morton, "What Ever Happened to the Men of Hawk Hill?" *Air & Space Magazine*, December 2015.

DeBakey, Michael E., and Florindo A. Simeone, "Battle Injuries of the Arteries in World War II: An Analysis of 2,471 Cases," *Annals of Surgery*, Vol. 123, No. 4, April 1946.

Defense Advanced Research Projects Agency, "Revolutionizing Prosthetics," webpage, undated.

———, "DARPA Provides Mobius Bionics LUKE Arms to Walter Reed," press release, Washington, D.C., December 22, 2016.

———, "Giving the Gift of Independence on the Fourth of July: Veterans Receive DARPA's LUKE Arm," press release, June 30, 2017.

Defense Casualty Analysis System, "U.S. Military Casualties, Operation Enduring Freedom: Casualty Summary by Casualty Category," Alexandria, Va.: Defense Manpower Data Center, February 2, 2017.

Defense Centers of Excellence for Psychological Health and Traumatic Brain Injury, "Centers of Excellence Align Under Defense Health Agency," Military Health System website, November 1, 2017.

Defense Health Board, *Combat Trauma Lessons Learned from Military Operations of 2001–2013*, Falls Church, Va.: Office of the Assistant Secretary of Defense for Health Affairs, March 9, 2015.

Defense Health Board Task Force on Mental Health, *An Achievable Vision: Report of the Department of Defense Task Force on Mental Health*, Falls Church, Va.: Defense Health Board, June 2007.

Defense Manpower Data Center, "DoD Personnel, Workforce Reports & Publications: Historical Reports—FY 1954–1993," Washington, D.C.: Department of Defense, May 28, 2015.

———, *U.S. Military Casualties—Operation Enduring Freedom (OEF) Casualty Summary by Month and Service*, database, Monterey, Calif.: Defense Casualty Analysis System, as of May 23, 2016.

Dennison, Robert L., Arthur S. Abramson, and Howard A. Rusk, *Report to the President from the Committee on Veterans' Medical Services*, Washington, D.C.: U.S. Government Printing Office, 1950.

Department of the Air Force, Office of the Surgeon General, *A Concise History of the USAF Aeromedical Evacuation System*, Washington, D.C.: U.S. Government Printing Office, 1976.

Department of Defense Directive 6000.12, *Health Services Operations and Readiness*, Washington, D.C.: Office of the Secretary of Defense, incorporating change 1, January 20, 1998.

Department of Defense Instruction 6000.11, *Patient Movement*, September 9, 1998.

Department of Defense Instruction 6490.11, *DoD Policy Guidance for Management of Mild Traumatic Brain Injury/Concussion in the Deployed Setting*, Washington, D.C., September 18, 2012.

Department of Defense Regulation 4515.13-R, *Air Transportation Eligibility*, Change 3, April 9, 1998.

Department of War, "War Department Demobilization Plan After the Defeat of Germany," Washington, D.C., September 6, 1944.

DeVries, Larry G., "General History of the Deployment of Reserve Forces in Southeast Asia," Department of Minnesota Reserve Officers Association website, March 22, 2009.

Director U.S. Veterans' Bureau, *Annual Report for the Fiscal Year Ended June 30, 1930*, Washington, D.C.: Veterans Administration, December 1, 1930.

"Disabled Soldier Support System," *Soldiers Magazine*, May 1, 2005.

DMDC—*See* Defense Manpower Data Center.

DoD—*See* U.S. Department of Defense.

DoD IG—*See* U.S. Department of Defense Inspector General.

DoD Task Force on Mental Health—*See* Department of Defense Task Force on Mental Health.

Dole, Bob, *One Soldier's Story: A Memoir*, New York: Harper Collins Publishers, 2005.

Dole-Shalala Commission—*See* President's Commission on Care for America's Returning Wounded Warriors.

Dominguez, Michael, "Prepared Statement of the Honorable Michael Dominguez Before the House Committee on Oversight and Government Reform, Subcommittee on National Security and Foreign Affairs," Washington, D.C.: Department of Defense, April 17, 2007.

Donnelly, William M., *Transforming an Army at War: Designing the Modular Force 1991–2005*, Washington, D.C.: U.S. Army Center of Military History, 2007.

Dorland, Peter, and James Nanney, *Dust Off: Army Aeromedical Evacuation in Vietnam*, Washington, D.C.: U.S. Army Center of Military History, 1982.

Dougan, Clark, and Stephen Weiss, *The Vietnam Experience: Nineteen Sixty-Eight*, Boston: Boston Publishing Company, 1983.

Dougherty, Paul J., "Wartime Amputations," *Military Medicine*, Vol. 158, No. 12, December 1993, pp. 755–763.

Dougherty, Paul J., Lynne V. McFarland, Douglas G. Smith, Alberto Esquenazi, Donna Jo Blake, and Gayle E. Reiber, "Multiple Traumatic Limb Loss: A Comparison of Vietnam Veterans to OIF/OEF Servicemembers," *Journal of Rehabilitation Research & Development*, Vol. 47, No. 4, 2010, pp. 333–348.

Doukas, William C., "Amputee Care Center: Summary of Current Plan for Battle Casualty Research at WRAMC," information paper, Washington, D.C.: Walter Reed Medical Center, May 31, 2003a.

———, "U.S. Army Amputee Care Program Board of Directors Minutes," memorandum for the record, Washington, D.C.: Walter Reed Medical Center, September 24, 2003b.

Draper, Debra A., *DOD and VA Health Care: Action Needed to Strengthen Integration Across Care Coordination and Case Management Programs*, Washington, D.C.: U.S. Government Accountability Office, GAO-12-129T, October 6, 2011.

Drayer, Calvin S., and Albert J. Glass, "Italian Campaign (9 September 1943–1 March 1944), Psychiatry Established at Army Level," in William S. Mullins, ed., *Medical Department, United States Army in World War II: Neuropsychiatry in World War II*, Vol. II: *Overseas Theaters*, Washington, D.C.: Office of the Surgeon General, Department of the Army, 1973.

Driscoll, Robert S., "U.S. Army Medical Helicopters in the Korean War," *Military Medicine*, Vol. 166, No. 4, April 2001, pp. 290–296.

Dupuy, Trevor N., *The Evolution of Weapons and Warfare*, New York: The Bobbs-Merrill Company, Inc., 1980.

Dursa, Erin K., Shannon K. Barth, Aaron I. Schneiderman, and Robert M. Bossarte, "Physical and Mental Health Status of Gulf War and Gulf Era Veterans: Results from a Large Population-Based Epidemiological Study," *Journal of Occupational and Environmental Medicine*, Vol. 58, No. 1, January 2016, pp. 41–46.

DVA—*See* U.S. Department of Veterans Affairs.

DVA and DoD—*See* U.S. Department of Veterans Affairs and U.S. Department of Defense.

Eastridge, Brian, "Prologue," in Eric Savitsky and Brian Eastridge, eds., *Combat Casualty Care: Lessons Learned from OEF and OIF*, Fort Detrick, Md.: Office of the Surgeon General, Borden Institute, 2012.

Eastridge, Brian J., Donald Jenkins, Stephen Flaherty, Henry Schiller, and John B. Holcomb, "Trauma System Development in a Theater of War: Experiences from Operation Iraqi Freedom and Operation Enduring Freedom," *Journal of Trauma: Injury, Infection, and Critical Care*, Vol. 61, December 2006, pp. 1366–1373.

Eastridge, Brian J., Robert L. Mabry, Peter Seguin, Joyce Cantrell, Terrill Tops, Paul Uribe, Olga Mallett, Tamara Zubko, Lynne Oetjen-Gerdes, Todd E. Rasmussen, Frank K. Butler, Russell S. Kotwal, John B. Holcomb, Charles Wade, Howard Champion, Mimi Lawnick, Leon Moores, and Lorne H. Blackbourne, "Death on the Battlefield (2001–2011): Implications for the Future of Combat Casualty Care," *Journal of Trauma and Acute Care Surgery*, Vol. 73, No. 6, Supp. 5, 2012, pp. S431–S437.

Egendorf, Arthur, Charles Kadushin, Robert S. Laufer, George Rothbart, and Lee Sloan, *Legacies of Vietnam: Comparative Adjustment of Veterans and Their Peers*, New York: Center for Policy Research, 1981.

Eibner, Christine, and Heather Krull, eds., *Current and Projected Characteristics and Unique Health Care Needs of the Patient Population Served by the Department of Veterans Affairs*, Santa Monica, Calif.: RAND Corporation, 2015.

Eilon, Lindsey, and Jack Lyon, *Evolution of Department of Defense Directive 5100.1, "Functions of the Department of Defense and Its Major Components,"* white paper, Washington, D.C.: Office of the Secretary of Defense, Director, Administration & Management, Organizational Management & Planning, April 2010.

Einstein, Albert, and Sigmund Freud, *The Einstein-Freud Correspondence (1931–32)*, The Modern World, 1931–1932.

Eisen, Seth A., Han K. Kang, Frances M. Murphy, Melvin S. Blanchard, Domenic J. Reda, William G. Henderson, Rosemary Toomey, Leila W. Jackson, Renee Alpern, Becky J. Parks, Nancy Klimas, Coleen Hall, Hon S. Pak, Joyce Hunter, Joel Karlinsky, Michael J. Battistone, and Michael J. Lyons, "Gulf War Veterans' Health: Medical Evaluation of a U.S. Cohort," *Annals of Internal Medicine*, Vol. 142, No. 11, June 7, 2005, pp. 881–890.

Eisenhower, Dwight David, "Letter to Chairman, President's Commission on Veterans' Pensions, Concerning a Study of Veterans' Benefits," to Omar N. Bradley, Washington, D.C., March 5, 1955.

———, "President Eisenhower's News Conference, April 7, 1954," *The Pentagon Papers*, Boston: Beacon Press, 1971, pp. 597–598.

Embrey, Ellen, "Statement by Ms. Ellen Embrey, Deputy Assistant Secretary of Defense for Force Health Protection and Readiness before the House Committee on Veterans Affairs, Subcommittee on Health," Washington, D.C.: U.S. Department of Defense, January 24, 2002.

Emrey-Arras, Melissa, *Gulf War Illness: Improvements Needed for VA to Better Understand, Process, and Communicate Decisions on Claims*, Washington, D.C.: U.S. Government Accountability Office, GAO-17-511, June 2017.

England, Gordon, "Senior Oversight Committee," memorandum for Secretaries of the Military Departments et al., Washington, D.C.: U.S. Department of Defense, May 3, 2007a.

———, "Statement of the Honorable Gordon England, Deputy Secretary of Defense, Before the Senate Armed Services Committee and the Senate Veterans Affairs Committee," Washington, D.C.: Department of Defense, April 12, 2007b.

Englehardt, Joseph P., *Desert Shield and Desert Storm: A Chronology and Troop List for the 1990–1991 Persian Gulf Crisis*, Carlisle Barracks, Pa.: U.S. Army War College, Strategic Studies Institute, AD-A234 743, March 25, 1991.

Environmental Agents Service, "Persian Gulf Registry Program Approved," *Persian Gulf Review*, Vol. 1, No. 1, October 1992.

EO—*See* Executive Order.

Epidemiology Program, Post-Deployment Health Group, *Report on VA Facility Specific Operation Enduring Freedom (OEF), Operation Iraqi Freedom (OIF), and Operation New Dawn (OND) Veterans Diagnosed with Potential or Provisional PTSD*, Washington, D.C.: U.S. Department of Veterans Affairs, Office of Patient Care Services, January 2017.

Executive Order 10122, *Regulations Governing Payment of Disability Retirement Pay, Hospitalization, and Re-Examination of Members and Former Members of the Uniformed Services*, Washington, D.C.: The White House, April 14, 1950.

Executive Order 10400, *Amending Executive Order No. 10122 of April 14, 1950, entitled "Regulations Governing Payment of Disability Retirement Pay, Hospitalization, and Re-Examination of Members and Former Members of the Uniformed Services,"* Washington, D.C.: The White House, September 27, 1952.

Executive Order 10588, *Establishing the President's Commission on Veterans' Pensions*, Washington, D.C.: The White House, January 14, 1955.

Executive Order 10631, *Code of Conduct for Members of the Armed Forces of the United States*, Washington, D.C.: The White House, August 17, 1955.

Executive Order 12961, *Presidential Advisory Committee on Gulf War Veterans' Illnesses*, Washington, D.C.: The White House, May 26, 1995.

Executive Order 13075, *Special Oversight Board for Department of Defense Investigations of Gulf War Chemical and Biological Incidents*, February 19, 1998.

Executive Order 13426, *Establishing a Commission on Care for America's Returning Wounded Warriors and a Task Force on Returning Global War on Terror Heroes*, Washington, D.C.: The White House, March 6, 2007.

Executive Order 13625, *Improving Access to Mental Health Services for Veterans, Service Members, and Military Families*, Washington, D.C.: The White House, August 31, 2012.

Extremity Trauma and Amputation Center of Excellence, "About Us," Military Health System website, undated.

Fackler, Martin L., *Effects of Small Arms on the Human Body*, Presidio of San Francisco, Calif.: Wound Ballistics Laboratory, Letterman Army Institute of Research, undated.

Fandos, Nicholas, "Veterans Affairs Shake-Up Stirs New Fears of Privatized Care," *New York Times*, March 29, 2018.

Farmer, Carrie M., Susan D. Hosek, and David M. Adamson, eds., *Balancing Demand and Supply for Veterans' Health Care: A Summary of Three RAND Assessments Conducted Under the Veterans Choice Act*, Santa Monica, Calif.: RAND Corporation, RR-1165/4-RC, 2016.

Farmer, Carrie M., Heather Krull, Thomas W. Concannon, Molly Simmons, Francesca Pillemer, Teague Ruder, Andrew M. Parker, Maulik P. Purohit, Liisa Hiatt, Benjamin Batorsky, and Kimberly A. Hepner, *Understanding Treatment of Mild Traumatic Brain Injury in the Military Health System*, Santa Monica, Calif.: RAND Corporation, RR-844-OSD, 2016.

Farmer, Kenneth L., "Medical Care of Injured and Wounded Service Members," statement before the Senate Committee on Veterans' Affairs, 109th Cong., 1st Sess., March 15, 2005.

Farrell, Brenda S., *Military Personnel: DOD Is Expanding Combat Service Opportunities for Women, but Should Monitor Long-Term Integration Progress*, Washington, D.C.: U.S. Government Accountability Office, GAO-15-589, July 2015.

————, *Human Capital: Additional Actions Needed to Enhance DOD's Efforts to Address Mental Health Care Stigma*, Washington, D.C.: U.S. Government Accountability Office, GAO-16-404, April 2016a.

————, *Military Health Care: Army Needs to Improve Oversight of Warrior Transition Units*, Washington, D.C.: U.S. Government Accountability Office, GAO-16-583, July 2016b.

Faust, Drew Gilpin, *This Republic of Suffering: Death and the American Civil War*, New York: Alfred A. Knopf, 2008.

Feickert, Andrew, *Mine-Resistant, Ambush-Protected (MRAP) Vehicles: Background and Issues for Congress*, Congressional Research Service, January 18, 2011.

Feller, Carolyn M., and Constance J. Moore, eds., *Highlights in the History of the Army Nurse Corps*, Washington, D.C.: U.S. Army Center of Military History, 1995.

Field Manual 4-02.25 (FM 8-10-25), *Employment of Forward Surgical Teams: Tactics, Techniques, and Procedures*, Washington, D.C.: Headquarters, Department of the Army, March 2003.

Field Manual 4-02.51 (FM 8-51), *Combat and Operational Stress Control*, Washington, D.C.: Headquarters, Department of the Army, 2006.

Field Manual 8-5, *Medical Field Manual: Mobile Units of the Medical Department*, Washington, D.C.: War Department, January 12, 1942, Change 2, April 20, 1944.

Field Manual 8-10-6, *Medical Evacuation in a Theater of Operations: Tactics, Techniques, and Procedures*, Washington, D.C.: Headquarters, Department of the Army, April 14, 2000.

Field Manual 8-10-25, *Employment of Forward Surgical Teams Tactics, Techniques, and Procedures*, Washington, D.C.: Headquarters, Department of the Army, 1997.

Finn, Belinda J., *Audit of the Veterans Health Administration's Outpatient Waiting Times*, Washington, D.C.: Department of Veterans Affairs, Office of Inspector General, Report No. 07-00616-199, September 10, 2007.

————, *Audit of Alleged Manipulation of Waiting Times in Veterans Integrated Service Network 3*, Washington, D.C.: Department of Veterans Affairs, Office of Inspector General, Report No. 07-03505-129, May 19, 2008.

Fischer, Scott H., *The Forward Surgical Team Experience in Contemporary Operations: Impetus for Change*, Fort Leavenworth, Kan.: U.S. Army Command and General Staff College, 2003.

Fisher, Kenneth Edward, *A Comparative Analysis of Selected Congressional Documents Related to Educational Benefits Legislation for the Veterans of World War II, the Korean Conflict, and the Vietnam Era Under the G.I. Bill*, Tallahassee, Fla.: Florida State University, College of Education, 1975.

Flood, Katherine M., and Sheila Saliman, "Rehabilitation Following Amputation," in Susan H. Mather and Neil S. Otchin, eds., *Traumatic Amputation and Prosthetics*, Washington, D.C.: Department of Veterans Affairs, 2002, pp. 18–27.

Flynn, George Q., *The Draft, 1940–1973*, Lawrence, Kan.: University Press of Kansas, 1993.

Flynn, Maranda, "Combat Lifesaver Course Trains Soldiers to Save Lives on, off Battlefield," U.S. Army website, July 31, 2014.

FM—*See* Field Manual.

Fogel, Richard L., *Vietnam Veterans: A Profile of VA's Readjustment Counseling Program*, Washington, D.C.: U.S. General Accounting Office, GAO/HEHS-87-63, August 1987.

Forman, Sidney, "Why the United States Military Academy Was Established in 1802," *Military Affairs*, Vol. 29, No. 1, Spring 1965, pp. 16–28.

Forsten, Robert D., Brett J. Schneider, Sharette Kirsten Gray, Colin Daniels, and Gary J. Drouillard, "Provision of Behavioral Health Services During Operation Iraqi Freedom One," in Elspeth Cameron Ritchie, ed., *Combat and Operational Behavioral Health*, Washington, D.C.: Borden Institute, Walter Reed Army Medical Center, 2011.

Frank, Benis M., and Henry I. Shaw, Jr., *History of U.S. Marine Corps Operations in World War II*, Vol. V: *Victory and Occupation*, Washington, D.C.: Headquarters, U.S. Marine Corps, Historical Branch, G-3 Division, 1968.

Franks, Tommy, *American Soldier*, New York: Regan Books, 2004.

Friedman, Matthew J., "Literature in *DSM-5* and *ICD-11*," *PTSD Research Quarterly*, Vol. 25, No. 2, 2014a.

———, *PTSD History and Overview*, Washington, D.C.: National Center for PTSD, U.S. Department of Veterans Affairs, March 24, 2014b.

Frostenson, Sarah, and Jeremy C. F. Lin, "Trump Will Increase Troops in Afghanistan. Here's How U.S. Troop Levels Have Changed Since 2001," *Politico*, August 22, 2017.

Fukuyama, Francis, *The End of History and the Last Man*, New York: Free Press, 1992.

Futrell, Robert F., *The United States Air Force in Korea 1950–1953*, rev. ed., Washington, D.C.: U.S. Air Force, Office of Air Force History, 1983.

Gailey, Robert, Lynne V. McFarland, Rory A. Cooper, Joseph Czerniecki, Jeffrey M. Gambel, Sharon Hubbard, Charles Maynard, Douglas G. Smith, Michele Raya, and Gayle E. Reiber, "Unilateral Lower-Limb Loss: Prosthetic Device Use and Functional Outcomes in Servicemembers from Vietnam War and OIF/OEF Conflicts," *Journal of Rehabilitation Research & Development*, Vol. 47, No. 4, 2010, pp. 317–332.

Gambel, Jeff, "The Process of Returning to Duty or Not After Limb Loss," in Amputee Coalition, ed., *Military In-Step*, 2014.

Gambone, Michael D., *The Greatest Generation Comes Home: The Veteran in American Society*, College Station, Tex.: Texas A&M University Press, 2005.

Gammons, Stephen L. Y., *The Korean War: The UN Offensive, 16 September–2 November 1950*, Washington, D.C.: U.S. Army Center of Military History, 2006.

GAO—*See* U.S. General Accounting Office (the name changed to U.S. Government Accountability Office in 2004).

Gardella, Rich, Talesha Reynolds, and Andrew Blankstein, "VA Whistleblowers Describe Alleged 'Cooking' of the Books," NBC News, May 9, 2014.

Garrett, John, *Task Force Smith: The Lesson Never Learned*, Fort Leavenworth, Kan.: School of Advanced Military Studies, U.S. Army Command and General Staff College, 1999.

Garrison, Fielding H., *Notes on the History of Military Medicine*, Washington, D.C.: Association of Military Surgeons, 1922.

Gasko, Oded, "Surgery in the Field During the Lebanon War, 1982: Doctrine, Experience and Prospects for Future Changes," *Israel Journal of Medical Science*, Vol. 20, No. 4, April 1984, pp. 350–354.

Gates, Robert M., *Quadrennial Defense Review Report*, Washington, D.C.: Department of Defense, 2010.

———, *Duty: Memoirs of a Secretary at War*, New York: Alfred A. Knopf, 2014.

Gates, Thomas, Thomas Curtis, Frederick Dent, Milton Friedman, Crawford Greenewalt, Alan Greenspan, Alfred Gruenther, Stephen Herbits, Theodore Hesburgh, Jerome Holland, John Kemper, Jeanne Noble, W. Allen Walis, and Roy Wilkins, *The Report of the President's Commission on an All-Volunteer Armed Force*, Washington, D.C.: U.S. Government Printing Office, February 1970.

Gawande, Atul, "Casualties of War—Military Care for the Wounded from Iraq and Afghanistan," *New England Journal of Medicine*, Vol. 351, No. 24, December 9, 2004, pp. 2471–2475.

Gebicke, Mark E., *Operation Desert Storm: Problems with Air Force Medical Readiness*, Washington, D.C.: U.S. General Accounting Office, December 1993.

———, *Wartime Medical Care: Aligning Sound Requirements with New Combat Care Approach Is Key to Restructuring Force*, Washington, D.C.: U.S. General Accounting Office, GAO/T-NSIAD-95-129, March 30, 1995.

———, *Wartime Medical Care: DOD Is Addressing Capability Shortfalls, but Challenges Remain*, Washington, D.C.: U.S. General Accounting Office, GAO/NSIAD-96-224, December 1996.

———, *Medical Readiness: Efforts Are Underway for DOD Training in Civilian Trauma Centers*, Washington, D.C.: U.S. General Accounting Office, GAO/NSIAD-98-75, April 1998.

Gehring, Stephen P., *From the Fulda Gap to Kuwait: U.S. Army Europe and the Gulf War*, Washington, D.C.: Department of the Army, 2002.

Gentzler, Doreen, "New Technology Allows Amputees to Feel Through Artificial Limbs," NBC News, October 8, 2019.

"Gen. Vessey Sees Women as Biggest Military Change," *Washington Post*, February 3, 1984.

Geren, Pete, and George W. Casey, Jr., *2009 U.S. Army Posture Statement: Army Force Generation (ARFORGEN)*, Washington, D.C., May 2009.

Gerhardt, Robert T., Robert L. Mabry, Robert A. De Lorenzo, and Frank K. Butler, "Fundamentals of Combat Casualty Care," in Eric Savitsky and Brian Eastridge, eds., *Combat Casualty Care: Lessons Learned from OEF and OIF*, Falls Church, Va.: Office of the Surgeon General, Department of the Army, 2012.

Gibson, Sloan D., and Laura Junor, *VA/DoD Joint Executive Committee Annual Report Fiscal Year 2014*, Washington, D.C.: Department of Veterans Affairs and Department of Defense, September 30, 2014.

Gibson, Sloan D., and Jessica L. Wright, *VA/DoD Joint Executive Committee Annual Report Fiscal Year 2013*, Washington, D.C.: Department of Veterans Affairs and Department of Defense, September 30, 2013.

Gillett, Mary C., *The Army Medical Department: 1775–1818*, Washington, D.C.: U.S. Government Printing Office, 1981.

Ginn, Richard Van Ness, *The History of the U.S. Army Medical Service Corps*, Washington, D.C.: U.S. Army Medical Department, Office of Medical History, 1997.

Glass, Albert J., "Psychiatry in the Korean Campaign: A Historical Review," *U.S. Armed Forces Medical Journal*, Vol. 4, No. 10, October 1952, pp. 1387–1401.

———, "History and Organization of a Theater Psychiatric Service Before and After 30 June 1951," in Frank L. Bauer, ed., *Recent Advances in Medicine and Surgery (19–30 April 1954), Based on Professional Medical Experiences in Japan and Korea, 1950–1953*, Vol. II, Washington, D.C.: U.S. Army Medical Service Graduate School, Walter Reed Army Medical Center, 1954.

———, "Army Psychiatry Before World War II," in Albert J. Glass and Robert J. Bernucci, eds., *Neuropsychiatry in World War II*, Vol. I: *Zone of Interior*, Washington, D.C.: Department of the Army, 1966, pp. 3–23.

Glass, Albert J., and Franklin D. Jones, *Psychiatry in the U.S. Army: Lessons for Community Psychiatry*, Bethesda, Md.: Uniformed Services University of the Health Sciences, 2005.

Glass, Andrew J., "Defense Report: Draftees Shoulder Burden of Fighting and Dying in Vietnam," *National Journal*, August 15, 1970, pp. 1747–1755.

Glasson, William H., *History of Military Pension Legislation in the United States*, New York: The Columbia University Press, 1900.

Goldberg, Matthew S., "Comparing the Costs of the Veterans' Health Care System with Private-Sector Costs," testimony before the Subcommittee on Health of the Committee on Veterans' Affairs, U.S. House of Representatives, Washington, D.C.: Congressional Budget Office, January 28, 2015.

———, "Casualty Rates of US Military Personnel During the Wars in Iraq and Afghanistan," *Defence and Peace Economics*, 2016, pp. 1–21.

Golding, Heidi, and Adebayo Adedeji, *The All-Volunteer Military: Issues and Performance*, Washington, D.C.: Congressional Budget Office, July 2007.

Gordon, Suzanne, "Yes, Trump Is Privatizing the VA," *The Hill*, June 16, 2017.

Gornick, Marian, "Trends and Regional Variations in Hospital Use Under Medicare, *Health Care Financing Review*, Vol. 3, No. 3, 1982, pp. 41–73.

Gough, Terrence J., *U.S. Army Mobilization and Logistics in the Korean War: A Research Approach*, Washington, D.C.: U.S. Army Center of Military History, 1987.

Gould, W. Scott, and Gail H. McGinn, *VA/DoD Joint Executive Council Annual Report Fiscal Year 2009*, Washington, D.C.: Department of Veterans Affairs and Department of Defense, September 30, 2009.

Gould, W. Scott, and Jo Ann Rooney, *VA/DoD Joint Executive Council Annual Report Fiscal Year 2011*, Washington, D.C.: Department of Veterans Affairs and Department of Defense, December 2011.

Gould, W. Scott, and Clifford L. Stanley, *VA/DoD Joint Executive Council Annual Report Fiscal Year 2010*, Washington, D.C.: Department of Veterans Affairs and Department of Defense, September 30, 2010.

Gould, W. Scott, and Jessica L. Wright, *VA/DoD Joint Executive Committee Annual Report Fiscal Year 2012*, Washington, D.C.: Department of Veterans Affairs and Department of Defense, September 30, 2012.

Graves, Clifford L., *Front Line Surgeons: A History of The Third Auxiliary Surgical Group*, San Diego, Calif.: Frye & Smith, 1950.

Gray, Carl R., Jr., *Annual Report of the Administrator of Veterans' Affairs for the Fiscal Year 1952*, Washington, D.C.: Veterans' Administration, January 7, 1953.

Green, Charles B., Suzanne Crockett-Jones, and Karen Guice, *Department of Defense Recovering Warrior Task Force 2010-2011 Annual Report*, Alexandria, Va.: Department of Defense Task Force on the Care, Management, and Transition of Recovering Wounded, Ill, and Injured Members of the Armed Forces, September 2, 2011.

Greene-Shortridge, Tiffany M., Thomas W. Britt, and Carl Andrew Castro, "The Stigma of Mental Health Problems in the Military," *Military Medicine*, Vol. 172, No. 2, February 2007, pp. 157–161.

Greenstein, Fred I., and Richard H. Immerman, "What Did Eisenhower Tell Kennedy About Indochina? The Politics of Misperception," *Journal of American History*, Vol. 79, No. 2, September 1992, pp. 568–587.

Greenwood, John T., "Portable Surgical Hospitals," webpage, August 30, 2013.

Greenwood, John T., and F. Clifton Berry, Jr., *Medics at War: Military Medicine from Colonial Times to the 21st Century*, Annapolis, Md.: Naval Institute Press, 2005.

Greer, Gordon B., *What Price Security?* Lincoln, Neb.: iUniverse, Inc., 2005.

Griffin, Richard J., *Veterans Health Administration: Review of Patient Wait Times, Scheduling Practices, and Alleged Patient Deaths at the Phoenix Health Care System*, Washington, D.C.: Office of Inspector General, Department of Veterans Affairs, Report No. 14-02603-267, August 26, 2014.

Grissmer, David, and Bernard D. Rostker, "Military Personnel in a Changing World," in Joseph Kruzel, ed., *American Defense Annual: 1991–1992*, New York: Lexington Books, 1992, pp. 127–145.

Grob, Gerald N., "Origins of DSM-I: A Study in Appearance and Reality," *American Journal of Psychiatry*, Vol. 148, No. 4, April 1991, pp. 421–431.

Gulf War Veterans' Illnesses Task Force, *2012–13 Report of the Department of Veterans Affairs Gulf War Veterans' Illnesses Task Force to the Secretary of Veterans Affairs*, Washington, D.C.: U.S. Department of Veterans Affairs, January 2014.

Hafner, Brian J., Laura L. Willingham, Noelle C. Buell, Katheryn J. Allyn, and Douglas G. Smith, "Evaluation of Function, Performance, and Preference as Transfemoral Amputees Transition from Mechanical to Microprocessor Control of the Prosthetic Knee," *Archives of Physical Medical Rehabilitation*, Vol. 88, February 2007, pp. 207–217.

Haley, Sarah A., "When the Patient Reports Atrocities: Specific Treatment Considerations of the Vietnam Veteran," *Archives of General Psychiatry*, Vol. 30, No. 2, February 1, 1974, pp. 191–196.

Hall, Wilford F., "Air Evacuation," *Journal of the American Medical Association*, Vol. 147, No. 11, November 10, 1951, pp. 1026–1028.

Hall, Wilford F., and Joseph D. Nolan, "Advantages of Air Transportation of Patients," *United States Armed Forces Medical Journal*, Vol. 1, No. 1, January 1950, pp. 115–118.

Hampton, Oscar P., Jr., "Orthopedic Surgery in the Mediterranean Theater of Operations," in John Boyd Coates, ed., *Medical Department of the United States Army in World War II: Surgery in World War II*, Washington, D.C.: U.S. Army Medical Department, Office of Medical History, 1957.

Hansen, John C., "The Vietnam Veterans vs. Agent Orange: The War That Lingers," *GAO Review*, Spring 1981, pp. 29–36.

Hanson, Frederick R., ed., *Combat Psychiatry: Experiences in the North African and Mediterranean Theaters of Operation, American Ground Forces, World War II*, Washington, D.C.: U.S. Army Medical Department, 1949.

Hanson, Thomas E., *Combat Ready? The Eighth U.S. Army on the Eve of the Korean War*, College Station, Tex.: Texas A&M University Press, 2010.

Hardaway, Robert M., "Viet Nam Wound Analysis," *Journal of Trauma*, Vol. 18, No. 9, September 1978, pp. 635–643.

———, "The Wounded Patient," in Robert M. Hardaway, ed., *Care of the Wounded in Vietnam*, Manhattan, Kan.: Sunflower University Press, 1988.

———, "200 Years of Military Surgery," *Injury: International Journal of the Care of the Injured*, Vol. 30, 1999, pp. 387–397.

———, "Wound Shock: A History of Its Study and Treatment by Military Surgeons," *Military Medicine*, Vol. 169, No. 4, April 2004, pp. 265–269.

Hartenstein, Ingo, *Medical Evacuation in Afghanistan: Lessons Identified! Lessons Learned?* Brussels, Belgium: North Atlantic Treaty Organization, Research and Technology, RTO-MP-HFM-157, December 2008.

Hauret, Keith G., Laura Pacha, Bonnie J. Taylor, and Bruce H. Jones, "Surveillance of Disease and Nonbattle Injuries During US Army Operations in Afghanistan and Iraq," *Army Medical Department Journal*, April–September 2016, pp. 15–23.

Hayes, David K., "Weapons and Mechanism of Injury in Operation Iraqi Freedom and Operation Enduring Freedom," in Joseph A. Brennan, G. Richard Holt, and Richard W. Thomas, eds., *Otolaryngology/Head and Neck Surgery Combat Casualty Care in Operation Iraqi Freedom and Operation Enduring Freedom*, Fort Sam Houston, Tex.: Borden Institute, 2015.

Hayes, James H., "The Valiant Die Once," self-published, 1999.

Henning, Charles A., *Military Retirement: Major Legislative Issues*, Washington, D.C.: Congressional Research Service, IB85159, January 3, 2006.

Herget, Carl H., George B. Coe, and James C. Beyer, "Wound Ballistics and Body Armor in Korea," in James C. Beyer, ed., *Wound Ballistics*, Washington, D.C.: U.S. Army Medical Department, Office of Medical History, 1962.

Hernandez, Lyla M., Jane S. Durch, Dan G. Blazer II, and Isabel V. Hoverman, eds., *Gulf War Veterans: Measuring Health*, Washington, D.C.: National Academies Press, 1999.

Hershey, Lewis B., *Selective Service Under the 1948 Act Extended: July 9, 1950–June 19, 1951*, Washington, D.C.: U.S. Government Printing Office, 1953.

Hinton, Harold B., "Doctor Draft Bill Goes to President," *New York Times*, September 2, 1950.

Hoge, Charles W., Jennifer L. Auchterlonie, and Charles S. Milliken, "Mental Health Problems, Use of Mental Health Services, and Attrition From Military Service After Returning from Deployment to Iraq or Afghanistan," *Journal of the American Medical Association,* Vol. 295, No. 9, March 1, 2006, pp. 1023–1032.

Hoge, Charles W., Carl A. Castro, Stephen C. Messer, Dennis McGurk, Dave I. Cotting, and Robert L. Koffman, "Combat Duty in Iraq and Afghanistan, Mental Health Problems, and Barriers to Care," *New England Journal of Medicine*, Vol. 351, No. 1, July 1, 2004, pp. 13–22.

Hoge, Charles W., Dennis McGurk, Jeffrey L. Thomas, Anthony L. Cox, Charles C. Engel, and Carl A. Castro, "Mild Traumatic Brain Injury in U.S. Soldiers Returning from Iraq," *New England Journal of Medicine*, Vol. 358, No. 5, January 31, 2008, pp. 453–463.

Hoge, Charles W., Christopher G. Ivany, Edward A. Brusher, Millard D. Brown III, John C. Shero, Amy B. Adler, Christopher H. Warner, and David T. Orman, "Transformation of Mental Health Care for U.S. Soldiers and Families During the Iraq and Afghanistan Wars: Where Science and Politics Intersect," *American Journal of Psychiatry*, Vol. 173, No. 4, April 2016, pp. 1–10.

Holcomb, John B., Frank K. Butler, and Peter Rhee, "Hemorrhage Control Devices: Tourniquets and Hemostatic Dressings," *The Bulletin (American College of Surgeons)*, Vol. 100, No. 1, Supplement, September 2015, pp. 66–70.

Holcomb, John B., Neil R. McMullin, Lisa Pearse, Jim Caruso, Charles E. Wade, Lynne Oetjen-Gerdes, Howard R. Champion, Mimi Lawnick, Warner Farr, Sam Rodriguez, and Frank K. Butler, "Causes of Death in U.S. Special Operations Forces in the Global War on Terrorism, 2001–2004," *Annals of Surgery*, Vol. 245, No. 6, June 2007, pp. 986–991.

Holcomb, John B., Lynn G. Stansbury, Howard R. Champion, Charles Wade, and Ronald F. Bellamy, "Understanding Combat Casualty Care Statistics," *Journal of Trauma: Injury, Infection, and Critical Care*, Vol. 60, February 2006, pp. 397–401.

Holmes, Robert H., "Wound Ballistics and Body Armor," *Journal of the American Medical Association*, Vol. 150, No. 2, September 13, 1952, pp. 73–78.

Holmes, Robert H., William F. Enos, Jr., and James C. Beyer, "Medical Aspects of Body Armor in Korea," in Frank L. Bauer, ed., *Recent Advances in Medicine and Surgery (19–30 April 1954), Based on Professional Medical Experiences in Japan and Korea 1950–1953*, Vol. I, Washington, D.C.: U.S. Army Medical Service Graduate School, Walter Reed Army Medical Center, 1954.

Holt, G. Richard, and Timothy K. Jones, "Evacuation and Roles of Care," in Joseph A. Brennan, G. Richard Holt, and Richard W. Thomas, eds., *Otolaryngology/Head and Neck Surgery Combat Casualty Care in Operation Iraqi Freedom and Operation Enduring Freedom*, Fort Sam Houston, Tex.: Borden Institute, 2015.

Hooker, Richard, *MASH: A Novel About Three Army Doctors*, New York: William Morrow, 1968.

Hooper, [Rebecca S.], "Center for the Intrepid at Brooke Army Medical Center," information paper, Washington, D.C.: Office of the Surgeon General, Department of the Army, May 8, 2007.

Horn, Kenneth, Kimberlie Biever, Kenneth Burkman, Paul DeLuca, Lewis Jamison, Michael Kolb, and Aatif Sheikh, *Lightening Body Armor: Arroyo Support to the Army Response to Section 125 of the National Defense Authorization Act for Fiscal Year 2011*, Santa Monica, Calif.: RAND Corporation, TR-1136-A, 2012.

House Committee on Veterans' Affairs, "Veterans' Health Care Eligibility Reform Act of 1996: Report to Accompany H.R. 3118," 104th Cong., 2nd Sess., Washington, D.C.: U.S. Government Printing Office, July 18, 1996.

House Resolution 1735, *FY 16 National Defense Authorization Bill: Title VII—Health Care Provisions Items of Special Interest—Comptroller General Report on Army Warrior Transition Units*, Washington, D.C.: House Armed Services Committee, Subcommittee on Military Personnel, 2015.

Howard, John M., "Historical Vignettes of Arterial Repair: Recollections of Korea 1951–1953," *Annals of Surgery*, Vol. 228, No. 5, November 1998, pp. 716–718.

Howard, William G., *History of Aeromedical Evacuation in the Korean War and Vietnam War*, thesis, Fort Leavenworth, Kan.: U.S. Army Command and General Staff College, 2003.

Howe, Edmund G., and Franklin D. Jones, "Ethical Issues in Combat Psychiatry," in Franklin D. Jones, ed., *Military Psychiatry: Preparing in Peace for War*, Washington, D.C.: Borden Institute, Walter Reed Army Medical Center, 1994.

Howes, Lori, "Annex Q (Medical Holdover Operations) to HQDA OPORD 04-01," message forwarded to multiple recipients, January 20, 2004.

H.R.—*See* House Resolution.

Huang, Grace, Sharon Kim, Joseph Gasper, Yiling Xu, Thomas Bosworth, and Laurie May, *2016 Survey of Veteran Enrollees' Health and Use of Health Care*, Rockville, Md.: Westat, March 2017.

Hudak, Ronald P., Christine Morrison, Mary Carstensen, James S. Rice, and Brent R. Jurgersen, "The U.S. Army Wounded Warrior Program (AW2): A Case Study in Designing a Nonmedical Case Management Program for Severely Wounded, Injured, and Ill Service Members and Their Families," *Military Medicine*, Vol. 174, No. 6, 2009, pp. 566–571.

Hughes, Carl W., "Acute Vascular Trauma in Korean War Casualties: An Analysis of 80 Cases," *Surgery, Gynecology and Obstetrics*, Vol. 99, 1954a, pp. 91–100.

———, "Primary Surgery of Blood Vessels in Korea: An Analysis of Major Artery Repairs in Korea During 1953," in Frank L. Bauer, ed., *Recent Advances in Medicine and Surgery (19–30 April 1954) Based on Professional Medical Experiences in Japan and Korea, 1950–1953*, Vol. I, Washington, D.C.: U.S. Army Medical Service Graduate School, Walter Reed Army Medical Center, 1954b.

———, "Arterial Repair During the Korean War," *Annals of Surgery*, Vol. 147, No. 4, April 1958, pp. 555–561.

Hull, Anne, and Dana Priest, "The Hotel Aftermath: Inside Mologne House, the Survivors of War Wrestle with Military Bureaucracy and Personal Demons," *Washington Post*, February 19, 2007.

Hurd, William W., and John G. Jernigan, "Introduction," in William W. Hurd and John G. Jernigan, eds., *Aeromedical Evacuation: Management of Acute and Stabilized Patients*, New York: Springer-Verlag, 2003.

Ingalls, Nichole, David Zonies, Jeffrey A. Bailey, Kathleen D. Martin, Bart O. Iddins, Paul K. Carlton, Dennis Hanseman, Richard Branson, Warren Dorlac, and Jay Johannigman, "A Review of the First 10 Years of Critical Care Aeromedical Transport During Operation Iraqi Freedom and Operation Enduring Freedom: The Importance of Evacuation Timing," *JAMA Surgery*, Vol. 149, No. 8, June 2014, pp. 807–813.

Inspectors General of the U.S. Department of Defense and U.S. Department of Veterans Affairs, *DoD/VA Care Transition Process for Service Members Injured in OIF/OEF*, Washington, D.C., June 12, 2008.

Intrepid Fallen Heroes Fund, "Rehabilitation and Advanced Training Skills Center," New York, undated.

Irey, Thomas R., "Soldiering, Suffering, and Dying in the Mexican War," *Journal of the West*, Vol. 11, No. 2, 1972.

Iserson, Kenneth V., and John C. Moskop, "Triage in Medicine, Part I: Concept, History, and Types," *Annals of Emergency Medicine*, Vol. 49, No. 3, March 2007, pp. 275–281.

Jaffin, Jonathan H., *Medical Support for the American Expeditionary Forces in France During the First World War* Fort Leavenworth, Kan.: U.S. Army Command and General Staff College, 1990.

Jahke, Edward J., Jr., and Sam F. Seeley, "Acute Vascular Injuries in the Korean War," *Annals of Surgery*, Vol. 138, No. 2, August 1953, pp. 158–177.

Jahner, Kyle, "House Subcommittee Requests GAO Report on WTUs," *Army Times*, May 6, 2015.

Jernigan, John G., "Aircraft Considerations for Aeromedical Evacuation," in William W. Hurd and John G. Jernigan, eds., *Aeromedical Evacuation: Management of Acute and Stabilized Patients*, New York: Springer-Verlag, 2003.

Joellenbeck, Lois M., Philip K. Russell, and Samuel B. Guze, eds., *Strategies to Protect the Health of Deployed U.S. Forces: Medical Surveillance, Record Keeping, and Risk Reduction*, Washington, D.C.: National Academies Press, 1999.

Johns Hopkins Applied Physics Laboratory, "Prosthetics: The Program," webpage, undated.

Joint Commission on Mental Illness and Health, *Action for Mental Health: Final Report*, New York: Basic Books, Inc., Publishers, 1961.

Joint Publication 3-24, *Counterinsurgency*, Washington, D.C.: Office of the Joint Chiefs of Staff, November 22, 2013.

Joint Publication 4-02.2, *Joint Tactics, Techniques and Procedures for Patient Movement in Joint Operations*, Washington, D.C.: Office of the Joint Chiefs of Staff, December 30, 1996.

Joint Staff, *Focused Logistics Roadmap*, Washington, D.C.: Office of the Joint Chiefs of Staff, 1997.

Jones, Edgar, and Simon Wessely, "'Forward Psychiatry' in the Military: Its Origins and Effectiveness," *Journal of Traumatic Stress*, Vol. 16, No. 4, August 2003, pp. 411–419.

———, *Shell Shock to PTSD: Military Psychiatry from 1900 to the Gulf War*, New York: Psychology Press, 2005.

Jones, Franklin D., "Chronic Post-Traumatic Stress Disorders," in Franklin D. Jones, ed., *War Psychiatry*, Washington, D.C.: Borden Institute, Walter Reed Army Medical Center, 1995a.

———, "Psychiatric Principles in Future Warfare," in Franklin D. Jones, Linette R. Sparacino, Victoria L. Wilcox, Joseph M. Rothberg, and James W. Stokes, eds., *War Psychiatry*, Washington, D.C.: Borden Institute, Walter Reed Army Medical Center, 1995b.

———, "Military Psychiatry Since World War II," in Roy W. Menninger and John C. Nemiah, eds., *American Psychiatry After World War II*, Washington, D.C.: American Psychiatric Press, 2000.

———, "Military Psychiatry After the First Year of the Korean War," in Albert J. Glass and Franklin D. Jones, eds., *Psychiatry in the U.S. Army: Lessons for Community Psychiatry*, Bethesda, Md.: Uniformed Services University of the Health Sciences, 2005.

Jones, Franklin D., Linette R. Sparacino, Victoria L. Wilcox, and Joseph M. Rothberg, eds., *Military Psychiatry: Preparing in Peace for War*, Falls Church, Va.: Office of the Surgeon General, Department of the Army, 1994.

Jones, Franklin D., Linette R. Sparacino, Victoria L. Wilcox, Joseph M. Rothberg, and James W. Stoke, *War Psychiatry*, Textbook of Military Medicine, Washington, D.C.: Borden Institute, Walter Reed Army Medical Center, 1995.

Jones, Franklin Del, and Arnold W. Johnson, Jr., "Medical and Psychiatric Treatment Policy and Practice in Vietnam," *Journal of Social Issues*, Vol. 31, No. 4, Fall 1975, pp. 49–65.

Jones, Toby Craig, "America, Oil, and War in the Middle East," *Journal of American History*, Vol. 99, No. 1, June 2012, pp. 208–218.

Joseph, Stephen C., *Medical Readiness Strategic Plan 1995–2001*, Washington, D.C.: Office of the Assistant Secretary of Defense for Health Affairs, March 20, 1995.

Joseph, Stephen C., and the Comprehensive Clinical Evaluation Program Evaluation Team, "A Comprehensive Clinical Evaluation of 20,000 Persian Gulf War Veterans," *Military Medicine*, Vol. 162, No. 3, March 1997, pp. 149–155.

JP—*See* Joint Publication.

Julian, Dave, "Military Severely Injured Center: Briefing for the Veterans' Disability Benefits Commission," briefing slides, Washington, D.C.: U.S. Department of Defense, 2005.

Kalasinsky, Victor F., and Robert J. Jaeger, *Annual Summary: Federally Sponsored Research on Gulf War Veterans' Illnesses for 2015*, Washington, D.C.: U.S. Department of Veterans Affairs, 2016.

Kang, Han K., Clare M. Mahan, Kyung Y. Lee, Carol A. Magee, and Frances M. Murphy, "Illnesses Among United States Veterans of the Gulf War: A Population-Based Survey of 30,000 Veterans," *Journal of Occupational and Environmental Medicine*, Vol. 42, No. 5, May 2000, pp. 491–501.

Kapp, Susan, and Joseph A. Miller, "Lower Limb Prosthetics," in Paul F. Pasquina and Rory A. Cooper, eds., *Care of the Combat Amputee*, Washington, D.C.: Borden Institute, Walter Reed Army Medical Center, 2009, pp. 553–580.

Karter, Thomas, "Veterans' Pension Act of 1959," *Social Security Bulletin*, December 1959, pp. 18–21.

Katzman, Kenneth, *Afghanistan: Post-Taliban Governance, Security, and U.S. Policy*, Washington, D.C.: Congressional Research Service, RL30588, June 6, 2016.

Keeley, Lawrence H., *War Before Civilization: The Myth of the Peaceful Savage*, New York: Oxford University Press, 1996.

Keen, W. W., "Military Surgery in 1861 and 1918," *Rehabilitation of the Wounded: The Annals*, Vol. 80, November 1918.

Keener, Mary Lou, "Aid & Attendance Allowance for Improved Pension Purposes," memorandum to Chairman, Board of Veterans' Appeals, Department of Veterans Affairs, Washington, D.C., December 13, 1994.

Kelly, Joseph F., Amber E. Ritenour, Daniel F. McLaughlin, Karen A. Bagg, Amy N. Apodaca, Craig T. Mallak, Lisa Pearse, Mary M. Lawnick, Howard R. Champion, Charles E. Wade, and John B. Holcomb, "Injury Severity and Causes of Death from Operation Iraqi Freedom and Operation Enduring Freedom: 2003–2004 Versus 2006," *Journal of Trauma: Injury, Infection, and Critical Care*, Vol. 64, No. 2, February Supplement, 2008, pp. S21–S27.

Kennedy, John F., "Inaugural Address," January 20, 1961.

"Kennedy's Vision for Mental Health Never Realized," *USA Today*, October 20, 2013.

Keyes, Charley, "Steep Cost of Military Vehicles Outlined in Army Report," CNN, January 27, 2011.

Kiley, Kevin C., "Walter Reed Army Medical Center Outpatient Care," statement before the Senate Armed Services Committee, Washington, D.C.: Department of the Army, March 6, 2007.

King, Ludlow, "Lightweight Body Armor," *Quartermaster Review*, March–April 1953.

Kinkead, Eugene, *In Every War But One*, New York: W.W. Norton & Company, 1959.

Kirkpatrick, Charles E., *Building the Army for Desert Storm*, Arlington, Va.: Association of the United States Army, Institute of Land Warfare, November 1991.

Kishbaugh, David, Timothy R. Dillingham, Robin S. Howard, Melissa W. Sinnott, and Praxedes V. Belandres, "Amputee Soldiers and Their Return to Active Duty," *Military Medicine*, Vol. 160, No. 2, February 1995, pp. 82–84.

Kitchens, John W., *Cargo Helicopters in the Korean Conflict*, U.S. Army Aviation Museum Foundation website, 2003.

Klesius, Mike, "The Flying Emergency Room: One Reason More Soldiers Are Making It Home Alive," *Air & Space Magazine*, November 2012.

Knuth, Tom, Peter B. Letarte, Geoffrey Ling, Leon E. Moores, Peter Rhee, David Tauber, and Art Trask, *Guidelines for the Field Management of Combat-Related Head Trauma*, New York: Brain Trauma Foundation, 2005.

Koebler, Jason, "New Prosthetics Keep Amputee Soldiers on Active Duty," *U.S. News and World Report*, May 25, 2012.

Kolb, Richard K., "Korea's 'Invisible Veterans' Return to an Ambivalent America," *Veterans of Foreign Wars Magazine*, Vol. 85, No. 3, November 1997, pp. 24–32.

Kotwal, Russ S., Frank K. Butler, Erin P. Edgar, Stacy A. Shackelford, Donald R. Bennett, and Jeffrey A. Bailey, *Saving Lives on the Battlefield: A Joint Trauma System Review of Pre-Hospital Trauma Care in Combined Joint Operating Area–Afghanistan (CJOA-A)*, MacDill Air Force Base, Fla.: U.S. Central Command, January 30, 2013a.

Kotwal, Russ S., Frank K. Butler, Harold R. Montgomery, Tyson J. Brunstetter, George Y. Diaz, James W. Kirkpatrick, Nancy L. Summers, Stacy A. Shackelford, John B. Holcomb, and Jeffrey A. Bailey, *The Tactical Combat Casualty Care Casualty Card: TCCC Guidelines—Proposed Change 1301*, Fort Sam Houston, Tex.: Department of Defense Joint Trauma System Committee on Tactical Combat Casualty Care, April 30, 2013b.

Kotwal, Russ S., Jeffrey T. Howard, Jean A. Orman, Bruce W. Tarpey, Jeffrey A. Bailey, Howard R. Champion, Robert L. Mabry, John B. Holcomb, and Kirby R. Gross, "The Effect of a Golden Hour Policy on the Morbidity and Mortality of Combat Casualties," *JAMA Surgery*, Vol. 151, No. 1, January 2016, pp. 15–24.

Kotwal, Russ S., Harold R. Montgomery, Bari M. Kotwal, Howard R. Champion, Frank K. Butler, Jr., Robert L. Mabry, Jeffrey S. Cain, Lorne H. Blackbourne, Kathy K. Mechler, and John B. Holcomb, "Eliminating Preventable Death on the Battlefield," *Archives of Surgery*, Vol. 146, No. 12, December 2011, pp. 1350–1358.

Kragh, John F., Jr., Michelle L. Littrel, John A. Jones, Thomas J. Walters, David G. Baer, Charles E. Wade, and John B. Holcomb, "Battle Casualty Survival with Emergency Tourniquet Use to Stop Limb Bleeding," *Journal of Emergency Medicine*, Vol. 20, No. 10, 2009.

Kragh, John F., Jr., Kenneth G. Swan, Dale C. Smith, Robert L. Mabry, and Lorne H. Blackbourne, "Historical Review of Emergency Tourniquet Use to Stop Bleeding," *American Journal of Surgery*, Vol. 203, No. 2, February 2012, pp. 242–252.

Kragh, John F., Jr., Thomas J. Walters, Ted Westmoreland, Robert M. Miller, Robert L. Mabry, Russ S. Kotwal, Brandi A. Ritter, Douglas C. Hodge, Dominique J. Greydanus, Jeffrey S. Cain, Donald L. Parsons, Erin P. Edgar, H. Theodore Harcke, David G. Baer, Michael A. Dubick, Lorne H. Blackbourne, Harold R. Montgomery, John B. Holcomb, and Frank K. Butler, "Tragedy into Drama: An American History of Tourniquet Use in the Current War," *Journal of Special Operations Medicine*, Vol. 13, No. 3, Fall 2013.

Krepinevich, Andrew F., Jr., *The Army and Vietnam*, Baltimore, Md.: Johns Hopkins University Press, 1986.

Krueger, Chad A., Joseph C. Wenke, and James R. Ficke, "Ten Years at War: Comprehensive Analysis of Amputation Trends," *Journal of Trauma and Acute Care Surgery*, Vol. 73, No. 6, Supplement 5, 2012, pp. S438–S444.

Kulka, Richard A., William E. Schlenger, John A. Fairbank, Richard L. Hough, B. Kathleen Jordan, Charles R. Marmar, and David A. Grady, *Trauma and the Vietnam War Generation: Report of Findings from the National Vietnam Veterans Readjustment Study*, New York: Brunner/Mazel Publishers, 1990.

Kulka, Richard A., William E. Schlenger, John A. Fairbank, Richard L. Hough, B. Kathleen Jordan, Charles R. Marmar, and Daniel S. Weiss, *Contractual Report of Findings from the National Vietnam Veterans Readjustment Study*, Vol. I: *Executive Summary, Description of Findings, and Technical Appendices*, Research Triangle Park, N.C.: Research Triangle Institute, November 7, 1988.

Kurtzleben, Danielle, "How the U.S. Troop Levels in Afghanistan Have Changed Under Obama," chart, National Public Radio website, July 6, 2016.

Landler, Mark, "Obama Says He Will Slow Troop Reductions in Afghanistan," *New York Times*, July 7, 2016.

LaNoue, Alcide M., *Care and Disposition of Amputee War Casualties*, Leavenworth, Kan.: U.S. Army Command and General Staff College, 1971.

Larrey, D. J. [Dominique Jean], *Memoirs of Military Surgery and Campaigns of the French Armies*, trans. Richard Willmott Hall, Baltimore: Joseph Cushing, 1814.

Laver, Harry S., "Preemption and the Evolution of America's Strategic Defense," *Parameters*, Vol. 35, No. 2, Summer 2005.

Lead Inspector General for Overseas Contingency Operations, *Operation Freedom's Sentinel Report to the United States Congress: October 1, 2017–December 31, 2017*, Washington, D.C.: U.S. Department of Defense, U.S. Department of State, and U.S. Agency for International Development, 2017.

Ledford, Frank F., Jr., "From the Surgeon General of the Army: Medical Support for Operation Desert Storm," *Journal of the U.S. Army Medical Department*, January/February 1992, pp. 3–6.

Lee, Gus C., and Geoffrey Y. Parker, *Ending the Draft: The Story of the All Volunteer Force*, Washington, D.C.: Human Resources Research Organization, April 1977.

Lee, Jongsoo James, *The Partition of Korea After World War II: A Global History*, New York: Palgrave Macmillan, 2006.

Lerner, E. Brooke, and Ronald M. Moscati, "The Golden Hour: Scientific Fact or Medical 'Urban Legend'?" *Academic Emergency Medicine*, Vol. 8, No. 7, July 2001.

Lifton, Robert Jay, statement before the Subcommittee on Veterans Affairs of the Committee on Labor and Public Welfare, U.S. Senate, 91st Cong., 1st and 2nd Sess, hearing on the Examination of the Problems of the Veterans Wounded in Vietnam, Washington, D.C.: U.S. Government Printing Office, 1970.

———, "Home from the War: The Psychology of Survival," *Atlantic Monthly*, Vol. 230, November 1972, pp. 56–72.

Lindsey, Douglas, "Professional Considerations of Patient Evacuation," in Frank L. Bauer, ed., *Recent Advances in Medicine and Surgery (19–30 April 1954), Based on Professional Medical Experiences in Japan and Korea 1950–1953*, Vol. I, Washington, D.C.: U.S. Army Medical Service Graduate School, Walter Reed Army Medical Center, 1954.

Link, Mae Mills, and Hubert A. Coleman, *Medical Support: Army Air Forces in World War II*, Washington, D.C.: U.S. Government Printing Office, 1955.

Little, Donald D., *Combat Crew Rotation: World War II and Korean War*, Maxwell Air Force Base, Ala.: Historical Studies Branch, USAF Historical Division, Aerospace Studies Institute, Air University, January 1968.

Little, Robert, "Modern Combat Lacking in Old Medical Supply," *Baltimore Sun*, March 6, 2005a.

———, "Probe Urged of Policy on Tourniquets," *Baltimore Sun*, March 10, 2005b.

———, "Stanching Wounds," *Baltimore Sun*, November 20, 2005c.

———, "Investigation Reveals Army's Risky Medical Practices," *Baltimore Sun*, March 28, 2009.

Ludmerer, Kenneth M., *Time to Heal: American Medical Education from the Turn of the Century to the Era of Managed Care*, New York: Oxford University Press, 1999.

Lyle, Amaani, "Panetta Discusses Efforts to Tackle Suicide," American Forces Press Service, September 24, 2012.

Lynch, Charles, Frank W. Weed, and Loy McAfee, eds., *The Medical Department of the United States Army in the World War*, Vol. I: *The Surgeon General's Office*, Washington, D.C.: War Department, 1923.

Lynch, Charles, Joseph Ford, and Frank W. Weed, *The Medical Department of the United States Army in the World War*, Vol. VIII: *Field Operations*, Washington, D.C.: U.S. Army Medical Department, Office of Medical History, 1925.

Lyons, Richard D., "How Release of Mental Patients Began," *New York Times*, October 30, 1984.

Mabry, Earl W., Robert A. Munson, and Londe A. Richardson, "The Wartime Need for Aeromedical Evacuation Physicians: The U.S. Air Force Experience During Operation Desert Storm," *Aviation, Space, and Environmental Medicine*, Vol. 64, No. 10, October 1993, pp. 941–946.

Mabry, Robert L., "Tourniquet Use on the Battlefield," *Military Medicine*, Vol. 171, No. 5, May 2006.

Maisel, Albert Q., "Third Rate Medicine for First Rate Men," *Cosmopolitan*, March and May 1945.

Management of Post-Traumatic Stress Working Group, *VA/DoD Clinical Practice Guideline for the Management of Post-Traumatic Stress*, Vers. 1.0, Washington, D.C.: U.S. Department of Veterans Affairs and U.S. Department of Defense, January 2004.

———, *VA/DoD Clinical Practice Guideline for Management of Post-Traumatic Stress*, Vers. 2.0, Washington, D.C.: U.S. Department of Veterans Affairs and U.S. Department of Defense, 2010.

Management of Upper Extremity Amputation Rehabilitation Working Group, *VA/DoD Clinical Practice Guideline for Management of Upper Extremity Amputation Rehabilitation*, Department of Veterans Affairs and Department of Defense, 2014.

Manring, M. M., Alan Hawk, Jason H. Calhoun, and Romney C. Andersen, "Treatment of War Wounds: A Historical Review," *Clinical Orthopaedics and Related Research*, Vol. 467, No. 8, August 2009, pp. 2168–2191.

Marble, Sanders, *Rehabilitating the Wounded: Historical Perspective on Army Policy*, Washington, D.C.: Office of Medical History, Office of the Surgeon General, Department of the Army, 2008.

———, "Mobile Hospitals Saved Lives in WWII," *Mercury Newsletter*, October 2009.

———, "Forward Surgery and Combat Hospitals: The Origins of the MASH," *Journal of the History of Medicine and Allied Sciences*, Vol. 69, No. 1, 2012.

———, "The Evolution and Demise of the MASH, 1946–2006: Organizing to Perform Forward Surgery as Medicine and the Military Change," *Army History*, Summer 2014, pp. 23–39.

———, "US Military Drawdowns 1970–1999: Army Medical Department and Military Health System Responses," *U.S. Army Medical Department Journal*, October–December 2015, pp. 38–47.

Marcum, Cheryl Y., Robert M. Emmerichs, Jennifer Sloan McCombs, and Harry J. Thie, *Methods and Actions for Improving Performance of the Department of Defense Disability Evaluation System*, Santa Monica, Calif.: RAND Corporation, MR-1228-OSD, 2002.

Marren, John J., "Psychiatric Problems in Troops in Korea During and Following Combat," *U.S. Armed Forces Medical Journal*, Vol. 7, No. 5, May 1956, pp. 715–726.

Marshall, George C., "Transition from the Point System to a Length-of-Service Policy," memorandum to the President of the United States, Washington, D.C., October 31, 1945.

Marshall, S. L. A., *Pork Chop Hill: The American Fighting Man in Action, Korea, Spring, 1953*, New York: William Morrow and Company, 1956.

Marshall, Scott A., Randy Bell, Rocco A. Armonda, Eric Savitsky, and Geoffrey S. F. Ling, "Traumatic Brain Injury," in Eric Savitsky and Brian Eastridge, eds., *Combat Casualty Care: Lessons Learned from OEF and OIF*, Falls Church, Va.: Office of the Surgeon General, Department of the Army, 2012.

Marshall, Tyrone C., Jr., "Hagel Issues Guidance for Veterans' Discharge Upgrade Requests," press release, Washington, D.C.: U.S. Department of Defense, September 3, 2014.

Martin, James A., "Combat Psychiatry: Lessons from the War in Southwest Asia," *Journal of the U.S. Army Medical Department*, January/February 1992, pp. 40–44.

Maughon, J. S., "An Inquiry into the Nature of Wounds Resulting in Killed in Action in Vietnam," *Military Medicine*, Vol. 135, January 1970, pp. 8–13.

Mayer, William E., "Brainwashing: The Ultimate Weapon," paper presented at transcription of address given at the San Francisco Naval Shipyard in the Naval Radiological Defense Laboratory, San Francisco, October 4, 1956.

———, "Military Cold War Education and Speech Review Policies, Part 3," testimony before the Special Preparedness Subcommittee of the Committee on Armed Services, U.S. Senate, April 3, 1962, pp. 1148–1198.

———, "A Guide to the William E. Mayer P.O.W. Brainwashing Audio," Austin: University of Texas, Briscoe Center for American History, 2014.

Mayfield, Gerald W., "Vietnam War Amputees," in William E. Burkhalter, ed., *Orthopedic Surgery in Vietnam*, Washington, D.C.: U.S. Army Medical Department, Office of Medical History, 1994.

McCarl, J. R., and Lurtin R. Ginn, *Decisions of the Comptroller General of the United States, Vol. 4, July 1, 1924 to June 30, 1925*, Vol. 4, Washington, D.C.: U.S. Government Printing Office, 1925.

McClellan, George B., "General Orders No. 147: Organization of the Ambulance Corps and the Management of Ambulance Trains," near Harrison's Landing, Va.: Headquarters Army of the Potomac, August 2, 1862.

McFarland, Lynne V., Sandra L. Hubbard Winkler, Allen W. Heinemann, Melissa Jones, and Alberto Esquenazi, "Unilateral Upper-Limb Loss: Satisfaction and Prosthetic-Device Use in Veterans and Servicemembers from Vietnam and OIF/OEF Conflicts," *Journal of Rehabilitation Research & Development*, Vol. 47, No. 4, 2010, pp. 299–316.

McGrath, John J., *The Korean War: Restoring the Balance, 25 January–8 July 1951*, Washington, D.C.: U.S. Army Center of Military History, 2003.

McHale, Kathleen A., "Care of War Amputees [Amputee Care in Combat Zone Hospitals and Amputee Care in Conus]," memorandum for the Surgeon General, Falls Church, Va., October 11, 2001a.

McHale, Kathleen A., "Care of War Amputees," proposal for care memorandum to LTG James Peake, Surgeon General, U.S. Army, Falls Church, Va., October 11, 2001b.

McMinn, John H., and Max Levin, *The Medical Department: Personnel in World War II*, Washington, D.C.: Office of the Surgeon General, Department of the Army, 1963.

Medical Readiness Division, J-4, *Force Health Protection*, Washington, D.C.: Office of the Joint Chiefs of Staff, 1997.

"Medical Treatment in World War II," Olive-Drab website, undated.

Mendez, Bryce H. P., Alan Ott, Kristy N. Kamarck, Barbara Salaar Torreon, and Lawrence Kapp, *FY2020 National Defense Authorization Act: Selected Military Personnel Issues*, Washington, D.C.: Congressional Research Service, R46107, February 25, 2020.

Menninger, William C., "Neuropsychiatric Problems in the Army," memorandum for Gen. Kirk through Gen. Hillman, dated June 15, 1944, reproduced in Albert J. Glass and Robert J. Bernucci, eds., *Neuropsychiatry in World War I*, Vol. I: *Zone of Interior*, Washington, D.C.: U.S. Government Printing Office, 1966, pp. 807–816.

———, *Psychiatry in a Troubled World: Yesterday's War and Today's Challenge*, New York: The Macmillan Company, 1948.

Menninger, William C., Malcolm J. Farrell, and Henry W. Brosin, "The Consultant System," in Albert J. Glass, and Robert J. Bernucci, eds., *Neuropsychiatry in World War II, Vol. I: Zone of Interior*, Washington, D.C.: U.S. Government Printing Office, 1966, pp. 67–96.

Mental Health Advisory Team IV, *Mental Health Advisory Team (MHAT) IV: Operation Enduring Freedom 05-07*, Fort Sam Houston, Tex.: Office of the Surgeon General, U.S. Army Medical Command, November 17, 2006.

Meredith, Lisa S., Cathy D. Sherbourne, Sarah Gaillot, Lydia Hansell, Hans V. Ritschard, Andrew M. Parker, and Glenda Wrenn, *Promoting Psychological Resilience in the U.S. Military*, Santa Monica, Calif.: RAND Corporation, MG-996-OSD, 2011.

"Mickey Mouse Boots," Olive-Drab website, undated.

Miles, Donna, "Disabled Soldier Support System Helping Wounded Troops," American Forces Press Service, October 20, 2004.

Miller, John C., "Combat Life Saver, Lesson 16: Overview of Combat Life Saver Tasks and Equipment," U.S. Army, 2018.

Miller, Joseph A., "Executive Summary: Advanced Prosthetic Technologies," Washington, D.C.: Walter Reed Medical Center, U.S. Army Amputee Patient Care Program, November 8, 2004.

Miller, Paul D., "Bush on Nation Building and Afghanistan," *Foreign Policy*, November 17, 2010.

Miller, Thomas W., ed., *The Praeger Handbook of Veterans' Health-History, Challenges, Issues, and Developments*, Vol. I: *History, Eras, and Global Healthcare*, Santa Barbara, Calif.: Praeger, 2012.

Milliken, Charles S., Jennifer L. Auchterlonie, and Charles W. Hoge, "Longitudinal Assessment of Mental Health Problems Among Active and Reserve Component Soldiers Returning from the Iraq War," *Journal of the American Medical Association*, Vol. 298, No. 18, November 14, 2007, pp. 2141–2148.

Milner, Samuel, "Trouble Decade: The U.S. Army Medical Service in the Post-World War II and Korea Era," Washington, D.C., U.S. Army Military History Institute, 1964.

Montgomery, G. V. (Sonny), "The Last Thing We Need Now Is to Go Back to the Military Draft," *Washington Post*, December 4, 1990, p. A17.

Moorefield, Kenneth P., *Assessment of DOD Wounded Warrior Matters—Fort Drum*, Washington, D.C.: Deputy Inspector General for Special Plans & Operations, Department of Defense Inspector General, SPO-2011-010, September 30, 2011.

———, *Assessment of DOD Wounded Warrior Matters—Joint Base Lewis-McChord*, Washington, D.C.: Deputy Inspector General for Special Plans & Operations, Department of Defense Inspector General, DODIG-2013-087, May 31, 2013.

Moskos, Charles C., Jr., *The American Enlisted Man: The Rank and File in Today's Military*, New York: Russell Sage Foundation, 1970.

Mullins, Richard J., "A Historical Perspective of Trauma System Development in the United States," *Journal of Trauma: Injury, Infection, and Critical Care*, Vol. 47, No. 3, September Supplement 1999, pp. S8–S14.

Murray, Clinton K., Scott R. Hitter, and Stephen L. Jones, "Army Medical Department at War: Lessons Learned," *Army Medical Department Journal*, April–September 2016, pp. 1–3.

Nathan, Matthew L., and Suzanne Crockett-Jones, *Department of Defense Recovering Warrior Task Force 2013–2014 Annual Report*, Alexandria, Va.: Department of Defense Task Force on the Care, Management, and Transition of Recovering Wounded, Ill, and Injured Members of the Armed Forces, September 2, 2014.

National Academies of Sciences, Engineering, and Medicine, *Veterans and Agent Orange: Update 2014*, Washington, D.C.: National Academies Press, 2016.

National Archives, *Vietnam War U.S. Military Fatal Casualty Statistics: Electronic Records Reference Report*, webpage, as of August 2013.

National Center for PTSD, "Mission and Overview," webpage, undated.

National Center for Veterans Analysis and Statistics, *Profile of Sheltered Homeless Veterans for Fiscal Years 2009 and 2010*, Washington, D.C.: U.S. Department of Veterans Affairs, September 2012.

———, "Unique Veteran Users Profile FY 2015," briefing slides, Washington, D.C.: U.S. Department of Veterans Affairs, December 2016.

———, "VETPOP2016 Living Veterans by Period of Service, Gender, 2015–2045," table, Washington, D.C.: U.S. Department of Veterans Affairs, 2018.

National Military Family Association, "Fact Sheet: Resources for Wounded or Injured Servicemembers and their Families," Alexandria, Va., July 2006.

National Research Council, *Study of Health Care for American Veterans*, Washington, D.C.: U.S. Government Printing Office, June 7, 1977.

Navy Medical Center San Diego, "Comprehensive Combat and Complex Casualty Care," webpage, undated.

Nededog, Jethro, "The 20 Most-Watched TV Show Finales of All Time, Ranked," *Business Insider*, May 16, 2017.

Neel, Spurgeon, *Vietnam Studies: Medical Support of the U.S. Army in Vietnam, 1965–1970*, Washington, D.C.: U.S. Army Medical Department, Office of History, 1991.

Nelson, Colleen McCain, and Ben Kesling, "White House Review of VA Finds 'Corrosive Culture,' Poor Management," *Wall Street Journal*, June 27, 2014.

Nelson, Thomas J., Travis Clark, Eric T. Stedje-Larsen, Christopher T. Lewis, James M. Grueskin, Eddy L. Echols, Derek B. Wall, Erin A. Felger, and Harold R. Bohman, "Close Proximity Blast Injury Patterns from Improvised Explosive Devices in Iraq: A Report of 18 Cases," *Journal of Trauma: Injury, Infection, and Critical Care*, Vol. 65, No. 1, July 2008, pp. 212–217.

Nehmer v. U.S. Veterans Admin., 712 F. Supp. 1404, N.D. Cal., May 3, 1989.

Nichiporuk, Brian, and Carl H. Builder, *Information Technologies and the Future of Land Warfare*, Santa Monica, Calif.: RAND Corporation, MR-560-A, 1995.

Nicosia, Gerald, *Home to War: A History of the Vietnam Veterans' Movement*, New York: Crown Publishers, 2001.

Nixon, Richard M., "The All-Volunteer Armed Force," transcript of a radio address, Washington, D.C.: Republican National Committee, October 17, 1968.

Nolan, David L., "Airborne Tactical Medical Support in Grenada," *Military Medicine*, Vol. 155, No. 3, March 1990, pp. 104–111.

Nunn, Sam, "Remarks by U.S. Senator Sam Nunn Before the Georgia General Assembly," Washington, D.C.: Office of Senator Sam Nunn, March 5, 1973.

———, "Defense Budget Blanks," *Congressional Record*, Vol. 136, No. 32, March 22, 1990.

Obama, Barack, "Statement by the President," Washington, D.C.: The White House, May 30, 2014.

O'Connell, Karen M., Marguerite T. Littleton-Kearney, Elizabeth Bridges, and Sandra C. Bibb, "Evaluating the Joint Theater Trauma Registry as a Data Source to Benchmark Casualty Care," *Military Medicine*, Vol. 177, No. 5, May 2012, pp. 546–552.

Odom, Charles B., "Third U.S. Army," in John Boyde Coates, Jr., ed., *Medical Department of the United States Army in World War II: Activities of Surgical Consultants*, Part II: *Surgical Consultants to Field Armies in Theaters of Operations*, Washington, D.C.: U.S. Army Medical Department, Office of Medical History, 1961.

Office of the Assistant Secretary of Defense for Health Affairs, "Traumatic Brain Injury: Definition and Reporting," memorandum, October 1, 2007.

Office of Management and Budget, "Historical Tables, Budget of the United States Government, Fiscal Year 2015: Gross Domestic Product and Deflators Used in the Historical Tables: 1940–2019," Washington, D.C.: U.S. Government Printing Office, 2015.

Office of the Assistant Secretary of Defense for Force Management and Personnel, *Population Representation in the Military Services: Fiscal Year 1991*, Washington, D.C.: U.S. Department of Defense, October 1992.

Office of the Assistant Secretary of Defense for Manpower, Reserve Affairs and Logistics, *America's Volunteers: A Report on the All-Volunteer Armed Forces*, Washington, D.C., December 31, 1978.

Office of the Assistant Secretary of Defense for Public Affairs, "Use of the Draft Has Ended," press release, Washington, D.C., January 27, 1973.

Office of the Press Secretary, "U.S. Policy on Viet-Nam," press release, Washington, D.C.: The White House, October 3, 1963.

———, "Fact Sheet: Keeping America's Promise to Those Who Have Defended Our Freedom," Washington, D.C.: The White House, November 8, 2007.

———, "Readout of the President's Meeting with Acting Veterans Affairs Secretary Sloan Gibson and Rob Nabors," Washington, D.C.: The White House, June 27, 2014.

Office of the Special Assistant to the Deputy Secretary of Defense for Gulf War Illnesses, GulfLINK website, undated.

———, *Annual Report: November 1996–November 1997*, Washington, D.C.: U.S. Department of Defense, January 6, 1998.

———, *Third Report: November 1998–November 1999*, Washington, D.C.: U.S. Department of Defense, 2000.

Office of the Surgeon General, "Army Returns Handicapped Veterans to Full Duty Position," Washington, D.C.: U.S. Department of Defense, October 12, 1951.

Office of the Surgeon General, Army Service Forces, "Nomenclature of Psychiatric Disorders and Reactions," *Journal of Clinical Psychology*, Vol. 57, No. 7, [1946] 2000, pp. 925–934.

Office of the Surgeon General, Department of the Army, "Infrastructure Improvement for the U.S. Army Amputee Patient Care Program," report to Congress, Falls Church, Va., January 20, 2004.

Office of the Surgeon General, U.S. Army Medical Command, *Joint Mental Health Advisory Team 7 (J-MHAT 7): Operation Enduring Freedom 2010 Afghanistan*, Fort Sam Houston, Tex., February 22, 2011.

———, *Mental Health Advisory Team 9 (J-MHAT 9): Operation Enduring Freedom 2013 Afghanistan*, Fort Sam Houston, Tex., October 10, 2013.

Office of the Under Secretary of Defense for Personnel and Readiness, *Population Representation in the Military Services: Fiscal Year 2001*, Washington, D.C., March 2003.

———, *Population Representation in the Military Services: Fiscal Year 2014*, Washington, D.C., March 2016.

Official Data Foundation/Alioth LLC, CPI Inflation Calculator website, 2019.

O'Hanlon, Michael E., "History Will Credit Shinseki," *Japan Times*, June 19, 2003.

Okie, Susan, "Traumatic Brain Injury in the War Zone," *New England Journal of Medicine*, Vol. 352, No. 20, May 19, 2005, pp. 2043–2047.

Operation Iraqi Freedom Mental Health Advisory Team, *Report to the U.S. Army Surgeon General & HQDA G-1*, December 16, 2003.

Oritz, Jose M., "The Revolutionary Flying Ambulance of Napoleon's Surgeon," *Army Medical Department Journal*, October–December 1998, pp. 17–25.

OSAGWI—*See* Office of the Special Assistant to the Deputy Secretary of Defense for Gulf War Illnesses.

Otis, George A., and D. L. Huntington, *The Medical and Surgical History of the War of the Rebellion*, Part III, Vol. II: *Surgical History*, Washington, D.C.: U.S. Government Printing Office, 1883.

Owens, Brett D., John F. Kragh, Jr., Joseph C. Wenke, Joseph Macaitis, Charles E. Wade, and John B. Holcomb, "Combat Wounds in Operation Iraqi Freedom and Operation Enduring Freedom," *Journal of Trauma: Injury, Infection, and Critical Care*, Vol. 64, No. 2, 2008, pp. 295–299.

PAC—*See* Presidential Advisory Committee on Gulf War Veterans' Illnesses.

Page, Thomas N., and Spurgeon H. Neel, "Army Aeromedical Evacuation," *U.S. Armed Forces Medical Journal*, Vol. 8, No. 8, August 1957, pp. 1195–1200.

Palmer, Robert R., Bell I. Wiley, and William R. Keast, "The Army Specialized Training Program and the Army Ground Forces," *The Army Ground Forces: The Procurement and Training of Ground Combat Troops*, reprint, Washington, D.C.: Historical Section, Army Ground Forces Historical Division, Department of the Army, 1948, pp. 28–39.

Panangala, Sidath Viranga, *Veterans' Health Care Issues in the 109th Congress*, Washington, D.C.: Congressional Research Service, RL32961, October 26, 2006.

———, *The Veterans Choice Program (VCP): Program Implementation*, Washington, D.C.: Congressional Research Service, R44562, January 5, 2017.

Panangala, Sidath Viranga, and Daniel T. Shedd, *Veterans Exposed to Agent Orange: Legislative History, Litigation, and Current Issues*, Washington, D.C.: Congressional Research Service, R43790, November 18, 2014.

Panangala, Sidath Viranga, Daniel T. Shedd, and Umar Moulta-Ali, *Veterans Affairs: Presumptive Service Connection and Disability Compensation*, Washington, D.C.: Congressional Research Service, R41405, November 18, 2014.

Panangala, Sidath Viranga, and Jared S. Sussman, "Introduction to Veterans Health Care," information sheet, Washington, D.C.: Congressional Research Service, updated October 24, 2019.

Parker, Gary W., and Frank M. Batha, Jr., *A History of Marine Observation Squadron Six*, Washington, D.C.: Headquarters, U.S. Marine Corps, History and Museums Division, 1982.

Pash, Melinda L., *In the Shadow of the Greatest Generation: The Americans Who Fought the Korean War*, New York: New York University Press, 2012.

Pasquina, Paul F., "DOD Paradigm Shift in Care of Servicemembers with Major Limb Loss," *Journal of Rehabilitation Research & Development*, Vol. 47, No. 4, 2010, pp. xi–xiv.

Pasquina, Paul F., Charles R. Scoville, Brian Belnap, and Rory A. Cooper, "Introduction: Developing a System of Care for the Combat Amputee," in Paul F. Pasquina and Rory A. Cooper, eds., *Care of the Combat Amputee*, Washington, D.C.: Borden Institute, Walter Reed Army Medical Center, 2009.

Patel, Tarak H., Kimberly A. Wenner, Shaun A. Price, Michael A. Weber, Autumn Leveridge, and Scott J. McAtee, "A U.S. Army Forward Surgical Team's Experience in Operation Iraqi Freedom," *Journal of Trauma: Injury, Infection, and Critical Care*, Vol. 57, No. 2, August 2004, pp. 201–207.

Peoples, George E., Tad Gerlinger, Robert Craig, and Brian Burlingame, "The 274th Forward Surgical Team Experience During Operation Enduring Freedom," *Military Medicine*, Vol. 170, No. 6, June 2005a, pp. 451–459.

———, "Combat Casualties in Afghanistan Cared for by a Single Forward Surgical Team During the Initial Phases of Operation Enduring Freedom," *Military Medicine*, Vol. 170, No. 6, June 2005b, pp. 462–468.

Pereira, Bruno M. T., Mark L. Ryan, Michael P. Ogilvie, Juan Carlos Gomez-Rodriguez, Patrick McAndrew, George D. Garcia, and Kenneth G. Proctor, "Predeployment Mass Casualty and Clinical Trauma Training for US Army Forward Surgical Teams," *Journal of Craniofacial Surgery*, Vol. 21, No. 4, July 2010, pp. 982–986.

Perkins, Jeremy G., and Alec C. Beekley, "Damage Control Resuscitation," in Eric Savitsky and Brian Eastridge, eds., *Combat Casualty Care: Lessons Learned from OEF and OIF*, Falls Church, Va.: Department of the Army, Office of the Surgeon General, 2012.

Perry, Walter L., Richard E. Darilek, Laurinda L. Rohn, and Jerry M. Sollinger, *Operation Iraqi Freedom: Decisive War, Elusive Peace*, Santa Monica, Calif.: RAND Corporation, RR-1214-A, 2015.

Peters, Heidi M., Moshe Schwartz, and Lawrence Kapp, *Department of Defense Contractor and Troop Levels in Iraq and Afghanistan: 2007–2016*, Washington, D.C.: Congressional Research Service, R44116, August 15, 2016.

Peterson, Donald B., and Rawley B. Chambers, "Restatement of Combat Psychiatry," *American Journal of Psychiatry*, Vol. 109, No. 4, October 1952, pp. 249–254.

Peterson, Leonard T., "Orthopedic Surgery," in John Boyd Coates, Jr., and B. Noland Carter, eds., *Medical Department of United States Army Surgery in World War II: Activities of Surgical Consultants*, Vol. I, Washington, D.C.: Office of the Surgeon General, Department of the Army, 1962, pp. 49–64.

Peterson, Robert A., *Summary of Statement of Robert A. Peterson, Senior Associate Director, Human Resources Division, Before the United States Senate on Agent Orange*, Washington, D.C.: U.S. General Accounting Office, November 18, 1981.

Philipps, Dave, "Pattern of Misconduct: Psychological Screenings Prompt Call for More Reforms," *Colorado Springs Gazette*, October 7, 2013.

———, "Veterans Want Past Discharges to Recognize Post-Traumatic Stress," *New York Times*, February 22, 2016, p. A9.

Philipps, Dave, and Nicholas Fandos, "Intrigue at V.A. as Secretary Says He Is Being Forced Out," *New York Times*, February 18, 2018.

Phillips, R. Cody, *Operation Joint Guardian: The U.S. Army in Kosovo*, Washington, D.C.: U.S. Army Center of Military History, 2007.

Philpott, Tom, "Group 8 Vets Invited Back to VA," American Legion website, September 16, 2009.

Place, Ronald J., Robert M. Rush, Jr., and Edward D. Arrington, "Forward Surgical Team (FST) Workload in a Special Operations Environment: The 250th FST in Operation Enduring Freedom," *Current Surgery*, Vol. 60, No. 4, July/August 2003, pp. 418–422.

Place, Ronald J., Clifford A. Porter, Kenneth Azarow, and Alan L. Beitler, "Trauma Experience Comparison of Army Forward Surgical Team Surgeons at Ben Taub Hospital and Madigan Army Medical Center," *Current Surgery*, Vol. 58, No. 1, January/February 2001, pp. 90–93.

Pleeter, Saul, *Military Compensation Background Papers*, 6th ed., Washington, D.C.: Office of the Under Secretary for Personnel and Readiness, 2005.

Polly, David W., "Amputee Care Center: Summary of Current Plan for Battle Casualty Research at WRAMC," information paper, Washington, D.C.: Walter Reed Medical Center, Amputee Care Center, June 7, 2003.

Polly, David W., Tamara J. LaFrancois, Jeff M. Gambel, Barbara J. Birnesser, and Joseph A. Miller, "The U.S. Army Amputee Care Program," Washington, D.C.: Walter Reed Medical Center, Amputee Care Center, August 7, 2003.

Polo, James A., *Reform of the Army Physical Disability Evaluation System*, Carlisle Barracks, Pa.: U.S. Army War College, 2009.

Poston, Walker S. C., Christopher K. Haddock, Sara A. Jahnke, and Nattinee Jitnarin, "What Do Veterans Service Organizations' Web Sites Say About Tobacco Control?" *American Journal of Health Promotion*, Vol. 28, No. 2, November/December 2013, pp. 88–96.

Pratt, Jerry W., and Robert M. Rush, Jr., "The Military Surgeon and the War on Terrorism: A Zollinger Legacy," *American Journal of Surgery*, Vol. 186, 2003, pp. 292–295.

"President Signs Legislation Authorizing Priority Treatment," *Persian Gulf Review*, Vol. 2, No. 1, September 1994, p. 4.

Presidential Advisory Committee on Gulf War Veterans' Illnesses, *Final Report*, Washington, D.C.: U.S. Government Printing Office, December 1996.

———, *Special Report*, Washington, D.C., October 31, 1997.

President's Commission on Care for America's Returning Wounded Warriors [Dole-Shalala Commission], *Serve, Support, Simplify*, July 2007a.

———, *Serve, Support, Simplify: Subcommittee Reports & Survey Findings*, July 30, 2007b.

President's Commission on Veterans' Pensions [Bradley Commission], *Findings and Recommendations: Veterans' Benefits in the United States*, Washington, D.C., April 1956a.

———, *The Historical Development of Veterans' Benefits in the United States: A Report on Veterans' Benefits in the United States*, Washington, D.C.: U.S. Government Printing Office, Staff Report 1, May 9, 1956b.

———, *Veterans in Our Society: Data on the Conditions of Military Service and on the Status of the Veteran*, Washington, D.C.: U.S. Government Printing Office, Staff Report 4, June 21, 1956c.

———, *The Veterans' Administration Disability Rating Schedule: Historical Development and Medical Appraisal—A Report on Veterans' Benefits in the United States*, Washington, D.C.: U.S. Government Printing Office, Staff Report 8, Part B, July 18, 1956d.

———, *Compensation for Service-Connected Disabilities: A Report on Veterans' Benefits in the United States*, Washington, D.C.: U.S. Government Printing Office, Staff Report 8, Part A, August 3, 1956e.

————, *Veterans' Non–Service-Connected Pensions: A Report on Veterans' Benefits in the United States*, Washington, D.C.: U.S. Government Printing House, Staff Report 10, August 27, 1956f.

President's New Freedom Commission on Mental Health, *Achieving the Promise: Transforming Mental Health Care in America*, Rockville, Md., July 22, 2003.

Priest, Dana, and Anne Hull, "Soldiers Face Neglect, Frustration at Army's Top Medical Facility," *Washington Post*, February 18, 2007.

Principi, Anthony J., "Illnesses Not Associated with Service in the Gulf During the Gulf War," *Federal Register*, Vol. 66, No. 130, 2001, pp. 35702–35710.

Pruitt, Basil A., Jr., "The Symbiosis of Combat Casualty Care and Civilian Trauma Care: 1914–2007," *Journal of Trauma: Injury, Infection, and Critical Care*, Vol. 64, No. 2, February Supplement 2008, pp. S4–S8.

"Psychologists, MH Groups Attack Vietnam War," *Psychiatric News*, July 5, 1972.

Pub. L.—*See* Public Law.

Public Law 66-190, *An Act to Revise and Equalize Rates of Pension to Certain Soldiers, Sailors, and Marines of the Civil War and the War with Mexico, to Certain Widows, Including Widows of the War of 1812, Former Widows, Dependent Parents, and Children of Such Soldiers, Sailors, and Marines, and to Certain Army Nurses, and Granting Pensions and Increase of Pensions in Certain Cases*, May 1, 1920.

Public Law 67-47, *Veterans' Bureau Act*, August 9, 1921.

Public Law 68-242, *World War Veterans Act of 1924*, June 7, 1924.

Public Law 77-140, *To Provide for the Discharge or Retirement of Enlisted Men of the Regular Army and of the Philippine Scouts in Certain Cases*, June 30, 1941.

Public Law 78-346, *Servicemen's Readjustment Act of 1944*, June 22, 1944.

Public Law 80-253, *National Security Act of 1947*, July 26, 1947.

Public Law 81-351, *Career Compensation Act of 1949*, October 12, 1949.

Public Law 81-779, *Selective Service Act of 1948, Amendment*, September 9, 1950.

Public Law 82-28, *Joint Resolution to Provide Certain Benefits for Certain Persons Who Shall Have Served in the Armed Forces of the United States on and After June 27, 1950*, May 11, 1951.

Public Law 82-488, *Department of Defense Appropriation Act, 1953*, Title VII, *Combat Duty Pay Act of 1952*, July 10, 1952.

Public Law 82-550, *Veterans Readjustment Assistance Act of 1952*, July 16, 1952.

Public Law 84-182, *Mental Health Study Act of 1955*, July 28, 1955.

Public Law 86-211, *Veterans' Pension Act of 1959*, August 29, 1959.

Public Law 86-639, *Veterans Medical Services Act*, July 12, 1960.

Public Law 88-408, *Joint Resolution to Promote the Maintenance of International Peace and Security in Southeast Asia [Gulf of Tonkin Resolution]*, August 10, 1964.

Public Law 89-358, *Veterans' Readjustment Benefits Act of 1966*, March 3, 1966.

Public Law 90-77, *Veterans' Pension and Readjustment Assistance Act of 1967*, August 31, 1967.

Public Law 91-441, *Armed Forces: Appropriation Authorization, 1971*, October 7, 1970.

Public Law 92-129, *Military Selective Service Act of 1967 Amendments*, September 28, 1971.

Public Law 92-426, *Uniformed Services Health Professionals Act of 1972*, September 21, 1972.

Public Law 93-274, *Uniformed Services, Medical Officers, Revised Pay Structure [Uniformed Services Variable Incentive Pay Act for Physicians]*, May 6, 1974.

Public Law 96-22, *Veterans' Health Care Amendments of 1979*, June 13, 1979.

Public Law 97-72, *Veterans' Health Care, Training, and Small Business Loan Act of 1981*, November 3, 1981.

Public Law 98-223, *Veterans' Compensation and Program Improvement Amendments of 1984*, March 2, 1984.

Public Law 98-528, *Veterans' Health Care Act of 1984*, October 19, 1984.

Public Law 98-542, *Veterans' Dioxin and Radiation Exposure Compensation Standards Act*, October 24, 1984.

Public Law 99-433, *Goldwater-Nichols Department of Defense Reorganization Act of 1986*, October 1, 1986.

Public Law 102-4, *Agent Orange Act of 1991*, February 6, 1991.

Pulbic Law 102-585, *Veterans Health Care Act of 1992*, November 4, 1992.

Public Law 103-210, *An Act to Amend Title 38, United States Code, to Provide Additional Authority for the Secretary of Veterans Affairs to Provide Health Care for Veterans of the Persian Gulf War*, December 20, 1993.

Public Law 103-446, *Veterans' Benefits Improvement Act of 1994*, November 2, 1994.

Public Law 104-106, *National Defense Authorization Act for Fiscal Year 1996*, February 10, 1996.

Public Law 104-262, *Veterans' Health Care Eligibility Reform Act of 1996*, October 9, 1996.

Public Law 107-103, *Veterans Education and Benefits Expansion Act of 2001*, December 27, 2001.

Public Law 108-136, *National Defense Authorization Act for Fiscal Year 2004*, November 24, 2003.

Public Law 109-163, *National Defense Authorization Act for Fiscal Year 2006*, January 6, 2006.

Public Law 110-181, *National Defense Authorization Act for Fiscal Year 2008*, January 28, 2008.

Public Law 110-417, *Duncan Hunter National Defense Authorization Act for Fiscal Year 2009*, October 14, 2008.

Public Law 111-84, *National Defense Authorization Act for Fiscal Year 2010*, October 28, 2009.

Public Law 111-163, *Caregivers and Veterans Omnibus Health Services Act of 2010*, May 5, 2010.

Public Law 113-146, *Veterans' Access, Choice, and Accountability Act of 2014*, August 7, 2014.

Public Law 114-92, *National Defense Authorization Act for Fiscal Year 2016*, November 25, 2015.

Public Law 115-182, *John S. McCain III, Daniel K. Akaka, and Samuel R. Johnson VA Maintaining Internal Systems and Strengthening Integrated Outside Networks Act of 2018 [VA MISSION Act of 2018]*, June 6, 2018.

Quigley, Samantha L., "Troops, Families to Benefit from New Center for Injured," *American Forces Press Service*, February 2, 2005.

"R-4 Sikorsky Helicopter," Olive-Drab website, undated.

Ramchand, Rajeev, Rena Rudavsky, Sean Grant, Terri Tanielian, and Lisa Jaycox, "Prevalence of, Risk Factors for, and Consequences of Posttraumatic Stress Disorder and Other Mental Health Problems in Military Populations Deployed to Iraq and Afghanistan," *Current Psychiatry Reports*, Vol. 17, No. 5, May 2015.

Ramchand, Rajeev, Terri Tanielian, Michael P. Fisher, Christine Anne Vaughan, Thomas E. Trail, Caroline Epley, Phoenix Voorhies, Michael William Robbins, Eric Robinson, and Bonnie Ghosh-Dastidar, *Hidden Heroes: America's Military Caregivers*, Santa Monica, Calif.: RAND Corporation, RR-499-TEDF, 2014.

RAND Corporation, "Gulf War Illness," webpage, undated.

Rasmussen, Todd E., David G. Baer, Andrew P. Cap, and Brian C. Lein, "Ahead of the Curve: Sustained Innovation for Future Combat Casualty Care," *Journal of Trauma and Acute Care Surgery*, Vol. 79, No. 4, Supplement 1, 2015, pp. S61–S63.

Rasmussen, Todd E., and Kenneth J. Cherry, Jr., "Historical Perspectives in Vascular Surgery, Military Vascular Surgery," in John W. Hallett, Jr., Joseph L. Mills, Sr., Jonothan J. Earnshaw, Jim A. Reekers, and Thom W. Rooke, eds., *Comprehensive Vascular and Endovascular Surgery*, Amsterdam: Elsevier, 2009.

Ravage, Barbara, "As Real as It Gets: The Evolution of Trauma Care and Emergency Medicine," *Safety Net*, Vol. 20, No. 1, Spring 2006, pp. 14–17.

Rearden, Steven L., *The Formative Years: 1947–1950*, Washington, D.C.: Office of the Secretary of Defense, 1984.

Recovering Warrior Task Force, *Charter of the Department of Defense Task Force on the Care, Management, and Transition of Recovering Wounded, Ill, and Injured Members of the Armed Forces*, Washington, D.C.: U.S. Department of Defense, November 20, 2012.

Rehabilitation of Lower Limb Amputation Working Group, *VA/DoD Clinical Practice Guideline for Rehabilitation of Lower Limb Amputation*, Washington, D.C.: Department of Veterans Affairs and Department of Defense, 2007.

Reiber, Gayle E., Lynne V. McFarland, Sharon Hubbard, Charles Maynard, David K. Blough, Jeffrey M. Gambel, and Douglas G. Smith, "Servicemembers and Veterans with Major Traumatic Limb Loss from Vietnam War and OIF/OEF Conflicts: Survey Methods, Participants, and Summary Findings," *Journal of Rehabilitation Research & Development*, Vol. 47, No. 4, 2010, pp. 275–297.

Reister, Frank A., *Battle Casualties and Medical Statistics: U.S. Army Experience in the Korea War*, Washington, D.C.: U.S. Army Medical Department, Office of Medical History, 1973.

———, *Medical Statistics in World War II*, Washington, D.C.: Office of the Surgeon General, Department of the Army, 1975.

Remick, Kyle N., "The Surgical Resuscitation Team: Surgical Trauma Support U.S. Army Special Operations Forces," *Journal of Special Operations Medicine*, Vol. 9, No. 4, Fall 2009, pp. 20–25.

Research Advisory Committee on Gulf War Veterans' Illnesses, *Gulf War Illness and the Health of Gulf War Veterans: Scientific Findings and Recommendations*, Washington, D.C.: U.S. Government Printing Office, November 2008.

Reston, James, "The Meaning of Vienna," *New York Times*, June 10, 1979.

Reynolds, Gary K., *U.S. Prisoners of War and Civilian American Citizens Captured and Interned by Japan in World War II: The Issue of Compensation by Japan*, Washington, D.C.: Congressional Research Service, RL30606, December 17, 2002.

Reznick, Jeffrey S., Jeff Gambel, and Alan J. Hawk, "Historical Perspectives on the Care of Service Members with Limb Amputations," in Paul F. Pasquina and Rory A. Cooper, eds., *Care of the Combat Amputee*, Washington, D.C.: Borden Institute, Walter Reed Army Medical Center, 2009.

Rice, Donald B., *Defense Resource Management Study: Final Report*, Washington, D.C.: U.S. Government Printing Office, February 1979.

Ricks, Thomas E., and Walter Pincus, "Pentagon Plans Major Changes in U.S. Strategy; Rumsfeld Envisions Shift in Size, Focus of Military," *Washington Post*, May 7, 2001.

Ritchie, Elspeth Cameron, "Psychiatry in the Korean War: Perils, PIES, and Prisoners of War," *Military Medicine*, Vol. 167, No. 11, November 2002, pp. 898–903.

———, "Foreword," in Elspeth Cameron Ritchie, ed., *Combat and Operational Behavioral Health* Washington, D.C.: Borden Institute, Walter Reed Army Medical Center, 2011.

Rivera, Mario A., "Eagle DUSTOFF and JTTS Make Army Medicine History in Afghanistan," webpage, U.S. Army, 2014.

Robertson, Robert E., *Military Disability System: Improved Oversight Needed to Ensure Consistent and Timely Outcomes for Reserve and Active Duty Service Members*, Washington, D.C.: U.S. Government Accountability Office, GAO-06-362, March 2006.

Rogers, Frederick B., and Katelyn Rittenhouse, "The Golden Hour in Trauma: Dogma or Medical Folklore?" *Journal of Lancaster General Hospital*, No. 9, Spring 2014, p. 1.

Roosevelt, Franklin Delano, "Medical Discharge from the Armed Forces," memorandum to the Secretary of War, Washington, D.C.: The White House, December 4, 1944.

Ross, James W., *Study of Vehicle Transportation Requirements for Hospitals at the Corps Level*, thesis, Wright-Patterson Air Force Base, Ohio: Air Force Institute of Technology, Air University, 1990.

Rostker, Bernard D., *Air Reserve Forces Personnel Study*: Vol. I, *The Personnel Structure and Posture of the Air National Guard and the Air Force Reserve*, Santa Monica: RAND Corporation, R-1049-PR, 1973, p. 37.

———, *I Want You: The Evolution of the All-Volunteer Force*, Santa Monica, Calif.: RAND Corporation, MG-265-RC, 2007.

———, *Providing for the Casualties of War: The American Experience Through World War II*, Santa Monica, Calif.: RAND Corporation, MG-1164-OSD, 2013.

Rudman, Warren B., *Special Oversight Board for Defense Department Investigation of Gulf War Chemical and Biological Incidents: Final Report*, Washington, D.C.: Executive Office of the President, December 20, 2000.

Rumsfeld, Donald H., "Defense Strategy Review," testimony before the Senate Armed Services Committee," transcript, ProQuest Congressional website, June 21, 2001.

———, *Known and Unknown: A Memoir*, New York: Sentinel, 2011.

Rush, Robert M., Jr., Neil R. Stockmaster, Harry K. Stinger, Edward D. Arrington, John G. Devine, Linda Atteberry, Benjamin W. Starnes, and Ronald J. Place, "Supporting the Global War on Terror: A Tale of Two Campaigns Featuring the 250th Forward Surgical Team (Airborne)," *American Journal of Surgery*, Vol. 189, 2005, pp. 564–570.

Rusk, Howard A., "'Doctor Draft' Law Change to Confront New Congress: Current Legislation, Held Discriminatory by Medical Association, Terminates on July 1," *New York Times*, November 9, 1952.

Salmon, Thomas W., *The Care and Treatment of Mental Diseases and War Neuroses ("Shell Shock") in the British Army*, New York: War Work Committee of the National Committee for Mental Hygiene, Inc., 1917.

Salmon, Thomas W., and Norman Fenton, "Neuropsychiatry in the American Expeditionary Forces," in Frank W. Weed, ed., *The Medical Department of the United States Army in the World War*, Vol. X: *Neuropsychiatry*, Washington, D.C.: Office of the Surgeon General, Department of the Army, 1929.

Samet, Jonathan M., and Catherine C. Bodurow, eds., *Improving the Presumptive Disability Decision-Making Process for Veterans*, Washington, D.C.: National Academies Press, 2008.

Sanchez, Justin, "Revolutionizing Prosthetics," Defense Advanced Research Projects Agency website, undated.

Sandler, Stanley, *The Korean War: No Victors, No Vanquished*, Lexington, Ky.: University Press of Kentucky, 1999.

Sarka, Rudolph A., "Evacuation at Soksa-ri," in John G. Westover, ed., *Combat Support in Korea*, Part V: *Medical Support*, Washington, D.C.: U.S. Army Center of Military History, 955 (online version of 1987, 1990 reprint).

Scales, Robert H., Jr., *Certain Victory: United States Army in the Gulf War*, Washington, D.C.: Office of the Chief of Staff, U.S. Army 1993.

Schell, Terry L., and Grant N. Marshall, "Survey of Individuals Previously Deployed for OEF/OIF," in Terri Tanielian and Lisa H. Jaycox, eds., *Invisible Wounds of War: Psychological and Cognitive Injuries, Their Consequences, and Services to Assist Recovery*, Santa Monica, Calif.: RAND Corporation, 2008, pp. 87–115.

Schneider, Brett J., John C. Bradley, and David M. Benedek, "Psychiatric Medications for Deployment: An Update," *Military Medicine*, Vol. 172, No. 7, July 2007, pp. 681–685.

Schneider, Brett J., John C. Bradley, Christopher H. Warner, and David M. Benedek, "Psychiatric Medications in Military Operations," in Elspeth Cameron Ritchie, ed., *Combat and Operational Behavioral Health*, Washington, D.C.: Borden Institute, Walter Reed Army Medical Center, 2011.

Schoenfeld, Andrew J., "The Combat Experience of Military Surgical Assets in Iraq and Afghanistan: A Historical Review," *American Journal of Surgery*, Vol. 204, No. 3, September 2012, pp. 377–383.

Schoenhard, William, "Inappropriate Scheduling Practices," memorandum to Network Director (10N1-23), Washington, D.C., April 26, 2010.

Scholten, Joel, and Douglas Bidelspach, "VA TBI Screening and Evaluation Program," briefing slides, Washington, D.C.: Veterans Health Administration, 2016.

Schubert, Frank N., and Theresa L. Kraus, eds., *The Whirlwind War: The United States Army in Operations Desert Shield and Desert Storm*, Washington, D.C.: U.S. Army Center of Military History, 1995.

Schuck, Peter H., *Agent Orange on Trial: Mass Toxic Disaster in the Courts*, Cambridge, Mass.: Belknap Press, 1986.

Scott, Christine, *Veterans Affairs: Historical Budget Authority, FY 1940–FY 2012*, Washington, D.C.: Congressional Research Service, RS22897, June 13, 2012.

Scott, Christine, Sidath Viranga Panangala, Sarah A. Lister, and Charles A. Henning, *Disability Evaluation of Military Servicemembers*, Washington, D.C.: Congressional Research Service, RL33991, May 7, 2007.

Scott, Wilbur J., *Vietnam Veterans Since the War: The Politics of PTSD, Agent Orange and the National Memorial*, Norman, Okla.: University of Oklahoma Press, 1993.

Scoville, Charles, "Amputee Care: Summary of Current Plan for the Care of Amputee Patients," information paper, Falls Church, Va., Office of the Surgeon General of the Army, November 29, 2001a.

———, "Recommendations for Care of War Amputees," draft executive summary, Washington, D.C.: Office of the Surgeon General of the Army, October 16, 2001b.

———, "Care of Active Duty Persons with Lower Limb Amputations at a MEDCEN," table, Washington, D.C.: Walter Reed Medical Center, Amputee Patient Care Center, April 5, 2002a.

———, "Guidelines for Managements of War Amputees: To Establish a Uniform Approach to Treatment of Patients Requiring Amputation of an Extremity Following War Trauma," Washington, D.C.: Walter Reed Medical Center, Amputee Patient Care Center, April 4, 2002b.

———, "Amputee Care Center—Updated Information to the Amputee Patient Care Board of Directors," information paper, Washington, D.C.: Walter Reed Medical Center, Amputee Patient Care Center, November 13, 2003a.

———, "Amputee Care Center: Update on the Care of Amputee Patients at Walter Reed Army Medical Center," information paper, Washington, D.C.: Walter Reed Medical Center, Amputee Care Center, October 21, 2003b.

———, "Amputee Patient Registry and Follow Up Programs " information paper, Washington, D.C.: Walter Reed Medical Center, Amputee Care Center, October 30, 2003c.

———, "Army and VA Collaboration on Amputee Care," information paper, Washington, D.C.: Walter Reed Medical Center, Amputee Care Center, September 26, 2003d.

———, "The Team Approach to Amputee Rehabilitation," information paper, Washington, D.C.: Walter Reed Medical Center, Amputee Care Center, October 29, 2003e.

———, "US Army Amputee Patient Care Program Update," information paper, Washington, D.C.: Walter Reed Medical Center, Amputee Patient Care Center, December 11, 2003f.

———, "Walter Reed Amputee Center Infrastructure Improvement Plan," information paper, Washington, D.C.: Walter Reed Medical Center, Amputee Patient Care Center, December 31, 2003g.

———, "Wounding Patterns Resulting from Military Conflict," information paper, Washington, D.C.: Walter Reed Medical Center, Amputee Patient Care Center, November 26, 2003h.

———, "The Military Amputee Patient Care Program," information paper, Washington, D.C.: Walter Reed Medical Center, Amputee Patient Care Center, March 26, 2004a.

———, "Military Amputee Patient Care Program—Update on Amputee Patient Care," information paper, Washington, D.C.: Walter Reed Medical Center, Amputee Patient Care Center, March 26, 2004b.

———, "Prosthetic Costs," Washington, D.C.: Walter Reed Medical Center, Amputee Patient Care Center, June 17, 2004c.

———, "Current Information on the Amputee Patient Care Program " information paper, Washington, D.C.: Walter Reed Medical Center, Amputee Care Center, March 1, 2005a.

———, "Fisher Foundation," executive summary, Washington, D.C.: Walter Reed Medical Center, Amputee Care Center, June 2, 2005b.

———, "Fisher Foundation II," executive summary, Washington, D.C.: Walter Reed Medical Center, Amputee Care Center, June 28, 2005c.

———, "Walter Reed Army Medical Center Military Amputee Training Center," information paper, Washington, D.C.: Walter Reed Medical Center, Amputee Care Center, September 14, 2005d.

———, "Amputee Patient Care," Washington, D.C.: Office of the Surgeon General of the Army, 2006a.

———, "Military Amputee Training Center (MATC) Project and BRAC," information paper, Washington, D.C.: Walter Reed Medical Center, Amputee Care Center, January 26, 2006b.

———, "Military Amputee Training Center (MATC) Project and BRAC II," information paper, Washington, D.C.: Walter Reed Medical Center, Amputee Care Center, August 24, 2006c.

———, "Armed Forces Amputee Patient Care Program: Briefing Presented at the Annual Meeting of the American College of Sports Medicine," Washington, D.C.: Walter Reed Army Medical Center, May 31, 2007a.

———, "Current Information on the Amputee Patient Care," information paper, Washington, D.C.: Walter Reed Medical Center, Amputee Care Center, March 20, 2007b.

———, "Military Advanced Training Center, Walter Reed Army Medical Center," information paper, Washington, D.C.: Walter Reed Medical Center, Amputee Care Center, March 5, 2007c.

"Secretary Brown Establishes 'Blue Ribbon' Panel; Group Met in May to Consider Medical Problems Faced by Persian Gulf Veterans," *Persian Gulf Review*, Vol. 1, No. 3, September 1993, p. 1.

"Secretary Brown Praises Congress for Passage of Persian Gulf Legislation," *Persian Gulf Review*, Vol. 3, No. 1, January 1995, p. 1.

Secretary of War, "Statement by the Secretary of War on War Department Demobilization Plan," Washington, D.C.: Department of War, May 10, 1945.

Selective Service System, "Induction Statistics," webpage, undated.

"Senator Credits UPI Report on Poor GI Care," United Press International, November 6, 2003.

Shambora, William, "What Changes of a Basic Nature, if any, Should Be Made in the American Division and Corps Medical Regiments, and in the American Type Army Medical Service," Ft. Leavenworth, Kan., U.S. Army Command and General Staff School, March 29, 1935.

Shane, Leo, III, "Once a Fixed Issue, the VA Disability Claims Backlog Is on the Rise Again," *Military Times*, March 24, 2017.

Shanker, Thom, "Gates Seeks to Improve Battlefield Trauma Care in Afghanistan," *New York Times*, January 27, 2009.

Shatan, Chaim F., "Post-Vietnam Syndrome," *New York Times*, May 6, 1972, p. 35.

———, "The Grief of Soldiers: Vietnam Combat Veterans' Self-Help Movement," *American Journal of Orthopsychiatry*, Vol. 43, No. 4, July 1973.

———, "Stress Disorder and DSM-III," memorandum to Vietnam Veterans Working Group, March 5, 1978.

Shay, Jonathan, *Achilles in Vietnam: Combat Trauma and the Undoing of Character*, New York: Atheneum, 1994.

———, *Odysseus in America: Combat Trauma and the Trials of Homecoming*, New York: Scribner, 2002.

Shephard, Ben, *A War of Nerves: Soldiers and Psychiatrists in the Twentieth Century*, Cambridge, Mass.: Harvard University Press, 2001.

Shulkin, David J., "Beyond the VA Crisis—Becoming a High-Performance Network," *New England Journal of Medicine*, Vol. 374, No. 11, March 17, 2016, pp. 1003–1005.

———, "Privatizing the V.A. Will Hurt Veterans," *New York Times*, March 28, 2018.

Sigford, Barbara J., "Paradigm Shift for VA Amputation Care," *Journal of Rehabilitation Research & Development*, Vol. 47, No. 4, 2010, pp. xv–xix.

Silas, Sharon M., "Veterans Health Care: VA Needs to Address Challenges as It Implements the Veterans Community Care Program," testimony before the Committee on Veteran's Affairs, U.S. Senate, April 10, 2019.

Sinitski, Emily H., Edward D. Lemaire, and Natalie Baddour, "Evaluation of Motion Platform Embedded with Force Plate-Instrumented Treadmill," *Journal of Rehabilitation Research & Development*, Vol. 52, No. 2, 2015, pp. 221–234.

Sisk, Richard, "A Million Veterans Have Looked Into Private Care Since Mission Act Rollout," Military.com website, September 25, 2019.

Sisson Mobility Restoration Center, "C-Leg," undated.

Smith, Clarence McKittrick, *The Medical Department: Hospitalization and Evacuation, Zone of Interior*, Washington, D.C.: Office of the Chief of Military History, Department of the Army, 1956.

Smith, Douglas G., and Gayle E. Reiber, "VA Paradigm Shift in Care of Veterans with Limb Loss," *Journal of Rehabilitation Research & Development*, Vol. 47, No. 4, 2010, pp. vii–x.

Smith, John Russell, "Rap Groups and Group Therapy for Viet Nam Veterans," in Stephen M. Sonnenberg, Arthur S. Blank, Jr., and John A. Talbott, eds., *The Trauma of War: Stress and Recovery in Vietnam Veterans*, Washington, D.C.: American Psychiatric Press, 1985.

Smith, Ray, "Casualties—US vs NVA/VC," webpage, January 23, 2000.

Smith, Robert Ross, *Triumph in the Philippines*, Washington, D.C.: U.S. Army Center of Military History, 1993.

Snyder, Holly, Ihor Y. Gawdiak, and Robert Worden, *Veterans Benefits and Judicial Review: Historical Antecedents and the Development of the American System: A Study Prepared for the United States Court of Veterans Appeals*, Washington, D.C.: Federal Research Division, Library of Congress, August 8, 1991.

Solomon, Zahava, *Combat Stress Reaction: The Enduring Toll of War*, New York: Plenum Press, 1993.

Solomon, Zahava, Rami Benbenishty, and Mario Mikulincer, "A Follow-Up of the Israel Casualties of Combat Stress Reaction ('Battle Shock') in the 1982 Lebanon War," *British Journal of Clinical Psychology*, Vol. 27, May 1988, pp. 125–135.

Sosa, Ingeborg, "The Journal Interview—MG Michael J. Scott, Jr., MC, Commanding General, 7th Medical Command, Europe," *Journal of the U.S. Army Medical Department*, January/February 1992.

Sparrow, John C., *History of Personnel Demobilization in the United States Army*, Washington, D.C.: Department of the Army, July 1952.

Spencer, Frank C., "Historical Vignette: The Introduction of Arterial Repair into the US Marine Corps, US Naval Hospital, in July–August 1952," *Journal of Trauma: Injury, Infection, and Critical Care*, Vol. 60, No. 4, April 2006, pp. 906–909.

Staedler, Steve, "The 36th Aeromedical Evacuation Squadron's First Mission," Air Force Print News Today website, June 6, 2009.

Staley, Michael L., *Audit of the Veterans Health Administration's Outpatient Scheduling Procedures*, Washington, D.C.: Department of Veterans Affairs, Office of Inspector General, Report No. 04-02887-169, July 8, 2005.

Steinman, Ron, ed., *Women in Vietnam: The Oral History*, New York: TV Books, 2000.

Steinweg, Kenneth K., "Mobile Surgical Hospital Design: Lessons from 5th MASH Surgical Packages for Operations Desert Shield/Desert Storm," *Military Medicine*, Vol. 158, No. 11, November 1993, pp. 733–739.

Stephenson, Jeffrey C., "Echelons of Care and Aeromedical Evacuation from the Middle East Area of Operations," *ADF Health*, Vol. 9, June 2008, pp. 9–14.

Stern, Seth, "Body Armor Could Be a Technological Hero of War in Iraq," *Christian Science Monitor*, April 2, 2003.

Stewart, Richard W., *The Korean War: The Chinese Intervention, 3 November 1950–24 January 1951*, Washington, D.C.: U.S. Army Center of Military History, 2003.

———, ed., *American Military History*, Vol. II: *The United States Army in a Global Era, 1917–2003*, 2nd ed., Washington, D.C.: U.S. Army Center of Military History, 2005.

Stille, Charles J., *History of the Sanitary Commission Being the General Report of Its Work During the War of the Rebellion*, Philadelphia: J.B. Lippincott & Co., 1866.

Stillwaugh, Elva, "Personnel Policies in the Korean Conflict," unpublished draft, Washington, D.C., U.S. Army Center of Military History, undated.

Stinger, Harry, and Robert Rush, "The Army Forward Surgical Team: Update and Lessons Learned, 1997–2004," *Military Medicine*, Vol. 171, No. 4, April 2006, pp. 269–272.

Stinner, Daniel J., Travis C. Burns, Kevin L. Kirk, and James R. Ficke, "Return to Duty Rate of Amputee Soldiers in the Current Conflicts in Afghanistan and Iraq," *Journal of Trauma: Injury, Infection, and Critical Care*, Vol. 68, No. 6, June 2010, pp. 1476–1479.

Stork, Joe, and Ann M. Lesch, "Background to the Crisis: Why War?" *Middle East Report*, No. 167, November–December 1990, pp. 11–18.

Strassman, Harvey D., Margaret B. Thaler, and Edgar H. Schein, "A Prisoner of War Syndrome: Apathy as a Reaction to Severe Stress," *American Journal of Psychiatry*, Vol. 112, June 1956, pp. 998–1003.

Strite, Charles H., "Equipping the Combat Support Hospital: A Case Study," *Army Sustainment*, Vol. 42, No. 5, September–October 2010.

Sullivan, Gordon, "No More Task Force Smiths," *Army Magazine*, January 1992.

Sullivan, Michael J., *Rapid Acquisition of MRAP Vehicles*, Washington, D.C.: U.S. Government Accountability Office, GAO-10-155T, October 8, 2009.

Summerall, E. Lanier, "Traumatic Brain Injury and PTSD: Focus on Veterans," Washington, D.C.: U.S. Department of Veterans Affairs, National Center for PTSD, November 6, 2017.

Tangredi, Sam J., *All Possible Wars? Toward a Consensus View of the Future Security Environment, 2001–2025*, Washington, D.C.: Institute for National Strategic Studies, National Defense University, 2000.

Tanielian, Terri, and Lisa H. Jaycox, eds., *Invisible Wounds of War: Psychological and Cognitive Injuries, Their Consequences, and Services to Assist Recovery*, Santa Monica, Calif.: RAND Corporation, MG-720-CCF, 2008.

Tarrant, David, Scott Friedman, and Eva Parks, "Injured Heroes, Broken Promises, Part 1: The War After the War," *Dallas Morning News*, November 22, 2014a.

———, "Injured Heroes, Broken Promises, Part 2: Insulted by Treatment," *Dallas Morning News*, November 22, 2014b.

———, "Injured Heroes, Broken Promises, Part 5: Far More Wait than Hurry Up in Army Mental Care," *Dallas Morning News*, September 3, 2015.

Task Force on Returning Global War on Terror Heroes, *Report of the Task Force on Returning Global War on Terror Heroes*, Washington, D.C., April 9, 2007.

Technical Manual 9-803, *1/4-Ton 4x4 Truck*, Washington, D.C.: War Department, 1944.

"Tet Offensive: Turning Point in Vietnam War," *New York Times*, January 31, 1988.

Thomas, Jeffrey L., "Summary of Key Findings from the Mental Health Advisory Team 6 (MHAT 6): OEF and OIF," briefing slides, Washington, D.C.: Department of Military Psychiatry, Walter Reed Army Institute of Research, January 15, 2010.

Thorson, Chad M., Joseph J. Dubose, Peter Rhee, Thomas E. Knuth, Warren C. Dorlac, Jeffrey A. Bailey, George D. Garcia, Mark L. Ryan, Robert M. Van Haren, and Kenneth G. Proctor, "Military Trauma Training at Civilian Centers: A Decade of Advancements," *Journal of Trauma and Acute Care Surgery*, Vol. 73, No. 6, Supplement 5, 2012, pp. S483–S489.

Tiffany, William J., Jr., and William S. Allerton, "Army Psychiatry in the Mid-'60s," *American Journal of Psychiatry*, Vol. 1234, No. 7, January 1967, pp. 810–821.

Timberg, Robert, *The Nightingale's Song*, New York: Simon and Schuster, 1995.

Tolchin, Martin, "Length of Average Hospital Stay Drops 22%," *New York Times*, May 25, 1988.

Tolson, John J., *Vietnam Studies: Airmobility 1961–1971*, online reprint, Washington, D.C.: Department of the Army, 1989.

Tompkins, Harvey J., "Korean Veterans with Psychiatric Disabilities," *Military Medicine*, Vol. 117, No. 1, July 1955, pp. 34–38.

Tong, Darryl, and Ross Beirne, "Combat Body Armor and Injuries to the Head, Face, and Neck Region: A Systematic Review," *Military Medicine*, Vol. 178, No. 4, April 2013, pp. 421–426.

Towell, Pat, *Forging The Sword: Unit Manning in the US Army*, Washington, D.C.: Center for Strategic and Budgetary Assessments, September 2004.

Trunkey, Donald, "Changes in Combat Casualty Care," *Journal of the American College of Surgeons*, Vol. 214, No. 6, June 2012, pp. 879–891.

Tucker, Spencer, "Fact Sheet: Task Force Smith," 1992.

U.S. Army, *2013 Weapons Systems Handbook*, Washington, D.C., 2013.

U.S. Army Center of Military History, *Korea—1950*, Washington, D.C.: U.S. Government Printing Office, 1997.

———, "Pork Chop Hill," webpage, 2010.

U.S. Army Institute of Surgical Research, "Tactical Combat Casualty Care Guidelines," Fort Sam Houston, Tex.: U.S. Army Medical Department Center and School, June 2, 2014.

———, "Joint Trauma System: The Department of Defense Center of Excellence for Trauma," database, August 8, 2016a.

———, "TCCC Journal Watch List," webpage, August 8, 2016b

U.S. Army Medical Service Historical Unit, *Annual Report: The Surgeon General, United States Army, Fiscal Year 1964*, Washington, D.C., 1964.

———, *Annual Report: The Surgeon General, United States Army, Fiscal Year 1965*, Washington, D.C., 1965.

———, *Annual Report: The Surgeon General, United States Army, Fiscal Year 1966*, Washington, D.C., 1966.

———, *Annual Report: The Surgeon General, United States Army, Fiscal Year 1967*, Washington, D.C., 1967.

———, *Annual Report: The Surgeon General, United States Army, Fiscal Year 1968*, Washington, D.C., 1968.

———, *Annual Report: The Surgeon General, United States Army, Fiscal Year 1969*, Washington, D.C., 1969.

———, *Annual Report: The Surgeon General, United States Army, Fiscal Year 1970*, Washington, D.C., 1970.

———, *Annual Report: The Surgeon General, United States Army, Fiscal Year 1971*, Washington, D.C., 1971.

———, *Annual Report: The Surgeon General, United States Army, Fiscal Year 1972*, Washington, D.C., 1972.

———, *Annual Report: The Surgeon General, United States Army, Fiscal Year 1973*, Washington, D.C., 1973.

U.S. Army Transportation Museum, "The Bell H-13 SIOUX Helicopter," undated.

U.S.C.—*See* U.S. Code.

U.S. Code, Title 38, Veterans' Benefits, Part II, General Benefits, Chapter 11, Compensation for Service-Connected Disability or Death, Subchapter II, Wartime Disability Compensation, Sec. 1117, Compensation for Disabilities Occurring in Persian Gulf War Veterans, as of June 15, 2006.

U.S. Code, Title 38, Veterans' Benefits, Part II, General Benefits, Chapter 11, Compensation for Service-Connected Disability or Death, Subchapter VI, General Compensation Provisions, Sec. 1151, Benefits for Persons Disabled by Treatment or Vocational Rehabilitation, as of December 10, 2004.

U.S. Department of Defense, "About the Office of Warrior Care Policy: Background," webpage, undated.

———, *Conduct of the Persian Gulf War: Final Report to Congress*, Washington, D.C.: U.S. Department of Defense, April 1992a. Digitized version with appendixes, courtesy of Google and Hathi Trust.

———, *National Military Strategy of the United States*, Washington, D.C., January 1992b.

———, *National Military Strategy of the United States of America: A Strategy of Flexible and Selective Engagement*, Washington, D.C., 1995.

———, *National Military Strategy of the United States of America—Shape, Respond, Prepare Now: A Military Strategy for a New Era*, Washington, D.C.: Department of Defense, 1997.

———, *Quadrennial Defense Review Report*, Washington, D.C., September 30, 2001.

———, "Army Surgeon General Kiley Submits Retirement Request," Washington, D.C.: American Forces Press Service, March 12, 2007.

———, *Measuring Stability and Security in Iraq*, Washington, D.C., March 2009.

U.S. Department of Defense Inspector General, *Medical Mobilization Planning and Execution: Inspection Report*, Washington, D.C., 93-INS-13, September 1993.

———, *DoD Testing Requirements for Body Armor*, Arlington, Va., January 29, 2009.

U.S. Department of Defense Warrior Care, "Integrated Disability Evaluation System (IDES)," brochure, undated.

U.S. Department of State, "U.S. Involvement in the Vietnam War: The Tet Offensive, 1968," webpage, 2015.

U.S. Department of State, Office of the Historian, "Kennan and Containment, 1947," webpage, undated, c. 2010.

———, "Milestones: 1961–1968: U.S. Involvement in the Vietnam War: the Gulf of Tonkin and Escalation, 1964," undated.

U.S. Department of Veterans Affairs, "Summary: Veterans Access, Choice and Accountability Act of 2014 ("Choice Act")," fact sheet, Washington, D.C.: Office of Public Affairs, undated a.

———, "Vet Center Program," webpage, undated b.

———, *Analysis of Presumptions of Service Connection*, Washington, D.C., December 23, 1993.

———, "Pension: Aid & Attendance and Housebound," webpage, December 8, 2015.

———, "About Gulf War Veterans," in *VA Research on Gulf War Veterans*, Washington, D.C., September 2016a.

———, *Federal Benefits for Veterans, Dependents, and Survivors: Chapter 2 Service-Connected Disabilities—2014 VA Disability Compensation*, U.S. Department of Veterans Affairs, February 4, 2016b.

———, *FY 2016 Agency Financial Report (AFR): Honoring the Past, Inspiring the Future*, Washington, D.C., 2016c.

———, "VA Social Work: Fisher House Program," webpage, November 17, 2016d.

———, "Budget in Brief," *2018 Congressional Submission*, Washington, D.C., 2017a.

———, "Returning Servicemembers (OEF/OIF/OND)," webpage, October 17, 2017b.

———, "VA Caregiver Support: Care for Veterans," webpage, July 5, 2017c.

———, "VA Caregiver Support: Caring for Seriously Injured Post-9/11 Veterans," fact sheet, July 20, 2017d.

———, "Vet Center Program," webpage, January 19, 2018.

U.S. Department of Veterans Affairs and U.S. Department of Defense, "DoD and VA Take New Steps to Support the Mental Health Needs of Service Members and Veterans," joint fact sheet, undated.

———, "VA/DoD Clinical Practice Guideline for the Management of Concussion-Mild Traumatic Brain Injury," Vers. 2.0, Washington, D.C., February 2016.

U.S. Department of Veterans Affairs, Office of Research and Development, "VA Research on Vietnam Veterans," webpage, undated.

U.S. General Accounting Office, *Agent Orange: Poor Contracting Practices at Centers for Disease Control Increased Costs*, Washington, D.C., GAO/GGD-99-122BR, September 1990.

———, *Operation Desert Storm: Full Army Medical Capability Not Achieved*, Washington, D.C., GAO/NSIAD-92-175, August 1992.

————, *Agent Orange: Actions Needed to Improve Communications of Air Force Ranch Hand Study Data and Results*, Washington, D.C., GAO/NSIAD-00-31, December 1999.

Usher, Chad, "Forward Surgical Team," video, Bala Maghrab, Afghanistan: 126th FST, October 6, 2011.

U.S. House of Representatives, Committee on Veterans' Affairs, "Findings of the Veterans' Disability Benefits Commission," hearing, 110th Cong., 1st Sess., Washington, D.C., October 10, 2007.

————, "A Continued Assessment of Delays in VA Medical Care and Preventable Veterans Deaths," hearing, 113th Cong., 2nd Sess., Washington, D.C.: U.S. Government Publishing Office, April 9, 2014.

U.S. Senate, Armed Services Subcommittee on Manpower and Personnel, "Costs of the All-Volunteer Force," hearing, 95th Cong., 2nd Sess., Washington, D.C.: U.S. Government Printing Office, February 6, 1978.

U.S. Senate Committee on Finance, "Veteran's Pensions," hearing, 86th Cong., 1st Sess., Washington, D.C., July 28–29, 1959.

U.S. Special Operations Command, *United States Special Operations Command History*, MacDill Air Force Base, Fla.: History and Research Office, 2007.

USSOCOM—*See* U.S. Special Operations Command.

VA Employee Education System, "Guideline Summary for the VA/DoD Clinical Practice Guideline for Rehabilitation of Lower Limb Amputation," Department of Veterans Affairs and Department of Defense, January 2008.

Valdiri, Linda A., Virginia E. Andrews-Arce, and Jason M. Seery, "Training Forward Surgical Teams for Deployment: The US Army Trauma Training Center," *Critical Care Nurse*, Vol. 35, No. 2, April 2015, pp. e11–e17.

Vanderburg, Kathleen, "Aeromedical Evacuation: A Historical Perspective," in William W. Hurd and John G. Jernigan, eds., *Aeromedical Evacuation: Management of Acute and Stabilized Patients*, New York: Springer-Verlag, 2003.

Van Devanter, Lynda, *Home Before Morning: The Story of an Army Nurse in Vietnam*, New York: Warner Books, 1983.

Vandiver, John, "Vietnam Leads to the Death of the Draft and the Rise of the Professional Soldier," *Stars and Stripes*, November 11, 2014.

Veterans' Disability Benefits Commission, *Honoring the Call to Duty: Veterans' Disability Benefits in the 21st Century*, Washington, D.C., October 2007.

Veterans Health Administration, "TBI Screening and Evaluation Research," fact sheet, Washington, D.C.: U.S. Department of Veterans Affairs, Polytrauma and Blast-Related Injuries QUERI, July 28, 2014.

————, "Polytrauma/TBI System of CARE: Polytrauma System of Care Facilities," U.S. Department of Veterans Affairs website, June 3, 2015.

————, "Enrollment Priority Groups," Washington, D.C., December 2016a.

————, *Restoring Trust in Veterans Health Care: Fiscal Year 2016 Annual Report*, Washington, D.C., December 2016b.

————, "Gulf War Presumptives," *Gulf War Newsletter*, Winter 2016c, pp. 6–7.

Veterans of the Vietnam War and the Veterans Coalition, "A Brief History of the Agent Orange Class Action Lawsuit," webpage, undated.

VHA—*See* Veterans Health Administration.

Vickers, George R., "U.S. Strategy and the Vietnam War," in Jayne S. Werner and Luu Doan Huynh, eds., *The Vietnam War: Vietnamese and American Perspectives*, Armonk, N.Y.: M.E. Sharpe, Inc., 1993.

Vietnam Veterans Against the War, "VVAW: Where We Came from, Who We Are," webpage, 2015.

Vietnam Veterans of America, "A Short History of VVA," webpage, 2015.

"Vietnam War Statistics," LZ Sally website, 2015.

"The Vietnam War: Seeds of Conflict, 1945–1960," The History Place website, 1999.

Vogel, Steve, "Walter Reed Official Returned to Full Duty," *Washington Post*, May 26, 2007.

———, "Army Probing PTSD Diagnoses," *Washington Post*, May 16, 2012.

Vogel, Steve, and William Branigin, "Army Fires Commander of Walter Reed," *Washington Post*, March 2, 2007.

Walter Reed National Military Medical Center, "Welcome to the Amputee Service—Military Advanced Training Center (MATC)," webpage, undated.

Wanke, Paul, *Russian/Soviet Military Psychiatry: 1904–1945*, New York: Routledge, 2005.

Warner, Christopher H., George N. Appenzeller, Matthew J. Barry, Anthony Morton, and Thomas Grieger, "The Evolving Role of the Division Psychiatrist," *Military Medicine*, Vol. 172, No. 9, September 2007, pp. 918–924.

Warner, Christopher H., George N. Appenzeller, Todd Yosick, Matthew J. Barry, Anthony J. Morton, Jill E. Breitbach, Gabrielle Bryen, Angela Mobbs, Amanda Robbins, Jessica Parker, and Thomas Grieger, "The Division Psychiatrist and Brigade Behavioral Health Officers," in Elspeth Cameron Ritchie, ed., *Combat and Operational Behavioral Health*, Washington, D.C.: Borden Institute, Walter Reed Army Medical Center, 2011.

Warner, Christopher H., Jill E. Breitbach, George N. Appenzeller, Virginia Yates, Thomas Grieger, and William G. Webster, "Division Mental Health in the New Brigade Combat Team Structure, Part I: Predeployment and Deployment," *Military Medicine*, Vol. 172, No. 9, September 2007a, pp. 907–911.

———, "Division Mental Health in the New Brigade Combat Team Structure, Part II: Redeployment and Postdeployment," *Military Medicine*, Vol. 172, No. 9, September 2007b, pp. 912–917.

Watkins, Katherine E., Harold Alan Pincus, Brad Smith, Susan M. Paddock, Thomas E. Mannle, Jr., Abigail Woodroffe, Jake Solomon, Melony E. Sorbero, Carrie M. Farmer, Kimberly A. Hepner, David M. Adamson, Lanna Forrest, and Catherine Call, *Veterans Health Administration Mental Health Program Evaluation: Capstone Report*, Santa Monica, Calif.: RAND Corporation and Altarum Institute, TR-956-VHA, 2011.

Webb, William J., *The Outbreak 27 June–15 September 1950*, Washington, D.C.: U.S. Army Center of Military History, CMH Pub 19-6, 2006.

Weinstein, Edwin A., "The Fifth U.S. Army Neuropsychiatry Center—'601st,'" in William S. Mullins, ed., *Medical Department, United States Army in World War II: Neuropsychiatry in World War II*, Vol. II: *Overseas Theaters*, Washington, D.C.: Office of the Surgeon General, Department of the Army, 1973.

Weisfeld, Neil E., Victoria D. Weisfeld, and Catharyn T. Liverman, *Military Medical Ethics: Issues Regarding Dual Loyalties—Workshop Summary*, Washington, D.C.: National Academies Press, 2009.

Wenger, Jennie W., Caolionn O'Connell, and Linda Cottrell, *Examination of Recent Deployment Experience Across the Services and Components*, Santa Monica, Calif.: RAND Corporation, RR-1928-A, 2018.

West, Iris J., *The Women of the Army Nurse Corps During the Vietnam War*, Washington, D.C.: U.S. Army Center of Military History, undated.

West, Nadja Y., and Steve Jones, eds., "US Army Medical Department at War: Lessons Learned 2001–2015," *United States Army Medical Department Journal*, April–September 2016.

West, Togo, John O. Marsh, John J. H. Schwarz, James Bacchus, Arnold Fisher, John P. Jumper, Charles H. Roadman II, Kathleen L. Martin, and Lawrence W. Holland, *Rebuilding the Trust: Independent Review Group Report on Rehabilitative Care and Administrative Processes at Walter Reed Army Medical Center and National Naval Medical Center*, Washington, D.C.: U.S. Department of Defense, April 2007.

Whelan, Thomas J., Jr., statement before the Subcommittee on Veterans Affairs of the Committee on Labor and Public Welfare, U.S. Senate, 91st Cong., 1st and 2nd Sess., hearing on the Examination of the Problems of the Veterans Wounded in Vietnam, Washington, D.C.: U.S. Government Printing Office, 1969.

Willbanks, James H., "Shock and Awe of Tet Offensive Shattered U.S. Illusions," *U.S. News & World Report*, January 29, 2009.

Willenz, June A., *Women Veterans: America's Forgotten Heroines*, New York: Continuum, 1983.

Williams, Kayla, *Plenty of Time When We Get Home: Love and Recovery in the Aftermath of War*, New York: W.W. Norton & Company, Inc, 2014.

Williams, Kayla, and Michael E. Staub, *Love My Rifle More Than You: Young and Female in the U.S. Army*, New York: W.W. Norton & Company, 2005.

Williamson, Randall B., *Army Health Care: Progress Made in Staffing and Monitoring Units That Provide Outpatient Case Management, but Additional Steps Needed*, Washington, D.C.: U.S. Government Accountability Office, GAO-09-357, April 2009a.

———, *Recovering Servicemembers: DOD and VA Have Jointly Developed the Majority of Required Policies but Challenges Remain*, Washington, D.C.: U.S. Government Accountability Office, GAO-09-728, July 2009b.

———, *DoD and Va Health Care: Federal Recovery Coordination Program Continues to Expand but Faces Significant Challenges*, Washington, D.C.: U.S. Government Accountability Office, GAO-11-250, March 2011.

———, *Recovering Servicemembers and Veterans: Sustained Leadership Attention and Systematic Oversight Needed to Resolve Persistent Problems Affecting Care and Benefits*, Washington, D.C.: U.S. Government Accountability Office, GAO-13-5, November 2012.

———, *Actions Needed to Address Higher-Than-Expected Demand for the Family Caregiver Program*, Washington, D.C.: U.S. Government Accountability Office, GAO-14-675, September 2014.

———, *VA Health Care: Improved Monitoring Needed for Effective Oversight of Care for Women Veterans*, Washington, D.C.: U.S. Government Accountability Office, GAO-17-52, December 2016.

———, *Actions Needed to Ensure Post-Traumatic Stress Disorder and Traumatic Brain Injury Are Considered in Misconduct Separations*, Washington, D.C.: U.S. Government Accountability Office, GAO-17-260, May 2017.

Wilson, Clay, *Improvised Explosive Devices (IEDs) in Iraq and Afghanistan: Effects and Countermeasures*, Washington, D.C.: Congressional Research Service, RS22330, August 28, 2007.

Wilson, Tim, "The Prison of Hopelessness," *Air Force Print News Today* website, August 23, 2006.

Wiltse, Charles M., *The Medical Department: Medical Service in the Mediterranean and Minor Theaters*, Washington, D.C.: U.S. Government Printing Office, 1965.

Winkenwerder, William, Jr., "Statement by Dr. William Winkenwerder, Jr., Assistant Secretary of Defense for Health Affairs/Special Assistant for Gulf War Illnesses, Medical Readiness, and Military Deployments before the House Committee on Government Reform Subcommittee on National Security, Veterans Affairs, and International Relations," Washington, D.C.: U.S. Department of Defense, January 24, 2002.

———, "The Military Health System: Overview Statement," testimony before the U.S. House of Representatives, Armed Services Committee, Subcommittee on Military Personnel, 109th Cong., 1st Sess., October 19, 2005.

Wiersema, Richard E., *No More Bad Force Myths: A Tactical Study of Regimental Combat in Korea*, Fort Leavenworth, Kan.: School of Advanced Military Studies, U.S. Army Command and General Staff College, 1997.

Wolf, Jeffrey, "Army Secretary Steps Down in Wake of Walter Reed Scandal," Associated Press, March 2, 2007.

Wolfowitz, Paul, "Ribbon Cutting Ceremony for Military Severely Injured Joint Support Operations Center," remarks, Washington, D.C.: Department of Defense, February 1, 2005.

Woodard, Scott C., "The Story of the Mobile Army Surgical Hospital," *Military Medicine*, Vol. 168, No. 7, July 2003, pp. 503–513.

Woodward, J. J., *The Medical and Surgical History of the War of the Rebellion (1861–65)*, Vol. 1, Part I: *Medical History*, Washington, D.C.: Government Printing Office, 1870.

Wounded Warrior Project, "Wounded Warrior Project Launches Groundbreaking Warrior Care Network," press release, January 26, 2016.

World Health Organization, *International Classification of Diseases*, 9th rev., 1978.

WRAMC—*See* Walter Reed National Military Medical Center.

Wright, Donald P., James R. Bird, Steven E. Clay, Peter W. Connors, Scott C. Farquhar, Lynne Chandler Garcia, and Dennis F. Van Wey, *A Different Kind of War: The United States Army in Operation Enduring Freedom (OEF), October 2001–September 2005*, Fort Leavenworth, Kan.: Combat Studies Institute Press, 2010.

"WW II Helicopter Evacuation," Olive-Drab website, undated.

Zinni, Anthony C., "A Commander Reflects," *Proceedings: The U.S. Naval Institute*, Vol. 126, No. 7, July 2000, pp. 34–37.

Zwerdling, Daniel, "Do Soldiers Receive Adequate Mental Health Care?" transcript, *Talk of the Nation*, National Public Radio, December 7, 2006a.

———, "Pentagon to Investigate Mental Health Treatment," transcript, *Morning Edition*, National Public Radio, December 8, 2006b.

———, "Soldiers Face Obstacles to Mental Health Services," transcript, *Morning Edition*, National Public Radio, December 4, 2006c.

———, "Soldiers Say Army Ignores, Punishes Mental Anguish," transcript, *All Things Considered*, National Public Radio, December 4, 2006d.

———, "Gaps in Mental Care Persist for Fort Carson Soldiers," transcript, *All Things Considered*, National Public Radio, May 24, 2007a.

———, "Return to Fort Carson Raises More Questions," transcript, *All Things Considered*, National Public Radio, May 26, 2007b.

———, "Missed Treatment: Soldiers with Mental Health Issues Dismissed for 'Misconduct,'" transcript, *All Things Considered*, National Public Radio, October 28, 2015.